Clinics in Developmental Medicine

Spinal Cord Injury in the Child and Young Adult

Clinics in Developmental Medicine

Spinal Cord Injury in the Child and Young Adult

Edited by

LAWRENCE C VOGEL
Shriners Hospitals for Children;
Rush Medical College
Chicago, IL
USA

KATHY ZEBRACKI
Shriners Hospitals for Children;
Loyola University Chicago
Chicago, IL
USA

RANDAL R BETZ
Institute for Spine and Scoliosis
Lawrenceville, NJ
USA

MJ MULCAHEY
Jefferson School of Health Professions
Thomas Jefferson University
Philadelphia, PA
USA

2014
MAC KEITH PRESS

6 Market Road, London, N7 9PW

Editor: Hilary M. Hart
Managing Director: Ann-Marie Halligan
Production Manager: Udoka Ohuonu
Project Management: Prepress Projects Ltd

First published in this edition in 2014

British Library Cataloguing-in-Publication data
A catalogue record for this book is available from the British Library

Cover image: Dr Megan Wilson, DC

ISBN: 978-1-909962-34-7

Typeset by Prepress Projects Ltd, Perth, UK
Printed by TJ International, Padstow, Cornwall, UK

Mac Keith Press is supported by Scope

CONTENTS

AUTHORS' APPOINTMENTS

Nadia Barakat	Department of Clinical Research, Shriners Hospitals for Children; Department of Radiology, Temple University School of Medicine, Philadelphia, PA, USA
Andrea L Behrman	Kosair Charities Center for Pediatric Neurorecovery, Kentucky Spinal Cord Injury Research Center, Department of Neurological Surgery, University of Louisville, Louisville, KY, USA
Randal R Betz	Institute for Spine and Scoliosis, Lawrenceville, NJ, USA
Fin Biering-Sørensen	Department for Spinal Cord Injuries, Glostrup Hospital, University of Copenhagen, Copenhagen, Denmark
Glendaliz Bosques	Department of Physical Medicine and Rehabilitation, University of Texas, Health Science Center at Houston, Houston, TX, USA
Thomas N Bryce	Department of Rehabilitation Medicine, Icahn School of Medicine at Mount Sinai, NY, USA
Christina L Calhoun	Department of Occupational Therapy, Jefferson School of Health Professions, Thomas Jefferson University, Philadelphia, PA, USA
Shuyan Chen	Department of Anatomy and Neurobiology, Drexel University, Philadelphia, PA, USA
Yuying Chen	Department of Physical Medicine and Rehabilitation, University of Alabama at Birmingham, Birmingham, AL, USA

Zoë Chevalier	Department of Clinical Psychology, The National Spinal Injuries Centre, Stoke Mandeville Hospital, Aylesbury, UK
Kathleen Chlan	Spinal Cord Injury Research, Shriners Hospitals for Children, Chicago, IL, USA
Rory A Cooper	Department of Rehabilitation Science & Technology, University of Pittsburgh; US Department of Veterans Affairs, Human Engineering Research Laboratories, Pittsburgh, PA, USA
Loren T Davidson	Department of Physical Medicine and Rehabilitation, University of California, Davis; Shriners Hospitals for Children, Northern California, Sacramento, CA, USA
Gregory Dean	Department of Urology, Temple University, Philadelphia, PA, USA
Michael J DeVivo	Department of Physical Medicine and Rehabilitation, University of Alabama at Birmingham, Birmingham, AL, USA
Michael Dichiaro	Department of Physical Medicine and Rehabilitation, University of Colorado Health Sciences Center, Children's Hospital Colorado, Denver, CO, USA
Scott H Faro	Department of Radiology, Biomedical, Electrical and Computer Engineering, Department of Radiology, Temple University School of Medicine, Philadelphia, PA, USA
George Ghobrial	Department of Neurosurgery, Thomas Jefferson University, Philadelphia, PA, USA
Bridget Harrington	School of English, Media Studies and Art History, University of Queensland, Brisbane, QLD, Australia
Michael Harrington	School of Languages and Comparative Cultural Studies, University of Queensland, Brisbane, QLD, Australia
James S Harrop	Departments of Neurological and Orthopedic Surgery, Division of Spine and Peripheral Nerve Surgery, Delaware Valley SCI Center, Thomas Jefferson University, Philadelphia, PA, USA

Lisa A Harvey	Sydney Medical School/Northern, University of Sydney, Sydney, NSW, Australia
Dena R Howland	Kosair Charities Center for Pediatric Neurorecovery, Kentucky Spinal Cord Injury Research Center, Departments of Neurological Surgery, Anatomical Sciences and Neurobiology and Bioengineering, University of Louisville; Robley Rex Veterans Medical Center, Louisville, KY, USA
Miriam Hwang	Orthopaedic and Rehabilitation Engineering Center, Marquette University, Milwaukee, WI; Scientific Staff, Shriners Hospitals for Children, Chicago, IL, USA
Kelly M Johnson	Division of Nursing and Patient Care Services, Children's Hospital Colorado, Aurora, CO, USA
Kurt L Johnson	Department of Rehabilitation Medicine, School of Medicine, University of Washington, Seattle, WA, USA
Therese E Johnston	Department of Physical Therapy, Jefferson School of Health Professions, Thomas Jefferson University, Philadelphia, PA, USA
Kevin Jones	Department of Clinical Psychology, The National Spinal Injuries Centre, Stoke Mandeville Hospital, Aylesbury, UK
Deepan C Kamaraj	Department of Rehabilitation Science & Technology, School of Health and Rehabilitation Sciences, University of Pittsburgh, Pittsburgh, PA, USA
Michelle Kauffman-Lawson	Department of Ambulatory Nursing, Children's Hospital, Colorado, Aurora, CO, USA
Erin H Kelly	Spinal Cord Injury Research, Shriners Hospitals for Children; Department of Disability and Human Development, University of Illinois, Chicago, IL, USA
Sara J Klaas	Director of Business Development, Shriners Hospital for Children, Chicago, IL, USA
Scott H Kozin	Chief of Staff, Shriners Hospitals for Children, Philadelphia, PA, USA
Andrei Krassioukov	Department of Medicine, Divison of Physical Medicine and Rehabilation, University of British Columbia, Vancouver, BC, Canada

James S Krause	College of Health Professions, Medical University of South Carolina, Charleston, SC, USA
John Kuluz	Department of Pediatric Neurosurgery, Miami Children's Hospital, Miami, FL, USA
Kerry A Lavan	South Campus Orthopedics & Rehabilitation Specialty Clinics, Children's Hospital Colorado, Aurora, CO, USA
Jan McCreary	UQ Advantage Office, University of Queensland, Brisbane, QLD, Australia
Craig M McDonald	Department of Physical Medicine and Rehabilitation, University of California, Davis; Shriners Hospitals for Children, Northern California, Sacramento, CA, USA
Teresa L Massagli	Department of Rehabilitation Medicine, University of Washington and Seattle Children's Hospital, Seattle, WA, USA
Dennis J Matthews	Department of Physical Medicine and Rehabilitation, University of Colorado School of Medicine, Aurora, CO, USA
Lisa Merenda	Clinical Editor, Wolters Kluwer Health, Philadelphia, PA, USA
James W Middleton	Rehabilitation Studies Unit, Northern Clinical School, Sydney, Medical School, The University of Sydney, Sydney, NSW, Australia
Feroze B Mohamed	Department of Radiology, Biomedical, Electrical and Computer Engineering, Department of Radiology, Temple University School of Medicine, Philadelphia, PA, USA
MJ Mulcahey	Department of Occupational Therapy, Jefferson School of Health Professions, Thomas Jefferson University, Philadelphia, PA, USA
H Herndon Murray	Spinal Cord Injury Service, Orthopedic Surgery, Shepherd Center, Peachtree Orthopedic Clinic, Atlanta, GA, USA
Virginia Simson Nelson	Department of Physical Medicine and Rehabilitation, University of Michigan Medical School, Ann Arbor, MI, USA

Joyce Oleszek	Department of Physical Medicine and Rehabilitation, University of Colorado School of Medicine, Aurora, CO, USA
Joshua M Pahys	Department of Orthopaedic Surgery, Shriners Hospital for Children, Philadelphia, PA, USA
Tonya M Palermo	Anesthesiology and Pain Medicine, University of Washington and Seattle Children's Research Institute, Seattle, WA, USA
Nigel Price	Department of Orthopedic Surgery, University of Missouri Kansas City, Division of Orthopedic Surgery, Children's Mercy Hospital, Kansas City, MO, USA
David W Pruitt	Division of Physical Medicine & Rehabilitation, Cincinnati Children's Hospital Medical Center, Cincinnati, OH, USA
Karla S Reed	College of Health Professions, Medical University of South Carolina, Charleston, SC, USA
Maria R Reyes	Department of Rehabilitation Medicine, University of Washington, Seattle, WA, USA
Heather Russell	Shriners Hospitals for Children, Philadelphia, PA, USA
Amer F Samdani	Department of Surgery, Shriners Hospitals for Children, Philadelphia, PA, USA
Michael E Selzer	Center for Neural Repair and Rehabilitation, Shriners Hospitals for Children Pediatric Research Center; Temple University School of Medicine, Philadelphia, PA, USA
Shelley A Trimble	University of Louisville Kosair Charities Center for Pediatric Neurorecovery, Frazier Rehabilitation Institute, Louisville, KY, USA
Lawrence C Vogel	Department of Pediatrics, Shriners Hospitals for Children; Department of Pediatrics, Rush Medical College, Chicago, IL, USA
Pamela Wilson	Department of Physical Medicine and Rehabilitation, University of Colorado Health Sciences Center, Children's Hospital Colorado, Denver, CO, USA

Kathy Zebracki	Department of Psychology, Shriners Hospitals for Children; Department of Psychology, Loyola University Chicago, Chicago, IL, USA
Dan A Zlotolow	Department of Orthopaedic Surgery, Temple University School of Medicine; Department of Orthopaedic Surgery, Shriners Hospitals for Children, Philadelphia, PA, USA

FOREWORD

Twenty-nine years ago, a 3-year-old boy was run over by a bicycle while playing near the beach. He sustained a spinal cord injury (SCI) and suffered tetraplegia. In the years after the incident, he attended numerous rehabilitation and medical facilities and overcame one complication after another. Today, he is married, a father of two children, and working as a computer programmer. His story shows what is possible when a child or young adult sustains an SCI. However, this cannot happen without a lot of dedicated care, as demonstrated clearly in the story of Bridget Harrington in the first chapter of this book.

Spinal Cord Injury in the Child and Young Adult is a proper and timely addition to the *The Child with a Spinal Cord Injury*, published in 1996 and edited by Randal Betz and MJ Mulcahey, who, with Lawrence Vogel and Kathy Zebracki, share the editorship of this new volume.

Real progress has been made in improving the knowledge and understanding of SCI in recent decades, and this book contains information on all aspects of comprehensive care.

Children and young adults are distinct from adults with SCI in one major respect: they will, as all children do, develop physically and psychologically as they age. An SCI, however, will influence the maturation process in various ways. This ongoing 'double evolution' means that, over 10 or more years, the limitations caused by the SCI will change and new challenges for care will develop. The purposes of care will evolve as children develop into adulthood and will present an extra challenge for both achieving specific goals and management.

Section 1 of this volume gives an overview of SCI, looking at epidemiology, assessment, and life care planning, and includes the International Spinal Cord Injury data sets. Children and young adults are a minority of the overall population with SCI, and they represent an age-specific incidence of under 10 new cases per million children (age 0 to 15 years) and about 20 to 25 new cases per million children (age 0 to 19 years) in the USA. This still results in hundreds of new cases per year.

Section 2 gives specific information on the early management of SCI, focusing on pathophysiology, acute management, and principles of treatment of spine stability in children. Early management is of upmost importance, as it always has consequences for future care.

Section 3 provides unique perspectives on non-traumatic causes of pediatric SCI, the management of high tetraplegia, and concomitant brain injury.

Valuable information on medical management, including nutrition, is given in Section 4, including for the bladder and bowel, spasticity, autonomic dysfunction, medical complications, skin integrity, pain, and metabolic complications. These are major factors affecting a person's quality of life and frequently resulting in re-admission during follow-up. Children differ from adults in all these areas and the knowledge needed to offer proper care is well presented in the chapters of this section.

Section 5 focuses on neuromusculoskeletal management, including upper extremity function and orthopedic complications unique to children, such as neuromuscular scoliosis and hip subluxation.

Section 6 focuses on all aspects of physical rehabilitation, describing precisely and practically the recommendations on how to implement specific rehabilitation treatment. The psychosocial aspects of SCI are discussed in Section 7, including education, emotions, leisure/ recreation, and long-term outcomes.

The final section deliberates on research priorities and future directions.

This volume provides a thorough examination of the current knowledge on SCI. It will be a great help for emergency services, healthcare providers, rehabilitation physicians, neurosurgeons, orthopedic surgeons, and allied professionals, such as nurses, physical therapists, occupational therapists, and psychologists involved in the care of children and young adults with SCI. It will be a useful resource for clinical researchers, teachers, and students interested in this topic. It is a must for libraries in specialized services.

The book is easy to read, with comprehensive information presented in an attractive and understandable way. The case vignettes illustrate the challenges experienced by specific groups of individuals with SCI and those who care for them. The headings make quick consulting of the content possible. The tables contain useful extra information; the figures help clarify specific topics.

The evolution of the treatment of SCI will continue and one can hope that further achievements will improve the quality of life and life expectancy of this group of individuals with SCI.

The editors and the contributors are to be congratulated for this fine work.

Professor Jean Jacques Wyndaele
President of the International Spinal Cord Society

PREFACE

Since the publication of *The Child with a Spinal Cord Injury* in 1996 (Betz and Mulcahey 1996), there have been significant advances in the management of young people with spinal cord injuries (SCIs). These advances have enhanced functional abilities and have facilitated greater community-wide participation, which have improved the lives of young people with SCIs and their families. Since the mid-1990s, the management of young people with an SCI has become more comprehensive, embodying the principles of the World Health Organization's International Classification of Functioning, Disability and Health model. Emphasis has shifted toward activity and participation within young people's environments, taking into account personal factors such as family values and culture. For example, the goal of upper extremity interventions such as therapy, bracing or reconstructive surgery expands beyond accomplishing a better grip to improve function and independence to effortless and spontaneous use of the hands for performance in play, school, chores, and self-care activities. Another example is that the goals of ambulation or wheelchair training are not merely to move by walking or wheeling, but to increase community access and participation and to improve ergonomics to prevent future secondary health conditions such as chronic shoulder pain and dysfunction.

Since the mid-1990s, we have also seen a steady increase in pediatric SCI research and scholarly activities associated with evidence-based pediatric SCI care. Notable examples include the development and validation of SCI pediatric-specific evaluation tools such as the Needs Assessment Checklist and large item-banks of daily routines; inclusion of pediatric considerations in the development of International SCI Core Data Sets and International Perspectives on SCI pediatric psychometric testing of the International Standards for Neurological Classification of Spinal Cord Injury and other notable adult SCI measures; systematic reviews and reports on pediatric SCI epidemiology; and the gathering of data on the psychosocial outcomes of children and adolescents with an SCI along with their caregivers and on the long-term outcomes of adults who sustained pediatric injuries and the implication of these outcomes on pediatric SCI rehabilitation and habilitation.

Despite all of the advances since the 1990s, of which many will be discussed in this book, there are several major areas that need to be addressed in the future. It is the editors' hope that this book will stimulate young clinicians and researchers to take the progress made and build on this further in the future. There is a compelling need for our interventions to be more evidence based and to be accessible and affordable for all young people with SCI worldwide. Increased efforts must be made to prevent SCIs. This requires a thorough understanding of the epidemiology of SCI throughout the world and attention to be paid to emerging technologies that will facilitate prevention, as well as those that cause SCI, such as the mobile phone and distracted driving. Greater emphasis must be put on preventing premature death and secondary health conditions. Management of young people with SCI must include comprehensive transition planning that assures successful passage from adolescence into adulthood. Because of the relatively long lifespan of young people with SCI, the issue of aging must be addressed in the lives of young people with SCI to avoid overuse syndromes and premature cardiovascular disease so that they may enjoy a full, healthy, and satisfying life.

This book, *Spinal Cord Injury in the Child and Young Adult*, will address a variety of topics relevant to pediatric-onset SCI including epidemiology, medical, surgical, urologic, rehabilitative and psychosocial issues, and future directions. Our intended audience is those in the myriad disciplines who constitute the interprofessional teams that care for young people with SCI from the scene of a crash, through acute care and initial rehabilitation, to long-term follow-up. We hope this book will benefit both students and senior clinicians, as well as the professional who regularly or infrequently cares for young people with SCI. The first chapter sets the tempo by providing an insight from a young adult with pediatric-onset SCI and her family; this perspective should uphold our focus on this book's central theme, namely young people with SCI and their success as individuals and family and community members.

Lawrence C Vogel, Kathy Zebracki, Randal R Betz and MJ Mulcahey
September 2014

REFERENCE

Betz RR, Mulcahey MJ (eds) (1996) *The Child with a Spinal Cord Injury*. Rosemont, IL: American Academy of Orthopaedic Surgeons.

ACKNOWLEDGMENTS

The editors recognize that pediatric spinal cord injury is relatively rare and therefore requires a concerted effort for all to work as one. We would like to acknowledge the individuals and organizations who have supported clinical care, educational activities, and research in pediatric spinal cord injury and who have developed pivotal collaborations for advancing excellence in pediatric spinal cord injury. We owe a great deal of gratitude to the authors of each chapter of *Spinal Cord Injury in the Child and Young Adult* and to our many external reviewers. Finally, we would like to acknowledge our current and past patients and their families from whom we derive our inspiration and energy as clinicians, educators, researchers, and advocates.

The author of Chapter 6 would like to acknowledge Glenda Bosques, MD; Manuel Gonzalez-Brito, DO; Nigel Price, MD; Dave Pruitt, MD; John Ragheb, MD; Laure Rutter, RN; and Lawrence C Vogel, MD, for their contributions to the manuscript.

The author of Chapter 10 greatly appreciates the contribution of Alicia M January, PhD (Marquette University, Shriners Hospitals for Children, Chicago, IL, USA) in providing Table 10.1, 'Neuropsychological assessment instruments for children'.

The authors of Chapter 15 would like to thank Meghan Birkholz, MSPH Epidemiology/ Outcomes, Children's Hospital Colorado, for analysis of Pediatric Health Information Systems data for this chapter; Marisa Dzarnoski, RD, CNSC, Registered Dietitian, Children's Hospital Colorado, for the nutritional recommendations table; and Theresa Capaci, PA-C, WCC, Department of Plastic Surgery, University of Colorado/Children's Hospital Colorado (author of the 'Surgical Intervention' section).

The authors of Chapter 20 would like to thank Jillian Strober Horowitz (Thomas Jefferson University, School of Health Professions, Philadelphia) for her contributions to this chapter.

The authors of Chapter 23 wish to acknowledge the review and information provided by John Cobb, BScOT, Acute Spine Program, Vancouver General Hospital, Vancouver, BC, Canada; and Curt Johnson, MS, CRC, ATP, University of Washington Medical Center, Seattle, WA, USA.

The authors of Chapter 28 acknowledge support from the Craig H. Neilsen Foundation, the Christopher and Dana Reeve Foundation through a cooperative agreement with the Centers for Disease Control (Award No 1U59DD000838), Commonwealth of Kentucky Challenge for Excellence, Kentucky Spinal Cord and Head Injury Research Trust, and the Rebecca F. Hammond Trust.

The editors of this book would like to thank Hilary Hart, Anne-Marie Halligan, Udoka Ohuonu, and Alessy Beaver for their thoughtful reviews and critiques of this book and guidance along the process.

Section 1 Overview

1
LIFE WITH A SPINAL CORD INJURY: FROM THE PARENTS', DAUGHTER'S, AND CLINICIAN'S PERSPECTIVE

Bridget Harrington, Michael Harrington, Jan McCreary and Heather Russell

Case vignette

Bridget is a 21-year-old female with a T1 American Spinal Injury Association Impairment Scale (AIS) C spinal cord injury as a consequence of a brain and spinal cord abscess at the age of 14 years. Bridget was otherwise healthy until the age of 14 years when she developed a frontal lobe brain abscess with right hemiplegia subsequent to a sinus infection while she was living abroad with her parents owing to her father's sabbatical. She underwent neurosurgical repair to drain the abscess, and subsequently demonstrated some improvement of the right hemiplegia. Approximately two weeks later, she experienced further deterioration, at which time computed tomography demonstrated an occipital lobe abscess, necessitating a second neurosurgical procedure. Postoperatively, Bridget experienced visual problems along with upper and lower extremity paralysis. After this second surgery, Bridget remained in the intensive care unit for 7 weeks, requiring ventilator support and a tracheotomy. After being weaned off the ventilator, she received in-patient rehabilitation and, approximately 10 weeks after onset of her symptoms, she was transferred back home for further in-patient rehabilitation in Australia in a children's hospital. Her diagnosis at that time was an incomplete spinal cord injury (C5 sensory level, C7 motor level) with neurogenic bladder and bowel, neuropathic pain, and spasticity. She remained hospitalized for rehabilitation for approximately 9 months and during that time underwent placement of an intrathecal baclofen pump, and tendo-achilles and hamstring lengthenings. She has since also undergone Mitrofanoff (appendicovesicostomy) and Malone antegrade continent enema procedures. Bridget has experienced slow but continued recovery in her upper extremities, with her right arm functioning more strongly than her left. In addition, she has some functioning in her lower extremities (i.e. her left leg being stronger than her right leg). Her current presentation suggests an incomplete T1 spinal cord injury AIS C. Bridget's primary mode of mobility is a power wheelchair, although she also has a manual wheelchair. Prior to the onset of her illness, Bridget was a high-functioning student with excellent grades. Her premorbid level of functioning was estimated to be within the high average to superior range. Repeated neuropsychological assessments have demonstrated cognitive improvements across all domains relative to her initial performance after illness onset; however, she continues to be adversely impacted by an impairment in speed of mental/motor processing and, to a modest extent, weakness in perceptual reasoning ability.

The parents' perspective

Introduction

Bridget's illness, surgery, and ensuing recovery over the past 6 years has gone through several phases. There was the initial acute phase in the Netherlands that lasted 3 months, followed by the return to Australia and 9 months of hospitalization. Upon her release from hospital, we had a challenging 2-year period in which she completed high school and attempted to re-establish the life she had before the illness. The fourth, and current, phase has centered on university life and ongoing rehabilitation, including periodic visits to the USA for treatment. As she is physically stronger and increasingly independent, for Bridget it has been a time of developing new interests, passions, and friends.

Coping

Treatment of Bridget's brain injury required two operations, the second of which left her totally paralyzed from the head down. Over 7 weeks in intensive care she regained enough function to speak, eat, and use her right hand. The severity of her condition meant we were in a state of near shock, and this was compounded by the fact that we were on our own in a foreign country. The initial diagnosis was a myopathy and prognosis of an ultimately successful recovery, and we were thus driven by a level of hope that might not have been there in different circumstances, for example following a severe car crash.

Once we arrived back in Australia, Bridget's neurologist confirmed that she did in fact have a spinal cord injury (SCI) and one that would lead to other medical issues, including tight tendons, spasticity, and the need to insert a baclofen pump. In addition, she needed to undergo a cranial reconstruction for the previous surgery. In the early days our emotional energy was focused on these matters but, after a time, life started to return to some routine, as we balanced work with a constant presence at the hospital. It was at this time that the life-changing nature of Bridget's condition began to be felt. Jan was overcome by profound guilt for what had happened to Bridget and grief for the impact the injury was having, and possibly would have on her for the rest of her life. Speaking to social workers helped but she found she needed to deal with her grief more privately. For his part, Michael coped largely by focusing on the immediate medical condition and by explicitly avoiding thinking about the future. The present was enough to deal with. Family, friends, colleagues, and employers provided tremendous emotional and financial support. But, on perhaps too many occasions, well-meaning individuals would attempt to assure us with the observation 'It must have happened for a reason'. Words intended to comfort instead provoked the most visceral of emotional reactions. Jan often wanted to scream: 'This hasn't happened to your child. What possible reason could there be for it happening to mine?'. One of the most comforting comments for Jan came from one of Bridget's specialists who simply and quite dispassionately pointed out that no one was to blame, that these things happen. (His actual words were 'It is not your fault. Shit happens and this is a lot of shit'.)

The trauma of Bridget's injury and the demands of the recovery process placed an enormous stress on our relationship. During the initial phase in the Netherlands, a social worker warned us that marriages are often a casualty in these situations and that we should be aware of the toll the stress will take. Our experience certainly bore that out, as we went through a long period when it felt like our daily lives were totally defined and absorbed by Bridget's recovery. In retrospect, we realize how important it was that we each had time and space to come to terms with the huge change in our life in our own ways.

Bridget has made huge improvements over the last 6 years. She has been studying part time at university for the past 3 years and is doing well in her classes. She has gone from being completely paralyzed from the neck down to being able to use both hands (including writing), get in and out of bed and her wheelchair using a frame, and even walk 30 feet with the aid of parallel bars or a walker. After being dropped off at university, she is completely independent and, in the last 6 months, she has started going to town on the bus on her own.

It is still difficult to come to terms with the consequences of her illness. But, at the same time, there is always hope that she will continue to become more independent.

Dealing with the Healthcare System

Over the course of Bridget's treatment, recovery, and rehabilitation, we have had experience with the Dutch, Australian, and American healthcare systems. Bridget was initially treated at a major university hospital in the Netherlands. Overall, we felt we received excellent care. Despite not speaking Dutch, we never felt that language was an issue and every effort was made to keep us informed. However, we did feel great frustration at not knowing what caused the paralysis after the second operation. An SCI was ruled out in favor of a myopathy or neuropathy arising from the second surgery, although neither diagnosis was conclusive. When we returned to Australia, the issue had still not been resolved and, indeed, follow-up tests in Australia indicated that she did sustain a high-level SCI as result of the infection, the surgery, or a combination thereof.

Upon our return to Australia, Bridget was treated by a complex care team in a local children's hospital. The complexity and severity of Bridget's condition meant that rehabilitation could only be undertaken after the more pressing medical issues had been addressed. Working with a large team was frustrating. Despite the team leader working very hard to keep us and the team on the same page, we often felt that communication only happened when we pushed it. In retrospect, we feel that we were not adequately prepared for the wide-ranging medical, physical, and psychological consequences of an SCI. Vital information, particularly regarding the long-term bowel and bladder issues experienced by patients suffering from an SCI, was either mentioned in passing or ignored. We would have preferred to have been given too much information, even if at times it was difficult to deal with, than to have been left, as we were, unaware of issues that may (and did) develop later.

Dealing with a complex care team and then with a large out-patient rehabilitation program meant we interacted with a number of therapists, working both as teams and as individuals. There was limited continuity in personnel and the interactions came to take on a predictable pattern. At the initial encounter, the first question was invariably 'What are your goals?'. Our first instinctive reaction was 'We have a daughter with an incomplete SCI of unknown etiology. We want her to walk, to be independent. That is our goal. What other goal could there be?'. Of course the person posing the question wanted to identify specific needs relevant to her current condition. The frustration we often felt was that we didn't know what was possible. We found it frustrating and quite stressful to be asked to identify goals without having any idea of what might be useful and achievable. After about the third such encounter we also learned that there would never be any attempt to monitor or assess whether the goals are met, or any attempt to provide us with tools to do that monitoring and assessment ourselves.

Healthcare in Australia is provided jointly by the state and federal governments. On Bridget's 18th birthday, her care was transferred to the adult spinal cord unit at another hospital in our city. In Queensland, there are no out-patient SCI rehabilitation services. However, funding is provided for biweekly treatment from a private provider as well as for in-home care, both of which we manage. We have been lucky to have a neurophysiotherapist who has been a perfect fit for Bridget both professionally and personally.

Bridget has a support worker who comes to the house for about 25 hours a week, funded by the state disability agency. The support worker helps get Bridget up, showered, and dressed in the morning, takes her to her physiotherapy sessions, and then drops her off at university for the rest of the day. The support worker makes an enormous difference to our lives. It has allowed Jan to continue working full time and has reduced the physical demands on both of us that caring for someone with an SCI brings. We have also received funding for home modifications, transportation, and medical supplies. The complexity of her case has meant we have interacted with many agencies and our experience has confirmed the importance of a patient having a strong advocate who is persistent, and on occasion insistent, that her voice is heard.

Since 2008, Bridget has also been extremely fortunate to be able to receive treatment periodically from an adolescent SCI unit in a children's hospital in the USA. We have made five visits over the past 3 years for in-patient rehabilitation treatment for periods of 2 to 3 weeks each. The program complements and reinforces her therapy treatment in Australia, provides her with the chance to interact with other patients her age suffering from an SCI, and provides us with some peace of mind that comes with having an additional informed perspective on her rehabilitation.

In conclusion, having a child with an SCI is a life-changing experience in the literal sense of the phrase. The change is continuous and the end is uncertain. We have often been told that our journey with Bridget is like running a marathon and not a 100-m dash. You need to take each day as it comes.

The daughter's perspective

Introduction

When people see someone in a wheelchair, they assume that the worst part of sustaining an SCI is not being able to walk. As someone with an SCI, I can tell you that there are many other aspects of the injury that are far more challenging. Sustaining an SCI can mean that everything in your body below the level of your injury can be affected. One of my greatest physical challenges is bladder and bowel dysfunction. The incomplete nature of my injury is another aspect of my condition that is hard to come to terms with. Finally, my SCI has greatly affected my relationships with my parents and my friends.

Physical Challenges

The most obvious aspect of an SCI is the physical changes to your body. For me, the most frustrating aspect of my injury has been my bladder and bowel dysfunction. At the end of 2009, I underwent a Mitrofanoff procedure to allow me to catheterize through a hole in my navel. Prior to the surgery, I managed my bladder with an in-dwelling catheter and a leg bag. The Mitrofanoff has been fantastic, as it has given me independence and control over at least one aspect of my life.

During the Mitrofanoff operation I also received a Malone antegrade continent enema (MACE) to allow me to manage my bowels more effectively. The MACE was promised as an effective and relatively efficient means to manage a process that had, up to that point, been neither. In fact, the MACE experience has been an extremely frustrating one. At the best of times it has worked adequately, but at the worst of times it has been hellish. My day is dominated by sitting on the toilet, and the procedure itself has at times made me feel so ill I have had to lie down for half an hour. The unpredictability of the process keeps me constantly on edge; consequently, I often feel as though my bowels are holding me captive.

Before sustaining an SCI I always thought that it simply meant you lost leg function. I know now how incredibly complex SCIs are. The location of your injury and whether it is incomplete or complete can drastically change your level of functioning. Having an incomplete SCI is both a good and bad thing. It has been around six and a half years since I sustained my injury, and I am still making considerable, albeit painfully slow, physical improvements, where I have gone from being paralyzed from the neck down on a ventilator to being able to step with my left leg. I know this would not be happening if I had sustained a complete injury. At the same time, however, is the uncertainty of whether the progress will continue. One of my doctors recently told me he expects I will walk again aided in some capacity and, while I have great confidence in his expertise, deep down I am no more certain of this than the doctor who told me in 2006 that I would probably never walk again. I know there are probably some people who have complete SCIs who would read this and consider me ungrateful for not appreciating the improvements I have made, but it is hard to always feel positive when I know that any given improvement could be my last.

Social Realities

As an only child of two parents who work full time I have always been independent. My parents and I have always had a close relationship but when I sustained my SCI that relationship changed. I was forced back into a dependence on my parents that I had never had, at least not since infancy. In the past 6 years I have spent most of my time in close contact with my parents and I feel as though this forced closeness has strained our relationship. At my age many people are considering moving out of home, but I know that, physically speaking, that is not something that is possible for me right now. I still feel close to my parents but my physical dependence on them has meant that I do not have the same chance for space when I am in a bad mood.

Sustaining an SCI at 14 years of age has meant that not only did I have to spend a year in hospital recovering from and trying to accept my injury, but I also missed out on a year of school and socializing with my friends. This loss meant that, when I went back to school a year after my injury, I felt as though I was suspended in time. I did not have the space to grow as a person because of my injury and my unwanted 'celebrity' status at school. Everyone, even students and teachers I did not know, knew my name and what had happened to me. Although my friends had been very supportive during my hospital stay, once I was back at school I felt a distance between us. I do not know if this distance came from my feeling that everything in my life had changed irrevocably or that my friends were treating me differently given the change in my physical situation; I suspect it was a combination of the two. It was an incredibly lonely time.

While I still keep in contact with some of my friends from high school (and not just through Facebook), I have also made a number of new friends through the clubs and societies on campus. I have noticed that I approach my friendships with these people very differently to those I had with people who knew me before my injury. The most obvious difference is that very few of my friends at university know why I am in a wheelchair. It probably should not matter, but the fact that I do not talk about it makes me feel as though I am holding something back from these people. I think this reservation partly stems from the desire to be known as more than 'Bridget in a wheelchair'; I would rather be remembered as 'Bridget the psych major who cares about the environment and just happens to be in a wheelchair'. Despite my conscious choice to distance my university self from my injury, I sometimes feel as though I have created a barrier and this barrier means I do not feel as close to my university friends as I might otherwise.

Since 2008, I have made periodic visits to a children's hospital in Chicago that specializes in pediatric SCI rehabilitation. During these visits I undergo intensive in-patient rehabilitation for a period of 2 to 3 weeks. The staff and the rehabilitation program are fantastic, but the best thing about the experience has been the chance to interact with other people my own age with SCIs because in Australia I do not have that opportunity.

Meeting and interacting with other young people has helped me to better come to terms with my injury. The people I have met are dealing with similar physical challenges and – in psychosocial terms – are at similar points in their lives. At the same time, the experience has also made me realize how different my SCI is, caused as it was by a brain infection and its treatment. Many of the young people I have met have a complete SCI caused by trauma.

This difference affected how connected I felt to the others, even though when we have talked about our injuries and our lives we all seem to be going through similar problems at school and feel the same insecurities.

I do not think I have ever really 'come to terms' with my SCI. Part of the reason is because the effects of my injury have been constantly changing as I have regained function, but part of it comes down to the fact that I spent 14 years living without an SCI. During this time I developed close relationships with many people and my injury changed all of that. Two years after I sustained my injury someone who had received their SCI decades before told me that, one day, I would see my SCI as the best thing that ever happened to me. After six and a half years of living with an SCI, I doubt I will ever feel this way. My SCI changed me physically and psychologically, and has left its mark on all of my relationships. However, it has happened and it is something I cannot change. All I can do is make the best life I can.

The clinician's perspective

Introduction

The profound life changes involved in pediatric SCIs are clearly illustrated in the story of Bridget and her parents, Jan and Michael. Like Bridget's family, most families coping with an SCI report that things are never quite the same after the injury. It is important to note, however, that, overall, young people living with an SCI do not experience poor psychological outcomes (Anderson et al 2009). Young people are highly resilient and adaptive. Children often view themselves as differently abled rather than disabled and, although things may never be 'normal' again, for most young people with an SCI, they find a 'new normal' that can be rich and satisfying. In fact, after a child's SCI, it is often the parents or caregivers who experience the most distress (Kelly et al 2011). The job of the pediatric rehabilitation professional, therefore, is to help families cope with the changes brought about by an SCI, adapt to them successfully, and manage expectations for the future. The story of Bridget and her parents highlights a number of key points to be addressed in this process. These will be discussed in three sections: (1) the concerns shared by both Bridget and her parents; (2) the concerns presented by her parents; and (3) Bridget's individual concerns.

Shared Concerns

Bridget and her parents describe frustration with uncertainty about her prognosis, an issue that is commonly distressing to children and families after an SCI. Making matters more difficult for this particular family is that the etiology of Bridget's injury was unclear. As a result, medical personnel were not always able to provide straightforward answers and explanations. From experience, families want to know what they can expect in the future, whether this comes in the form of good or bad news. Indeed, Jan 'would have preferred to have been given too much information, even if at times it was difficult to deal with, than to have been left, as we were, unaware of issues that may (and did) develop later'. Concerns about the lack of information run through each account. For example, Jan and Michael describe being asked what their rehabilitation 'goals' for Bridget were without knowing what was possible. An SCI was uncharted terrain for them and they did not always feel they were given a usable map.

For Bridget, she expressed feeling unprepared for the new realities of her life and a lack of clarity on the part of the medical staff providing care. The conflicting needs of patients and medical professionals are visible here. For example, information regarding specific strategies for management of SCI complications may be viewed as immediate concerns by medical staff, but are sometimes seen as secondary to patients and families who want to know more of the 'big picture' of what daily life with an SCI will look like. Although the family felt they had generally received excellent care, it is clear that they struggled with uncertainties in what to expect from the future.

The perception of a lack of information on the part of Bridget's family has important implications for the rehabilitation professional. Of course, there are simply no answers to some questions. Pediatric SCIs are complex and recovery is highly variable. Families and medical professionals may have different perspectives regarding information needs. Knowing that anxious families are likely to have trouble remembering detailed information, medical personnel are rightly hesitant to offer speculation about the future. However, the entire team can work together to foster acceptance of the unknown in each family member and in the family as a whole over time.

A corollary concern also shared by both Bridget and her parents is the difficulty in contending with the complexities of the medical system. An SCI in a child is a multifaceted condition that requires input from numerous specialists of a various disciplines. As a result, families unfamiliar with the medical system may feel lost in the shuffle, with the unfortunate effect of constantly shifting the locus of control in a child's recovery amongst a cast of peripheral characters not well known to the family. Because Bridget needed medical care in several different countries, her experience may fall on the extreme end of this spectrum. However, Bridget's and Jan's accounts bring up issues commonly encountered: Jan describes 'limited continuity in personnel' and Bridget was told to expect very different outcomes depending on the clinician. This is understandably confusing and frustrating to all family members. Furthermore, many families, especially those of low socio-economic status and/or those who do not speak the predominant language of the hospital, may feel intimidated by medical staff and reticent to ask questions. In short, the patient and the family may perceive barriers between themselves and medical professionals that may interfere with treatment and increase uncertainty and anxiety. In this context, it is most important that the treatment team makes itself available to answer questions and to repeat information as needed.

A further area of difficulty presented by both Bridget and her parents could perhaps best be described as isolation. SCIs are life altering and all family members are likely to experience a period of grieving for the former life that was lost. Although Jan and Michael state that their extended family was extremely supportive, they also recall that 'well-meaning individuals would attempt to assure' them with unhelpful comments, including that the injury 'must have happened for a reason'. Support from other parents who had gone through similar situations would have been helpful. For Bridget, sustaining an SCI in adolescence 'meant that not only did [she] have to spend a year in hospital recovering from and trying to accept [her] injury, but [she] also missed out on a year of school and socializing'. Furthermore, she notes that, when she returned to school, she 'felt a distance' with her peers. These concerns are shared by other young people after an SCI (Mulcahey 1991). Children's social worlds move quickly, such that any time away can seem like an eternity. When a return to normative social activities is possible, the presence of noticeable physical limitations can feel highly isolating. Bridget wants to be defined by her peers as Bridget 'who just happens to be in a wheelchair', but the barrier of difference in a child's development often feels insurmountable. Bridget regrets the limited opportunities to interact with people her own age who are living with an SCI. Furthermore, she notes some intragroup isolation; although the young adults she knows with SCI 'are dealing with similar physical challenges and... are at similar points in their lives', her SCI is 'different'. Because the etiology of her SCI is uncommon, she does not feel complete kinship with her peers with spinal cord lesions. Nevertheless, Bridget illustrates the resilience of many young people in her description of successfully seeking out new friendships after her injury and developing a rewarding social circle. Members of the treatment team can facilitate this socialization process by connecting the family with other families who have undergone similar experiences.

Finally, although Bridget's entrance into university is a success story, both Bridget and her parents struggle with issues surrounding independence and future goals. In typical development, generally, parents expect children and children expect themselves to become more independent as they get older. Unfortunately, SCI subverts that process. The emotion surrounding these issues for both Bridget and her parents is clear in their individual accounts; Jan and Michael state 'we want her to walk, to be independent', while Bridget notes that she was 'forced back into a dependence on her parents that [she] had never had, at least not since infancy'. It is clear that neither Bridget nor her parents had pictured living with what Bridget calls 'forced closeness' at this stage of their lives. Moreover, it should be noted that this is in the context of a health aide who helps Bridget approximately 25 hours a week; many families without this resource are likely to experience much more uncomfortable 'closeness'.

Some families experience a rather opposing challenge, in terms of independence, than that described by Bridget's family. That is, many parents of children with SCI become uncomfortable with a child's normative needs for separation and autonomy; it is difficult for parents to let go of children they may have come to view, through years of caregiving and medical treatment, as frail and delicate. Some parents want to protect their children from the realities of life with a disability. Furthermore, in their own lives, parents have not had the benefit of knowing individuals with SCI who lead full and rich lives with positive outcomes (e.g. attaining higher levels of formal education than able-bodied peers; Zebracki et al 2010). As a result, parents may not encourage their children to pursue opportunities (educational, occupational, social) outside of the home, and children may feel guilty about their desire to separate from their parents. Conversely, a child may become enmeshed with their well-meaning but over-protective parents such that they are reluctant to consider opportunities to live a fuller life. They may come to internalize their parents' views of their disability or subconsciously fear hurting their parents by beginning to separate during late adolescence and adulthood. As part of the rehabilitation process, the team can work with the family to help set reasonable goals and expectations, provide encouragement, access educational and occupational resources, and assist families with tracking progress.

Parents' Concerns

Although Jan and Michael note that their family was blessed with 'tremendous' financial support from family and friends, it is hard to overemphasize the financial burden of pediatric SCI. This burden usually is a primary focus of the parents when more pressing concerns (e.g. the child's immediate health and treatment) should be the focus of attention. Often, one or both parents must take time off work in order to care for the child, further compounding the family's monetary worries. In addition to acute care costs, children with SCI require a lifetime of specialized medical care to prevent secondary complications and address self-care needs. As full-time SCI caregiving by family members can result in decrements in family members' mental and physical health (Nogueira et al 2012), hiring a health aide may be necessary. Jan and Michael state that even a part-time health aide has made 'an enormous difference' in their lives, allowing both parents to maintain full-time work.

Jan and Michael also report substantial marital strain in the aftermath of Bridget's injury. Very perceptively, they note their different coping styles, stating that Michael tended to 'focus on the immediate medical condition' while Jan needed to 'deal with her grief more privately'. In addition to shock and grief following a child's SCI, parents may report a great deal of guilt surrounding a child's injury. Although a parent can cognitively understand that a child's injury was either unavoidable or an unintended accident, parents often experience significant trauma when their child sustains an SCI. The tendency for parents to become completely absorbed in the child's recovery, to the exclusion of maintaining the committed partnership, may also contribute to distance between the partners. These factors, when combined with differing coping styles and financial strain, can create a tenuous relationship.

On the other hand, a committed partnership or marriage can be an extraordinary support system for dealing with the distress of a child's SCI. The team should make every effort to help parents make decisions together about a child's treatment and needs, and work on communication skills between the couple. There is a tendency after a child's injury for one parent to become the primary caregiver. Although this may be unavoidable, the 'non-primary' parent should still take an active role in decision making. All decisions and care being the designated provenance of one individual is a pattern that should not become engrained. Additionally, frustrations caused by differing coping styles can be addressed with the goal of helping each partner understand that grief and trauma responses can take many different forms.

Jan and Michael's account of their marital progress since Bridget's injury speaks of their strengthened relationship. This is an ideal outcome. The couple speaks with mutual sympathy, perceptiveness, and understanding. It is important to note that many parents of children with SCI are no longer involved in a romantic partnership with each other. In these cases, fostering mutual understanding and a team approach to managing the child's care can be difficult. Both parents should be advised that effective teamwork is vital to the child's physical and mental health. If necessary, family counseling should be recommended to achieve this goal. Finally, in working with single-parent or non-traditional families, it is desirable to bring in other family members for support. Raising a child with an SCI is a team effort.

Patient's Concerns

In addition to grief, shock, and loss, children may be traumatized by the circumstances of the injury. Furthermore, some children are injured in circumstances that result in serious injury and/or loss of life to loved ones, immeasurably compounding challenges to recovery and adjustment. Bridget, fortunately, was not one of these children, but notes a number of adverse emotional consequences of her injury. Bridget is sensitive to the interruption of her emotional development, stating 'I did not have the space to grow as a person because of my injury'. She astutely observes an extremely important point in pediatric SCI recovery: adjustment changes as the child changes. Children are not static physically or emotionally and the child's world is constantly changing. Although Bridget does not specifically mention this factor, as a child enters adolescence, dating, sexuality, and fertility are often confusing in the best of circumstances. For a child with SCI, this can be compounded immeasurably.

Acceptance of different abilities is extremely important to a child's adjustment. Bridget is clearly a young woman with a wide range of problem-solving skills at her disposal, but this is not true of all children who sustain an SCI. Research suggests that some coping strategies, specifically cognitive restructuring, are related to positive mental health outcomes in adults with SCI (Kennedy et al 2003). Proficiency in evaluating negative cognitions and accurately reframing challenges are extremely helpful skills for the child with SCI. Simple psychoeducation – for example helping the child to understand that behavioral activation works wonders for a depressed mood – can have wide-ranging benefits. Children with SCI tend to be isolated socially. It is important that they feel able to seek and obtain social support from peers and family members. These skills are likely to benefit the child in adulthood, as research suggests that adults with SCI are at a higher risk of mental health difficulties (Fann et al 2011). As in any other child, seeking professional help when necessary cannot be overstated.

In conclusion, on behalf of myself, the editors, and SCI rehabilitation professionals everywhere, I offer my deepest gratitude to Bridget, Jan, and Michael for sharing their story. In doing so, they have provided a wealth of information to introduce this book. More importantly, they are a wonderful example of the willingness of families who have 'been there' to share their stories – even the most troubling parts – to help other families in similar situations. It is important for rehabilitation professionals to remember that people with SCI and their families are truly at the front lines of rehabilitation research. They are our most important resource in learning how to better treat SCI. Their strength, courage, and resilience inspire me every day, and I am continuously grateful to work with these extraordinary children and families.

REFERENCES

Anderson CJ, Kelly EH, Klaas SJ, Russell H, Daharsh E, Vogel LC (2009) Anxiety and depression in children and adolescents with spinal cord injuries. *Dev Med Child Neurol* 51: 826–32. http://dx.doi.org/10.1111/j.1469-8749.2009.03268.x

Fann JR, Bombardier CH, Richards JS, Tate DG, Wilson CS, Temkin N (2011) Depression after spinal cord injury: comorbidities, mental health service use, and adequacy of treatment. *Arch Phys Med Rehabil* 92: 352–60. http://dx.doi.org/10.1016/j.apmr.2010.05.016

Kelly EH, Anderson CJ, Garma S et al (2011) Relationships between the psychological characteristics of youth with spinal cord injury and their primary caregivers. *Spinal Cord* 49: 200–5. http://dx.doi.org/10.1038/sc.2010.78

Kennedy P, Duff J, Evans M, Beedie A (2003) Coping effectiveness training reduces depression and anxiety following traumatic spinal cord injuries. *Br J Clin Psychol* 42: 41–52. http://dx.doi.org/10.1348/014466503762842002

Mulcahey MJ (1991) Returning to school after a spinal cord injury: perspectives from four adolescents. *Am J Occup Ther* 46: 305–11. http://dx.doi.org/10.5014/ajot.46.4.305

Nogueira PC, Rabeh SA, Caliri MH, Dantas RA, Haas VJ (2012) Burden of care and its impact on health-related quality of life of caregivers of individuals with spinal cord injury. *Rev Lat Am Enfermagem* 20: 1048–56. http://dx.doi.org/10.1590/S0104-11692012000600006

Zebracki K, Anderson C, Chlan K, Vogel L (2010) Outcomes of adults with pediatric-onset spinal cord injury: longitudinal findings and implications on transition to adulthood. *Top Spinal Cord Inj Rehab* 16: 17–25. http://dx.doi.org/10.1310/sci1601-17

2
EPIDEMIOLOGY

Yuying Chen and Michael J DeVivo

Injury is the leading cause of death for children and adolescents in the USA (Centers for Disease Control and Prevention 2009). Millions of young people, aged 0 to 19 years, suffer injuries requiring treatment in the emergency department every year. Spinal cord injury (SCI) accounts for only a small proportion of all injuries in children; however, its physical and psychosocial consequences are devastating. Very few people experience complete neurologic recovery after SCI (Fawcett et al 2007). A significant proportion of SCIs result in neurologically complete and tetraplegic deficits. Managing an SCI and the related health conditions costs several million dollars throughout the life (Cao et al 2011, National Spinal Cord Injury Statistical Center 2013), which poses a significant burden to individuals with SCI, their families, and society. The adverse impact and preventability of SCI highlights the need for public health action.

Understanding the epidemiologic profile of SCI is essential for prevention and control as well as for strategic planning for clinical and supportive services specific for the region and country. The goal of this chapter is to provide an overview of the quantitative and qualitative features of SCI in children, in contrast to adults with SCI. In addition to reviewing worldwide literature, etiologic and demographic profiles and the mortality experience of persons who were enrolled in the National SCI Database (NSCID) (Stover et al 1999) and National Shriners SCI Database (NSSCID) (DeVivo and Vogel 2004) in the USA will be presented.

Incidence: new injuries

Annual incidence measures the number of new injuries that occur during a 1-year period. The global mapping project, launched by the International Spinal Cord Society, reported an annual SCI incidence rate of 39 new cases per million population in the USA, which is close to that of Canada (35 per million in 2006 and 52 per million in 2010), but considerably higher than the figures reported in Western Europe (16 per million) and Australia (15 per million) (Cripps et al 2011, Lee et al 2014). International variation can largely be explained by the differences in methodology (i.e. case definition, eligibility, reporting procedures, and completeness of case ascertainment) and differences in population characteristics, environmental factors, and pre-hospital mortality rates. Interestingly, a higher percentage of violence-related SCIs was reported in North America (16%) than in Western Europe (6%) and Australia (2%) (Lee et al 2014).

Within the USA, SCIs also vary geographically, which, to some extent, is due to the different research methodology and population characteristics. Data from the USA SCI registries in the 1980s and 1990s showed that the annual rates (per million population) were 25 new cases in West Virginia (Woodruff and Baron 1994), 28 in Arkansas (Acton et al 1993), 30 in Virginia (Virginia Department of Rehabilitation Services 1993), 39 in Utah (Thurman et al 1994), 40 in Oklahoma (Price et al 1994), 43 in New York (Relethford et al 1991), 45 in Colorado (Colorado Department of Public Health and Environment 1997), 46 in Louisiana (Bayakly and Lawrence 1992), 46 in Georgia (Johnson 1992), 56 in Rhode Island (Buechner et al 2000), 59 in Mississippi (Surkin et al 2000), and 83 in Alaska (Warren et al 1995). Previous population-based studies at the regional (Clifton 1983, Burke et al 2001) and national level (Kalsbeek et al 1980, Bracken et al 1981, Vitale et al 2006) in the USA showed similar figures, ranging from 25 to 60 new cases per million per year. Taken together, excluding those who die at the scene of the accident, SCI incidence on average is about 40 new cases per million population per year. Given the current population size in the USA of 313 million people, there are approximately 12 500 new SCIs each year.

There have not been any national population-based incidence studies of SCI in the USA since the 1990s. As a result, it is not clear whether the number of new injuries every year has increased, decreased, or remained the same in recent years.

How Many Children Sustain a Spinal Cord Injury Every Year?

Population-based incidence studies of children with SCI are limited in the literature; however, virtually all of those that do exist support the idea that the risk of getting an SCI is lowest for children younger than 16 years. The age-specific incidence rate is typically less than 10 new cases per million children aged 0 to 15 years and about 20 to 25 new cases per million children aged 0 to 19 years in the USA, which also varies by regions and countries (Table 2.1) (Kewalramani et al 1980, Bracken et al 1981, Acton et al 1993, Dixon et al 1993, Price et al 1994, Thurman et al 1994, Woodruff and Baron 1994, Warren et al 1995, Martins et al 1998, Buechner et al 2000, Surkin et al 2000, Augutis and Levi 2003, Vitale et al 2006, Puisto et al 2010, van den Berg et al 2010, Noonan et al 2012). Children younger than 16 years account for about 3% to 5% of total SCIs that occur each year (Table 2.1), resulting in approximately 375 to 625 new cases given the annual total of 12 500 SCIs per year in the USA. People younger than 20 years account for approximately 15% to 20% of new SCIs, or 1875 to 2500 cases every year in the USA.

Males experience a higher risk of SCI than females. When all ages are considered, the male to female ratio is about 4.0 (Acton et al 1993, Price et al 1994, Thurman et al 1994, Woodruff and Baron 1994, Surkin et al 2000). This sex difference is much smaller among children and adolescents, where the male to female ratio was reported to be between 1.0 and 2.4 (Table 2.1). The higher incidence in males is presumably related to the increased risk-taking behavior they exhibit after early childhood. For example, males may be more likely to participate in acts of violence and contact sports, as well as own and/or drive a car, than their female counterparts as they grow into adulthood.

In the USA, the incidence rates are higher for black people than for white people, especially among males and for violence-related SCI. The black to white incidence rate ratio is

TABLE 2.1
Age-specific annual incidence rate of spinal cord injury

Population	Study period	Age group (years)	% total spinal cord injuries	Age-specific rate (per million children)	Male to female rate ratio	Incidence rate, all ages (per million population)
USA						
National Hospital Discharge Survey (Bracken et al 1981)	1970–1977	0–14	5.5	–	–	40.1
		0–19	–	21.2	–	
		20–24	–	68.0	–	
Healthcare Cost and Utilization Project Kid's Inpatient Database (Vitale et al 2006)	1997, 2000	0–18	–	19.9	2.4	–
Northern California (Kewalramani et al 1980)	1970–1971	0–15	4.8 and 9.4[a]	8.9 and 18.2[a]	1.7[a]	32.2 and 53.4[a]
Arkansas (Acton et al 1993, Augutis and Levi 2003)	1980–1989	0–14	–	5.0	–	28.5
West Virginia (Woodruff and Baron 1994)	1985–1988	0–14	–	1.0	1.0	25.0
		15–24	–	46.0	3.0	
Oklahoma (Price et al 1994)	1988–1990	0–14	3.2	6.0	1.8	40.0
		15–19	17.5	94.0	2.7	
		20–24	15.2	85.0	6.0	
Utah (Thurman et al 1994, Augutis and Levi 2003)	1989–1991	0–14	12.1[a]	16.7[a]	–	39.0 and 43.0[a]
Alaska (Warren et al 1995)	1991–1993	0–4	0	0.0	–	83.0
		5–14	2.8	14.0	2.9	
		15–24	20.9	120.0	3.2	
Mississippi (Surkin et al 2000)	1992–1994	0–14	3.5[a]	11.3[a]	2.4[a]	59.0 and 77.0[a]
		15–19	13.2[a]	116.7[a]	9.2[a]	
		20–24	15.2[a]	152.6[a]	5.2[a]	
Rhode Island (Buechner et al 2000)	1994–1998	0–14	–	9.0	–	56.0
Canada						
Noonan et al 2012	2010			Male / Female		53.0[a]
		0–4	0.3[a]	3.8[a] / 1.9[a]	2.0[a]	
		5–9	1.8[a]	22.0[a] / 14.4[a]	1.5[a]	
		10–14	2.0[a]	22.0[a] / 14.4[a]	1.5[a]	
		15–19	9.5[a]	91.0[a] / 62.5[a]	1.5[a]	
		20–24	11.2[a]	132.1[a] / 38.3[a]	3.4[a]	

TABLE 2.1
(Continued)

Population	Study period	Age group (years)	% total spinal cord injuries	Age-specific rate (per million children)	Male to female rate ratio	Incidence rate, all ages (per million population)
Sweden						
Augutis and Levi 2003	1985–1996	0–14	–	1.9 and 3.8[a]	–	15.0[a]
		0–15	–	2.4 and 4.6[a]	–	
Finland						
Puisto et al 2010	1997–2006	0–18	–	1.9 and 4.3[a]	–	–
Portugal						
Martins et al 1998	1989–1992	0–14	–	27.0[a]	–	57.8[a]
New Zealand						
Dixon et al 1993	1979–1988	0–14	–	8.6	–	43.3

[a]Including pre-hospital deaths.

between 1.4 and 2.0 overall (Bracken et al 1981, Acton et al 1993, Price et al 1994, Surkin et al 2000, Burke et al 2001), but ranges from 6.3 to 17.8 for violence-related SCI (Bayakly and Lawrence 1992, Acton et al 1993, Price et al 1994, Surkin et al 2000). A similar difference in ethnic groups in the risk of getting an SCI was also noted in children and adolescents (Kewalramani et al 1980, Vitale et al 2006).

Etiologies and Risk Factors

External causes of SCI are often grouped into five categories: motor vehicle crashes, acts of violence, sports/recreational activities, falls, and all other causes (such as pedestrian injuries, machinery accidents, natural disasters). Some studies also reported the impairment of spinal cord function resulting from adverse effects of medical, surgical, or diagnostic procedures and treatments for non-spinal cord conditions as the sixth category (DeVivo and Vogel 2004). Motor vehicle crashes are the leading cause of SCI across all ages except persons older than 65 years, for whom falls rank first (Acton et al 1993, Price et al 1994, Jackson et al 2004). A breakdown of etiology as a function of age at injury among 35 080 persons with SCI enrolled in the NSCID and NSSCID between 1973 and 2002 is shown in Table 2.2. The five age groupings included preschool children (aged 0–5y), school-aged children (aged 6–12y), younger adolescents (aged 13–15y), older adolescents (aged 16–21y), and adults (aged >21y) (DeVivo and Vogel 2004). Motor vehicle crashes were shown to cause approximately 50%

TABLE 2.2
Etiologic and neurologic profile of persons with spinal cord injury reported to the National Spinal Cord Injury Database and National Shriners Spinal Cord Injury Database

Year of injury	2005–2011					1973–2002 (DeVivo and Vogel 2004)				
Age at injury (y)	**0–5**	**6–12**	**13–15**	**16–21**	**>22**	**0–5**	**6–12**	**13–15**	**16–21**	**>22**
Sample size	80	107	197	1535	5914	416	464	1417	8988	23 795
Etiology (%)										
Vehicular	60.0	57.0	41.1	51.8	41.5	65.2	51.7	40.7	49.1	44.3
Violence	5.0	3.7	12.2	20.4	9.4	8.7	21.6	18.9	21.6	15.8
Sports	0.0	9.4	25.9	17.3	8.5	0.2	10.6	28.2	18.3	7.6
Falls	7.5	7.5	7.6	6.8	31.2	6.5	6.5	7.9	8.1	24.1
Medical/surgical	16.3	18.7	8.1	0.8	4.6	11.6	4.9	2.8	0.6	3.1
Other	11.2	3.7	5.1	2.9	4.8	7.7	4.7	1.5	2.2	5.1
Injury level (%)										
C1–C4	23.3	12.5	17.1	24.0	33.2	11.7	15.8	18.1	15.7	20.7
C5–C8	21.7	24.0	34.8	28.9	27.1	20.2	18.2	36.1	35.9	33.2
T1–T6	23.3	28.1	20.9	19.0	13.6	–	–	–	–	–
T7–S5	31.7	34.4	26.7	27.8	25.4	–	–	–	–	–
T1–S5	–	–	–	–	–	66.3	64.2	43.9	46.9	44.7
Healthy	0.0	1.0	0.5	0.4	0.7	1.7	1.7	1.9	1.5	1.4
Injury completeness (%)										
AIS A	80.7	68.4	55.6	56.8	39.1	67.9	62.1	54.9	56.3	47.3
AIS B	8.8	8.4	13.3	15.5	13.0	–	–	–	–	–
AIS C	3.5	7.4	10.6	11.5	17.0	–	–	–	–	–
AIS D	7.0	14.7	20.0	15.9	30.3	–	–	–	–	–
AIS E	0.0	1.1	0.6	0.4	0.7	1.7	1.7	1.9	1.5	1.4

AIS, American Spinal Injury Association Impairment Scale.

of all injuries. The next most common etiologies for the preschool children were medical and surgical complications (11.6%) and violence (8.7%). Among young people aged 6 to 21 years, sports and violence were the next most common causes. Among adults, in contrast, falls were the second (24.1%) and violence (15.8%) was the third leading cause.

A recent analysis of NSCID and NSSCID participants who were injured between 2005 and 2011 showed that vehicle crashes remain the leading cause across all age groups (Chen et al 2013). Violence, however, has declined regardless of age and now ranks fifth among young people aged 0 to 12 years (Table 2.2). The top 10 specific etiologies among children aged 0 to 15 years were automobile (40.1%), medical and surgical complications (12.8%), gunshots (8.1%), falls (7.6%), diving (5.7%), other sport injuries (4.2%), all-terrain vehicle or cycle (3.9%), pedestrian injuries (3.1%), motorcycle (2.3%), hits by falling objects (1.8%), and bicycle (1.8%).

Vehicle crashes are the leading cause of SCI for both males and females (Acton et al 1993, Price et al 1994, Jackson et al 2004). The major sex difference in etiologic profile is in the proportion of gunshot wounds, motorcycle crashes, and diving injuries that cause more SCIs in males than females (Chen et al 2013). Acts of violence are a common cause of SCI among black people, and this cause has a similar share of total injuries to vehicle crashes (Price et al 1994). Among white people, violence is usually reported as the fourth leading cause, after vehicle crashes, falls, and sports. The differences between sexes and ethnic groups are true regardless of age groups (DeVivo and Vogel 2004).

Seasonal variation has been described, with the highest number of new SCIs occurring from May to August (Acton et al 1993, Chen et al 2013), which is in parallel with the increase in motorcycle crashes, diving injuries, and other recreational sport mishaps in the warmer months. Such seasonal trends, however, are less obvious among children under 6 years of age (Fig. 2.1). More SCIs occurred on Saturdays and Sundays than on any other day (Acton et al 1993), which was most probably attributable to a higher number of motorcycle crashes and diving incidents during the weekends (Chen et al 2013). In contrast, medical and surgical complications as a cause of SCI are more common on Mondays and Tuesdays than during the weekends (Chen et al 2013), which is consistent with the finding of a higher number of SCIs on Mondays among children under 6 years of age (Fig. 2.2), for whom medical and surgical complications are the second leading cause of SCI.

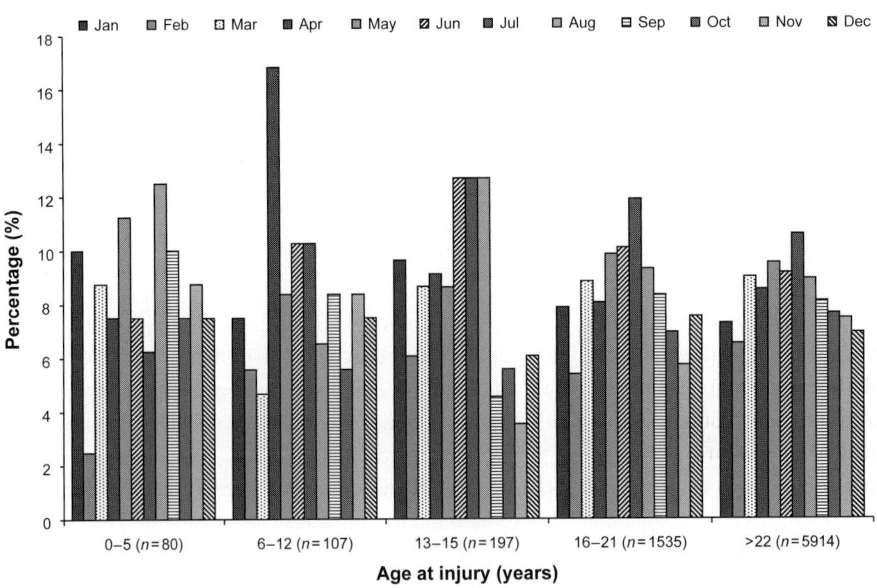

Fig. 2.1 Seasonal variation: percentage of reported cases by month of injury between 2005 and 2011.

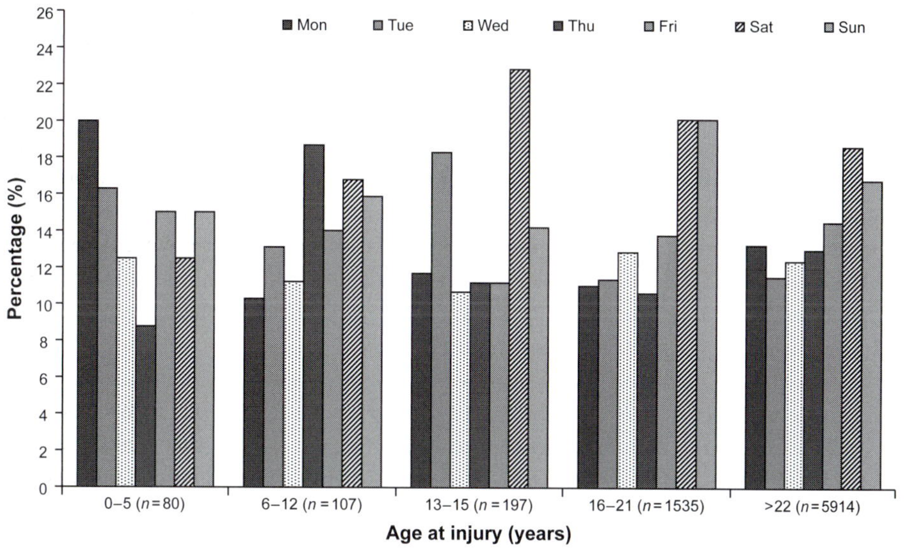

Fig. 2.2 Percentage of reported cases by day of week between 2005 and 2011.

The reported proportion of SCIs across different etiologies is a function of the frequency of participation in each activity and the risk of SCI for each activity, both of which vary substantially by age and other personal and environmental factors. For example, the lack of sport-related SCI reported among children younger than 6 years (Table 2.2) does not necessarily suggest that sport is safer for this age group than for others, but is probably a result of the fact that participation in sport/recreational activity is not as common during early childhood and that the intensity and breadth of activities differ by age groups. Similarly, the increase of SCIs related to medical/surgical complications on Mondays and Tuesdays might simply be because more complicated procedures are scheduled for those days.

Alcohol use at the time of injury is reported or patients are tested positive for alcohol in 22% to 50% of new SCIs (Acton et al 1993, Price et al 1994, Thurman et al 1994, Woodruff and Baron 1994, Warren et al 1995, Surkin et al 2000, Burke et al 2001, Garrison et al 2004, Vitale et al 2006), and it is particularly common among Native Americans, injuries occurring between 10 p.m. and 4 a.m., pedestrian injuries, and cervical injuries (Price et al 1994, Warren et al 1995, Garrison et al 2004). Analyzing data from the National Trauma Data Bank in the USA in 1997 and 2000, Vitale et al reported that alcohol and drug consumption were involved in 30% of all pediatric SCI cases (age <19y) and a seat belt was not worn by 68% of children with SCI injured in vehicle crashes (Vitale et al 2006).

Level and Completeness of Injury

The preserved neurologic function after SCI, classified by the International Standards for Neurological Classification of Spinal Cord Injury (Kirshblum et al 2011) is largely determined by the etiology and mechanism of injury. The physiological and skeletal maturity of the spine also influences the level and completeness of injury in children.

With little age variation, gunshot wounds and medical/surgical complications typically result in paraplegia, whereas diving incidents usually lead to tetraplegic injuries (DeVivo and Vogel 2004, Chen et al 2013). DeVivo and Vogel reported that vehicular crashes typically resulted in paraplegia in children younger than 13 years, but caused more tetraplegic than paraplegic injuries in adults (DeVivo and Vogel 2004). This finding, however, may not be applicable to acute SCIs, particularly regarding individuals who did not survive the first few months after injury, as the study sample largely represented delayed admissions to a Shriners Hospitals for Children and the mortality was known to be much higher among young children with tetraplegic and vehicular injuries than other ages and injuries (Kewalramani et al 1980, Vitale et al 2006, Parent et al 2011). Furthermore, the reliability of neurologic assessment among children under 5 years of age is limited (Mulcahey et al 2007).

Falls seem to cause more tetraplegic injuries in preschool children and adults, but more paraplegic injuries in children aged 6 to 12 years and 16 to 21 years (DeVivo and Vogel 2004). A previous study noted a substantial number of falls and medical/surgical complications resulting in motor functional incomplete injuries (American Spinal Injury Association Impairment Scale [AIS] D), whereas the majority of gunshot wounds and motorcycle crashes resulted in a complete injury (AIS A) (Chen et al 2013).

Level and completeness of injury by age groups among the NSCID and NSSCID participants is depicted in Table 2.2, which largely reflects the etiologies of SCI that predominate in different age groups. Compared with the previous 1973 to 2002 injury cohort (DeVivo and Vogel 2004), the proportion of high cervical injuries has increased among children below 6 years of age (11.7% vs 23.3%), aged 16 to 21 years (15.7% vs 24.0%), and aged more than 22 years (20.7% vs 33.2%). Paraplegic injuries have decreased from 66.3% to 55.0% for young people aged 0 to 5 years and from 44.7% to 39.0% for adults. Complete injuries (AIS A) have increased from 67.9% to 80.7% for young people aged 0 to 5 years and from 62.1% to 68.4% for young people aged 6 to 12 years, but have decreased from 47.3% to 39.1% for adults. Some of the findings, however, are inconsistent compared with other case series. For example, previous findings of a higher percentage of cervical injuries in children, in particular those below 8 years of age (Puisto et al 2010, Parent et al 2011), are not noted in the NSCID and NSSCID case series. This discrepancy could be partially explained by the differences in population characteristics, mechanisms of injury, and study samples (early vs late admissions).

The presence of SCI without radiographic abnormality has been well described among skeletally immature children. The percentage of SCI without radiographic abnormality varied by different case series and diagnostic tools from 5% to 72% (Augutis and Levi 2003, DeVivo and Vogel 2004, Parent et al 2011, Schottler et al 2012). The percentage was also found to decrease with increasing age, from 72% among preschool children (Schottler et al 2012) to 20% among older adolescents (aged 16–21y) (DeVivo and Vogel 2004).

The NSCID and NSSCID combined database represents the largest series of persons with SCI available to date and provides valuable insight into the demographics and etiology of SCIs in children. Nonetheless, both databases are hospital based rather than population based. It is therefore not feasible to identify appropriate denominator data to calculate actual incidence rates of SCI and estimate the risks across groups. The findings from the combined databases are influenced by the locations of the centers that contributed data to the NSCID and NSSCID during the study period, which might not be applicable to all SCIs occurring in the USA or other countries.

Mortality

Based on the discharge records from the National Data Bank in the USA in 1997 and 2000, 10% of pediatric SCI cases (aged <19y) were deceased before discharge from acute hospital care. Including those who died at the scene of injury, the mortality rate during the first year after injury among young people aged 0 to 15 years was reported to be as high as 59% in Northern California in 1970 to 1971 (Kewalramani et al 1980) and 60% in Sweden in 1985 to 1996 (Augutis and Levi 2003). Mortality during the acute phase is most often associated with motor vehicular crashes, upper cervical injuries, very young age, and a low Glasgow Coma Scale score presenting to the emergency department (Kewalramani et al 1980, Vitale et al 2006, Parent, et al 2011).

The NSCID and NSSCID data show that the overall mortality after the first year of injury is approximately 2% per year (National Spinal Cord Injury Statistical Center 2011), but certainly varies considerably by current age, age at injury, neurologic impairment, and other factors (DeVivo et al 1999, Krause et al 2004, Shavelle et al 2007). For persons with SCI who are currently aged 20 years or younger, annual mortality is approximately 0.6%, compared with 0.01% for the general population (DeVivo and Chen 2011). For the 20 to 24 years age group, annual mortality is 0.7% for persons with SCI and 0.1% for the general population. Given the same current age and comparable demographic and neurologic characteristics, people who sustain an SCI at a younger age (<16y) seem to have a higher annual mortality (30% greater) than those injured when 16 years or older (Shavelle et al 2007). Several possible explanations have been proposed, including the long-term deleterious effects of an SCI and medical complications unique to persons with pediatric-onset SCI that contribute to the excess in morbidity and mortality.

Mortality odds during the first year of injury have continued to improve since the 1970s (having improved by approximately 74%), regardless of age groups (Table 2.3) (Strauss et al 2006). However, among those surviving the first year of injury, annual mortality has remained relatively constant since the 1980s for both children and adults. As a result, life expectancy of persons with SCI remains below average. Recent estimates of life expectancy from the NSCID and NSSCID are depicted by severity of injury, age at injury, and ventilator dependency in Table 2.4.

Prevalence: how many children live with spinal cord injury?

Prevalence measures the number of persons with an SCI who are alive during a given point in or period of time. It reflects a function of incidence (number of new cases each year) and mortality (number of deceased cases each year). The prevalence of SCI has been estimated by applying the mathematical relationship between incidence, survival, and prevalence; extrapolating data from a regional disability survey; using data from a national surveillance system; and using a national probability sample of small geographic areas and institutions.

TABLE 2.3

Trends in mortality odds ratios among 48 586 participants enrolled in the National Spinal Cord Injury Database and National Shriners Spinal Cord Injury Database

	Mortality odds ratio	
Calendar year	**During the first year of injury**	**Year 2 after injury or later**
Age at injury: 0–21y		
1970–1979 (reference group)	1.00	1.00
1980–1989	0.72	0.66
1990–1999	0.70	0.69
2000–2006	0.42	0.71
2007–2012	0.26	0.63
Age at injury: >21y		
1970–1979 (reference group)	1.00	1.00
1980–1989	0.72	0.86
1990–1999	0.57	0.81
2000–2006	0.46	0.89
2007–2012	0.27	0.82

TABLE 2.4

Life expectancy for persons with spinal cord injury surviving at least 1 year after injury

	Life expectancy (y)					
		Non-ventilator dependent				Ventilator dependent
		AIS D	AIS A, B, or C			
Current age (y)	**2008 US population**	**Any level**	**Paraplegia**	**C5–C8**	**C1–C4**	**Any level**
10	68.8	62.0	54.6	49.6	45.7	33.1
15	63.8	57.1	49.7	44.8	40.9	28.5
20	59.0	52.4	45.1	40.4	36.6	24.9
25	54.3	47.8	40.8	36.2	32.7	21.9
30	49.5	43.2	36.4	32.0	28.7	18.7
50	31.0	25.4	19.7	16.3	13.8	7.1

AIS, American Spinal Injury Association Impairment Scale.

The range of prevalence reported worldwide is between 236 cases per million in India in 1986 and 1184 per million in Canada (Lee et al 2014). In the USA, utilizing a complex mathematical model, Lasfargues et al projected that the number of persons living with

SCI would increase to 276281 in 2014 in the USA because of improved life expectancy (Lasfargues et al 1995).

The current mean age of persons living with SCI, including new and existing cases, has been estimated to be between 41 and 45 years in the USA (Berkowitz et al 1992, DeVivo and Chen 2011, DeVivo 2012). Approximately 5.4% were below 25 years of age, that is approximately 15 000 children and young adults, given the projected 276 281 persons with SCI in 2014. In Canada, the percentage of children and young adults living with SCI in 2010 was estimated to be 0.03% for persons below 5 years of age, 0.22% for persons between 5 and 9 years, 0.54% for persons between 10 and 14 years, 1.63% for persons between 15 and 19 years, and 3.23% for persons between 20 and 24 years (Noonan et al 2012).

Characteristics of prevalence in an SCI population were recently estimated by analyzing data from the NSCID and NSSCID (DeVivo and Chen 2011): 78.3% were male, 13.7% were at least 60 years of age, 48.8% had tetraplegia, and 51.3% had neurologically complete injuries, which is similar to previous findings in the USA in 1988 (Berkowitz et al 1992) and in Helsinki, Finland, in 1999 (Dahlberg et al 2005).

Summary

1 The annual incidence of SCI, excluding those who die at the scene of injury, is approximately 40 cases per million population or 12 500 new cases each year in the USA, given the current US population size of 313 million people. Of them, approximately 375 to 625 cases are younger than 15 years, and 1875 to 2500 are younger than 20 years.

2 It was estimated that, in 2014, approximately 276 000 people live with an SCI in the USA. Approximately 5.4% of them were below 25 years of age, that is about 15 000 children and young adults.

3 Life expectancy of persons with SCI improved until the early 1980s, but has not changed since then, remaining significantly below average. Injuries at a younger age (<16y) seem to increase the risk of early mortality.

4 The risk and external cause of SCI varies by age, ethnic group, and sex. Age and the mechanism of injury have a major impact on the level and extent of the preserved neurologic function after SCI.

5 Prevention of SCI must be multifaceted in consideration of personal characteristics and mechanical causes as well as the social and political context of the injury. As prevention programs probably compete for recognition of benefits and costs against other regional and national agendas and resource priorities, strategies should be aimed at the targeted population and major causes that are likely to be successful and have a meaningful impact on reducing the incidence of SCI.

REFERENCES

Acton PA, Farley T, Freni LW, Ilegbodu VA, Sniezek JE, Wohlleb JC (1993) Traumatic spinal cord injury in Arkansas, 1980 to 1989. *Arch Phys Med Rehabil* 74: 1035–40. doi: 10.1016/0003-9993(93)90058-I

Augutis M, Levi R (2003) Pediatric spinal cord injury in Sweden: incidence, etiology and outcome. *Spinal Cord* 41: 328–36. doi: 10.1038/sj.sc.3101478

Bayakly AR, Lawrence DW (1992) *Spinal Cord Injury in Louisiana 1991 Annual Report*. New Orleans, LA: Louisiana Office of Public Health.

Berkowitz M, Harvey C, Greene C, Wilson SE (1992) *The Economic Consequences of Traumatic Spinal Cord Injury*. New York, NY: Demos Publications.

Bracken MB, Freeman DH Jr, Hellenbrand K (1981) Incidence of acute traumatic hospitalized spinal cord injury in the United States, 1970–1977. *Am J Epidemiol* 113: 615–22.

Buechner JS, Speare MC, Fontes J (2000) Hospitalizations for spinal cord injuries, 1994–1998. *Med Health R I* 83: 92–3.

Burke DA, Linden RD, Zhang YP, Maiste AC, Shields CB (2001) Incidence rates and populations at risk for spinal cord injury: a regional study. *Spinal Cord* 39: 274–8. doi: 10.1038/sj.sc.3101158

Cao Y, Chen Y, DeVivo MJ (2011) Lifetime direct cost after spinal cord injury. *Top Spinal Cord Inj Rehab* 16: 10–16. doi: 10.1310/sci1604-10

Centers for Disease Control and Prevention (2009) *Web-based Injury Statistics Query and Reporting System (WISQARS)*. Atlanta, GA: US Department of Health and Human Services CDC. Available at: http://www.cdc.gov/injury/wisqars/ (accessed 1 April 2013).

Chen Y, Tang Y, Vogel LC, DeVivo MJ (2013) Causes of spinal cord injury. *Top Spinal Cord Inj Rehab* 19: 1–8. doi: 10.1310/sci1901-1

Clifton GL (1983) Spinal cord injury in the houston-galveston area. *Tex Med* 79: 55–7.

Colorado Department of Public Health and Environment (1997), *1996 Annual Report of the Traumatic Spinal Cord Injury Early Notification System*. Denver, CO: Colorado Department of Transportation Printing Office.

Cripps RA, Lee BB, Wing P, Weerts E, Mackay J, Brown D (2011) A global map for traumatic spinal cord injury epidemiology: towards a living data repository for injury prevention. *Spinal Cord* 49: 493–501. doi: 10.1038/sc.2010.146

Dahlberg A, Kotila M, Leppanen P, Kautiainen H, Alaranta H (2005) Prevalence of spinal cord injury in Helsinki. *Spinal Cord* 43: 47–50. doi: 10.1038/sj.sc.3101616

DeVivo MJ (2012) Epidemiology of traumatic spinal cord injury: trends and future implications. *Spinal Cord* 50: 365–72. doi: 10.1038/sc.2011.178

DeVivo MJ, Chen Y (2011) Trends in new injuries, prevalent cases, and aging with spinal cord injury. *Arch Phys Med Rehabil* 92: 332–8. doi: 10.1016/j.apmr.2010.08.031

DeVivo MJ, Vogel LC (2004) Epidemiology of spinal cord injury in children and adolescents. *J Spinal Cord Med* 27(Suppl 1): S4–10.

DeVivo MJ, Krause JS, Lammertse DP (1999) Recent trends in mortality and causes of death among persons with spinal cord injury. *Arch Phys Med Rehabil* 80: 1411–19. http://dx.doi.org/10.1016/S0003-9993(99)90252-6

Dixon GS, Danesh JN, Caradoc-Davies TH (1993) Epidemiology of spinal cord injury in New Zealand. *Neuroepidemiology* 12: 88–95. doi: 10.1159/000110305

Fawcett JW, Curt A, Steeves JD et al (2007) Guidelines for the conduct of clinical trials for spinal cord injury as developed by the ICCP panel: spontaneous recovery after spinal cord injury and statistical power needed for therapeutic clinical trials. *Spinal Cord* 45: 190–205. doi: 10.1038/sj.sc.3102007

Garrison A, Clifford K, Gleason SF, Tun CG, Brown R, Garshick E (2004) Alcohol use associated with cervical spinal cord injury. *J Spinal Cord Med* 27: 111–15.

Jackson AB, Dijkers M, DeVivo MJ, Poczatek RB (2004) A demographic profile of new traumatic spinal cord injuries: change and stability over 30 years. *Arch Phys Med Rehabil* 85: 1740–8. doi: 10.1016/j.apmr.2004.04.035

Johnson SC (1992) *Georgia Central Registry: Spinal Cord Disabilities and Traumatic Brain Injury*. Warm Springs, GA: Roosevelt Warm Springs Institute for Rehabilitation.

Kalsbeek WD, McLaurin RL, Harris BS, III, Miller JD (1980) The National Head and Spinal Cord Injury Survey: major findings. *J Neurosurg* Suppl: S19–S31.

Kewalramani LS, Kraus JF, Sterling HM (1980) Acute spinal-cord lesions in a pediatric population: epidemiological and clinical features. *Paraplegia* 18: 206–19. doi: 10.1038/sc.1980.36

Kirshblum SC, Burns SP, Biering-Sørensen F et al (2011) International standards for neurological classification of spinal cord injury (revised 2011). *J Spinal Cord Med* 34: 535–46. http://dx.doi.org/10.1179/204577211X13207446293695

Krause JS, DeVivo MJ, Jackson AB (2004) Health status, community integration, and economic risk factors for mortality after spinal cord injury. *Arch Phys Med Rehabil* 85: 1764–73. doi: 10.1016/j.apmr.2004.06.062

Lasfargues JE, Custis D, Morrone F, Carswell J, Nguyen T (1995) A model for estimating spinal cord injury prevalence in the United States. *Paraplegia* 33: 62–8. http://dx.doi.org/10.1038/sc.1995.16

Lee B, Cripps R, Fitzharris M, Wing P (2014) The global map for traumatic spinal cord injury epidemiology: update 2011, global incidence rate. *Spinal Cord* 52: 110–16. doi:10.1038/sc.2012.158

Martins F, Freitas F, Martins L, Dartigues JF, Barat M (1998) Spinal cord injuries--epidemiology in Portugal's central region. *Spinal Cord* 36: 574–8. doi: 10.1038/sj.sc.3100657

Mulcahey MJ, Gaughan J, Betz RR, Johansen KJ (2007) The International Standards for Neurological Classification of Spinal Cord Injury: reliability of data when applied to children and youths. *Spinal Cord* 45: 452–9. doi: 10.1038/sj.sc.3101987

National Spinal Cord Injury Statistical Center (2011) *2011 Annual Statistical Report for the Spinal Cord Injury Model Systems, Public Version*. Birmingham, AL: University of Alabama at Birmingham. Available at: https://www.nscisc.uab.edu/reports.aspx

National Spinal Cord Injury Statistical Center (2013) Spinal Cord Injury Facts and Figures at a Glance. Birmingham, AL: University of Alabama at Birmingham. Available at: https://www.nscisc.uab.edu/reports.aspx (accessed 24 May 2013).

Noonan VK, Fingas M, Farry A et al (2012) Incidence and prevalence of spinal cord injury in Canada: a national perspective. *Neuroepidemiology* 38: 219–26. doi: 10.1159/000336014

Parent S, Mac-Thiong JM, Roy-Beaudry M, Sosa JF, Labelle H (2011) Spinal cord injury in the pediatric population: a systematic review of the literature. *J Neurotrauma* 28: 1515–24. doi: 10.1089/neu.2009.1153

Price C, Makintubee S, Herndon W, Istre GR (1994) Epidemiology of traumatic spinal cord injury and acute hospitalization and rehabilitation charges for spinal cord injuries in Oklahoma, 1988–1990. *Am J Epidemiol* 139: 37–47.

Puisto V, Kaariainen S, Impinen A et al (2010) Incidence of spinal and spinal cord injuries and their surgical treatment in children and adolescents: a population-based study. *Spine (Phila Pa 1976)* 35: 104–7. doi: 10.1097/BRS.0b013e3181c64423

Relethford JH, Standfast SJ, Morse DL (1991) Trends in traumatic spinal cord injury – New York, 1982–1988. *MMWR Morb Mortal Wkly Rep* 40: 535–7, 543.

Schottler J, Vogel LC, Sturm P (2012) Spinal cord injuries in young children: a review of children injured at 5 years of age and younger. *Dev Med Child Neurol* 54: 1138–43. doi: 10.1111/j.1469-8749.2012.04411.x

Shavelle RM, DeVivo MJ, Paculdo DR, Vogel LC, Strauss DJ (2007) Long-term survival after childhood spinal cord injury. *J Spinal Cord Med* 30(Suppl 1): S48–S54.

Stover SL, DeVivo MJ, Go BK (1999) History, implementation, and current status of the National Spinal Cord Injury Database. *Arch Phys Med Rehabil* 80: 1365–71. doi: 10.1016/S0003-9993(99)90246-0

Strauss DJ, DeVivo MJ, Paculdo DR, Shavelle RM (2006) Trends in life expectancy after spinal cord injury. *Arch Phys Med Rehabil* 87: 1079–85. doi: 10.1016/j.apmr.2006.04.022

Surkin J, Gilbert BJ, Harkey HL, III, Sniezek J, Currier M (2000) Spinal cord injury in Mississippi. Findings and evaluation, 1992–1994. *Spine (Phila Pa 1976)* 25: 716–21. doi: 10.1097/00007632-200003150-00011

Thurman DJ, Burnett CL, Jeppson L, Beaudoin DE, Sniezek JE (1994) Surveillance of spinal cord injuries in Utah, USA. *Paraplegia* 32: 665-9. doi: 10.1038/sc.1994.107

van den Berg ME, Castellote JM, Mahillo-Fernandez I, de Pedro-Cuesta J (2010) Incidence of spinal cord injury worldwide: a systematic review. *Neuroepidemiology* 34: 184–92. doi: 10.1159/000279335

Virginia Department of Rehabilitation Services (1993) *Spinal Cord Injury in Virginia: A Statistical Fact Sheet*. Fishersville, VA: Virginia Spinal Cord Injury System.

Vitale MG, Goss JM, Matsumoto H, Roye DP Jr (2006) Epidemiology of pediatric spinal cord injury in the United States: years 1997 and 2000. *J Pediatr Orthop* 26: 745–9. doi: 10.1097/01.bpo.0000235400.49536.83

Warren S, Moore M, Johnson MS (1995) Traumatic head and spinal cord injuries in Alaska (1991–1993). *Alaska Med* 37: 11–19.

Woodruff BA, Baron RC (1994) A description of nonfatal spinal cord injury using a hospital-based registry. *Am J Prev Med* 10: 10–14.

3
LIFE CARE PLANNING

Lawrence C Vogel, Karla S Reed and James S Krause

> **Case vignette**
> Heather is a 14-year-old female who sustained a complete (American Spinal Injury Association Impairment Scale A) C6 spinal cord injury while diving into a 4-foot-deep above-ground pool when she was 12 years old. She has had minimal neurologic recovery since her injury; she uses a power-assisted wheelchair, she is on an intermittent catheterization program performed by her mother or school nurse, and her bowel program is performed daily by her mother. She is an excellent student and hopes to become a psychologist. A life care plan has been requested in order to determine her future needs and the associated costs.

The goal of this chapter is to provide an overview of the life care planning process for children (from birth to 12y of age) and adolescents (13–21y) with spinal cord injuries (SCIs). This will include defining a life care plan, describing its underlying principles, discussing its purpose, and outlining the process of developing a life care plan. The unique features of pediatric-onset SCI that impact life care planning, such as developmental milestones, musculoskeletal complications, and relatively long lifespan, will be highlighted. Finally, issues related to estimating life expectancy in pediatric-onset SCI will be discussed.

Definition of a life care plan

The current definition provided by the International Academy of Life Care Planners is 'The life care plan is a dynamic document based upon published standards of practice, comprehensive assessment, data analysis, and research, which provides an organized, concise plan for current and future needs with associated costs for individuals who have experienced catastrophic injury or have chronic health care needs' (International Academy of Life Care Planners 2012). The life care plan is a needs-based assessment used to generate estimates of the cost of providing for those needs. Because it is based solely on needs, it does not consider the availability of resources in developing the estimates (Deutsch et al 2005). A major principle of life care planning is that it employs a consistent methodology to analyze the individual needs resulting from SCI and throughout the lifespan. The life care plan is distinct to each adolescent with SCI in view of the uniqueness of each individual in respect to psychosocial, environmental, familial, cultural, and medical factors, as well as personal preferences (Deutsch et al 2005).

Purposes of a life care plan

Life care plans serve a variety of purposes. They provide young people with SCI and their families with a concise summary of a future plan as a guideline and reference (Deutsch et al 2005). The life care plan forms the basis for case management, in which advanced planning and prevention are the guiding principles rather than crisis intervention. Life care plans are an integral component of litigation proceedings and are used by insurance carriers to determine the future needs of the adolescent with an SCI. They are generally initiated by attorneys when litigation is involved or by case managers of insurance carriers. Life care plans should be developed by a healthcare or rehabilitation professional with appropriate training, experience, and, ideally, country-specific certification if available, such as the International Commission on Health Care Certification in the USA (May 2002).

Development of a life care plan

The development of a sound life care plan is dependent upon having a strong basis for making predictions regarding current and future needs. Identification of appropriate research is essential to establishing the foundation of the life care plan (Blackwell et al 2001). The types of research used vary widely. For instance, research on function establishes the probable outcomes related to a particular type or severity of injury. Studies of secondary health conditions and hospitalizations help to identify and allocate resources for the likelihood of complications that typically occur after SCI, such as pressure sores. Aging studies may be used to identify increased needs for assistance or treatment. This is particularly important with pediatric-onset SCI, since complications may develop in the decades after SCI onset. Studies of mortality are essential to estimating life expectancy which, in turn, set the limit for the number of years for which the life care plan will be in effect.

The process of developing a life care plan begins with a thorough understanding of the young person with an SCI, including a comprehensive review of all the pertinent medical, therapy, nursing, home care, and school records, and depositions that relate to the young person's SCI and related complications. To obtain a comprehensive picture, the life care planner should evaluate the young person, and this should ideally take place at the young person's home with pertinent caregivers present. This allows the life care planner to view the adolescent with an SCI in their natural environment within the context of their family. In addition, the life care planner should discuss the current condition and future needs of the young person with all treating physicians, therapists, psychologists, nurses, teachers, durable medical equipment providers, home healthcare providers, and other pertinent professionals.

Developmental issues

Life care plans must take into account the unique developmental aspect of a pediatric-onset SCI in a variety of ways. From birth through to young adulthood, immense changes continuously occur in all spheres of an individual's life, including physical, physiological, psychosocial, and cognitive changes. The physical changes occurring as an individual ages result in the need to change the type and size of necessary equipment such as the size of catheters and wheelchairs (see Chapters 11 and 22). Physiological changes dictate when bladder and bowel programs are initiated and the frequency of interventions such as catheterization. Long-term outcomes such as employment, independent living, and life satisfaction for individuals with pediatric-onset SCI are most affected by psychosocial and cognitive issues and must be taken into account in preparing a life care plan (Anderson et al 2004) (see Chapter 25). Ages that are particularly marked by significant psychosocial and cognitive changes are the early school ages (5–7y), adolescence (13–16y), and emerging adulthood (18–25y) (Zebracki et al 2010). These are ages when additional interventions should be considered to maximize independence and successful mastery during these very important transitional times. Interventions may include physical, occupational, speech, and recreation therapy; nursing education; and nutritional and psychological counseling. The early school-aged child becomes increasingly independent in activities of daily living and self-care activities including dressing, grooming, wheelchair skills, and the ability to perform intermittent catheterization. Adolescence is arguably the most tumultuous developmental phase with the increased need to be independent superimposed on non-compliance, along with adolescent–parent conflict and changing roles of the young person and parents. Interventions at this stage should focus on body image, self-esteem and coping strategies, and the importance of proper SCI care to prevent complications such as pressure ulcers. Normative milestones for the emerging adult include education, employment, independent living, financial independence, and social and psychosocial functioning. Therefore, psychological and vocational counseling may be very helpful during this transitional period with the goal of independence and self-management. In addition, emerging adults face health system discontinuities, such as the transition from pediatric medical care to adult care and the transition from parent-controlled healthcare to self-management. During this period of late adolescence/emerging adulthood, coordinated provision of care by both pediatric and adult healthcare workers may be beneficial in achieving a successful healthcare transition and minimizing complications such as pressure ulcers or urinary tract infections.

The consequences of aging are significant concerns for adults both with and without disabilities. For individuals with SCI, much attention has been given to overuse syndromes, particularly degenerative processes of the upper extremities with associated pain as a result of excessive use of the upper extremities related to wheelchair propulsion and transfers (Sie et al 1992, Dalyan et al 1999, Figoni 2009). In view of the long lifespan of adolescents with SCI, this group of individuals may be especially susceptible to overuse syndromes at a relatively young age compared with individuals who sustained their SCI as adults. Therefore, compared with the adult-onset SCI population, individuals with pediatric-onset SCI are expected to develop overuse syndromes at a younger age and live with this secondary disability for a greater duration. There are no published data delineating the timeline of aging for those with pediatric-onset SCI. Presumably, it is a function of several factors, including the duration of injury; age at follow-up; upper extremity injuries that occurred before, at the time of, or after the SCI; and the individual's weight.

Components of a life care plan

Components of a life care plan are generally grouped in standardized categories with each item of the life care plan having a frequency and duration of need along with an associated cost (Weed 2002). Present-day costs of items use pricing appropriate for the geographic area where the young person resides, and, for more expensive items, three sources should be identified. An example of one way of categorizing a life care plan is demonstrated in Box 3.1. The following sections begin with discussions on mobility and developmental changes, followed by medical complications unique to pediatric-onset SCI; these two topics overlap with several of the categories outlined in Box 3.1. The subsequent two sections will discuss medical evaluations and treatments and home or facility care. The last section will address the remaining life care plan categories.

Box 3.1 Components of a life care plan

- Projected non-physician evaluations
- Projected therapeutic modalities
- Future medical care – routine
- Future medical care – surgical or aggressive treatment
- Diagnostic testing and educational assessment
- Wheelchairs, including accessories and maintenance
- Transportation
- Aids for independent functioning
- Orthotics/prosthetics
- Drugs and supplies
- Home/facility care
- Recreation/leisure time
- Health and strength management
- Architectural
- Home furnishings and accessories
- Vocational/educational plan
- Potential complications

Mobility

Mobility issues that should be addressed in a life care plan for a child with an SCI should include wheeled mobility, ambulation, standing, and motor vehicles (see Chapter 22). Using mobility as an example, physical growth necessitates that age- and size-appropriate wheelchairs be prescribed. As young people age, recreation-specific wheelchairs and/or hand-powered bicycles may also be prescribed. Finally, because of aging and the risk of overuse syndromes, preservation of upper extremity function may necessitate transition to powered mobility as the individual ages. Regarding the timing of the transition to powered mobility, there are no definitive data to predict when this switch should occur.

Children as young as 12 to 18 months of age (see Chapter 22) can be independent in the use of either manual or power wheelchairs. Until children reach skeletal maturity, prescribed wheelchairs should have growth potential with an estimated replacement every 3 years. For age-appropriate recreational activities such as bicycle riding, a hand-powered tricycle or bicycle would be appropriate with an estimated replacement every 3 to 5 years. For wheelchair sporting activities such as basketball or quad rugby, appropriate sports chairs would be prescribed with an estimated replacement every 3 to 5 years.

Given the same level and severity of injury, children and adolescents are more likely than adults to use a variety of standers and orthotics to ambulate. Children as young as 9 months of age who have adequate neck control can be placed in standers which may be static or, ideally, mobile; these are continually modified to accommodate growth and replaced as needed owing to growth and wear. Depending on the level and severity of injury, adolescents use a variety of orthoses ranging from ankle–foot orthoses and knee–ankle–foot orthoses to reciprocating gait orthoses (see Chapter 22); depending on the extent of their use, orthoses and assistive devices used for ambulation should be replaced as needed owing to growth.

Issues related to transportation in motor vehicles include proper child safety restraints, which vary by state law but generally relate to restraints for children from birth to weighing 27 to 36kg and encompass seats ranging from rear-facing infant and toddler seats for children 2 years of age and younger to forward-facing car seats and boosters for older children and those less than 145cm in height. For most children with SCI, there is no need to account for restraints beyond what they would have needed if they did not have an SCI. Special restraints are needed for those with poor head and trunk control or young people with ventilator-dependent SCIs, or more frequent replacement of standard car restraints may be required for those utilizing orthoses that cause increased wear and tear on the restraints (see Chapter 22). Children or adolescents in power chairs or those for whom transfers from their wheelchair to the motor vehicle seats are not feasible will require a wheelchair-accessible motor vehicle equipped with a lift and proper wheelchair tie downs. Adolescents of driving age should undergo a comprehensive adapted driver's evaluation to determine their ability to drive and to identify appropriate adaptions. Subsequently, the adolescent should undergo adapted driving training with a trained instructor. For adolescents who use a manual wheelchair, physical and occupational therapy evaluation and training is required for the transfer from a wheelchair to a motor vehicle seat and storage of the wheelchair. For adolescents with tetraplegia who use power wheelchairs, an adapted van will be required with a wheelchair lift, an automatic wheelchair locking system, and appropriate adaptions for driving.

Medical Complications

Individuals with pediatric-onset SCI are at risk of complications that are unique to this SCI population, such as neuromuscular scoliosis or hip dysplasia (Betz 1997). Among children who sustain their SCI prior to puberty, the vast majority will develop scoliosis and approximately two-thirds will require surgery (Dearolf et al 1990). Because of the risk of scoliosis, most patients will need to be followed up every 3 to 6 months before the onset of puberty and every 6 months to 1 year after puberty with spine radiographs and by a pediatric spine surgeon or SCI physician (see Chapter 18). Most young people will require thoracolumbosacral orthoses, which will need to be replaced every 1 to 2 years, depending on growth and curve progression. In addition, although progression to spine fusion is largely dependent upon the age at which the injury occurred (Mulcahey et al 2013), the majority of children injured before puberty, and many who are injured after puberty, will require surgical correction of their spine deformity, which would be included in the 'future medical care, surgical or aggressive treatment' section of the life care plan (Dearolf et al 1990). Another potential item in this category ('future medical care, surgical or aggressive treatment') could include a continent catheterizeable conduit (Mitrofanoff procedure), which helps the caregiver assist with emptying the bladder, particularly in females with poor hand function, and which facilitates independence in self-catheterization in females with C6 and lower level tetraplegia and in many females with paraplegia who have difficulty with catheterization in their wheelchair (see Chapter 11) (Mitrofanoff 1980).

Similar to adult-onset SCI, young people with SCI are at risk of developing a variety of serious complications, such as pressure ulcers, upper extremity pain, urinary tract infections, and stones. However, because of their relatively long lifespan and hence long duration of potential exposure, adolescents with SCI are at risk of recurrence of these complications and of long-term chronic problems (Vogel et al 2002a,b).

A major goal of a life care plan and case management is to provide optimal care for an individual throughout his or her lifespan to prevent complications and enhance functioning, participation, and quality of life. Some research has indeed suggested that certain conditions are unlikely to occur among those who are in late adulthood at the time of onset of SCI because there is not sufficient time for the conditions to develop (Krause et al 1990). Conversely, the longer someone lives with SCI, the greater the risk of multiple conditions including orthopedic complications, such as contractures and curvature of the spine. Kidney stones also were related to years after injury. All these complications are likely to be particularly acute among those with pediatric-onset SCI. Other examples include severe or recurrent pressure ulcers, chronic renal failure resulting from recurrent urinary tract infections or kidney stones, or severe restrictions in transfers or propeling a manual wheelchair because of severe upper extremity pain. In the case of preventing pressure ulcers, periodic routine care by an SCI team should provide appropriate education, evaluate wheelchair seating and transfers, and assess nutritional status.

Medical Evaluations and Treatments

Life care plans typically have separate categories for projected evaluations and treatments, which are further separated into non-physician and physician services. In the case of medical care or physician services, routine care is separated from 'surgical or aggressive treatment' (as discussed above for spine surgery and the Mitrofanoff procedure). Generally, young people with SCI are followed up every 6 months until they are 21 years of age by an interdisciplinary

SCI team which consists of physical, occupational, speech, and recreation therapists; social workers; psychologists; nurses; dietitians; orthotists; and an SCI physician. In addition to these SCI team visits, the adolescent with an SCI should be seen by a urologist every 6 months to 1 year and a spine surgeon once a year.

Projected therapeutic modalities will typically include physical and occupational therapy two or three times a week each during the first year after injury, and one or two times a week during the next 1 to 2 years. After the first 2 or 3 years after injury, the frequency of physical and occupational therapy will depend upon the specific needs of the young person. Additional therapy may be beneficial during developmentally sensitive periods, such as early school age, adolescence, and emerging adulthood; this could include 1 to 2 weeks of intensive out-patient or in-patient rehabilitation or physical and occupational therapy two or three times a week each for 2 to 4 weeks. When young people with SCI are in school, they may receive physical, occupational, and speech therapy (if needed) to support their educational program as defined in their individualized education program. Young people with an SCI should receive physical and/or occupational therapy whenever they receive new or replacement equipment such as wheelchairs, orthotics, or splints. The frequency, duration, and specifics of the therapy vary for these situations. An adolescent receiving a new orthoses, such as a reciprocating gait orthoses, for the first time may require 2 weeks of intensive out-patient or in-patient physical therapy followed by one or two sessions of physical therapy per week for 3 to 6 months. In contrast, a child receiving a replacement of an orthotic for ambulation or an upper extremity splint may simply need one additional session of physical therapy or occupational therapy, respectively.

Additional therapy would also be warranted if a young person undergoes a surgical procedure that enhances function such as upper extremity reconstruction or a Mitrofanoff procedure. In the case of upper extremity reconstruction surgery, they would benefit from 1 week of intensive out-patient or in-patient occupational and physical therapy followed by occupational therapy one or two times a week for 3 to 6 months.

Home or Facility Care

One of the largest expenses of a life care plan is home or facility care. The amount and type of care required is dependent upon a variety of factors, including the level and severity of the SCI; the need for specialized services such as ventilator care, catheterization, a bowel program, and tube feedings; and state regulations regarding licensure for the various specialized services. A variety of practical issues need to be considered in home care for individuals with pediatric-onset SCI.

The role of family members (particularly parents) as care providers needs to be defined, including developmental issues. For example, parents typically provide around-the-clock care for their infants and toddlers, whether they have an SCI or not. However, if the child is ventilator dependent, skilled nursing care would be needed for most (16h) to all of the day. Another example where nursing care would be needed is an adolescent with an SCI with tetraplegia who is not independent in activities such as bladder and bowel programs, bathing, dressing, or transfers.

A paid attendant or skilled nursing professional would be ideal from the perspective of privacy and independence issues for the adolescent, in addition to facilitating more normal family relationships. Depending upon the young person's needs and state laws, a home-health aide or a personal care attendant may also be utilized. Other important concepts in home care for adolescents with SCI are the importance of promoting their autonomy throughout their development, which should include promoting their independence in all of their daily activities and having them perform age-appropriate chores. Additionally, respite care for the young person's parents should be provided on a regular basis; for example, 2 weeks each year, the youth receives around-the-clock care so that the parents can be relieved of all of their responsibilities.

In contrast to adults, children and adolescents generally will receive nursing, attendants, therapy, and related services during school hours, as this care relates to their educational needs. For adolescents who are ventilator dependent or require specialized services throughout the day, skilled nursing care may be needed 24 hours a day, 7 days a week. When an adolescent goes away to college, the type and amount of care required is again dependent upon the level and severity of their injury. Because it is so important that a college-aged individual becomes as independent as possible, they need to assume the responsibility for this care, which may include the hiring, training, and supervision of personal care attendants.

Diagnostic Testing and Educational Assessment

In addition to spine radiography being performed every 6 months before skeletal maturity, pelvic radiography should also be performed every 6 months before the onset of puberty and then annually because of the high incidence of hip dysplasia in those injured at a young age (see Chapter 18). The vast majority of young people with SCI have a neurogenic bladder, so they should have baseline renal ultrasounds, voiding cystourethrogram, and urodynamics (see Chapter 11). Subsequently, they would have annual renal ultrasounds with urodynamics performed as needed if there are significant changes in their neurologic condition. Other diagnostic tests that should be performed annually include dual-energy X-ray absorptiometry scans to evaluate bone density and body composition, and comprehensive chemistry and lipid panels and 25-hydroxy vitamin D levels because of the high risk of metabolic syndrome and vitamin D deficiency, respectively (Zebracki et al 2013).

Health and Strength Management

Because of the relatively long lifespan of individuals with a pediatric-onset SCI and a relatively sedentary lifestyle, significant attention must be paid to their nutrition and fitness status to mitigate the increased risk of cardiovascular disease (Johnson and Klaas 2000, Liusuwan et al 2007). In addition to having dietary and recreation therapy evaluations as a part of the regular SCI team visits, fitness strategies should be implemented such as functional electrical stimulation cycling, participation in wheelchair sports, and arm-propeled bicycles.

Orthotics/Prosthetics

The frequency of replacing orthotics and splints depends upon the child's age and usage such that replacement frequency could be as frequent as every 6 months to 2 years in children who are growing and have daily use, and every 2 years thereafter.

Architectural

Major architectural modifications or acquisition of an accessible home should occur after a child sustains an SCI, and one or two additional times should be expected in the future as they become adults and acquire their own home.

Vocational/Educational Plan

Employment rates after SCI are substantially below those of the general population; however, employment is associated with better overall health, higher quality of life, and greater longevity (Krause et al 2012). Therefore, it is important to consider how it may impact other areas of life relevant to the life care plan. Furthermore, there are substantial costs associated with the education required after injury to find employment, retain employment, and maximize employment outcomes. Vocational rehabilitation evaluation should be performed by a rehabilitation counselor who has experience in evaluating children and adolescents who have not had any work history before their injury.

Those with pediatric-onset SCI have a distinct advantage vocationally, in that those who are younger have a significantly greater likelihood of becoming employed (Anderson and Vogel 2002, Hwang et al in press) (see Chapter 25). However, despite the fact that those with pediatric-onset SCI have greater educational achievement than the general population, they are significantly less likely to be employed. The most significant predictor of employment after SCI is the presence of education after injury (Krause and Reed 2009). Because terminal education is determined after SCI onset among those with pediatric SCI, there is by definition an advantage vocationally compared with those who are older and whose education predates the injury. Education after injury probably explains some of the advantage of being injured at a younger age, as the individual has time to assess their direction vocationally and to do so in a manner consistent with the SCI.

It is possible to calculate outcomes under different educational scenarios such as completion of a high school certificate, some education beyond high school, and completion of a 4-year degree or higher. These outcomes will affect key outcomes within the life care plan. It can be anticipated that those who are likely to obtain employment will also do better in other areas of life, including having a greater longevity. The life care plan should contain sufficient resources to ensure that there is the opportunity to maximize educational and vocational attainment. There should also be sufficient resources for added expenses of working.

Life expectancy

One of the most challenging aspects of the life care plan is to establish life expectancy, which is influenced by a wide array of factors, some of which are difficult to determine at the time of injury. The primary factors historically used in predicting life expectancy include demographic characteristics such as sex, ethnic group, and, particularly, age (see Chapter 2). Injury factors are also important, including the severity of the injury and etiology.

In terms of injury severity, both neurologic level of injury and neurologic completeness of injury factor into the life expectancy estimate. They may be used separately, with neurologic completeness measured according to the American Spinal Injury Association Impairment

Scale (AIS) grade (A–D), or in combination. When combined, neurologic completeness is often categorized by those who have functional recovery (the AIS D forming one group) and three additional groups formed as a function of neurologic level among those with AIS A–C. This breakdown includes high cervical (C1–C4), low cervical (C5–C8), and non-cervical (thoracic, lumbar, sacral) (Krause et al 1999).

A body of research has identified the relationship of these biographic and injury characteristics with life expectancy (DeVivo and Stover 1995, Yeo et al 1998, DeVivo et al 1999). General tables for life expectancy or examples of life expectancy for individuals with particular characteristics, such as age and injury severity, are typically presented. The time between SCI onset and determination of mortality status is important, particularly within the first year. It is typical in studies of life expectancy to provide different estimates for 1-day survivors (i.e. those who survived at least 1 day after SCI) and 1-year survivors (i.e. those who survived at least 1 year). For those who are ventilator dependent, the timing of the life expectancy estimate is particularly critical, as survival or life expectancy improves the longer individuals have survived. For instance, Shavelle et al (2006) found a higher rate of mortality in the first 3 years after injury among those who are ventilator dependent, with the odds of increased mortality dramatically declining after the third year after injury.

Life expectancy is greatest for those with motor functional recovery, who have only a modest reduction compared with the general population. For those who do not have motor functional recovery, life expectancy is generally inversely related to the level of injury and AIS grade. Therefore, life expectancy is greater for those with non-cervical injuries and those with neurologically incomplete injuries. Those with preserved motor function, even if not significant, have greater life expectancies than those with incomplete sensory only or neurologically complete injuries. Life expectancy is particularly low for those who are ventilator dependent. Those injured before the age of 16 have diminished life expectancy compared with those with adult-onset SCI (Shavelle et al 2007), when controlling for a number of factors that include age, sex, ethnic group, cause of injury, and severity of injury.

A growing body of research has indicated that there is a wide array of risk and protective factors for mortality. A theoretical risk and prevention model has outlined a sequence of predictive factors of mortality, treating biographic and injury characteristics as the most basic starting point for the estimation of life expectancy (Krause et al 2013). This model accounts for psychological, socio-environmental, behavioral, and health factors in relation to mortality and life expectancy.

Researchers indicated health factors have been the strongest predictors of mortality, followed by behavioral and socio-environmental factors (Krause et al 2009). For instance, Krause et al (2008) focused on general health and secondary health conditions and found that several types of health conditions were associated with mortality: probable major depression, surgeries to repair pressure ulcers, fractures and/or amputations, symptoms of infections, and days hospitalized. Two studies are of particular importance to life care planning, each of which emphasizes the importance of socio-economic factors (correlate of outcomes in litigation) and risk of mortality and/or life expectancy. In the first study (Krause and Saunders 2012), the risk of mortality associated with low income (socio-environmental factor) and smoking (behavioral factor) were higher for those with SCI than those previously reported in the literature for the general population, even after including multiple statistical comparisons. In the second study (Krause et al 2012), which utilized data from the SCI Model System, dramatic differences in life expectancy were observed as a function of three socio-economic indicators (work status, education, and income), with the life expectancy of those with favorable characteristics more than double that of those with unfavorable characteristics for some levels of injury. These findings have significant implications for the estimation of life expectancy, particularly the findings related to favorable economics. The life care plan itself is designed to ensure resources are available to meet the lifetime *needs* of the individual with SCI and this is typically done by the allocation of money to meet these needs. Therefore, if the life care plan is implemented, many factors that may ultimately lead to mortality may be prevented and life expectancy may be underestimated by not accounting for these factors. The ultimate cost of underestimating life expectancy is that the individual may run out of the resources necessary to pay for his or her healthcare needs.

Based on the aforementioned studies, it is reasonable to utilize the assumption of favorable economics in predicting life expectancy in life care plans. In cases of pediatric-onset SCI, it is reasonable to estimate future education based on academic accomplishment and life goals, at least among adolescents. If future education cannot be predicted, then life expectancy may be estimated at different educational levels to identify possible scenarios for the life care plan. Including assumptions regarding education and income can be done with the same types of statistical formulae used when estimating life expectancy using biographic and injury characteristics. The inclusion of favorable economics only ensures that the 'average' life expectancy estimate is in line with those with similar economics, as well as biographic and injury status.

Summary

The development of the life care plan is the process of identifying lifetime needs and the associated costs related to the development of a health condition, such as SCI. In pediatric cases, the life care plan must consider several specific characteristics of those who were injured prior to adulthood. These span a wide range of issues that relate to developmental needs.

REFERENCES

Anderson CJ, Vogel LC (2002) Employment outcomes of adults who sustained spinal cord injuries as children or adolescents. *Arch Phys Med Rehabil* 83: 791–801. http://dx.doi.org/10.1053/apmr.2002.32742

Anderson CJ, Vogel LC, Betz RR, Willis KM (2004) Overview of adult outcomes in pediatric-onset spinal cord injuries: implications for transition to adulthood. *J Spinal Cord Med* 27(Suppl 1): S98–106.

Betz RR (1997) Orthopaedic problems in the child with spinal cord injury. *Top Spinal Cord Inj Rehab* 3: 9–19.

Blackwell TL, Krause JS, Winkler T, Steins SA (2001) *Spinal Cord Injury Desk Reference: Guidelines for Life Care Planning and Case Management*. New York, NY: Demos Medical Publishing.

Dalyan M, Cardenas DD, Gerard B (1999) Upper extremity pain after spinal cord injury. *Spinal Cord* 37: 191–5. http://dx.doi.org/10.1038/sj.sc.3100802

Dearolf WW 3rd, Betz RR, Vogel LC, Levin J, Clancy M, Steel HH (1990) Scoliosis in pediatric spinal cord-injured patients. *J Pediatr Orthop* 10: 214–18. http://dx.doi.org/10.1097/01241398-199003000-00016

Deutsch PM, Allison L, Cimino-Ferguson S (2005) Life care planning assessments and their impact on quality of life in spinal cord injury. *Top Spinal Cord Inj Rehab* 10: 135–45. doi: 10.1310/Y7LA-OU70-2UHY-CUGF

DeVivo MJ, Stover SL (1995) Long term survival and causes of death. In: Stover SL, Delisa JA, Whitenec GG (eds). *Spinal Cord Injury: Clinical Outcomes from the Model Systems.* Gaithersburg, MD: Aspen.

DeVivo MJ, Krause JS, Lammertse DP (1999) Recent trends in mortality and causes of death among persons with spinal cord injury. *Arch Phys Med Rehabil* 80: 1411–19. http://dx.doi.org/10.1016/S0003-9993(99)90252-6

Figoni SF (2009) Overuse shoulder problems after spinal cord injury: a conceptual model of risk and protective factors. *Clinical Kinesiology* 63: 12–22.

Hwang M, Zebracki K, Chlan K, Vogel L (2014). Longitudinal employment outcomes in adults with pediatric-onset spinal cord injury. *Spinal Cord* 52: 477–82. doi: 10.1038/sc.2014.32

International Academy of Life Care Planners (2012) *Standards of Practice* [online]. Available at: http://www.rehabpro.org/sections/ialcp/focus/standards/IALCP,%20-%20Standards%20of%20Practice.pdf (accessed 26 April 2012).

Johnson KA, Klaas SJ (2000) Recreation involvement and play in pediatric spinal cord injury. *Top Spinal Cord Inj Rehab* 6: 105–9. doi: 10.1310/F7XL-F11F-JU26-GFTK 10.1310/F7XL-F11F-JU26-GFTK

Krause JS, Reed KS (2009) Obtaining employment after spinal cord injury: relationship with pre- and post-injury education. *Rehab Couns Bull* 53: 27–33. doi: 10.1177/0034355208329443

Krause JS, Saunders LL (2012) Socioeconomic and behavioral risk factors for mortality: do risk factors observed after spinal cord injury parallel those from the general USA population? *Spinal Cord* 50: 609–13. doi: 10.1038/sc.2012.24

Krause JS, Saari JM, Dykstra D (1990) Quality of life and survival after spinal cord injury. *SCI Psychosocial Process* 3: 4–8.

Krause JS, Kewman D, DeVivo MJ et al (1999) Employment after spinal cord injury: an analysis of cases from the Model Spinal Cord Injury Systems. *Arch Phys Med Rehabil* 80: 1492–500. http://dx.doi.org/10.1016/S0003-9993(99)90263-0

Krause JS, Carter RE, Pickelsimer E, Wilson D (2008) A prospective study of health and risk of mortality after spinal cord injury. *Arch Phys Med Rehabil* 89: 1482–91. doi: 10.1016/j.apmr.2007.11.062

Krause JS, Zhai Y, Saunders LL, Carter RE (2009) Risk of mortality after spinal cord injury: an 8-year prospective study. *Arch Phys Med Rehabil* 90: 1708–15. doi: 10.1016/j.apmr.2009.04.020

Krause JS, Saunders LL, Acuna J (2012) Gainful employment and risk of mortality after spinal cord injury: effects beyond that of demographic, injury and socioeconomic factors. *Spinal Cord* 50: 784–8. doi: 10.1038/sc.2012.49

Krause JS, Saunders LL, DiPiro ND, Reed KS (2013). Theoretical risk and prevention model for secondary health conditions and mortality: 15 years of research. *Top Spinal Cord Inj Rehab* 19: 15–24. doi: 10.1310/sci1901-15

Liusuwan RA, Widman LM, Abresch RT, Johnson AJ, McDonald CM (2007) Behavioral intervention, exercise, and nutrition education to improve health and fitness (BENEfit) in adolescents with mobility impairment due to spinal cord dysfunction. *J Spinal Cord Med* 30(Suppl 1): S119–26.

May VR (2002) Certification in life care planning service delivery. *Top Spinal Cord Inj Rehab* 7: 88–98. doi: 10.1310/FQX9-YVA3-CGH3-0YNC

Mitrofanoff P (1980) Trans-appendicular continent cystostomy in the management of the neurogenic bladder. *Chir Pediatr* 21: 297–305.

Mulcahey MJ, Gaughan JP, Betz RR, Samdani AF, Barakat N, Hunter LN (2013) Neuromuscular scoliosis in children with spinal cord injury. *Top Spinal Cord Inj Rehabil* 19: 96–103. doi: 10.1310/sci1902-96

Shavelle RM, DeVivo MJ, Strauss DJ, Paculdo DR, Lammertse DP, Day SM (2006) Long-term survival of persons ventilator dependent after spinal cord injury. *J Spinal Cord Med* 29: 511–519.

Shavelle RM, Devivo MJ, Paculdo DR, Vogel LC, Strauss DJ (2007) Long-term survival after childhood spinal cord injury. *J Spinal Cord Med* 30(Suppl 1): S48–54.

Sie IH, Waters RL, Adkins RH, Gellman H (1992) Upper extremity pain in the postrehabilitation spinal cord injured patient. *Arch Phys Med Rehabil* 73: 44–8.

Vogel LC, Krajci KA, Anderson CJ (2002a) Adults with pediatric-onset spinal cord injury: part 1: prevalence of medical complications. *J Spinal Cord Med* 25: 106–16.

Vogel LC, Krajci KA, Anderson CJ (2002b) Adults with pediatric-onset spinal cord injury: part 2: musculo-skeletal and neurological complications. *J Spinal Cord Med* 25: 117–23.

Weed R (2002) Life care plan development. *Top Spinal Cord Inj Rehab* 7: 5–20. doi: 10.1310/130T-5AJU-W88W-RFT9

Yeo JD, Walsh J, Rutkowski SB, Soden RJ, Craven M, Middleton J (1998) Mortality following spinal cord injury. *Spinal Cord* 36: 329–36. http://dx.doi.org/10.1038/sj.sc.3100628

Zebracki K, Anderson CJ, Chlan KM, Vogel LC (2010) Outcomes of adults with pediatric-onset spinal cord injury: longitudinal findings and implications on transition to adulthood. *Top Spinal Cord Inj Rehab* 16: 17–25. doi: 10.1310/sci1601-7

Zebracki K, Hwang M, Patt P, Vogel L (2013) Autonomic cardiovascular dysfunction and vitamin D deficiency in pediatric spinal cord injury. *J Pediatr Rehab Med* 6: 45–52. doi:10.3233/PRM-130236

4
ASSESSMENT OF CHILDREN WITH SPINAL CORD INJURY

MJ Mulcahey and Fin Biering-Sørensen

Case vignette

Joey had a cervical spinal cord injury after he dived into a 3-foot-deep above-ground back-yard pool approximately 16 months ago at the age of 5 years 9 months. He was managed acutely at the local children's hospital where he underwent imaging of his spine and subsequent stabilization with instrumentation. Multiple systems including the respiratory system, musculoskeletal system, skin, bowel, and bladder were addressed and, once medically cleared, he was transferred to the pediatric rehabilitation floor where he participated in a 4-week in-patient course of SCI education, physical and occupational therapy, and child life therapy. Appropriate consultations with counselors, school support, neuropsychology specialists, wheelchair and seating specialists, orthotics specialists, and speech and language specialists also occurred, as needed. The Child Needs Assessment Checklist was used to define goals and establish and monitor the in-patient rehabilitation program. The International Standards for Neurological Classification of Spinal Cord Injury (ISNCSCI) was not used during in-patient rehabilitation owing to Joey's young age but therapy evaluations consisting of observational motor assessment during therapy and play, manual strength testing, and informal sensory testing suggested good motor function through to C5 and sensation through to C6. As per standard operating procedures, the motor FIM®[a] was administered at admission and before discharge from in-patient rehabilitation; motor FIM at admission was 18 and motor FIM at discharge was 27. After discharge, at home, Joey was independently moving a power wheelchair on level surfaces with his mother as his only caregiver; he continued to participate in out-patient physical and occupational therapy for an additional 6 months. The ISNCSCI was attempted at the time of discharge from

a FIM is a trademark of Uniform Data System for Medical Rehabilitation (UDSMR), a division of UB Foundation Activities, Inc. The use of the FIM instrument to collect data for this research study was authorized and conducted in accordance with the terms of a special purpose license granted to the licensee by UDSMR. The patient data collected in the course of this research study have not been processed by UDSMR and there is no implication that such data have been or will be subjected to UDSMR's standard data processing procedures or that they are otherwise comparable to data processed by UDSMR.

out-patient therapy but only muscle testing was successful; Joey did not tolerate sensory testing and could not follow the test instructions for deep anal sensation pressure or anal contraction. Motor level was noted to be C6 bilaterally. The motor FIM score at discharge from out-patient therapy increased from 27 to 31 and progress was made regarding the out-patient therapy goals; illustration of goal attainment scaling for 3 of the 15 out-patient goals is shown in Table 4.1.

At 7 years of age, Joey was seen by the SCI rehabilitation team as an out-patient for routine follow-up evaluation. The ISNCSCI and the musculoskeletal basic data set were completed (Figs 4.1 and 4.2). An explanation about the results of the ISNCSCI, particularly related to the American Spinal Injury Association Impairment Scale classification 'B', was provided. The FIM was administered and showed a small improvement from 31 (score at discharge from out-patient therapy approximately 8 months before) to 33. Joey's mother requested additional out-patient therapy to work on activities associated with morning routines and school.

Joey, now 8 years of age, returned for routine follow-up. The ISNCSCI and the musculoskeletal core data set were completed. There was no change in ISNCSCI finding. The musculoskeletal basic data set is shown in Figure 4.3. The FIM was administered and showed no change from 1 year ago, despite improvements shown by goal attainment scaling (Table 4.1). Joey's mother inquired about tendon transfers for restoration of grasp and pinch (Mulcahey et al 1995, 1999). The International Classification for Surgery of the Hand in Tetraplegia (Mulcahey et al 2007) was used to define a plan for reconstructive hand surgery. The Graded Redefined Assessment of Strength, Sensibility and Prehension as well as the Capabilities of the Upper Extremity Test (Marino et al 2012) were used as baseline measures of hand function, and goals specifically related to tendon transfers were developed for goal attainment scaling. Joey was referred to an orthopedics specialist for hand surgery which will be followed by rehabilitation after reconstructive surgery for tendon transfer re-education (see Chapter 20).

Introduction

Excellence in pediatric spinal cord injury (SCI) rehabilitation is reliant upon competent team members who understand the implications of the interaction between SCI and growth and development, an organizational environment that is centered on the family and child and uses evidence-based practice, and the systematic and deliberate use of evidence-based assessment techniques and outcomes instruments. The rehabilitation assessment of children with SCI is a process that involves, among other techniques, the use of diagnostic testing, standardized performance measures, and patient-reported outcomes. More recently, standard data sets have also been advocated for the standardized documentation of outcomes. Purposes for assessment include screening and diagnoses; benchmarking and reimbursement; goal setting and prioritization of rehabilitation goals; aid in decision making about treatment by parents and children; planning for environmental adaptations; longitudinal monitoring for the purpose of preventing secondary complications; identifying the need for habilitation; building evidence in support of treatment; and evaluating and comparing outcomes of routine care.

There are excellent resources (www.scireproject.com), including evidence-based and systematic reviews of outcomes instruments in SCI rehabilitation (Anderson et al 2008, Jackson et al 2008, Magasi et al 2008, Alexander et al 2009, Hill et al 2010), that are highly recommended. Discussions on screening and diagnostic tools and several important pediatric outcomes instruments are beyond the scope of this chapter but can be found in various chapters throughout this book (Chapters 6, 11, 17, 18, 22, and 29) and in other notable material (Staas et al 1998, Zidek and Srinivasan 2003, Mulcahey et al 2007, Dumas et al 2009). This chapter will review relevant research related to evaluation methods and outcomes instruments that have particular relevance to pediatric SCI rehabilitation, introduce and describe the development of computer adaptive testing for pediatric SCI, and discuss the International Spinal Cord Injury Data Sets. Finally, recommendations for future research related to development and validation of outcomes instruments for pediatric SCI work will be defined.

Neurologic assessment

One of the greatest successes of the international SCI community of researchers and clinicians is the development and endorsement of the International Standards for Neurological Classification of Spinal Cord Injury (ISNCSCI) (American Spinal Injury Association 2011, Kirshblum et al 2011), because they provide uniformity and thus an opportunity to compare and pool neurologic data from around the world. The neurologic assessments of the ISNCSCI, which include the motor, sensory, and anorectal examinations, contribute to the classification of SCI according to the American Spinal Injury Association (ASIA) Impairment Scale (AIS) (Kirshblum et al 2011). The sensory examination involves testing of dermatomes (Fig. 4.4) on the right and left side of the body for sensitivity to sharp–dull discrimination and to light touch appreciation. The motor examination is completed by testing 10 muscle functions bilaterally. The strength of each muscle is graded on an ordinal scale between 0 (complete paralysis) and 5 (normal active movement, full range of motion against full resistance). The anorectal examination involves the evaluation of sensation and contraction of the external anal sphincter. For this, the examiner applies pressure with the index finger to the rectal wall to test for deep anal sensation pressure and makes the request of the person being examined to squeeze as if holding a bowel movement (anal contraction). Classification of the motor, sensory, and neurologic levels are determined based upon the motor and sensory examination findings (Fig. 4.4). As summarized in Figure 4.4, the AIS designation is, in part, based upon sensory and motor sparing at the sacral segments.

Recent work with children showed that the ISNCSCI motor and sensory scores can be obtained in children as young as 6 years of age with moderate to strong reliability (Mulcahey et al 2011). The utility of the anorectal examinations in children has not been as evident, with documented problems associated with the test instructions for anal contraction, particularly for children injured before achieving bowel continence (Mulcahey et al 2011), and with test validity (Vogel et al 2009, Samdani et al 2011). Despite the potential limitations of the ISNCSCI, its use is recommended for children 6 years of age and older (Mulcahey et al 2011). For children

TABLE 4.1

Goal attainment scaling for several out-patient therapy goals related to morning routine and school. The criteria for scaling were defined by the child and parent, with input from the occupational therapists, before the start of out-patient therapy

		Goal attainment scaling method and criteria					Out-patient therapy	
Concern	**Goal**	**–2**	**–1**	**0**	**1**	**2**	**Admission**	**Discharge**
Unable to assist with any morning routine, creating significant time burden on mother and causing Joey and other children to be late for school. Refuses to allow older sibling to assist with dressing	To be able to wash face and brush teeth after set-up and dress upper body within a 25-min time frame without complaint or frustration. Would like older brother to assist with morning routines	Unable to wash face, brush teeth, or dress upper body within 25min. Complains during process and/or becomes extremely frustrated (crying, screaming, throwing items, etc.)	Washes face, brushes teeth and dresses upper body within 45min with little frustration (only infrequent complaints, no crying, no throwing items)	Washes face, brushes teeth, and dresses upper body within 25min without complaint or frustration	Washes face, brushes teeth, and dresses upper body within 25min without complaint or frustration. Attempts to assist with remaining morning routine by preparing underwear and socks. With complaint and fighting, allows older brother to assist with lower body dressing and transfer from bed to wheelchair	Washes face, brushes teeth, and dresses upper body within 25min without complaint or frustration. Attempts to assist with remaining morning routine by preparing underwear and socks. Initiates asking brother for help when mother is delayed or busy with other children	–2	1

Unable to remove or replace material from school bag, resulting in frustration and dependency during school time routines	To be able to pack school material and books in book bag	Is unable to move books from table into book bag. Cannot place markers, pencils, or universal cuff in pencil case. Cannot zip or unzip school bag	Is able to slide light books from table into book bag with books falling on to floor less than 25% of the time. Needs help with heavy books. Slides pencils, markers, and universal cuff into pencil case with items falling on to floor less than 25% of the time. Cannot zip and unzip book bag. Can complete activity within an acceptable time frame (5–10min) with minimal frustration	Is able to slide the majority of books from table into book bag without books falling; may need help with heavy books. Picks up light pencils and markers and places them in pencil case with very infrequent falls. Uses adaptive equipment to zip and unzip bag. Completes activity within 5min without frustration	Is able to place all material, including books, into book bag from table within 5min without any difficulty. Can remove light objects from book bag and place them on home work table. Needs help with removing large books	Is able to place all material, including books, into book bag from table within 5min without any difficulty. Can remove all objects from book bag and place them on table. Shows no frustration with activity; activity is habituated as a typical routine	–2	0
Unable to negotiate lunch line in school cafeteria, limiting participation with peers in school time	To be able to move through lunch line in school cafeteria and carry lunch on wheelchair tray to lunch table	Unable to move power wheelchair through lunch line without hitting other children or walls. Unable to move food to table without spilling	Can move power wheelchair along lunch line in the absence of other children, without hitting walls and without spilling food. Time to complete activity is unacceptably long (>10min)	Can move power wheelchair along lunch line when first in line without hitting children and without hitting the walls. Has difficulty with carrying food to table with many children in lunch room (some food spills, especially soup, mild) and fruit rolls off tray. Time to complete activity is longer than preferred (up to 5min)	Can move power wheelchair along lunch line when first in line without hitting children and without hitting the walls. When given a table close to lunch line, able to carry food to table without difficulty. Time to complete activity is acceptable (2–4 min)	Can move power chair through lunch line and lunch room without difficulty, regardless of the number of children in line or in lunch room and regardless of where table is placed. Activity requires no more than 4min and there is little, if any, spillage	–2	–1

A score of '0' reflects the projected performance that was expected at the completion of the 6-month out-patient therapy, whereas scores of –2 and +2 reflect much less and much more than the expected outcome, respectively. As shown, for each of the three goals, improvement was made with therapy as shown by progression from negative to positive (with zero being the desired outcome).

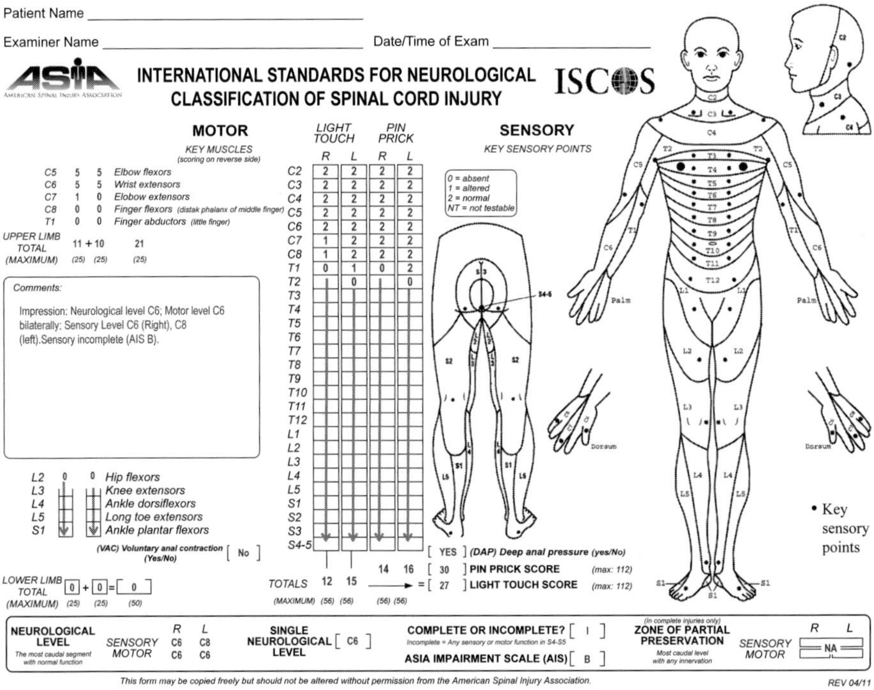
Patient Name
Examiner Name Date/Time of Exam
INTERNATIONAL STANDARDS FOR NEUROLOGICAL CLASSIFICATION OF SPINAL CORD INJURY
ASIA American Spinal Injury Association
ISCoS

MOTOR
KEY MUSCLES (scoring on reverse side)

	R	L	
C5	5	5	Elbow flexors
C6	5	5	Wrist extensors
C7	1	0	Elobow extensors
C8	0	0	Finger flexors (distak phalanx of middle finger)
T1	0	0	Finger abductors (little finger)

UPPER LIMB TOTAL (MAXIMUM) 11 + 10 = 21 (25) (25) (50)

Comments:
Impression: Neurological level C6; Motor level C6 bilaterally; Sensory Level C6 (Right), C8 (left).Sensory incomplete (AIS B).

	R	L	
L2	0	0	Hip flexors
L3	↓	↓	Knee extensors
L4			Ankle dorsiflexors
L5			Long toe extensors
S1			Ankle plantar flexors

(VAC) Voluntary anal contraction (Yes/No) [No]
LOWER LIMB TOTAL (MAXIMUM) 0 + 0 = 0 (25) (25) (50)

SENSORY
KEY SENSORY POINTS

	Light Touch R	Light Touch L	Pin Prick R	Pin Prick L
C2	2	2	2	2
C3	2	2	2	2
C4	2	2	2	2
C5	2	2	2	2
C6	2	2	2	2
C7	1	2	2	2
C8	1	2	2	2
T1	0	1	0	2
T2	↓	0	↓	0
T3–S4-5	↓	↓	↓	↓
TOTALS	12	15	14	16
(MAXIMUM)	(56)	(56)	(56)	(56)

0 = absent
1 = altered
2 = normal
NT = not testable

[YES] (DAP) Deep anal pressure (yes/No)
[30] PIN PRICK SCORE (max: 112)
[27] LIGHT TOUCH SCORE (max: 112)

• Key sensory points

NEUROLOGICAL LEVEL (The most caudal segment with normal function): SENSORY R C6, L C8; MOTOR R C6, L C6
SINGLE NEUROLOGICAL LEVEL [C6]
COMPLETE OR INCOMPLETE? [I] Incomplete = Any sensory or motor function in S4-S5
ASIA IMPAIRMENT SCALE (AIS) [B]
ZONE OF PARTIAL PRESERVATION (In complete injuries only) Most caudal level with any innervation: SENSORY, MOTOR R L NA
This form may be copied freely but should not be altered without permission from the American Spinal Injury Association.
REV 04/11

Fig. 4.1 Joey: 7 years of age. Completed 15 months after spinal cord injury; previous attempts unsuccessful owing to young age. Note, this form is the 2011 version; the 2013 version is shown in Fig. 4.4. Reproduced with permission from the American Spinal Injury Association.

younger than 6 years, observational motor assessment may facilitate the assessment of muscle strength and motor activity (Calhoun et al 2009a). Evaluation of severity (complete/incomplete) and classification using the AIS is not recommended for children between birth and 5 years of age; documentation in the medical record should specify that injury severity based on the ISNCSCI cannot be determined until at least 6 years of age (Mulcahey et al 2011). A thorough review of the ISNCSCI as it applies to children is available via an electronic learning module, the WeeSTep, through the ASIA (www.asia-spinalinjury.org).

The Graded Redefined Assessment of Strength, Sensibility and Prehension (GRASSP) is a recently developed impairment measure that is designed to evaluate neurologic function, particularly under conditions where change is expected (Kalsi-Ryan et al 2009, Rudhe and van Hedel 2009). The GRASSP creates an impairment profile of the upper limb using measures of sensation (via Semmes–Weinstein monofilaments), strength, and prehension (Kalsi-Ryan et al 2012a). Unlike the ISNCSCI, which is applicable for use with persons of any level of SCI, the GRASSP is designed to evaluate the neurologic impairment of persons with tetraplegia (C0–T1 injuries). Studies with adults with cervical-level SCI report strong reliability of GRASSP scores on repeated administrations, good concurrent validity, and better responsiveness than ISNCSCI examinations (Kalsi-Ryan et al 2012a,b). Future psychometric

Date performed: JOEY, 7 years old, 2.9 years following SCI

Neuro-Musculoskeletal history before spinal cord lesion (collected once):
Pre-existing congenital deformities of the spine and spinal cord
If yes, specify Diagnosis and Location____NA________________
If previous surgery due to this, description____NA________________
Date of surgery YYYYMMDD Unknown

Pre-existing degenerative spine disorders
If yes, specify Diagnosis and Location______NA________________
If previous surgery due to this, description___NA________________
Date of surgery YYYYMMDD Unknown

Pre-existing systemic neuro-degenerative disorders
If yes, specify Diagnosis and Location_NA________________
If previous surgery due to this, description______NA________________
Date of surgery YYYYMMDD Unknown

Presence of spasticity / spasms
No X Yes
Treatment for spasticity / spasms within the last four weeks?
No X Yes

Fractures, heterotopic ossifications, contractures, or degenerative changes/overuse:

	Fractures since spinal cord lesion (only those not documented previously)				Heterotopic ossification		Contracture		Degenerative changes / Overuse	
	Right	Left	Date of fracture YYYY/MM/DD	Fragility fracture	Right	Left	Right	Left	Right	Left
Neck / Cervical spine										
Shoulder / Humerus										
Elbow							X	X		
Forearm										
Wrist										
Hand										
Upper back / Thoracic spine										
Lower back / Lumbar spine										
Pelvis										
Hip / Femur							X	X		
Knee										
Tibia / Fibula										
Ankle										
Foot										

Method used to document heterotopic ossification, if present:
X-ray CT-scan Triple phase bone scan Other method, specify__________

Scoliosis
No **X** Yes
If scoliosis is present, method of assessment (check all that apply)
X Observation in sitting Observation in standing
X Plain radiographs in sitting Plain radiographs in standing
If scoliosis is present,
Surgically treated? If Yes: Date of surgery Unknown

X Other musculoskeletal problems; specify__bilateral hip subluxation

Do any of the above musculoskeletal challenges interfere with your activities of daily living (transfers, walking, dressing, showers, etc.)?
No – not at all X Yes, a little Yes

Fig. 4.2 International spinal cord injury musculoskeletal basic data set form (version 1.0). Completed as part of routine follow-up care. Reproduced with permission from the American Spinal Injury Association.

Date performed: JOEY, 8 years old, 3.9 years following SCI

Neuro-Musculoskeletal history before spinal cord lesion (collected once):
Pre-existing congenital deformities of the spine and spinal cord
If yes, specify Diagnosis and Location____NA________________
If previous surgery due to this, description____NA________________
Date of surgery YYYYMMDD Unknown

Pre-existing degenerative spine disorders
If yes, specify Diagnosis and Location______NA________________
If previous surgery due to this, description____NA________________
Date of surgery YYYYMMDD Unknown

Pre-existing systemic neuro-degenerative disorders
If yes, specify Diagnosis and Location_NA________________
If previous surgery due to this, description______NA________________
Date of surgery YYYYMMDD Unknown

Presence of spasticity / spasms
No X Yes
Treatment for spasticity / spasms within the last four weeks?
No X Yes

Fractures, heterotopic ossifications, contractures, or degenerative changes/overuse:

	Fractures since spinal cord lesion (only those not documented previously)				**Heterotopic ossification**		**Contracture**		**Degenerative changes / Overuse**	
	Right	Left	Date of fracture YYYY/ MM/DD	Fragility fracture	Right	Left	Right	Left	Right	Left
Neck / Cervical spine										
Shoulder / Humerus										
Elbow							X	X		
Forearm										
Wrist							X	X		
Hand										
Upper back / Thoracic spine										
Lower back / Lumbar spine										
Pelvis										
Hip / Femur							X	X		
Knee										
Tibia / Fibula	X		2014/03/03							
Ankle										
Foot										

Method used to document heterotopic ossification, if present:
X-ray CT-scan Triple phase bone scan Other method, specify__________

Scoliosis
No **X** Yes
If scoliosis is present, method of assessment (check all that apply)
X Observation in sitting Observation in standing
X Plain radiographs in sitting Plain radiographs in standing
If scoliosis is present,
Surgically treated? If Yes: Date of surgery Unknown

X Other musculoskeletal problems; specify__Right hip subluxation, Left hip dislocation

Do any of the above musculoskeletal challenges interfere with your activities of daily living (transfers, walking, dressing, showers, etc.)?
No – not at all X Yes, a little Yes

Fig. 4.3 International spinal cord injury musculoskeletal basic data set form (version 1.0). Completed as part of routine follow-up care. Note the change in data from last follow-up (see Fig. 4.2): tibia fracture; left hip dislocation. Reproduced with permission from the American Spinal Injury Association.

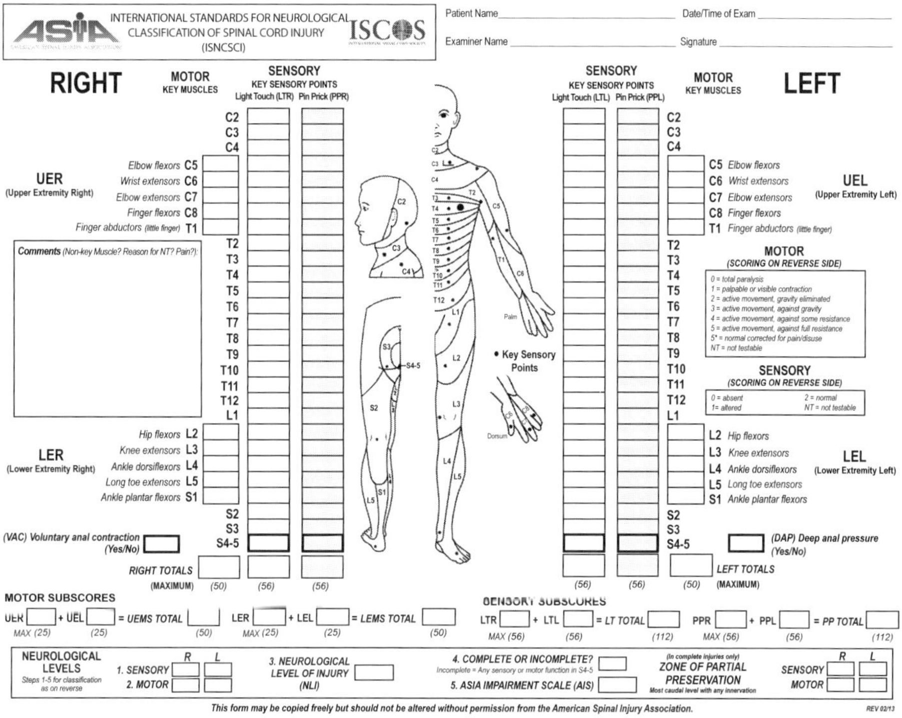

Fig. 4.4 Scoring form and classification guidelines for the International Standards for Neurological Classification of Spinal Cord Injury. Reprinted 2013 with permission from the American Spinal Injury Association: International Standards for Neurological Classification of Spinal Cord Injury, revised 2013; Atlanta, GA. Specific pediatric modifications are described in the electronic learning module, the WeeSTep, made available through the American Spinal Injury Association (http://www.asia-spinalinjury.org).

studies of the GRASSP should include children and young people. The GRASSP is available for purchase at http://grassptest.com/purchase.aspx.

Current research is under way to develop imaging techniques that may aid in the evaluation and classification of SCI in children who are too young to engage in the ISNCSCI or other impairment-based measures. Preliminary work on diffusion tensor imaging is very promising (see Chapter 29; Mohamed et al 2011, Mulcahey et al 2012a, Mulcahey 2013).

Assessment of activity

Functional Independence Measure for Children

Despite the concerted effort to understand the research in support of outcomes instruments for use in SCI rehabilitation and research (Magasi et al 2008, Alexander et al 2009), children have not been adequately considered. The FIM® (Uniform Data System for Medical Rehabilitation, Amherst, NY) (Hamilton et al 1987) may be the most widely used instrument to assess physical and cognitive dimensions of disability, but it has limitations when used with the population with SCI. Reported limitations include poor content range, gaps in content, ceiling and floor effects, inability to detect small but meaningful change, and a lack of items that are relevant for persons with SCI (Hall et al 1999, Garcia et al 2002, Furlan et al 2011). Limitations associated with ceiling effects and poor responsiveness have been documented when the FIM has been used with children with SCI (Mulcahey et al 1999, Garcia et al 2002). With additional mobility and walking items, content range and responsiveness of the FIM have been improved (Middleton et al 2006), but no psychometric work on the FIM with the additional items has been done with children. Despite these limitations, the FIM may have benefits for projecting economic burden (Cohen et al 2012), justifying therapy services (Riis et al 2011), and monitoring longitudinal changes in children with SCI (Allen et al 2009). One of the greatest limitations of the FIM with respect to outcomes is that it measures 'burden of care', which is a different construct than functional ability, activity performance, and participation (Anderson et al 2008). Like the FIM, the FIM for children (Wee FIM® Uniform Data System for Medical Rehabilitation, Amherst, NY) (Msall et al 1994) is an 18-item generic instrument that uses a seven-point rating scale ranging from 'complete independence' (score of 7) to 'total assistance' (score of 1). Generally, the WeeFIM is used with children 7 years of age and younger. The reported use of the WeeFIM in children with SCI is limited but indicates that it may be responsive to functional change during subacute in-patient rehabilitation (Garcia et al 2002) and after intensive treadmill training (Prosser 2007). The FIM and WeeFIM are proprietary and their use requires training, certification, and a fee (www.udsmr.org).

Spinal Cord Independence Measure

The Spinal Cord Independence Measure-III (SCIM-III) was developed as a 'disease'-specific instrument in response to the limitations of the FIM (Catz et al 1997). The SCIM-III, which contains items that evaluate self care, respiration, bladder and bowel management, and mobility, is gaining recognition as the instrument of choice for research and clinical applications (Anderson et al 2008, van Hedel et al 2009, Furlan et al 2011). Psychometric studies on the SCIM-III with adults with SCI have established moderate-to-strong reliability and validity indices and have shown that, when compared with the FIM, the SCIM-III has a broader content range and is more responsive to change (Itzkovich et al 2007, Anderson et al 2011, Bluvshtein et al 2011). There have been no large-scale studies of the SCIM-III with children with SCI, although there is evidence that field testing is occurring (Webster and Kennedy 2007, Calhoun and Mulcahey 2012). The SCIM-III is available at no cost (Catz et al 2007).

The Child Needs Assessment Checklist

The Child Needs Assessment Checklist (Berry and Kennedy 2003, Webster and Kennedy 2007) was developed based on the Adult Needs Assessment Checklist (Kennedy and Hamilton 1999) as a framework for SCI rehabilitation in children and goal setting in the context of treatment theory, growth, and development and a family-centered approach (Webster and Kennedy 2007). The checklist comprises 10 domains relevant to pediatric SCI rehabilitation (e.g. mobility, wheelchair and equipment, knowledge about spine) and 183 behavioral indicators that are scored on a scale of 0 to 3, where 0 reflects 'no independence' and 3 reflects 'full independence'. Scoring also includes a developmental consideration, such that children are not penalized for items where there is no independence owing to developmental age or level. Rehabilitation goals are established based on the results of the Child Needs Assessment Checklist and repeated administrations allow for evaluation of progress toward goals. Psychometric work on the Child Needs Assessment Checklist has been reported (Berry and Kennedy 2003, Webster and Kennedy 2007) and supports its use as a tool to define rehabilitation goals and to evaluate outcomes of pediatric rehabilitation programming.

Assessment of capacity and performance

There are several pediatric measures (Adair et al 2012) of mobility that have been used in children with a variety of diagnoses, including SCI. The psychometric work on the majority of these instruments has predominantly been with children with cerebral palsy. The Walking Index for Spinal Cord Injury (WISCI-II) has already gained recognition for adult SCI, and is a promising measure of walking capacity for children with SCI (Ditunno et al 2000). The WISCI-II uses an ordinal scale between 0 and 20 that reflects various levels of walking ability, taking into account the use of assistive devices, orthotic devices, and physical assistance. The assessment involves a 10-m (32.8-feet) walk, which is a distance often correlated with household ambulation (Catz et al 1997). The utility of the WISCI-II has been established in the adult population with SCI with evidence of good validity and reliability (van Hedel et al 2005, Ditunno et al 2007, Marino et al 2010, Burns et al 2011). Although its use with children has been limited (Prosser 2007, Fox et al 2010), there is preliminary evidence of strong inter- and intrarater reliability (intraclass correlation coefficient >0.98) when used with children with SCI (Calhoun and Mulcahey 2012).

Walking has also been evaluated as a function of speed and distance, using measures such as the Timed Up and Go Test (Mathias et al 1986) or indices such as the 6-m walk (American Thoracic Society 2002), 10-m walk (van Hedel et al 2005, 2006), or maximum walking distance (Johnston et al 2003, Behrman et al 2012); these methods are low cost and can be easily integrated into routine clinical practice (Poncumhak et al 2012). The WISCI-II and the 10-m walk have been recommended as the performance measures of choice for adult SCI (Jackson et al 2008) and are highly applicable to young people.

Patrick (2003) and Smith et al (2004) have proposed using standardized three-dimensional (3D) gait analysis with children with SCI, but access to motion analysis laboratories is difficult. In addition to barriers related to access, the financial cost of 3D gait analysis is relatively high. There is also an element of burden with respect to time and testing technique that may deter general acceptance of 3D motion analysis as a routine evaluation for children with SCI. Instrumented walkways such as the GaitMat-II (www.gaitmat.com) and GAITRite (www.gaitrite.com) have been reported as useful alternative methods to 3D motion analysis to evaluate walking speed, step length, stride length, and cadence (Fox et al 2010). These systems are portable, easily integrated into routine clinical practice, and, when compared with 3D motion analysis, are of a relatively low cost and burden.

Performance measures specific to upper extremity function of persons with SCI have been described (Stroh Wuolle et al 1994, Post et al 2006, Spooran et al 2006, Marino et al 2012) but to a lesser degree than lower extremity performance measures. None has gained widespread acceptance by adult SCI clinicians or researchers and only a few have been exposed to psychometric testing in children with SCI (Mulcahey et al 2004). The Jebsen Test of Hand Function (Jebsen et al 1969) is a commonly used upper extremity performance measure but lacks responsiveness to surgical tendon transfers for pinch and grasp in children (Mulcahey et al 1995). New initiatives hold promise for responsive and meaningful measures of upper extremity function (Coates et al 2011, Cornwell et al 2012, Kalsi-Ryan et al 2012a,b, Marino 2012); their development and validation should include children.

Even in the literature on adults, there is large inconsistency among current performance measures for wheeled mobility devices (Routhier et al 2003, Fliess-Douer et al 2010, Rushton et al 2012, Kirby 2002). Differences in scale levels (nominal, ordinal, interval, ratio) and scoring methods limit comparisons across studies (Fliess-Douer et al 2010, Kirby 2011). The Wheelchair Outcome Measure (Miller et al 2011) was developed specifically for SCI to evaluate the impact of wheelchair interventions on participation outcomes. Studies with adults with SCI show good to strong reliability and fair to moderate validity. Further research on the development and validation of outcomes measures for wheeled mobility for children with SCI is needed.

Assessment of participation and quality of life

A review of participation and quality of life measures relevant to SCI has been conducted, but it excluded children under 18 years of age and focused on three primary adult instruments (Magasi et al 2008, Hill et al 2010). The Craig Handicap Assessment and Reporting Technique (Whiteneck et al 1992), the Assessment of Life Habits (Fougeyrollas et al 1998), and the Impact on Participation and Autonomy (Cardol et al 2001) are recognized as useful assessments for adults with SCI (Hall et al 2001, Noonan et al 2009, Magasi and Post 2010). However, both the Craig Handicap Assessment and Reporting Technique and the Impact on Participation and Autonomy contain items that are not intended for child response (Cardol et al 2001, Magasi and Post 2010) and the pediatric version of the Assessment of Life Habits (Noreau et al 2007) has had limited use with children with SCI. The widely used Pediatric Quality of Life Inventory has concepts related to participation but has limitations when used with children with SCI (Oladeji et al 2007). The Children's Assessment of Participation and Enjoyment is designed for young people aged 6 to 21 years (King et al 2006) and, although it is long (55 items), it has been used with children with SCI (Gorzkowski et al 2010, Klaas et al 2010). The Children's Assessment of Participation and Enjoyment, which considers five dimensions of participation (diversity, intensity, enjoyment, with whom, and where) is available along with the Preference for Activities by Children by Harcourt Assessment, Inc., San Antonio, TX, USA (www.harcourtassessment.com). Other instruments that may be useful for children with SCI include the Lifestyle Assessment Questionnaire (Mackie et al 1998), Activities Scale for Kids (Young et al 2000), and the pediatric version of the Assessment of Life Habits (Noreau et al 2007). Further research is needed.

Assessment using goal attainment scaling

Although goal attainment scaling (GAS) has not been described with children with SCI, it has been described with children with cerebral palsy (Hoare et al 2012, Mayson et al 2012) and autism (Schaaf et al 2012) and within the context of rehabilitation (Steenbeek et al 2007, Evans 2012) and geriatric care (Rockwood et al 1993, Gordon et al 1999). GAS is a technique for evaluating an individual's progress toward patient-defined goals that involves a sequential process that sets goals of treatment; assigns a weight for each goal based on the importance or priority of the patient; establishes a continuum of possible outcomes; assesses baseline function; provides intervention for a specified period of time; evaluates performance on each goal using specified possible outcomes; and evaluates the extent of goal attainment (Kiresuk et al 1994). Although the principal strength of GAS is the ability to evaluate individualized change (Mailloux et al 2007), under certain conditions (Kiresuk et al 1994), the data from multiple patients can be aggregated and a comparison across goals and patients can be made. Other advantages include the versatility of the GAS with respect to evaluating goals across the International Classification of Function, Disability and Health domains, responsiveness to change and psychometric rigor (Choate et al 1981, Heavlin et al 1982, Lewis et al 1987, Schlosser 2004). Given the lack of sensitive measures in pediatric rehabilitation and the limited exposure of adult measures to children, GAS has the potential to provide an effective method to evaluate treatment outcomes in children with SCI.

Assessment using computer adaptive testing

Owing to the inherent limitations of traditional fixed-length instruments, such as ceiling and floor effects, gaps in content, and length (number of items), contemporary instruments using computer adaptive testing (CAT) are available for a wide range of applications (www.nihpromis.org) and are being developed for SCI (Calhoun et al 2009b, Jette et al 2012, Mulcahey et al 2012b,c). The advantages of CAT over traditional fixed-length measures are being demonstrated consistently with a range of clinical populations, supporting the position that CAT provides an unprecedented means for a precise, efficient, and meaningful method for evaluating reported outcomes of patients (Rebollo et al 2010, Fries et al 2011, Hou et al 2012, Kirisci et al 2012, Smits et al 2012, Turner-Bowker et al 2012).

For children with SCI, CAT is uniquely positioned to monitor outcomes of SCI. With CAT, the same question, which is of average difficulty (not too hard and not too easy), is presented to every person first; subsequent questions are presented based on the response to previous test questions, such that, if the item is answered as 'being really hard', an easier test item appears and, if the item is answered as 'being easy', a harder question appears. Perhaps one of the most desirable characteristics of CAT for longitudinal monitoring of outcomes in young people with SCI is that different items can be administered at different points of time based on the child's developmental age and level as well as on the child's function. As an example, an item about being able to apply cosmetics has little relevance to young children and males, but is highly relevant to adolescent females; an age and sex filter provides the mechanism to withhold this item for younger children and males but make it available to older females. The ability to administer different items as a child ages, while still being able to compare past scores with current scores, is unique to CAT; there is no traditional fixed-length instrument that can be administered throughout childhood and adolescence and provide meaningful information at each administration and a mechanism to compare outcomes over that time period. Additionally, with CAT, the same items are not administered to every child; through the use of other filters such as those for sex, level of injury, mechanism of mobility, and use of equipment, only items that provide meaningful information about a child are administered. For example, a child who only uses a wheelchair would never be administered items that are associated with walking. Likewise, a child with paraplegia would never be administered an item associated with using adaptive equipment for meals. The specificity of the items to the individual child allows CAT to administer only a few items that provide highly relevant and meaningful information. In addition to developing and validating CATs for children with cerebral palsy (Gorton et al 2010, Haley et al 2010, Montepetit et al 2011), development and calibration of item banks of mobility, daily routines, and participation for children with SCI have been completed with studies demonstrating efficiency and reliability through simulated CATs (Figs 4.5 and 4.6) (Calhoun et al 2009b, Mulcahey et al 2009, 2012a,b, 2013, Bent et al 2013). The vision is to make these pediatric SCI CATs available for clinical use and link them to CATs being developed for adults with SCI (Jette et al 2012, Tian et al 2014).

International Spinal Cord Injury Data Sets

Although there are diligent efforts being made to develop responsive and valid outcome measures for SCI, minimal data sets and longitudinal registries remain important assessment methods. SCI data sets (Box 4.1) have been systematically developed by international workgroups and reviewed by content experts worldwide (Biering-Sørensen et al 2008a,b, 2009, 2011b, 2012a,b, 2014, Widerström-Noga et al 2008, Krogh et al 2009a,b, Krassioukov et al 2010, Alexander et al 2011a,b, Bauman et al 2011, Charlifue et al 2012, Dvorak et al 2012, in press, Karlsson et al 2012, New and Marshall et al 2012). The intent of the SCI data sets is threefold:

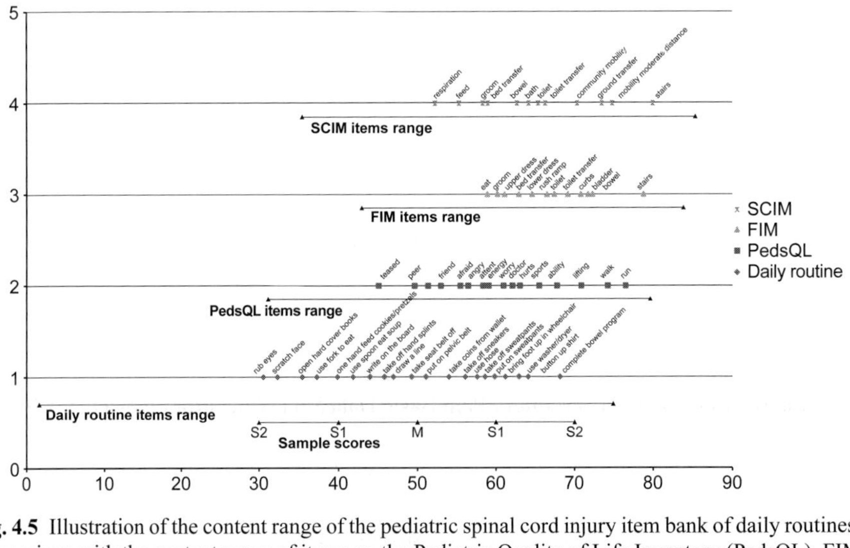

Fig. 4.5 Illustration of the content range of the pediatric spinal cord injury item bank of daily routines in comparison with the content range of items on the Pediatric Quality of Life Inventory (PedsQL), FIM®, and Spinal Cord Independence Measure (SCIM)-III. Note the floor effects on all three comparison measures and the gaps in content of the FIM and Pediatric Quality of Life Inventory.

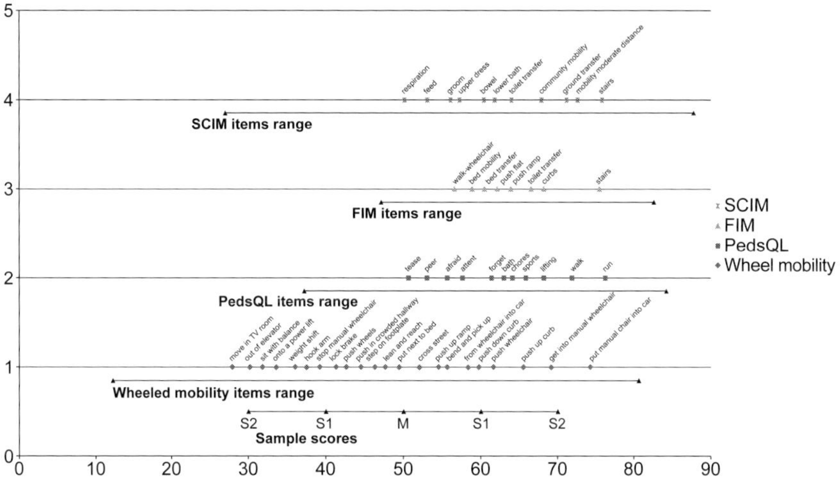

Fig. 4.6 Illustration of the content range of the pediatric spinal cord injury item bank of wheeled mobility in comparison with the content range of items on the Pediatric Quality of Life Inventory (PedsQL), FIM®, and Spinal Cord Independence Measure (SCIM)-III. Note the ceiling and floor effects on all three comparison measures and the gaps in content of the FIM and Pediatric Quality of Life Inventory.

Box 4.1 Listing of International Spinal Cord Injury Basic Data Sets. These data sets can be downloaded for free from http://www.iscos.org.uk/. Key references are provided

- International Spinal Cord Injury Spinal Column Injury Basic Data Set (Dvorak et al 2012)
- International Spinal Cord Injury Non-traumatic Data Sets (New and Marshall 2012)
- International Spinal Cord Injury Lower Urinary Tract Function Basic Data Set (Biering-Sørensen et al 2008a)
- International Spinal Cord Injury Urinary Tract Infection Basic Data Set (Goetz et al 2013)
- International Spinal Cord Injury Urodynamic Basic Data Set (Biering-Sørensen et al 2008b)
- International Spinal Cord Injury Urinary Tract Imaging Basic Data Set (Biering-Sørensen et al 2009)
- International Spinal Cord Injury Bowel Basic Data Set (Krogh et al 2009a)
- International Spinal Cord Injury Pain Basic Data Set (Widerström-Noga et al 2008, 2014)
- International Spinal Cord Injury Female Sexual and Reproductive Function Basic Data Set (Alexander et al 2011a)
- International Spinal Cord Injury Male Sexual Function Basic Data Set (Alexander et al 2011b)

Box 4.1 (Continued)

- International Spinal Cord Injury Cardiovascular Function Basic Data Set (Krassioukov et al 2010)
- International Spinal Cord Injury Pulmonary Function Basic Data Set (Biering-Sørensen et al 2012a)
- International Spinal Cord Injury Skin and Thermoregulation Function Basic Data Set (Karlsson et al 2012)
- International Spinal Cord Injury Endocrine and Metabolic Function Basic Data Set (Bauman et al 2011)
- International Spinal Cord Injury Musculoskeletal Basic Data Set (Biering-Sørensen et al 2012b)
- International Spinal Cord Injury Activity and Participation Basic Data Set
- International Spinal Cord Injury Quality of Life Basic Data Set (Charlifue et al 2012)
- International Spinal Cord Injury Upper Extremity Basic Data Set (Biering-Sørensen et al 2014)

to establish a common language across countries on clinical outcomes of SCI, to assist centers in developing new SCI databases, and to provide consistency for the design and publication of clinical research studies (Biering-Sørensen et al 2006). To facilitate ease of clinical implementation, the data sets, by design, are simple to use and relevant to clinicians. In addition, they are easily retrieved and available for use at no cost and without any specific restrictions (Biering-Sørensen et al 2006); they can be freely downloaded from the International Spinal Cord Society website: www.iscos.org.uk. The overall structure (Fig. 4.7) and terminology for the International SCI Data Sets have been developed within the framework of the International Classification of Function, Disability and Health (Biering-Sørensen et al 2006).

In addition to the SCI Basic Data Sets, there is the International SCI Core Data Set. The International SCI Core Data Set is designed to standardize the collection and reporting of a minimal amount of information after the first in-patient period and as a way to evaluate and compare current outcomes with results of published studies (DeVivo et al 2006). The SCI Core Data Set consists of 24 variables, including basic demographic characteristics, dates of admission and discharge from initial acute and rehabilitation care, cause of injury, place of discharge, presence of vertebral fractures and associated injuries, occurrence of spinal surgery, and measures of neurologic and ventilator status. There are recommended standards for reporting of the variables, including specifications associated with pediatric ages (DeVivo et al 2011, Biering-Sørensen et al 2012c). In contrast to the Core Data Set, the International SCI Basic Data Sets (listed in Table 4.2) define the minimal number of data elements that should be collected in routine clinical practice. The use of the Basic Data Sets by SCI practitioners creates a common structure worldwide. Currently there are also two SCI Extended Data Sets (Krogh et al 2009b, Lee et al 2010) that may be used for routine monitoring, but these were designed specifically to support research within particular areas. A third Extended Data Set is under development for pain, endocrine, and metabolic function.

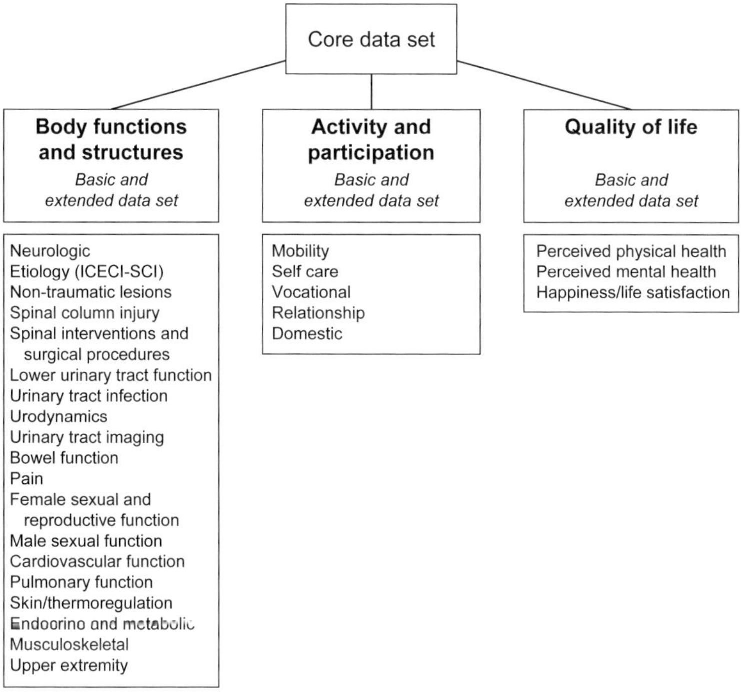

Fig. 4.7 Structure of the International Spinal Cord Injury Data Sets (www.iscos.org.uk). ICECI-SCI: WHO International Classification of External Causes of Injury – Spinal Cord Injury.

For the majority of SCI Core Data Sets and SCI Basic Data Sets, training cases are available through the website of the International Spinal Cord Society (www.iscos.org.uk). It is recommended that the training cases be reviewed before downloading and using a particular data set. Among other things, the training provides examples on how to code the data set form correctly. Recommendations for translation and reliability testing of the SCI Data Sets have also been developed (Biering-Sørensen et al 2011b). As a minimum requirement, it is recommended that the interrater reliability shall be tested by no fewer than two independent observers, and preferably in multiple countries (Biering-Sørensen et al 2011b).

The majority of variables on the SCI Data Sets are relevant to children. The SCI Data Sets provide a mechanism for pediatric centers to standardize the collection of key outcomes data for pooling, comparison, and benchmarking; this is particularly important in children, since no one institution sees a sufficient number of children with SCI to create a large enough data set.

Future research

There is a clear need for efficient, precise, and meaningful outcomes instruments in pediatric SCI. Currently, the SCI Data Sets offer pediatric institutions a framework for collecting minimal data sets on children with SCI. The ISNCSCI should be administered, in accordance with the guidelines, on all children with SCI 6 years of age and older. Although there has been no

TABLE 4.2

Illustration of goal attainment scaling using 3 of the 15 out-patient therapy goals. The criteria for scaling were defined before the start of out-patient therapy

		Goal attainment scaling method and criteria					6-month out-patient therapy	
Concern	**Goal**	**–2**	**–1**	**0**	**1**	**2**	**Admission**	**Discharge**
Unable to enjoy meal time with family owing to difficulty with feeding self and embarrassment about level of dependence and quality of self-feeding	To be able to eat dinner within a time frame comparable to the rest of the family with little effort and mess	Unable to finish meal on own within 45min. Meal is finished with physical help of another person. Highly frustrated (constant crying, refusal to feed self, refusal to eat)	Finishes meal within 10min after family is finished. Has multiple spills of food from utensil onto table and clothing. Shows some signs of frustration (asks for help once or twice, refuses to finish meal)	Finishes meal within 30min with minimal signs of frustration (complaining, asking for help, crying, refusing to eat) and with no more than two inadvertent spills of food from utensil	Finishes meal within 30min without frustration and without inadvertent spills of food from utensil	Finishes meal within 30min. Is pleasant and shows signs of enjoying meal time. May ask for second helpings of food	–2	0
Unable to move power wheelchair down ramps, limiting independent mobility in school and church	To be able to independently use wheelchair joystick to move down ramp while sitting in power chair without signs of fear and anxiety	Refuses to descend ramp. Shows significant signs of anxiety and fear (screaming, crying, refusing to participate in activity)	Descends ramp with someone's hand on shoulder (for security and sense of balance); person helping is walking alongside chair and providing verbal comfort and encouragement. Chair is on slow speed. There are some signs of anxiety and fear (verbalizing fear, asking for help, etc.)	Independently descends ramp on slow speed with little hesitancy (slight hesitation at top of ramp)	Independently descends ramp on slow speed with no hesitancy	Independently descends ramp on usual everyday speed with no hesitancy	–1	1

Unable to spend extended amounts of time at friends' homes or away from mother owing to bladder management routine	To be able to verbally instruct others in technique for intermittent catheterization with 100% accuracy	Unable to verbally describe the steps of self-catheterization	Is able to instruct others in technique for intermittent catheterization with 75% accuracy. Omits details about use of lubrication, hand washing, set-up, etc.	Is able to instruct others in technique for intermittent catheterization with 100% accuracy. Not able to physically assist with any aspect of activity	Is 100% accurate in verbal instruction for intermittent catheterization. Is able to assist with intermittent catheterization by helping guide insertion of catheter or removal of catheter. Assists with some clean-up. Physically participates in up to 25% of activity	Is 100% accurate in verbal instruction for intermittent catheterization. Is able to assist with intermittent catheterization by helping guide insertion of catheter or removal of catheter. Assists with some clean-up. Physically participates in up to 50% of activity	–1	0

A score of '0' reflects the projected performance that was expected at the completion of the 6-month out-patient therapy, whereas scores of –2 and +2 reflect much less and much more than the expected outcome, respectively.

work with children, the GRASSP may have utility in children once they are 6 years of age. GAS has demonstrated effectiveness in a variety of patient populations and would be an excellent tool to use with children with SCI. In the future, CAT will emerge as a primary method for child- and parent-reported outcomes. Regardless of the instrument used, particular attention must be paid to the child's cognitive development and ability; age range is one indicator. Additional work is needed to establish and evaluate instruments that measure motor recovery in children, wheeled mobility, upper limb function, activity performance, participation, and impact of pediatric SCI on carers and siblings.

Summary

This chapter provides an overview on instruments that may be useful in pediatric SCI rehabilitation. Prudence is recommended when selecting instruments, with particular consideration of psychometric properties, burden to the child and parent, and cost.

REFERENCES

Adair B, Said CM, Rodda J, Morris ME (2012) Psychometric properties of functional mobility tools in heredity spastic paraplegia and other childhood neurological conditions. *Dev Med Child Neurol* 54: 596–605. http://dx.doi.org/10.1111/j.1469-8749.2012.04284.x

Alexander M, Anderson K, Biering-Sørensen F et al (2009) Outcome measures in spinal cord injury. Recent assessment and recommendations for future directions. *Spinal Cord* 47: 582–91. http://dx.doi.org/10.1038/sc.2009.18

Alexander MS, Biering-Sørensen F, Elliott S, Kreuter M, Sønksen J (2011a) International spinal cord injury female sexual and reproductive function basic data set. *Spinal Cord* 49: 787–90. http://dx.doi.org/10.1038/sc.2011.7

Alexander MS, Biering-Sørensen F, Elliott S, Kreuter M, Sønksen J (2011b) International spinal cord injury male sexual function basic data set. *Spinal Cord* 49: 795–8. http://dx.doi.org/10.1038/sc.2010.192

Allen D, Mulcahey MJ, Haley SM et al (2009) Motor scores on the functional independence measure after pediatric spinal cord injury. *Spinal Cord* 47: 213–17. http://dx.doi.org/10.1038/sc.2008.94

American Spinal Injury Association (2011) *International Standards for the Neurologic Classification of Spinal Cord Injury Revised 2011* (booklet). Atlanta, GA: American Spinal Injury Association.

American Thoracic Society (2002) ATS Statement: Guideline for the Six-Minute Walk Test. *Am J Respir Crit Care Med* 166: 111–17. http://dx.doi.org/10.1164/ajrccm.166.1.at1102

Anderson K, Aito S, Atkins M et al; the Functional Recovery Outcome Measures Work Group (2008) Functional recovery measures for spinal cord injury: an evidence based review for clinical practice and research. *J Spinal Cord Med* 31: 133–44.

Anderson KD, Acuff ME, Arp BG et al (2011). United States (US) multicenter study to assess the validity and reliability of the spinal cord independence measure (SCIM-III). *Spinal Cord* 49: 880–5. http://dx.doi.org/10.1038/sc.2011.20

Bauman WA, Biering-Sørensen F, Krassioukov A (2011) The international spinal cord injury endocrine and metabolic function basic data set. *Spinal Cord* 49: 1068–72. http://dx.doi.org/10.1038/sc.2011.51

Behrman AL, Ardolino E, Vanhiel LR et al (2012) Assessment of functional improvement without compensation reduces variability of outcome measures after human spinal cord injury. *Arch Phys Med Rehabil* 93: 1518–29. http://dx.doi.org/10.1016/j.apmr.2011.04.027

Bent L, Mulcahey MJ, Kelly E et al (2013) Child- and parent- report computer-adaptive tests for assessing daily routines among youth with spinal cord injury. *Top Spinal Cord Inj Rehabil* 19: 104–13. http://dx.doi.org/10.1310/sci1902-104

Berry C, Kennedy P (2003) A psychometric analysis of the needs assessment checklist (NAC). *Spinal Cord* 41: 490–501. http://dx.doi.org/10.1038/sj.sc.3101460

Biering-Sørensen F, Charlifue S, DeVivo M et al (2006) International Spinal Cord Injury Data Sets. *Spinal Cord* 44: 530–4. http://dx.doi.org/10.1038/sj.sc.3101930

Biering-Sørensen F, Craggs M, Kennelly M, Schick E, Wyndaele JJ (2008a) International Lower Urinary Tract Function Basic Spinal Cord Injury Data Set. *Spinal Cord* 46: 325–30. http://dx.doi.org/10.1038/sj.sc.3102145

Biering-Sørensen F, Craggs M, Kennelly M, Schick E, Wyndaele JJ (2008b) International urodynamic basic spinal cord injury data set. *Spinal Cord* 46: 513–16. http://dx.doi.org/10.1038/sj.sc.3102174

Biering-Sørensen F, Craggs M, Kennelly M, Schick E, Wyndaele J-J (2009) International urinary tract imaging basic spinal cord injury data set. *Spinal Cord* 47: 379–83. http://dx.doi.org/10.1038/sc.2008.149.

Biering-Sørensen F, Charlifue S, Devivo MJ et al (2011a) Incorporation of the International Spinal Cord Injury Data Set elements into the National Institute of Neurological Disorders and Stroke Common Data Elements. *Spinal Cord* 49: 60–4. http://dx.doi.org/10.1038/sc.2010.90.

Biering-Sørensen F, Alexander MS, Burns S et al (2011b) Recommendations for translation and reliability testing of International Spinal Cord Injury Data Sets. *Spinal Cord* 49: 357–60. http://dx.doi.org/10.1038/sc.2010.153

Biering-Sørensen F, Krassioukov A, Alexander MS et al (2012a) International spinal cord injury pulmonary function basic data set. *Spinal Cord* 50: 418–21. http://dx.doi.org/10.1038/sc.2011.183

Biering-Sørensen F, Burns AS, Curt A et al (2012b) International spinal cord injury musculoskeletal basic data set. *Spinal Cord* 50: 797–802. http://dx.doi.org/10.1038/sc.2012.102

Biering-Sørensen F, Charlifue S, DeVivo MJ et al (2012c) Using the Spinal Cord Injury Common Data Elements. *Top Spinal Cord Inj Rehabil* 18: 23–7. http://dx.doi.org/10.1310/sci1801-23

Biering-Sørensen F, Bryden A, Curt A, Friden J, Harvey LA, Mulcahey MJ, Popovic MR, Prochazka A, Sinnott KA, Snoek G (2014) International spinal cord injury upper extremity basic data set. *Spinal Cord* [Epub ahead of print] doi: 10.1038/sc.2014.87

Bluvshtein V, Front L, Izkovich M et al (2011) SCIM III is reliable and valid in separate analysis for traumatic spinal cord lesions. *Spinal Cord* 49: 292–6. http://dx.doi.org/10.1038/sc.2010.111

Burns AS, Delparte JJ, Patrick M, Marino RJ, Ditunno JF (2011) The reproducibility and convergent validity of the walking index (WISCI) in chronic spinal cord injury. *Neurorehabil Neural Repair* 25: 149–57. http://dx.doi.org/10.1177/1545968310376756

Calhoun CL, Mulcahey MJ (2012) Pilot study of reliability and validity of the Walking Index for Spinal Cord Injury II (WISCI-II) in children and adolescents with spinal cord injury. *J Pediatr Rehabil Med* 5: 275–9. http://dx.doi.org/10.3233/PRM-2012-00224

Calhoun C, Chafetz R, Mulcahey MJ (2009a) A pilot study of observational motor assessment in infants and toddlers with spinal cord injury. *Pediatr Phys Ther* 21: 62–70. http://dx.doi.org/10.1097/PEP.0b013e31818f5bbd

Calhoun CL, Haley SM, Riley A, Vogel LC, McDonald CM, Mulcahey MJ (2009b) Development of items designed to evaluate activity performance and participation in children and adolescents with spinal cord injury. *Int J Pediatr* 2009: 854904. http://dx.doi.org/10.1155/2009/854904

Cardol M, de Haan RJ, de Jong BA, van den Bos GA, de Groot IJ (2001) Psychometric properties of the Impact on Participation and Autonomy Questionnaire. *Arch Phys Med Rehabil* 82: 210–16. http://dx.doi.org/10.1053/apmr.2001.18218

Catz A, Itzkovich M, Agranov E, Ring H, Tamir A (1997) SCIM – spinal cord independence measure: a new disability scale for patients with spinal cord lesions. *Spinal Cord* 35: 850–6. http://dx.doi.org/10.1038/sj.sc.3100504

Catz A, Itzkovich M, Tesio L et al (2007) A multicentre study on the spinal cord independence measure, version III: Rasch psychometric validation. *Spinal Cord* 45: 275–91. http://dx.doi.org/10.1038/sj.sc.3101960

Charlifue S, Post MW, Biering-Sørensen F et al (2012) International Spinal Cord Injury Quality of Life Basic Data Set. *Spinal Cord* 50: 672–5. http://dx.doi.org/10.1038/sc.2012.27

Choate R, Smith A, Cardillo JE, Thompson L (1981) Training in the use of goal attainment scaling. *Community Ment Health J* 17: 171–81. http://dx.doi.org/10.1007/BF00754364

Coates SK, Harvey LA, Dunlop SA, Allison GT (2011) The AUSpinal: a test of hand function for people with tetraplegia. *Spinal Cord* 49: 219–29. http://dx.doi.org/10.1038/sc.2010.86

Cohen JT, Marino RJ, Sacco P, Terrin N (2012) Association between the functional independence measure following spinal cord injury and long term outcomes. *Spinal Cord* 50: 728–33. doi: 10.1038/sc.2012.50

Cornwell AS, Liao JY, Bryden AM, Kirsch RF (2012) Standard task set for evaluating rehabilitation interventions for individuals with arm paralysis. *J Rehabil Res Dev* 49: 395–403. http://dx.doi.org/10.1682/JRRD.2011.03.0040

DeVivo M, Biering-Sørensen F, Charlifue S et al (2006) International Spinal Cord Injury Core Data Set. *Spinal Cord* 44: 535–40. http://dx.doi.org/10.1038/sj.sc.3101958

DeVivo MJ, Biering-Sørensen F, New P, Chen Y (2011) Standardization of data analysis and reporting of results from the International Spinal Cord Injury Core Data Set. *Spinal Cord* 49: 596–9. http://dx.doi.org/10.1038/sc.2010.172

Ditunno JF Jr, Ditunno PL, Graziani V et al (2000) Walking index for spinal cord injury (WISCI): an international multicenter validity and reliability study. *Spinal Cord* 38: 234–43. http://dx.doi.org/10.1038/sj.sc.3100993

Ditunno JF Jr, Barbeau H, Dobkin BH et al (2007) Validity of the walking scale for spinal cord injury and other domains of function in a multicenter clinical trial. *Neurorehabil Neural Repair* 21: 539–50. http://dx.doi.org/10.1177/1545968307301880

Dumas HM, Haley SM, Boyce ME, Peters CY, Mulcahey MJ (2009) Self-report measures of physical function for children with spinal cord injury: a review of current tools and an option for the future. *Dev Neurorehabil* 12: 113–18. http://dx.doi.org/10.1080/17518420902800936

Dvorak MF, Wing PC, Fehlings MG et al (2012) International spinal cord injury spinal column injury basic data set. *Spinal Cord* 50: 817–21. http://dx.doi.org/10.1038/sc.2012.60

Dvorak MF, Itshayek E, Fehlings MG, Vaccaro AR, Wing PC, Biering-Sorensen F, Noonan VK (in press) International spinal cord injury: spinal interventions and surgical procedures basic data set. *Spinal Cord.*

Evans JJ (2012) Goal attainment during rehabilitation early and late after acquired brain injury. *Curr Opin Neurol* 25: 651–5. http://dx.doi.org/10.1097/WCO.0b013e3283598f75

Fliess-Douer O, Vanlandewijck YC, Lubel Manor G, Van Der Woude LH (2010) A systematic review of wheelchair skills tests for manual wheelchair users with a spinal cord injury: towards a standardized outcome measure. *Clin Rehabil* 24: 867–86. http://dx.doi.org/10.1177/0269215510367981.

Fougeyrollas P, Noreau L, Bergeron H, Cloutier R, Dion SA, St Michel G (1998) Social consequences of long term impairments and disabilities: conceptual approach and assessment of handicap. *Int J Rehabil Res* 21: 127–41. http://dx.doi.org/10.1097/00004356-199806000-00002

Fox EJ, Tester NJ, Phadke CP et al (2010) Ongoing walking recovery 2 years after locomotor training in a child with severe incomplete spinal cord injury. *Phys Ther* 90: 793–802. http://dx.doi.org/10.3899/jrheum.110402

Fries J, Rose M, Krishnan E (2011) The PROMIS of better outcome assessment: responsiveness, floor and ceiling effects, and internet administration. *J Rheumatol* 38: 1759–64. doi: 10.3899/jrheum.110402

Furlan JC, Noonan V, Singh A, Fehlings MG (2011) Assessment of disability in patients with acute traumatic spinal cord injury: a systematic review of the literature. *J Neurotrauma* 28: 1413–30. http://dx.doi.org/10.1089/neu.2009.1148

Garcia RA, Gaebler-Spira D, Sisung C, Heinemann AW (2002) Functional improvement after pediatric spinal cord injury. *Am J Phys Med Rehabil* 81: 458–63. http://dx.doi.org/10.1097/00002060-200206000-00011

Goetz LL, Cardenas DD, Kennelly M et al (2013) International Spinal Cord Injury Urinary Tract Infection Basic Data Set. *Spinal Cord* 51: 700–4. http://dx.doi.org/10.1038/sc.2013.72

Gordon JE, Powell C, Rockwood K (1999) Goal attainment scaling as a measure of clinical important change in nursing home patients. *Age Ageing* 28: 275–81. http://dx.doi.org/10.1093/ageing/28.3.275

Gorton G, Watson K, Tucker C et al (2010) Precision and content range of a parent-reported item bank assessing lower extremity and mobility skills in children with cerebral palsy. *Dev Med Child Neurol* 52: 660–5. http://dx.doi.org/10.1111/j.1469-8749.2010.03615.x

Gorzkowski JA, Kelly EH, Klaas SJ, Vogel LC (2010) Girls with spinal cord injury: social and job-related participation and psychosocial outcomes. *Rehabil Psychol* 55: 58–67. http://dx.doi.org/10.1037/a0018275

Haley S, Chafetz RS, Tian R et al (2010) Validity and reliability of physical functioning computer adaptive tests for children with cerebral palsy. *J Pediatr Orthop* 30: 71–5. http://dx.doi.org/10.1097/BPO.0b013e3181c85453

Hall KM, Cohen ME, Wright J et al (1999) Characteristics of the functional independence measure in traumatic spinal cord injury. *Arch Phys Med Rehabil* 80: 1471–6. http://dx.doi.org/10.1016/S0003-9993(99)90260-5

Hall KM, Bushnik T, Lakisic-Kazazic B, Wright J, Cantagallo A (2001) Assessing traumatic brain injury outcome measures for long-term follow up of community-based individuals. *Arch Phys Med Rehabil* 82: 367–74. http://dx.doi.org/10.1053/apmr.2001.21525

Hamilton BB, Granger CV, Sherwin FS, Zielezny M, Tashman JS (1987) A uniform national data system for medical rehabilitation. In: Fuhrer MJ (ed.). *Rehabilitation Outcomes. Analysis and Measurement*. Baltimore, MD: Paul H. Brookes Publishing Co. pp. 137–47.

Heavlin WD, Lee-Merrow SW, Lewis VM (1982) The psychometric foundations of goal attainment scaling. *Community Ment Health J* 18: 230–41. http://dx.doi.org/10.1007/BF00754339

Hill MR, Noonan VK, Sakakibara BM, Miller WC; the SCIRE Research Team (2010) Quality of life instruments and definitions in individuals with spinal cord injury: a systematic review. *Spinal Cord* 48: 438–50. http://dx.doi.org/10.1038/sc.2009.164

Hoare B, Imms C, Villanueva E, Rawicki HB, Matyas T, Carey L (2012) Intensive therapy following upper limb botulinum toxin A injection in young children with unilateral cerebral palsy: a randomized trial. *Dev Med Child Neurol* 55: 238–47. http://dx.doi.org/10.1111/dmcn.12054

Hou WH, Shih CL, Chou YT et al (2012) Development of a computerized adaptive testing system of the Fugl-Meyer motor scale in stroke patients. *Arch Phys Med Rehabil* 93: 1014–20. http://dx.doi.org/10.1016/j.apmr.2011.12.005

Itzkovich M, Gelernter I, Biering-Sørensen F et al (2007) The spinal cord independence measure (SCIM) version III: reliability and validity in a multi-center international study. *Disability Rehabil* 29: 1926–33. http://dx.doi.org/10.1080/09638280601046302

Jackson AB, Camel CT, Ditunno JF et al (2008) Outcome measures for gait and ambulation in the spinal cord injury population. *J Spinal Cord Med* 31: 487–99.

Jebsen RH, Taylor N, Trieschmann RB, Trotter MH, Howard LA (1969) An objective and standardized test of hand function. *Arch Phys Med Rehabil* 50: 311–19.

Jette AM, Tulsky DS, Ni P et al (2012) Development and initial evaluation of the spinal cord injury- functional index. *Arch Phys Med Rehabil* 93: 1733–50. http://dx.doi.org/10.1016/j.apmr.2012.05.008

Johnston TE, Fison RL, Smith BT, Banarot DM, Betz RR, Mulcahey MJ (2003) Functional electrical stimulation for augmented walking in adolescents with incomplete spinal cord injury. *J Spinal Cord Med* 26: 390–400.

Kalsi-Ryan S, Curt A, Fehlings MG, Verrier MC (2009) Assessment of the hand in tetraplegia using the graded Redefined Assessment of Strength, Sensibility and Prehension (GRASSP): impairment versus function. *Top Spinal Cord Rehabil* 14: 34–46. http://dx.doi.org/10.1310/sci1404-34

Kalsi-Ryan S, Curt A, Verrier MC, Fehlings MG (2012a) Development of the Graded Redefined Assessment of Strength, Sensibility and Prehension (GRASSP): reviewing measurement specific to the upper limb in tetraplegia. *J Neurosurg Spine* 17(Suppl 1): S65–76. http://dx.doi.org/10.3171/2012.6.AOSPINE1258

Kalsi-Ryan S, Beaton D, Curt S et al (2012b) The Graded Redefined Assessment of Strength, Sensibility and Prehension (GRASSP): reliability and validity. *J Neurotrauma* 29. 905–14. http://dx.doi.org/10.1089/neu.2010.1504

Karlsson AK, Krassioukov A, Alexander MS, Donovan W, Biering-Sørensen F (2012) International spinal cord injury skin and thermoregulation function basic data set. *Spinal Cord* 50: 512–16. http://dx.doi.org/10.1038/sc.2011.167

Kennedy P, Hamilton LR (1999) The needs assessment checklist: a clinical approach to measuring outcome. *Spinal Cord* 37: 136–9. http://dx.doi.org/10.1038/sj.sc.3100745

King GA, Law M, King S et al (2006) Measuring children's participation in recreation and leisure activities: construct validation of the CAPE and PAC. *Child Care Health Dev* 33: 28–39. http://dx.doi.org/10.1111/j.1365-2214.2006.00613.x

Kirby RL (2011) Survey of wheelchair skills tests: making the case for broadening the search and assessment criteria. *Clin Rehabil* 25: 287. doi: 10.1177/0269215510380833

Kirby RL, Swuste J, Dupuis DJ, MacLeod DA, Monroe R (2002) The Wheelchair Skills Test: a pilot study of a new outcome measure. *Arch Phys Med Rehabil* 83: 10–18. http://dx.doi.org/10.1053/apmr.2002.26823

Kiresuk T, Smith A, Cardillo J (eds) (1994) Goal attainment scaling: applications, theory and measurement. London: Erlbaum.

Kirisci L, Tarter R, Reynolds M et al (2012) Computer adaptive testing of liability to addiction: identify individuals at risk. *Drug Alcohol Depend* 123(Suppl 1): S79–86. http://dx.doi.org/10.1016/j.drugalcdep.2012.01.016

Kirshblum SC, Burns SP, Biering-Sørensen F et al (2011) International standards for neurological classification of spinal cord injury (revised 2011). *J Spinal Cord Med* 34: 535–46. http://dx.doi.org/10.1179/204577211X13207446293695

Klaas SJ, Kelly EH, Gorzkowski J, Homko E, Vogel LC (2010) Assessing patterns of participation and enjoyment in children with spinal cord injury. *Dev Med Child Neurol* 52: 468–74. http://dx.doi.org/10.1111/j.1469-8749.2009.03552.x

Krassioukov A, Alexander MS, Karlsson AK, Donovan W, Mathias CJ, Biering-Sørensen F (2010) International spinal cord injury cardiovascular function basic data set. *Spinal Cord* 48: 586–90. http://dx.doi.org/10.1038/sc.2009.190

Krogh K, Perkash I, Stiens SA, Biering-Sørensen F (2009a) International bowel function basic spinal cord injury data set. *Spinal Cord* 47: 230–4. http://dx.doi.org/10.1038/sc.2008.102

Krogh K, Perkash I, Stiens SA, Biering-Sørensen F (2009b) International bowel function extended spinal cord injury data set. *Spinal Cord* 47: 235–41. http://dx.doi.org/10.1038/sc.2008.103

Lee BB, Cripps RA, Woodman RJ (2010) Development of an international spinal injury prevention module: application of the international classification of external cause of injury to spinal cord injury. *Spinal Cord* 48: 498–503. http://dx.doi.org/10.1038/sc.2009.168

Lewis AB, Spencer JH, Haas GL, DiVittis A (1987) Goal attainment scaling. Relevance and replicability in follow up inpatients. *J Nerv Ment Dis* 175: 408–18. http://dx.doi.org/10.1097/00005053-198707000-00004

Mackie PC, Jessen EC, Jarvis SN (1998) The lifestyle assessment questionnaire: an instrument to measure the impact of disability on the lives of children with cerebral palsy and their families. *Child Care Health Dev* 24: 473–86. http://dx.doi.org/10.1046/j.1365-2214.1998.00083.x

Magasi S, Post MW (2010) A comparative review of contemporary participation measures' psychometric properties and content coverage. *Arch Phys Med Rehabil* 91(Suppl 1): S17–28. http://dx.doi.org/10.1016/j.apmr.2010.07.011

Magasi S, Heinemann A, Whiteneck GG (2008) Participation following traumatic spinal cord injury: an evidence-based review of research. *J Spinal Cord Med* 31: 145–56.

Mailloux Z, May-Benson TA, Summers CA et al (2007) Goal attainment scaling as a measure of meaningful outcomes for children with sensory integration disorders. *Am J Occup Ther* 61: 254–9. http://dx.doi.org/10.5014/ajot.61.2.254

Marino RJ, Scivoletto G, Patrick M et al (2010) Walking index for spinal cord injury version 2 (WISCI-II) with repeatability of the 10-m walk time: inter- and intrarater reliabilities. *Am J Phys Med Rehabil* 89: 7–15. http://dx.doi.org/10.1097/PHM.0b013e3181c560eb

Marino RJ, Patrick M, Albrieght W et al (2012) Development of an objective test of upper limb function in tetraplegia: the capabilities of the upper extremity test. *Am J Phys Med Rehabil* 91: 478–86. http://dx.doi.org/10.1097/PHM.0b013e31824fa6cc

Mathias S, Nayak USL, Isaacs B (1986) Balance in the elderly patient: the 'Get-Up and Go' test. *Arch Phys Med Rehabil* 67: 387–9.

Mayson TA, Ward VJ, Harris SR (2012) Parent goals as outcome measures for child receiving treadmill training: a series of case reports. *Dev Neurorehabil* 15: 219–22. http://dx.doi.org/10.3109/17518423.2011.654282

Middleton JW, Harvey LA, Batty J, Cameron I, Quirk R, Winstanley J (2006) Five additional mobility and locomotor items to improve responsiveness of the FIM in wheelchair-dependent individuals with spinal cord injury. *Spinal Cord* 44: 495–504. http://dx.doi.org/10.1038/sj.sc.3101872

Miller WC, Garden J, Mortenson WB (2011) Measurement properties of the wheelchair outcome measure in individuals with spinal cord injury. *Spinal Cord* 49: 995–1000. http://dx.doi.org/10.1038/sc.2011.45

Mohamed F, Hunter L, Barakat N et al (2011) Diffusion tensor imaging of the pediatric spinal cord at 1.5 T: preliminary results. *Am J Neuroradiol* 32: 339–45. http://dx.doi.org/10.3174/ajnr.A2334

Montepetit K, Haley SM, Bilodeau N, Gorton G, Mulcahey MJ (2011) Content range and precision of a computer adaptive test of upper extremity function for children with CP. *Phys Occup Ther Pediatr* 31: 90–102. http://dx.doi.org/10.3109/01942638.2010.523449

Msall ME, DiGaudio K, Rogers BT et al (1994) The functional independence measure for children (WeeFIM). Conceptual basis and pilot use in children with disabilities. *Clin Pediatr* 33: 421–30.

Mulcahey MJ, Smith BT, Betz RR, Weiss AA (1995) Outcomes of tendon transfer surgery and occupational therapy in a child with tetraplegia secondary to spinal cord injury. *Am J Occup Ther* 49: 607–17. http://dx.doi.org/10.5014/ajot.49.7.607

Mulcahey MJ, Betz RR, Smith BT, Weiss AA (1999) A prospective study of the outcomes of tendon transfers with children with tetraplegia. *J Pediatr Orthop* 19: 319–28. http://dx.doi.org/10.1097/00004694-199905000-00008

Mulcahey MJ, Smith BT, Betz RR (2004) Psychometric rigor of the Grasp and Release Test for measuring functional limitation of persons with tetraplegia: a preliminary analysis. *J Spinal Cord Med* 27: 41–6.

Mulcahey MJ, Hutchinson D, Kozin S (2007) Assessment of the upper limb in tetraplegia: considerations in evaluation and outcomes research. *J Rehabil Res Dev* 44: 91–102. http://dx.doi.org/10.1682/JRRD.2005.10.0167

Mulcahey MJ, Calhoun C, Riley A, Haley S (2009) Children's reports of activity and participation after sustaining spinal cord injury: a cognitive interviewing study. *Dev Neurorehabil* 12: 191–200. http://dx.doi.org/10.1080/17518420902998177

Mulcahey MJ, Vogel L, Betz R, Samdani A, Chafetz R, Gaughan J (2011) The international standards for neurological classification of spinal cord injury: psychometric evaluation and guidelines for use with children and youth. *Phys Med Rehabil* 92: 1264–9. http://dx.doi.org/10.1016/j.apmr.2011.03.003

Mulcahey, MJ, Calhoun C, Tian F, Ni P, Vogel L, Haley S (2012a) Evaluation of newly developed item banks for child reported outcomes of participation following spinal cord injury. *Spinal Cord* 50: 915–19. doi: 10.1038/sc.2012.80

Mulcahey MJ, Calhoun CC, Tian F, Vogel L, Haley SM (2012b) Validity of the newly developed computer adaptive tests of mobility, activity and participation. *Topics in Spinal Cord Injury Rehab* 18(Suppl 1): 227.

Mulcahey, MJ, Samdani AF, Gaughan JP et al (2012c) Diffusion tensor imaging in pediatric spinal cord injury: preliminary examination of reliability and clinical correlation. *Spine* 37: 1–7. http://dx.doi.org/10.1097/BRS.0b013e3182470a08

Mulcahey MJ, Samdani AF, Gaughan JP et al (2013) Diagnostic accuracy of diffusion tensor imaging for pediatric cervical cord. *Spinal Cord* 51: 532–7. doi: 10.1038/sc.2013.36

New P, Marshall R (2014) International Spinal Cord Injury Data Sets for non-traumatic spinal cord injury. *Spinal Cord* 52: 123–32. doi: 10.1038/sc.2012.160

Noonan VK, Miller WC, Noreau L; SCIRE Research Team (2009) A review of instruments assessing participation in persons with spinal cord injury. *Spinal Cord* 47: 435–46. doi: 10.1038/sc.2008.171

Noreau L, Lepage C, Boissiere L et al (2007) Measuring participation in children with disabilities using the assessment of life habits. *Dev Med Child Neurol* 49: 666–71. http://dx.doi.org/10.1111/j.1469-8749.2007.00666.x

Oladeji O, Johnston T, Smith B, Mulcahey MJ, Betz RR, Lauer R (2007) Quality of life in children with spinal cord injury. *Phys Ther* 19: 296–300. http://dx/doi.org/10.1097/PEP.0b013e31815a12ef

Patrick JH (2003) Case for gait analysis as part of the management of incomplete spinal cord injury. *Spinal Cord* 41: 479–82. http://dx.doi.org/10.1038/sj.sc.3101524

Poncumhak P, Saengsuwan J, Kamruecha W, Amatachaya S (2013) Reliability and validity of three functional tests in ambulatory patients with spinal cord injury. *Spinal Cord* 51: 214–17. doi: 10.1038/sc.2012.126

Post MWM, van Lieshout F, Seelen HAM, Snoek GJ, IJzerman MJ, Pons C (2006) Measurement properties of the short version of the Van Lieshout test for arm/hand function of persons with tetraplegia after spinal cord injury. *Spinal Cord* 44: 763–71. http://dx.doi.org/10.1038/sj.sc.3101937

Prosser LA (2007) Locomotor training within an inpatient rehabilitation program after pediatric incomplete spinal cord injury. *Phys Ther* 87: 1224–32. http://dx.doi.org/10.2522/ptj.20060252

Rebollo P, Castejon I, Cuervo J et al (2010) Validation of a computer-adaptive test to evaluate generic health-related quality of life. *Health Qual Life Outcomes* 8: 147. doi:10.1186/1477-7525-8-147

Riis V, Jagial S, Boschen K, Verrier M (2011) Can administrative claim file review be used to gather physical therapy, occupational therapy and psychology payment data and functional independence measure scores? Implications for rehabilitation providers in the private health sector. *Physiother Can* 63: 324–33. http://dx.doi.org/10.3138/ptc.2010-25

Rockwood K, Stolee P, Fox RA (1993) Use of goal attainment scaling in measuring clinical important change in the frail elderly. *J Clin Epidemiol* 46: 1113–18. http://dx.doi.org/10.1016/0895-4356(93)90110-M

Routhier F, Vincent C, Desrosiers J, Nadeau S (2003) Mobility of wheelchair users: a proposed performance assessment framework. *Disabil Rehabil* 25: 19–34. http://dx.doi.org/10.1080/713813431

Rudhe C, van Hedel H (2009) Upper extremity function in persons with tetraplegia: relationships between strength, capacity and the SCIM. *Neurorehabil Neural Repair* 23: 413–21. http://dx.doi.org/10.1177/1545968308331143

Rushton PW, Miller WC, Kirby RL, Eng JJ (2012) Measure for assessment of confidence with manual wheelchair use (WheelCon-M) version 2.1: reliability and validity. *J Rehabil Med* 46: 61–7. http://dx.doi.org/10.2340/16501977-1069

Samdani A, Chafetz RS, Vogel LC, Betz RR, Gaughan JP, Mulcahey MJ (2011) The international standards for neurological classification of spinal cord injury: relationship between S4–5 dermatome testing and anorectal testing. *Spinal Cord* 49: 352–6. http://dx.doi.org/10.1038/sc.2010.144

Schaaf RC, Hunt J, Benevides T (2012) Occupational therapy using sensory integration to improve participation of a child with autism: a case report. *Am J Occup Ther* 66: 547–55. http://dx.doi.org/10.5014/ajot.2012.004473

Schlosser RW (2004) Goal attainment scaling as a clinical measurement technique in communication disorders: a critical review. *J Commun Disord* 37: 217–39. http://dx.doi.org/10.1016/j.jcomdis.2003.09.003

Smith PA, Hassani S, Reiners K, Vogel LC, Harris GF (2004) Gait analysis in children and adolescents with spinal cord injury. *J Spinal Cord Med* 27(Suppl 1): S44–9.

Smits N, Zitman FG, Cuijpers P et al (2012) A proof of principle for using adaptive testing for routines outcome monitoring: the efficiency of the Mood and Anxiety Symptoms Questionnaire – Anhedonic Depression CAT. *BMC Med Res Methodol* 12: 4. doi:10.1186/1471-2288-12-4

Spooren AI, Janssen-Potten YJ, Post MW, Kerckhofs E, Nene A, Seelen HA (2006) Measuring change in arm hand skilled performance in persons with a cervical spinal cord injury: responsiveness of the Van Lieshout Test. *Spinal Cord* 44: 772–9. http://dx.doi.org/10.1038/sj.sc.3101957

Staas WE, Formal CS, Freedman MK, Fried GW, Schmidt Read ME (1998) Spinal cord injury and spinal cord injury medicine. In: DeLisa JA, Gans BM (eds). *Rehabilitation Medicine: Principles and Practice*. 3rd Ed. Philadelphia, PA: Lippincott-Raven.

Steenbeek D, Ketelaar M, Galama K, Gorter JW (2007) Goal attainment scaling in pediatric rehabilitation: a critical review of the literature. *Dev Med Child Neurol* 49: 550–6. http://dx.doi.org/10.1111/j.1469-8749.2007.00550.x

Stroh Wuolle K, Van Doren CL, Thorpe GB, Keith MW, Peckham PH (1994) Development of quantitative hand grasp and release test for patients with tetraplegia using a hand neuroprosthesis. *J Hand Surg* 19: 209–18. http://dx.doi.org/10.1016/0363-5023(94)90008-6

Tian F, Ni P, Mulcahey MJ, Hambleton RK, Tulsky D, Haley SM, Jette AM (2014) Tracking functional status across the spinal cord injury lifespan: linking pediatric and adult patient reported outcome scores. *Arch Phys Med Rehabil* [Epub ahead of print]. doi: 10.1016/j.apmr.2014.05.023

Turner-Bowker DM, DeRosa MA, Saris-Baglama RN, Bjorner JB (2012) Development of a computerized adaptive test to assess health related quality of life in adults with asthma. *J Asthma* 49: 190–200. http://dx.doi.org/10.3109/02770903.2011.633674

van Hedel HJ, Wirz M, Dietz V (2005) Assessing walking ability in subjects with spinal cord injury: validity and reliability of 3 walking tests. *Arch Phys Med Rehabil* 86: 190–6. http://dx.doi.org/10.1016/j.apmr.2004.02.010

van Hedel HJA, Wirz M, Curt A (2006) Improving walking assessment in subjects with incomplete spinal cord injury: responsiveness. *Spinal Cord* 44: 352–6. http://dx.doi.org/10.1038/sj.sc.3101853

van Hedel HJ, Dietz V; European Multicenter Study on Human Spinal Cord Injury (EM-SCI) Study Group (2009) Walking during daily life can be validly and responsively assessed in subjects with spinal cord injury. *Neurorehabil Neural Repair* 23: 117–24. http://dx.doi.org/10.1177/1545968308320640

Vogel L, Samdani A, Chafetz R, Gaughan J, Betz RR, Mulcahey MJ (2009) Intra-rater reliability of the anorectal examination and classification of injury severity in children with spinal cord injury. *Spinal Cord* 47: 687–91. http://dx.doi.org/10.1038/sc.2008.180

Webster G, Kennedy P (2007) Addressing children's needs and evaluating rehabilitation outcomes after spinal cord injury: the Child Needs Assessment Checklist and goal planning program. *J Spinal Cord Med* 30(Suppl 1): S140–5.

Whiteneck GG, Charlifue SW, Gerhat KA, Overholser JD, Richardson GN (1992) Quantifying handicap: a new measure of long-term rehabilitation outcomes. *Arch Phys Med Rehabil* 73: 519–26.

Widerström-Noga E, Biering-Sørensen F, Bryce T et al (2008) The International Spinal Cord Injury Pain Basic Data Set. *Spinal Cord* 46: 818–23. http://dx.doi.org/10.1038/sc.2008.64

Widerström-Noga E, Biering-Sørensen F, Bryce TN, Cardenas DD, Finnerup NB, Jensen MP, Richards JS, Siddall PJ (2014) The International Spinal Cord Injury Pain Basic Data Set (version 2.0). *Spinal Cord* 52: 282–6. doi: 10.1038/sc.2014.4

Young NL, Williams JI, Yoshida KK, Wright JG (2000) Measurement properties of the activities scale for kids. *J Clin Epidemiol* 53: 125–37. http://dx.doi.org/10.1016/S0895-4356(99)00113-4

Zidek K, Srinivasan R (2003) Rehabilitation of a child with a spinal cord injury. *Semin Pediatr Neurol* 10: 140–50. http://dx.doi.org/10.1016/S1071-9091(03)00022-6

Section 2 Early Management of Spinal Cord Injury

5
PATHOPHYSIOLOGY OF SPINAL CORD INJURY

Shuyan Chen, Michael E Selzer and Amer F Samdani

Introduction

Each year, 12 to 58 persons per million population sustain a spinal cord injury (SCI), depending on the country (van den Berg et al 2010). Because it is so sensitive to trauma, the spinal cord is ordinarily protected by a strong, boney spine. Even a mild concussive injury can sometimes give rise to severe neural destruction. The reasons for this extreme sensitivity are not completely understood. Moreover, it is not known whether the sensitivity to trauma and the underlying mechanisms in pediatric SCI are different from those in adult SCI. Thus, most of this chapter will be based on pathophysiological data from adult humans and adult animals.

Human spinal cord injury pathology

If an injury is severe enough, a hemorrhagic lesion is formed that eventually includes a large cystic cavity surrounded by a fibrotic capsule. Similarly, laceration injuries produce open scar-lined lesions. This chapter will focus on more graded, contusive injuries, which involve impact without laceration or persistent compression, in which cellular mechanisms that lead to physical interruption of nerve fibers (axotomy) and secondary neuronal death can be studied. In general, the pathologic processes following SCI are divided into two events: the primary injury and the secondary injury. Norenberg et al (2004) divided the histologic changes in SCI into four phases: immediate (first 1–2h after injury), acute (2h–2d), intermediate (days to weeks), and late (weeks to years). We will summarize these phases, but will not go into detail about the histopathology here.

Immediate and Acute Spinal Cord Injury

Immediately after SCI, pathology is limited to the anatomical disruption owing to direct contact of the cord with either a causative projectile or the spinal canal. This can include hemorrhage, surface contusion, tissue laceration with axon tract interruption, and neuronal maceration. In the immediate and acute phases after a concussive SCI, the cord may appear relatively normally on magnetic resonance imaging (MRI). However, often by the time the patient is studied (usually in the acute phase), MRI changes may include edema, swelling, and even hemorrhage in the central gray matter. This is seen also in children (Dare et al 2002). Even if conventional MRI is normal, edema may be detected as an increased signal on diffusion-weighted imaging. However, during the first 1 to 2 hours, routine histology may be normal, consistent with the modern understanding that the ultimate pathology is a consequence of secondary injury. How this evolves into a large cystic scar (Fig. 5.1) is very complex. Shortly after SCI, systemic effects may make a contribution. Often there is reflexive hypotension and bradycardia and a condition called 'neurogenic shock', which can cause underperfusion of tissues, including the already injured cord. Exactly how the pathologic changes occur is not clear, but it is reasonable to assume that at least a major part of the secondary injury is the result of these systemic processes. From 2 hours to 2 days (the acute phase), the cord shows progressive changes secondary to a vicious cycle of vascular damage and inflammation. Leaky blood vessels give rise to vasogenic edema. This causes compression of those same venules and arterioles, which causes microhemorrhages, mainly in the central gray matter (central hemorrhagic necrosis). The extravasated blood gives rise to inflammation, primarily by neutrophils, which in humans is relatively mild and lasts only about 3 days. The hypoxia and inflammation can cause neuronal swelling (cytotoxic edema), early myelin breakdown, and neuronal death. There are two broad categories of cell death: necrosis and apoptosis (Lipton 1999). Necrosis is the familiar process whereby cells that are physically or chemically damaged by infection, toxins, trauma, or other environmental factors lose the integrity of their surface membranes and membrane-bound internal organelles such as mitochondria, at first swelling and then discharging their contents into the cytoplasm and extracellular space. Necrosis can be considered a mostly passive process, in which energy is dissipated and not adequate to repair the damaged cell. The cellular debris triggers a local inflammatory reaction, which can be seen by the appearance of white blood cells and macrophages in the affected area. In contrast, apoptosis is a process of programmed cell death, in

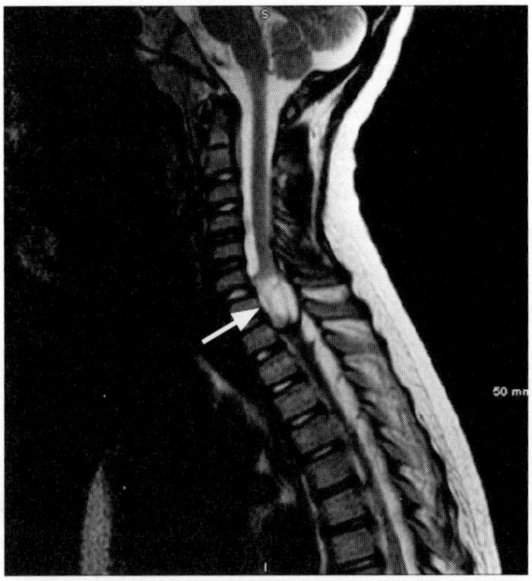

Fig. 5.1 Cyst formation after spinal cord injury. Sagittal T2-weighted cervical spine magnetic resonance image in an 11-year-old male who had sustained a low cervical spinal cord injury from a motor vehicle crash 5 years previously. His injury is now C8 American Spinal Injury Association Impairment Scale (AIS) grade A. This is consistent with the magnetic resonance image, which demonstrates a large cystic cavity (arrow) posterior to the C7 and T1 vertebral bodies.

which a stereotyped sequence of biochemical events, of which caspase enzymatic proteolysis cascades are the hallmark, results in orderly degradation of DNA and its neat packaging into membrane-bound nuclear fragments. The dying cell shrinks, does not discharge its contents into the extracellular space, and does not trigger inflammation. Apoptosis is an active, energy-requiring process and is often constructive, for example in the naturally occurring reduction in the number of motor neurons during embryonic development. During the acute phase, neuronal death occurs primarily by necrosis with eosinophilia. Although animal research suggests extensive apoptosis of neurons and glia, including oligodendrocytes (Beattie et al 2000), this has not been observed in human SCI (Kakulas 1999). Thus, the human literature has not included descriptions of the large-scale primary demyelination (as opposed to loss of myelin secondary to axon degeneration), as was described in acute SCI in animals. Like neuronal death, secondary loss of oligodendrocytes is mostly by necrosis, but apoptosis has also been seen in animals (Li et al 1996) and humans (Emery et al 1998). As in animals, injured axons develop swellings along their length and at their severed tips (retraction bulbs). These are filled with cytoskeletal elements such as neurofilaments, but they also stain for amyloid precursor protein (Norenberg et al 2004).

Intermediate Phase of Spinal Cord Injury

Beginning around 2 to 3 days, microglial cells become reactive, meaning they swell and begin to clear degenerative debris. Macrophages from the blood invade the spinal cord and become the predominant reactive monocytes. The role of these cells as promoters and inhibitors of neuronal survival, axon regeneration, and sprouting has been studied mostly in animals and will be discussed below, but their most obvious function is phagocytosis. The intermediate phase is also characterized by reactive gliosis (i.e. astrocytes proliferate, enlarge, and become filled with glial fibrillary acidic protein). This begins several days after the injury (Eddleston and Mucke 1993). Initially, these reactive astrocytes secrete a variety of trophic factors that probably help protect the remaining spinal cord tissue and may promote axon repair and plasticity (White and Jakeman 2008), but over the next 2 to 3 weeks they form a glial scar that lines the injured tissue. Although the scar helps to maintain the integrity of the spinal cord, it also acts as a barrier to axon regeneration, but the density of the glial scar is overestimated. It is believed that reactive astrocytes secrete chondroitin sulfate proteoglycans, which are increasingly viewed as major inhibitors of axon growth (Sharma et al 2012), but it is not clear to what degree the astrocytic elements themselves and the density of the glial scar contribute to the regeneration barrier.

Beginning 7 to 10 days after injury, new capillaries invade the injured spinal cord. These are leaky at first, but as they mature, a blood–spinal cord barrier is gradually reformed. There is debate about whether the re-establishment of microvasculature is a limiting factor in the ability of spinal cord axons to regenerate and restore connectivity across the injury. This is important because, if it were true, it would imply that an important approach to restoring functional connectivity after SCI is to increase the rate and magnitude of new capillary formation in the lesion. It is logical that axons might not be able to grow into areas that lack a sufficient blood supply to nourish them. Indeed, after SCI in rats, new capillaries invaded the zone of injury in advance of axons, which appeared in close apposition to the new capillaries at the edges of the lesion (Loy et al 2002). Although axons invade the injury area, they do not grow very far. On the other hand, normal central nervous system (CNS) capillaries have anatomic and molecular features that form a blood–brain/spinal cord barrier, and this reflects the need to protect the neurons from some blood constituents while promoting the transport of vital nutrients such as glucose. However, the new capillaries that form within the injured spinal cord are derived from angiogenic epithelial cells of meningeal origin and do not form a blood–CNS barrier. Instead, they are fenestrated, like peripheral capillaries, and mostly lack the GLUT-1 glucose transporter characteristic of CNS capillaries (Whetstone et al 2003).

Chronic Spinal Cord Injury

After the first few weeks, the injury site is invaded by fibroblasts and collagen. These are the main elements that cause the scar to become hard. Most people assume that the scar at the site of injury is composed mainly of astrocytes (i.e. the non-neuronal cells [glial cells]), referring to the 'astrocytic' or 'glial' scar, but this is not true. Although the astrocytes at the injury do undergo some proliferation and swelling, they form a relatively thin layer of cells lining the normal spinal cord. Unlike the astrocytic scar, which seems to have both trophic and inhibitory effects on axon regeneration, it is the mesenchymal elements of the scar (fibroblasts, collagen, etc., derived from tissues outside the CNS) that impart most of its dense mechanical properties and thus far appear to act only as physical barriers to re-establishing connectivity after SCI. Moreover, as necrotic tissue is cleared, the area of injury develops cystic cavities filled with cerebrospinal fluid and monocytic inflammatory cells (macrophages). Sometimes these cysts behave as though they are under pressure, becoming larger over time. These are called 'syrinxes' and may cause clinical worsening. The cause of syrinx development is not known, but the cavity may be in contact with the central canal, allowing accumulation of additional cerebrospinal fluid, and often the spinal cord is tethered by fibrous connective tissue to the surrounding spine. The only effective treatment is surgical drainage, and often the tethered cord is freed (Klekamp 2012), but no specific surgical approach has been shown to be superior to any other.

Another peculiar pathologic feature of many SCIs is the proliferation of Schwann cells and axons that entered the spinal cord from the nerve roots, particularly with a penetrating injury. The condition has been termed 'schwannosis' and it was seen in autopsies of 82% of patients who had survived more than 4 years after SCI (Bruce et al 2000). It is not clear whether schwannosis contributes to the delayed clinical deterioration seen in some patients (i.e. whether some patients experience further neurologic damage and disability owing to the mass effect produced by the proliferating Schwann cells and axons within the injured spinal cord).

Molecular pathophysiology of spinal cord injury: knowledge from animal studies

The basic pathologic features seen in human SCI have been observed in animal models, especially rats, although the animal literature does not fall neatly into Nordenberg stages for humans, which were described more recently. The two most commonly used models involve dorsal overhemisection and spinal cord contusion. Dorsal overhemisection is used because it interrupts the main corticospinal projection of rodents in the base of the dorsal columns and thus provides a controlled way to assess a discrete spinal cord projection that is important to motor function. The contusion model, although anatomically messier, is used to try to reproduce the mechanisms of the most common form of SCI in human patients and because it induces secondary mechanisms of neuronal injury that probably also occur in other forms of spinal cord injury (e.g. infarctions, traction, torsion). Other models, such as traction injury, have also been used, but these are not addressed here. In any model of traumatic SCI, mechanical forces applied at the site of the primary injury induce rupture of neuronal and endothelial cell membranes and axon tracts at the moment of the impact. This rupture of blood vessels and neurons creates a hemorrhagic zone of necrosis at and around the initial impact site. The reduction of blood flow and the disturbed membrane function cause ischemia and edema, further contributing to the necrosis. The initial direct tissue damage initiates a second phase of progressive tissue degeneration, which may take place over a period of weeks or even months. Over minutes to weeks, the lesion first spreads radially and rostrocaudally through the gray matter, then expands horizontally in the white matter. The proximal ends of damaged axons retract, while, distal to the injury, the axons undergo Wallerian degeneration. In the epicenter of the lesion, a cavity that is filled with fluid and necrotic debris of neurons and glial cells is formed. The cavity is surrounded by a glial scar, which is composed of reactive astrocytes, microglia, fibroblasts, and their depositions of extracellular matrix. Although the glial scar can prevent the further expansion of the lesion, as indicated above, this inhibitory environment also acts as a physical and, in particular, a chemical barrier to preclude the growth or repair of axon pathways. The overall expansion of tissue destruction from these secondary processes exacerbates the functional deficits caused by the initial impact. It is noteworthy here that many mouse strains have much less prominent excitotoxic secondary neural injury and scar formation after SCI than do other species, such as rats and humans, and these differences cannot be ascribed to size alone (Inman and Steward 2003). This is especially important because of the increasing tendency to use mice instead of rats to take advantage of the genetic tools available in mice. Nevertheless, SCI in mice leads to permanent paralysis, just as it does in rats and humans, although the quality of behavioral measures of SCI for mice is still primitive compared with those for rats.

Multiple molecular events (i.e. phospholipids breakdown, cytokine/chemokines production, lytic enzymes, reactive oxygen species [Fig. 5.2]) and cellular processes (excitotoxicity, microglia/macrophage activation, astrocyte reaction, leukocyte recruitment) can influence each other reciprocally and are responsible for most of the secondary damage that occurs in the vicinity of the lesion (Beattie 2004).

Cellular Inflammatory Responses Following Spinal Cord Contusion

The neuroinflammatory responses are complex processes with the involvement of both peripheral blood-derived cells and glial cells from the spinal cord parenchyma (Donnelly and Popovich 2008). Immediately after blood vessel damage, platelets arriving at the lesion site secrete lytic enzymes such as phospholipase A2 enzymes (Zucker and Nachmias 1985). By 3 hours after onset, as the blood–brain barrier is compromised, neutrophils and monocytes

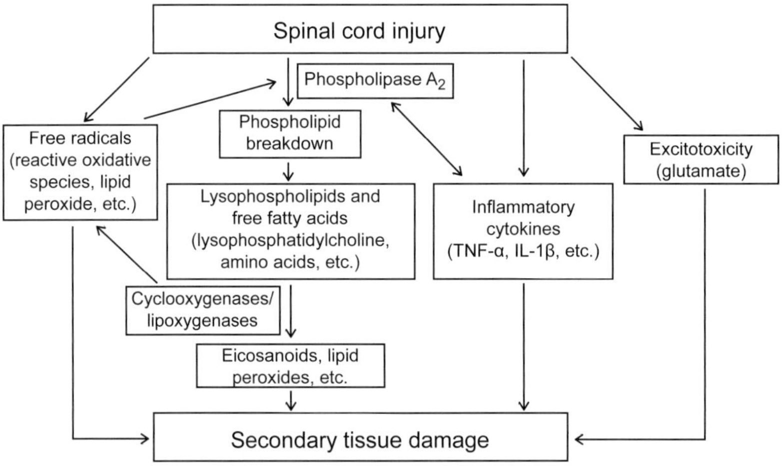

Fig. 5.2 Schematic molecular pathophysiology of spinal cord injury. The primary spinal cord injury initiates multiple molecular events including free radicals accumulation (such as reactive oxidative species), excitotoxicity (glutamate accumulation), elevation of the levels of inflammatory cytokines (such as TNF-α, IL-β), and phospholipids breakdown. The breakdown of phospholipids is elaborated here as an example of the complexity of those molecular pathways. The insult to the spinal cord leads to the hydrolysis of phospholipids, giving rise to lysophospholipids and free fatty acids. Arachidonic acid, the most prominent fatty acid, is then metabolized by cyclooxygenases (COX) and lipoxygenases (LOX) into a group of inflammatory mediators called eicosanoids. Moreover, these molecular events can influence each other reciprocally. For example, inflammatory cytokines interact with astrocytes, microglia, and macrophages and induce reactive oxidative species, adhesion molecules, cytokines, phospholipase enzymes, and eicosanoids in these cell types. Together, these molecular pathways are responsible for most of the secondary damage including the propagation of neuroinflammation and cell death.

extravasate out of the blood vessels into the CNS. At the same time, resident microglia and astrocytes from the spinal cord parenchyma are also activated. Invading macrophages replace the neutrophils after 2 to 3 days, whereas the lymphocytes enter the injury site after 1 week. The high level of activated microglia, macrophages, and astrocytes persist for weeks or even months (Donnelly and Popovich 2008). It appears that the principal function of the neutrophils and monocytes is the destruction of foreign organisms and the removal of degenerating debris. However, as part of this response, a plethora of cytokines, proteases, and reactive oxidative species are produced that can kill non-degenerating bystander cells and axons of passage and thereby exacerbate the functional deficits produced by the injury (Kury et al 2005).

Mediators of the inflammatory cascade therefore represent promising targets for pharmaceutical intervention. Indeed, a number of anti-inflammation strategies to deplete or neutralize neutrophils and macrophages, or to inhibit their functions, have provided consistent neuroprotection and improved neurologic recovery in experimental models (Iannotti et al 2011). In clinical work, the possible beneficial effects of the steroid methylprednisolone as a treatment for acute SCI may be partly the result of the suppression of inflammation near the site of injury (Chvatal et al 2008).

Toxins and Toxic Mediators

Reactive oxidative species such as superoxide (O_2^-), hydroxyl radical (•OH), and reactive nitrogen species are generated in all tissue injury, whether in the CNS or the periphery, as a consequence of insufficient blood supply and reperfusion of the damaged area (Lipton 1999) and affect all cell types, including the oligodendrocytes that produce myelin.

The other major source of toxicity following SCI is elevated extracellular glutamate levels. The glutamate released during synaptic transmission is cleared rapidly and is primarily taken up by astrocytes via active transport, so toxic levels usually do not accumulate. After SCI, glutamate is elevated to toxic levels, and expression of some (but not all) glutamate receptors is increased (Mills et al 2001). Excessive glutamate excitation results in cell death, probably owing to an accumulation of intracellular calcium.

Cytokines as Molecular Mediators of Inflammation

In spinal cord contusion models, the expression of the proinflammatory cytokines tumor necrosis factor α (TNF-α), interleukin 1β (IL-1β), and interleukin 6 (IL-6) from resident neurons, microglia, and astrocytes increases within 1 hour after severe injuries, and levels remain elevated for up to 2 days. The extent of secondary damage following SCI may partly depend on how the expression of different cytokines is balanced after the lesion. Indeed, the manipulation of cytokines was found to alter the inflammatory responses following SCI (Bethea et al 1999).

Lipids and Related Enzymes as Mediators of Inflammation

The hydrolysis of membrane glycerophospholipids and the generation of free fatty acids are among the first pathologic events that follow primary trauma to the spinal cord (Demediuk et al 1985, Girod et al 2011). Excessive hydrolysis of membrane phospholipids can lead to the alteration of membrane function, which can eventually lead to the functional failure of the membrane and necrotic cell death (Farooqui et al 2007).

Effects of growth-inhibitory molecules in preventing axon regeneration after spinal cord injury

Myelin-associated Growth Inhibitors

It has long been known that the ability of axons to regenerate is very different in the peripheral nervous system (PNS) and CNS. Whereas axons in the PNS can regenerate fairly long distances (in the order of centimeters), axons in the postnatal CNS cannot grow more than a few hundred micrometers. Insights into the causes of this difference were first suggested by Tello and Cajal and, in modern times, developed by Aguayo and colleagues, who discovered that injured CNS axons could grow for long distances into grafts of peripheral nerve (Richardson et al 1980). This suggested that the environment of the CNS might contain factors that inhibit axon growth and thus might account for the inability of axons to regenerate. Since then, it has been discovered that CNS myelin, but not PNS myelin, contains molecules that are inhibitory to axon growth in tissue culture. The most potent of these is Nogo-A (Chen et al 2000). Nogo binds to a receptor, NgR, which is complexed to two other receptors, one of which, P75, transmits the inhibitory signal across the neuronal membrane and activates the small GTPase

Rho-A (Yamashita and Tohyama 2003). Rho-A activates Rho kinase (ROCK), which in turn activates multiple intraneuronal reactions leading to growth cone collapse and inhibition of axon growth. Many studies that relied on neutralizing myelin-associated growth inhibitors (Schnell and Schwab 1990) or NgR (Lee et al 2004) have reported increased axon growth both proximal to and beyond the lesion, as well as enhanced functional recovery. This is true also for studies in which Nogo (Simonen et al 2003) or NgR (Kim et al 2004) have been knocked down in mutant mice. However, although these procedures enhanced collateral sprouting of spared axons, it is not clear to what degree true regeneration was enhanced in injured fibers, and most investigators now doubt that corticospinal tract axons regenerated.

Chondroitin Sulfate Proteoglycans

Another family of molecules that has been implicated in blocking axon regeneration in the CNS is the chondroitin sulfate proteoglycans (CSPGs) (Snow et al 1990). These molecules are secreted by both neurons and glia and are normally present in the extracellular matrix that surrounds many neurons (perineuronal nets) (Hartig et al 1994). CSPGs are secreted at the site of CNS injury and form part of the scar. Enzymatic digestion of CSPGs' sugar moieties has led to increased axon growth and enhanced functional recovery in partial injury models of SCI (Bradbury et al 2002, Fouad et al 2005, Houle et al 2006). As with the neutralization of myelin-associated growth inhibitors, the anatomical complexities of the mammalian CNS have made it difficult to know whether this axon growth represents true axon regeneration or only collateral sprouting by spared axons (see next paragraph).

Enhancing the cell-autonomous regenerative ability of neurons

Why Neurons Differ in their Regenerative Abilities

Although extracellular environmental cues may contribute to limiting axon growth after SCI, it is now clear that, during development, neurons undergo a reduction in their intrinsic regenerative abilities (Cai et al 2001, Goldberg et al 2002). Even within the same animal, different types of neurons appear to differ greatly in their intrinsic regenerative abilities. Corticospinal neurons appear to be especially poor regenerators, although their axons do undergo collateral sprouting (i.e. uninjured axons sprout collateral branches over short distances to innervate neurons that had lost their original innervation owing to the degeneration of the neighboring injured fibers).

Increasing a Cell's Intrinsic Regenerative Ability by Activating its Protein Synthesis Pathway

Cells respond to a variety of environmental stimuli, such as exposure to trophic factors, certain cytokines, and insulin, by activating an anabolic pathway. Central to this pathway is the activated form of the signaling molecule mammalian target of rapamycin (mTOR) (Fig. 5.3). The intrinsic ability of neurons to regenerate their axons has been enhanced in mice by conditional knockdown of the tumor suppressor gene phosphatase and tensin homolog (PTEN) in retinal ganglion cells, resulting in increased mTOR activity and improved regeneration of optic nerve fibers after optic nerve crush (Park et al 2008). Similarly, conditional knockdown of PTEN in

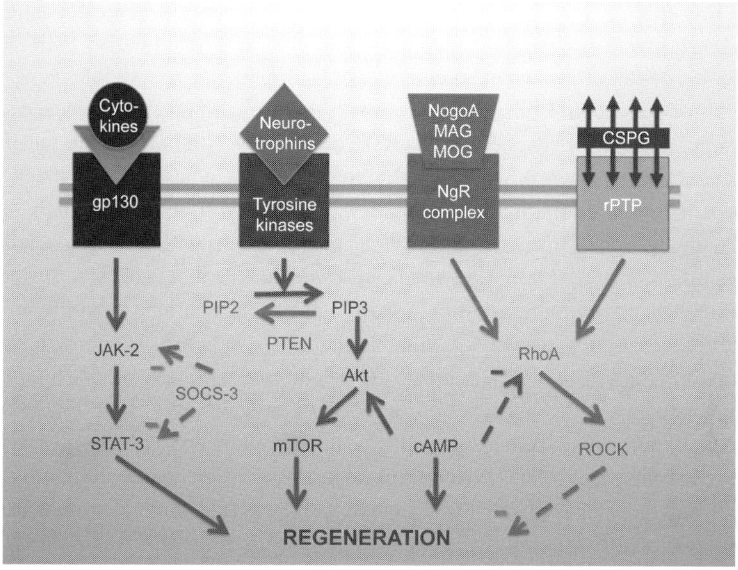

Fig. 5.3 Regeneration is controlled by parallel signaling pathways. Many environmental factors influence axon regeneration by binding to receptors on the neuronal surface. These receptors activate cascades of signaling molecules that link the receptors to downstream effects (e.g. gene activation via transcription factors). Growth-promoting cytokines of the interleukin-6 family bind to the gp130 receptor via specific linking receptors. This phosphorylates JAK-2, which activates the transcription factor STAT-3, triggering regeneration-promoting gene transcription. The JAK/STAT pathway is inhibited by SOCS 3. Thus, levels of SOCS-3 could be considered a neuron-intrinsic property that negatively influences the regenerative ability of neurons. Neurotrophins bind to receptor tyrosine kinases and activate inosine-3-phosphatase, which catalyzes the conversion of phosphatidylinositol (4,5)-biphosphate (PIP2) to phosphatidylinositol (3,4,5)-triphosphate (PIP3). This activates Akt (also called protein kinase B), which eventually leads to activation of mTOR, a key switch that promotes regeneration by activating protein synthesis. Phosphatase and tensin homolog (PTEN) converts PIP3 to PIP2, leading to reduced mTOR activation. Thus, levels of PTEN could be considered a neuron-intrinsic property that negatively influences the regenerative ability of neurons. The myelin-associated molecules NogoA, MAG, and MOG all bind to the Nogo receptor NgR, which, through complexing with the transmembrane receptors p75 and LINGO, activate the small GTPase RhoA, which, by activating Rho kinase (ROCK), leads to both short-term cytoskeletal breakdown and longer term transcriptional changes that inhibit regeneration. Similarly, chondroitin sulfate proteoglycans (CSPGs) bind to receptor protein tyrosine kinases (rPTP) and activate RhoA by unknown mechanisms. Activated rPTPs also inactivate Akt (not shown) by unknown mechanisms. Like activated rPTP, cAMP both inhibits RhoA activity and enhances activation of Akt. cAMP also activates the transcription factor cAMP response element-binding protein and thereby activates genes that promote regeneration. Thus, levels of cAMP could be considered a neuron-intrinsic property that positively influences the regenerative ability of neurons. A color version of this figure is available in the color plate section.

corticospinal tract neurons resulted in enhanced regeneration (or sprouting) of corticospinal axons and functional recovery after SCI (Liu et al 2010). Unfortunately, because mTOR activity also leads to cell proliferation, PTEN knockdown carries the risk of tumorigenesis. It is possible that manipulation of mTOR activity will be a means to enhance regeneration if a way can be found to dissociate the effect on protein synthesis from the effect on cell proliferation.

Stem cell therapies

In recent years, great hope has been placed on stem cells as a treatment for SCI. Despite the transplantation of stem cells and other cells cultured from human tissues into the spinal cords of thousands of patients in China and elsewhere, there is no convincing evidence so far that these therapies have had a beneficial effect (Harrop et al 2012). This does not mean that they will never work, and it is worthwhile considering why this field has drawn so much attention. The concept of a stem cell implies two properties: (1) it can proliferate indefinitely to generate new cells with identical properties; and (2) it can generate cells with more restricted potential fates (more differentiated). Embryonic stem cells have the potential to become any cell type in the body (i.e. they are pluripotent). After birth, groups of cells continue to proliferate, but they have more restricted fates, depending on their locations. These are called 'adult stem cells'. Those located in the CNS are called 'neural stem cells' and these can be induced to differentiate in vitro into any of the cell types of the CNS: neurons, astrocytes, or oligodendrocytes (Cao and Whittemore 2012). Stem-like cells that have become committed to a particular type of cell (e.g. neurons) are called 'progenitors'. Thus, there are neuronal progenitors and glial progenitors, and these can be further restricted in their fates (e.g. motor neuronal progenitors) before they stop proliferating. It was once thought that stages in differentiation are irreversible, but, in recent years, it has been possible to use molecular manipulations to generate less differentiated cells from more differentiated ones. Thus, even pluripotent embryonic stem-like cells (induced pluripotent stem cells) have been generated from adult somatic cells, such as mouse and human fibroblasts (Takahashi et al 2007). This was hailed as a major breakthrough because it provided a way to derive stem cells from a person's own somatic cells and avoided any ethical and religious concerns regarding the use of human embryos to derive stem cells.

Stem cells and other transplantable cells have several potential benefits in treating SCI. The most obvious benefit is being able to replace neurons that have been lost at the level of injury, owing to the direct impact of trauma or to secondary neuronal injury. This has been difficult to achieve because stem cells do not differentiate into neurons in the spinal cord. Consequently, the cells must be partially differentiated into neuronal precursors ex vivo, and then transplanted. Incorporation of the resulting neurons into electrophysiologically active synaptic relays has been reported (Bonner et al 2011, Lu et al 2012). A second benefit is that the cells can provide a supportive environment for neuroprotection or for injured axons to grow through. For example, mesenchymal stem cells derived from bone marrow have been transplanted into the spinal cord (Samdani et al 2009) and have been reported to enhance functional recovery, even if they do not become neurons or glial cells (Osaka et al 2010). Third, the cells can secrete trophic factors constitutively or be genetically engineered to deliver trophic factors and other growth-promoting molecules to protect neurons from axotomy-induced death and encourage axons to grow (Himes et al 2001, Sasaki et al 2009). Fourth, the cells can be used to replace lost astrocytes (Lepore et al 2006), which might have important trophic support functions. Fifth, they can replace killed oligodendrocytes to myelinate regenerated axons or remyelinate spared axons that have been demyelinated (reviewed in Cao and Whittemore [2012]). Despite the hopeful science, functional recovery in mammalian models of stem cell transplantation has not been truly impressive, and evidence for clinical improvement attributable to cell-based therapy is primitive. Most investigators agree that combination therapies will be required and that stem cell therapy still has a long way to go to prove its clinical value in SCI.

Summary

Spinal cord injury causes severe impairments because of complex cascading secondary neurodegenerative events associated with vascular reactions, excitotoxicity, neurotoxic cytokine release by macrophages/microglia, calcium-mediated activation of proteases and lipases, and generation of reactive oxygen species. At the same time, some of the cytokines released are growth promoting. A challenge for SCI research is to differentially suppress the neurotoxic signaling while enhancing the growth-promoting signaling. Moreover, we do not have effective methods of neuroprotection, and if we are to restore function to the large number of spinal cord-injured persons who are severely disabled, it will be necessary to promote axon regeneration and restoration of proper synaptic pathways. In part, this may involve neutralizing the growth-inhibitory molecules associated with CNS myelin and the matrix molecules secreted by injured neurons. However, although neutralizing NgR ligands and CSPGs have increased axon growth and promoted functional recovery in animals, it is not clear whether this was the result of collateral sprouting or true axon regeneration. Because some therapies appear to enhance sprouting but not regeneration by the same axons (e.g. corticospinal tract axons), it would seem that there are significant differences between these two processes. This would be especially important in treating patients with complete SCI (American Spinal Injury Association Impairment Scale [AIS] A) because there may be few, if any, spared axons to undergo compensatory sprouting. Therapeutic approaches that enhance the cell-autonomous regenerative abilities of neurons (e.g. by increasing cAMP, mTOR, or STAT-3 signaling) may also have important roles to play. However, no individual therapeutic intervention has thus far produced sufficiently robust regeneration to achieve sufficient functional recovery. Therefore, increasingly, combination therapies are being tried. Finally, almost all the information described above is based on studies of neurons (mostly embryonic, but in the case of dorsal root ganglia and retinal ganglion cells also postnatal) in culture or of adult rodents in vivo. More studies of neonatal and young animals are needed to determine if there are important differences in mechanisms that would suggest different therapeutic approaches for pediatric SCI. The very small sizes of young rodents and the fragility of their neural tissues make many experimental procedures difficult. A piglet model of SCI has been developed recently (Kuluz et al 2010), but it has not yet been exploited to elucidate basic pathophysiological mechanisms in the immature mammalian spinal cord.

REFERENCES

Beattie MS (2004) Inflammation and apoptosis: linked therapeutic targets in spinal cord injury. *Trends Mol Med* 10: 580–3. doi: 10.1016/j.molmed.2004.10.006

Beattie MS, Farooqui AA, Bresnahan JC (2000) Review of current evidence for apoptosis after spinal cord injury. *J Neurotrauma* 17: 915–25. doi: 10.1089/neu.2000.17.915

Bethea JR, Nagashima H, Acosta MC et al (1999) Systemically administered interleukin-10 reduces tumor necrosis factor-alpha production and significantly improves functional recovery following traumatic spinal cord injury in rats. *J Neurotrauma* 16: 851–63. http://dx.doi.org/10.1089/neu.1999.16.851

Bonner JF, Connors TM, Silverman WF, Kowalski DP, Lemay MA, Fischer I (2011) Grafted neural progenitors integrate and restore synaptic connectivity across the injured spinal cord. *J Neurosci* 31: 4675–86. http://dx.doi.org/10.1523/JNEUROSCI.4130-10.2011

Bradbury EJ, Moon LD, Popat RJ et al (2002) Chondroitinase ABC, promotes functional recovery after spinal cord injury. *Nature* 416: 636–40. doi: 10.1038/416636a

Bruce JH, Norenberg MD, Kraydieh S, Puckett W, Marcillo A, Dietrich D (2000) Schwannosis: role of gliosis and proteoglycan in human spinal cord injury. *J Neurotrauma* 17: 781–8. doi: 10.1089/neu.2000.17.781

Cai D, Qiu J, Cao Z, McAtee M, Bregman BS, Filbin MT (2001) Neuronal cyclic AMP, controls the developmental loss in ability of axons to regenerate. *J Neurosci* 21: 4731–9.

Cao Q, Whittemore SR (2012) Cell transplantation: stem cells and precursor cells. *Handb Clin Neurol* 109: 551–61. doi: 10.1177/1545968307308550

Chen MS, Huber AB, van der Haar ME et al (2000) Nogo-A, is a myelin-associated neurite outgrowth inhibitor and an antigen for monoclonal antibody IN-1. *Nature* 403: 434–9. http://dx.doi.org/10.1038/35000219

Chvatal SA, Kim YT, Bratt-Leal AM, Lee H, Bellamkonda RV (2008) Spatial distribution and acute anti-inflammatory effects of Methylprednisolone after sustained local delivery to the contused spinal cord. *Biomaterials* 29: 1967–75. doi: 10.1016/j.biomaterials.2008.01.002

Dare AO, Dias MS, Li V (2002) Magnetic resonance imaging correlation in pediatric spinal cord injury without radiographic abnormality. *J Neurosurg* 97(Suppl 1): 33–9. doi: 10.3171/spi.2002.97.1.0033

Demediuk P, Saunders RD, Anderson DK, Means ED, Horrocks LA (1985) Membrane lipid changes in laminectomized and traumatized cat spinal cord. *Proc Natl Acad Sci USA* 82: 7071–5. doi: 10.1073/pnas.82.20.7071

Donnelly DJ, Popovich PG (2008) Inflammation and its role in neuroprotection axonal regeneration and functional recovery after spinal cord injury. *Exp Neurol* 209: 378–88. doi: 10.1016/j.expneurol.2007.06.009

Eddleston M, Mucke L (1993) Molecular profile of reactive astrocytes--implications for their role in neurologic disease. *Neuroscience* 54: 15–36. doi: 10.1016/0306-4522(93)90380-X

Emery E, Aldana P, Bunge MB et al (1998) Apoptosis after traumatic human spinal cord injury. *J Neurosurg* 89: 911–20. doi: 10.3171/jns.1998.89.6.0911

Farooqui AA, Horrocks LA, Farooqui T (2007) Modulation of inflammation in brain: a matter of fat. *J Neurochem* 101: 577–99. doi: 10.1111/j.1471-4159.2006.04371.x

Fouad K, Schnell L, Bunge MB, Schwab ME, Liebscher T, Pearse DD (2005) Combining Schwann cell bridges and olfactory-ensheathing glia grafts with chondroitinase promotes locomotor recovery after complete transection of the spinal cord. *J Neurosci* 25: 1169–78. http://dx.doi.org/10.1523/JNEUROSCI.3562-04.2005

Girod M, Shi Y, Cheng JX, Cooks RG (2011) Mapping lipid alterations in traumatically injured rat spinal cord by desorption electrospray ionization imaging mass spectrometry. *Anal Chem* 83: 207–15. doi: 10.1021/ac102264z

Goldberg JL, Klassen MP, Hua Y, Barres BA (2002) Amacrine-signaled loss of intrinsic axon growth ability by retinal ganglion cells. *Science* 296: 1860–4. doi: 10.1126/science.1068428

Harrop JS, Hashimoto R, Norvell D et al (2012) Evaluation of clinical experience using cell-based therapies in patients with spinal cord injury: a systematic review. *J Neurosurg Spine* 17(Suppl 1): 230–46. doi: 10.3171/2012.5.AOSPINE12115

Hartig W, Brauer K, Bigl V, Bruckner G (1994) Chondroitin sulfate proteoglycan-immunoreactivity of lectin-labeled perineuronal nets around parvalbumin-containing neurons. *Brain Res* 635: 307–11. http://dx.doi.org/10.1016/0006-8993(94)91452-4

Himes BT, Liu Y, Solowska JM, Snyder EY, Fischer I, Tessler A (2001) Transplants of cells genetically modified to express neurotrophin-3 rescue axotomized Clarke's nucleus neurons after spinal cord hemisection in adult rats. *J Neurosci Res* 65: 549–64. http://dx.doi.org/10.1002/jnr.1185

Houle JD, Tom VJ, Mayes D, Wagoner G, Phillips N, Silver J (2006) Combining an autologous peripheral nervous system 'bridge' and matrix modification by chondroitinase allows robust functional regeneration beyond a hemisection lesion of the adult rat spinal cord. *J Neurosci* 26: 7405–15. http://dx.doi.org/10.1523/JNEUROSCI.1166-06.2006

Iannotti CA, Clark M, Horn KP, van Rooijen N, Silver J, Steinmetz MP (2011) A, combination immunomodulatory treatment promotes neuroprotection and locomotor recovery after contusion SCI. *Exp Neurol* 230: 3–15. doi: 10.1016/j.expneurol.2010.03.010

Inman DM, Steward O (2003) Physical size does not determine the unique histopathological response seen in the injured mouse spinal cord. *J Neurotrauma* 20: 33–42. doi: 10.1089/08977150360517164

Kakulas BA (1999) A review of the neuropathology of human spinal cord injury with emphasis on special features. *J Spinal Cord Med* 22: 119–24.

Kim JE, Liu BP, Park JH, Strittmatter SM (2004) Nogo-66 receptor prevents raphespinal and rubrospinal axon regeneration and limits functional recovery from spinal cord injury. *Neuron* 44: 439–51. doi: 10.1016/j.neuron.2004.10.015

Klekamp J (2012) Treatment of posttraumatic syringomyelia. *J Neurosurg Spine* 17: 199–211. doi: 10.3171/(2012)5.SPINE1(1904)

Kuluz J, Samdani A, Benglis D et al (2010) Pediatric spinal cord injury in infant piglets: description of a new large animal model and review of the literature. *J Spinal Cord Med* 33: 43–57.

Kury P, Zickler P, Stoll G, Hartung HP, Jander S (2005) Osteopontin a macrophage-derived matricellular glycoprotein inhibits axon outgrowth. *FASEB J* 19: 398–400. doi: 10.1096/fj.04-1777fje

Lee JK, Kim JE, Sivula M, Strittmatter SM (2004) Nogo receptor antagonism promotes stroke recovery by enhancing axonal plasticity. *J Neurosci* 24: 6209–17. doi: 10.1523/JNEUROSCI.1643-04.2004

Lepore AC, Neuhuber B, Connors TM et al (2006) Long-term fate of neural precursor cells following transplantation into developing and adult CNS. *Neuroscience* 142: 287–304. http://dx.doi.org/10.1016/j.neuroscience.2005.12.067

Li GL, Brodin G, Farooque M et al (1996) Apoptosis and expression of Bcl-2 after compression trauma to rat spinal cord. *J Neuropathol Exp Neurol* 55: 280–9. http://dx.doi.org/10.1097/00005072-199603000-00003

Lipton P (1999) Ischemic cell death in brain neurons. *Physiol Rev* 79: 1431–568.

Liu K, Lu Y, Lee JK et al (2010) PTEN, deletion enhances the regenerative ability of adult corticospinal neurons. *Nature Neurosci* 13: 1075–81. doi: 10.1038/nn.2603

Loy DN, Crawford CH, Darnall JB, Burke DA, Onifer SM, Whittemore SR (2002) Temporal progression of angiogenesis and basal lamina deposition after contusive spinal cord injury in the adult rat. *J Comp Neurol* 445: 308–24. doi: 10.1002/cne.10168

Lu P, Wang Y, Graham L et al (2012) Long-distance growth and connectivity of neural stem cells after severe spinal cord injury. *Cell* 150: 1264–73. http://dx.doi.org/10.1016/j.cell.2012.08.020

Mills CD, Fullwood SD, Hulsebosch CE (2001) Changes in metabotropic glutamate receptor expression following spinal cord injury. *Exp Neurol* 170: 244–57. doi: 10.1006/exnr.2001.7721

Norenberg MD, Smith J, Marcillo A (2004) The pathology of human spinal cord injury: defining the problems. *J Neurotrauma* 21: 429–40. doi: 10.1089/089771504323004575

Osaka M, Honmou O, Murakami T et al (2010) Intravenous administration of mesenchymal stem cells derived from bone marrow after contusive spinal cord injury improves functional outcome. *Brain Res* 1343: 226–35. http://dx.doi.org/10.1016/j.brainres.2010.05.011

Park KK, Liu K, Hu Y et al (2008) Promoting axon regeneration in the adult CNS by modulation of the PTEN/mTOR pathway. *Science* 322: 963–66. doi: 10.1126/science.1161566

Richardson PM, McGuinness UM, Aguayo AJ (1980) Axons from CNS neurons regenerate into PNS grafts. *Nature* 284: 264–5. doi: 10.1038/284264a0

Samdani AF, Paul C, Betz RR, Fischer I, Neuhuber B (2009) Transplantation of human marrow stromal cells and mono-nuclear bone marrow cells into the injured spinal cord: a comparative study. *Spine* 34: 2605–12. http://dx.doi.org/10.1097/BRS.0b013e3181bdca87

Sasaki M, Radtke C, Tan AM et al (2009) BDNF,-hypersecreting human mesenchymal stem cells promote functional recovery axonal sprouting and protection of corticospinal neurons after spinal cord injury. *J Neurosci* 29: 14932–41. http://dx.doi.org/10.1523/JNEUROSCI.2769-09.2009

Schnell L, Schwab ME (1990) Axonal regeneration in the rat spinal cord produced by an antibody against myelin-associated neurite growth inhibitors. *Nature* 343: 269–72. doi: 10.1038/343269a0

Sharma K, Selzer ME, Li S (2012) Scar-mediated inhibition and CSPG receptors in the CNS. *Exp Neurol* 237: 370–8. doi: 10.1016/j.expneurol.2012.07.009

Simonen M, Pedersen V, Weinmann O et al (2003) Systemic deletion of the myelin-associated outgrowth inhibitor Nogo-A improves regenerative and plastic responses after spinal cord injury. *Neuron* 38: 201–11. doi: 10.1016/S0896-6273(03)00226-5

Snow DM, Lemmon V, Carrino DA, Caplan AI, Silver J (1990) Sulfated proteoglycans in astroglial barriers inhibit neurite outgrowth in vitro. *Exp Neurol* 109: 111–30. doi: 10.1016/S0014-4886(05)80013-5

Takahashi K, Tanabe K, Ohnuki M et al (2007) Induction of pluripotent stem cells from adult human fibroblasts by defined factors. *Cell* 131: 861–72. http://dx.doi.org/10.1016/j.cell.2007.11.019

van den Berg ME, Castellote JM, Mahillo-Fernandez I, de Pedro-Cuesta J (2010) Incidence of spinal cord injury worldwide: a systematic review. *Neuroepidemiology* 34: 184–92; discussion 192. doi: 10.1159/000279335

Whetstone WD, Hsu JY, Eisenberg M, Werb Z, Noble-Haeusslein LJ (2003) Blood-spinal cord barrier after spinal cord injury: relation to revascularization and wound healing. *J Neurosci Res* 74: 227–39. doi: 10.1002/jnr.10759

White RE, Jakeman LB (2008) Don't fence me in: harnessing the beneficial roles of astrocytes for spinal cord repair. *Restor Neurol Neurosci* 26: 197–214.

Yamashita T, Tohyama M (2003) The p75 receptor acts as a displacement factor that releases Rho from Rho-GDI. *Nature Neurosci* 6: 461–7. doi: 10.1083/jcb.200202010

Zucker MB, Nachmias VT (1985) Platelet activation. *Arteriosclerosis* 5: 2–18. doi: 10.1161/01.ATV.5.1.2

6 ACUTE MANAGEMENT OF YOUNG PEOPLE WITH SPINAL CORD INJURY

John Kuluz

Case vignette

A 3-year-old male was admitted to the pediatric intensive care unit (PICU) after sustaining an acute cervical spinal cord injury from a fall. He was intubated in the trauma center because of hypoventilation. Computed tomography of the brain and spine were normal, and magnetic resonance imaging showed long segment swelling of the spinal cord from C2 to T4 without evidence of hemorrhage or ligamentous injury. He was immobilized with a Miami J collar. On admission he had hypotension and sinus bradycardia, which were managed with fluids and dopamine for the first 5 days. He was given high-dose methylprednisolone for 24 hours and stomach prophylaxis with ranitidine. Anticoagulation was not given. Nutrition was begun via nasogastric tube. Four days after admission his examination showed no sensory or motor function below C4. A Foley catheter was placed for urinary drainage and was removed after 1 week, after which intermittent catheterizations were conducted every 4 hours. The bowel program consisted of stool softeners and bisacodyl suppository every other day. Skin care included turning every 2 hours and close monitoring for pressure-related injuries. The child and his family were provided with pediatric psychology, social work, child life and speech, occupational, and physical therapy while in the PICU.

He had spontaneous respirations, and bilateral hemidiaphragm motion was demonstrated on fluoroscopy 1 week after injury, so sedation was reduced and weaning from mechanical ventilation was attempted. This was complicated by recurrent respiratory distress and atelectasis requiring increased ventilator settings. After several unsuccessful weaning attempts over 3 to 4 weeks, a tracheostomy was performed for chronic ventilator support. After 6 weeks in the PICU, he was transferred to the pediatric rehabilitation unit in a stable condition on a moderate level of ventilator support.

Introduction

Acute management of young people with new-onset spinal cord injury (SCI) is focused primarily on preventing secondary injury to the damaged and surrounding at-risk spinal cord. This management begins in the pre-hospital setting and extends along the continuum of care through trauma resuscitation, the operating room (in the event that surgical intervention is required), and the pediatric intensive care unit.

The respiratory and cardiovascular systems are the systems most commonly affected, and problems in these systems may be life threatening. Other associated traumatic injuries such as brain, pulmonary, cardiac, and abdominal injuries and long-bone fractures can intensify the challenges of caring for young people with SCI, especially in the first few weeks after injury. Achieving the best outcome for the child with an SCI requires an interprofessional team with input from pediatric trauma surgery, neurosurgery, orthopedics, critical care, physiatry, otolaryngology, pulmonology, gastroenterology, urology, psychology, nutrition, nursing, social work, speech and language pathology, and physical and occupational therapy. In this chapter, we review the issues that are most urgent to address in the first hours to days after acute SCI in young people. Other chapters of this book cover additional important acute care topics, such as assessment (Chapter 4), spine stabilization (Chapter 7), ventilator dependency (Chapter 9), bowel and bladder management (Chapter 11), autonomic dysfunctions (Chapter 13), medical complications (Chapter 14), and the skin (Chapter 15).

Pre-hospital care

Optimal pre-hospital care of young people with SCI requires that appropriate guidelines be developed and maintained through regional and state trauma systems regarding the evaluation, management, and transport of young people with SCI to trauma centers with the necessary resources to care for these children. Immobilization of the entire spine of all young people with the potential for SCI should be established by emergency medical service technicians at the injury scene and maintained until arrival at the trauma center. This is accomplished with the combination of a rigid cervical collar and supportive blocks on a backboard with straps to secure the entire spine. The method of immobilization must be suitable for the age and size of the child to maintain the spine in a neutral alignment. This is especially important in infants and toddlers because of their relatively large occiput, which tends to force the neck into flexion if placed flat on a rigid adult backboard; therefore, the back should be elevated relative to the occiput in young children to allow for occipital recess owing to their larger head size. This can be done simply with blankets or cushions on the backboard beneath the young person's trunk (Fig. 6.1a–d) (Herzenberg et al 1989).

Pre-hospital care should also ensure airway patency, adequate ventilation, oxygenation, and blood pressure. Supplemental oxygen and intravenous fluids should be started, and either invasive or non-invasive ventilation used for patients with hypercapnea or hypoxemia unresponsive to supplemental oxygen.

Imaging of young people with suspected spinal cord injury

The choice of imaging methods for cervical spine clearance has generated considerable debate (Hutchings and Willett 2009, Chung et al 2011, Easter et al 2011). For awake, cooperative patients without neck pain or neurologic deficits, a thorough history and physical examination is sufficient to clear the cervical spine (Viccellio et al 2001) (see Chapter 7, Box 7.1). In young people who are non-conversant, intoxicated, or have neck pain, altered mental status, neurologic deficits, midline tenderness, or a history of distracting injury, most protocols recommend

(a)

(b)

(c)

(d)

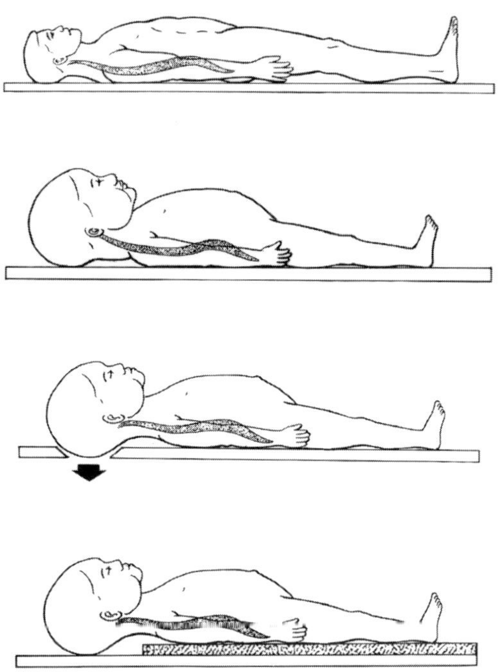

Fig. 6.1 Emergency transport and positioning of young children who have an injury of the cervical spine. The standard backboard may be hazardous. (a) Adult immobilized on a standard backboard. (b) Young child on a standard backboard; the relatively large head results in a kyphotic position of the neck. In (c), the child is on a modified backboard with a cut-out to recess the occiput, providing safe cervical positioning. In (d) the double mattress pad raises the chest, providing safe cervical positioning. Reproduced with permission from Herzenberg JK, Hensinger RN, Dedrick DK et al (1989) *J Bone Joint Surg* 71A: 15–22.

anteroposterior and lateral radiographs to assess the cervical spine from the skull base to T1. Cervical spine computed tomography is not generally recommended as first-line imaging, owing to concerns about radiation exposure in young people, and should be reserved for cases in which greater detail is needed in cases of suspected occult fractures or when plain films are inadequate. There are concerns about using computed tomography alone to clear the cervical spine, owing to its poor ability to assess soft tissues (Gebauer et al 2012), although some studies support this practice (Panczykowski et al 2011). The cervical spine should not be cleared for instability until dynamic flexion–extension radiographs are obtained. Flexion–extension radiographs should not be performed until the adolescent is stabilized from other injuries and should be performed under direct physician supervision. Finally, magnetic resonance imaging should be performed as soon as possible in young people with confirmed cervical SCI or unexplained hypotension to assess for ligamentous and soft tissue injury and to visualize the spinal cord (Frank et al 2002). In adults, as many as 13% of patients with cervical SCI will have concurrent non-contiguous spinal injuries, which appear to be more common in young people; therefore, imaging of the entire spine and spinal cord should be performed in young people with SCI at any level (Qaiyum et al 2001).

Finally, consideration should be given to performing early angiography in children with traumatic spinal injuries, looking particularly for aortic injuries associated with high-energy thoracic trauma and for vertebral artery or carotid injuries with cervical SCI, particularly in those with unexplained coma, ischemic changes on brain imaging, or clinical signs of stroke (Garg et al 1993). A prospective study in adults with blunt cervical trauma, skull base fractures, or severe facial fractures demonstrated vascular abnormalities in the carotids in 11% and vertebral arteries in 20% (Miller et al 2002). The appropriate imaging method for this endeavor, whether ultrasound, computed tomography, magnetic resonance imaging, or standard angiography, remains controversial.

Airway and respiratory support

Young people with SCI have a high incidence of respiratory failure, mainly owing to loss of function of the muscles of respiration. In cases of traumatic SCI, respiratory failure can be compounded by associated traumatic injuries to the brain, thorax, or abdomen. Airway management in young people with SCI is challenging owing to the hypotensive effects of anesthetics and because any movement of the spine during endotracheal intubation could result in secondary injury to the spinal cord. Vocal cord dysfunction, direct tracheal injury, and diaphragm weakness or paralysis are common with cervical SCI and predispose children to hypoxemia and overt respiratory failure. In these children, early endotracheal intubation can be life saving. For all young people with confirmed or suspected cervical SCI who require intubation, rapid sequence induction using cricoid pressure and manual inline stabilization for endotracheal intubation by an experienced clinician is required (Norwood et al 1994). Manual inline stabilization has been shown to reduce flexion, extension, and rotation of the cervical spine while providing maximal visualization for laryngoscopy (Heath 1994). Fiber-optic laryngoscopes have performed well in adult patient simulations but have not been shown to be better than or even equal to the standard Macintosh laryngoscope in pediatric patients undergoing intubation using cervical spine precautions and manual inline stabilization (Nileshwar and Garg 2010).

The choice of anesthetics for intubation of young people with SCI is influenced by the patient's cardiopulmonary status and potential for deterioration. As discussed below, patients with cervical and high thoracic SCI frequently present with neurogenic shock, which is characterized by low systemic vascular resistance, low blood pressure, and variable heart rates, with sinus bradycardia being the classic finding (Tator 1995) (see Chapter 13). This, coupled with other organ injuries, blood loss, and other stressors, such as hypothermia and systemic inflammatory response syndrome, increases the likelihood of profound hypotension and even cardiac arrest during anesthesia for intubation. For this reason, medications that lower systemic vascular resistance and blood pressure, such as thiopental and propofol, should be avoided, whereas ketamine, fentanyl, and etomidate offer better hemodynamic profiles. Regarding neuromuscular blockade, succinylcholine remains the agent of choice because of its rapid onset and short duration of action, although it should not be used more than 48 hours after injury because of the increased risk of hyperkalemia (Martyn and Richtsfeld 2006).

Young people with SCI should receive mechanical ventilatory support until it is clearly established that they have a stable, patent, and secure airway; are able to ventilate adequately; and have no other impediment to spontaneous ventilation such as lung or chest wall injury, or diaphragmatic injury or paralysis. Ventilator management should be guided by blood gas results following the guidelines for traumatic brain injury maintaining normocapnea and normoxia, as the spinal cord and cerebral vasculature respond similarly to changes in blood pressure, carbon dioxide, and hypoxia (Holtz et al 1988, 1989). Early tracheostomy in patients who fail extubation or fail to meet extubation criteria may improve respiratory mechanics and airway control enough to allow for weaning from mechanical ventilation, hastening the transition from acute care to the rehabilitation unit and thereby reducing costs (Seidl 2010). Children with cervical injuries should be evaluated completely for upper airway injury with laryngoscopy or bronchoscopy and diaphragmatic paresis or paralysis with fluoroscopy or ultrasound. In those with abnormal findings, a more conservative approach to weaning from mechanical ventilation and tracheal decannulation is required.

Compared with adults, young children have a more elastic and compliant chest wall, which predisposes them to greater loss of functional residual capacity, reduction in vital capacity, and development of atelectasis after SCI. This is especially important during the first days to weeks after SCI, when spinal shock causes the muscles of respiration to become flaccid, thereby greatly reducing vital capacity. Young people have fewer respiratory difficulties when SCI is at L1 or lower; however, when SCI is above L1, intercostal and abdominal muscle paralysis can lead to a weak cough, airway secretion build-up, and recurrent atelectasis (see also Chapters 9 and 14). Incentive spirometry, optimal positioning with an abdominal binder, chest physiotherapy, frequent suctioning, and early mobilization are the cornerstones of respiratory care (Ishikawa and Bach 2010). Other helpful mechanical strategies include the mechanical insufflator–exsufflator (CoughAssist™, Emerson, Cambridge, MA, USA) and the vibratory vest. The lungs and chest wall require a regular range of motion exercise and stretching to prevent chest wall contractures and lung restriction from muscle weakness and spasticity. Serial measurements of pulmonary function are helpful in determining the timing of extubation or the need to make changes in respiratory management.

Young people with upper cervical SCI may require long-term ventilatory support and may need to be transitioned to an intermediate care or respiratory care unit for extended periods of time before transfer to an acute rehabilitation center. Because rehabilitation centers may not be staffed or equipped to perform weaning protocols, the respiratory status of ventilator-dependent children should be stable before transfer. For young children and those with high cervical injuries, it is often better to achieve and maintain a stable level of ventilatory support that allows the child to avoid all periods of respiratory distress, hypoxemia, and recurrent atelectasis, rather than to liberate them completely from ventilatory support at the risk of serious complications (Padman 2003). Theophylline has been shown experimentally and anecdotally to improve diaphragmatic muscle function (by reducing breakdown of cyclic AMP) after cervical SCI, although insufficient evidence exists to recommend this for all patients (Bascom 2005, Nantwi and Goshgarian 2005). Theophylline may be beneficial for young people with partial or reduced diaphragm function who have failed weaning attempts.

Hemodynamics

During the acute phase of an SCI, particularly with injury at the cervical level, young people experience neurogenic shock manifested by hypotension and bradycardia, and as a result they are at risk of secondary spinal cord ischemia (Krassioukov and Claydon 2006, Furlan and Fehlings 2008) (see Chapter 13). The extent to which prolonged and severe hypotension requires vasopressor therapy to maintain mean arterial pressure (MAP) above 85 to 90mmHg correlates well with the severity of cervical or high-thoracic SCI, and can last up to 5 weeks after the injury (Lehmann et al 1987). In adults with SCI, Vale and colleagues found that 90% of those with complete cervical SCI required vasopressor therapy to maintain MAP at greater than 85mmHg for an average of 13 days, in contrast to 52% of those with incomplete cervical and 25% to 33% of those with complete or incomplete thoracic injuries (Vale et al 1997). Levi and colleagues invasively measured hemodynamics beginning 11±6 hours after complete and incomplete cervical SCI in adults and found that 82% required vasopressors for an average of 5.7 days after injury to maintain MAP at greater than 90mmHg (Levi et al 1993). These investigators demonstrated that hypotension was associated with decreased systemic and pulmonary vascular resistance.

Without aggressive management, hemodynamic instability can lead to delays in operative intervention after SCI and may worsen long-term outcomes by reducing spinal cord blood flow, which is already compromised by several vascular mechanisms, including primary injury to microvessels, intraluminal thrombosis, vasospasm, compression, edema, and endothelial injury (Tator and Fehlings 1991, Anthes et al 1996). Medical guidelines for the management of patients with SCI recommend maintenance of MAP in the high normal range (above 85–90mmHg) in adults for the first 7 days after injury or until stable (Congress of Neurological Surgeons 2002). Hemodynamic support of young people with neurogenic shock owing to SCI should begin with aggressive volume administration followed by catecholamine infusion if needed to maintain an adequate MAP and to increase systemic vascular resistance, heart rate, and cardiac output. Ideally, the mean arterial and systolic blood pressure should be maintained at or above the 50th centile for age in young people, for which the following equations are recommended: MAP=55 + (1.5 × age in years) and systolic blood pressure=85 + (2 × age in years) (Haque and Zaritsky 2007). Dopamine, epinephrine, and norepinephrine have both alpha and beta effects and have been used successfully in this setting, although epinephrine should be used with caution owing to its potential to cause tachyarrhythmias. Zahra and colleagues found that vasopressin concentrations increase acutely in response to severe cervical SCI in infant piglets, although the increase may be insufficient, suggesting that vasopressin could be helpful in stabilizing blood pressure after SCI (Zahra et al 2010).

One of the most dangerous hemodynamic complications of SCI is autonomic dysreflexia, which occurs in 48% to 85% of all individuals with SCI at T6 and above (see Chapter 13). Autonomic dysreflexia is manifested by a sudden exaggerated reflex increase in blood pressure, sometimes accompanied by bradycardia, in response to either a noxious or non-noxious stimulus originating below the level of injury. Although autonomic dysreflexia occurs more often in the chronic stage of SCI, it can also occur during the acute phase of SCI, but may be under-recognized (Silver 2000, Krassioukov et al 2009).

Venous thromboembolism

The incidence of venous thromboembolism in the pediatric population with SCI is less than that in the adult population (see Chapter 14). Deep venous thrombosis (DVT) is extremely rare in young people injured at 5 years of age and younger (0%) and in those injured between 6 and 12 years of age (2%) (Vogel et al 2011, Schottler et al 2012). In contrast, DVT was identified in 8% of those injured between 13 and 15 years of age and in 9% of those injured between 16 and 21 years of age. Venous thromboembolism in young people leading to pulmonary embolism is usually associated with prothrombotic disorders or other chronic conditions such as congenital heart disease, cancer, indwelling central catheters, burns, and major trauma. Hanson and colleagues recently described nine children younger than 18 years of age, six of whom were less than 12 years of age, with clinically significant venous thromboembolism out of a total of 144 young people admitted with trauma; the six prepubertal cases represent 4.2% of patients studied (Hanson et al 2010). Significant risk factors included parenteral nutrition, neuromuscular blockade, use of inotropes, and factor VII administration; only one patient had SCI (and had venous thromboembolism), so no conclusions could be made regarding SCI as a risk factor.

Because of the low incidence of DVT in young people injured before adolescence, prophylactic anticoagulation should be limited to those with other DVT risk factors, such as lower extremity or pelvic trauma and fractures. Prophylactic anticoagulation with low molecular weight heparin (LMWH) should start within 24 to 72 hours after injury if no active bleeding, other evidence of coagulopathy, or additional contraindications are present (see Chapter 14). Anticoagulation with LMWH should be adjusted to maintain anti-factor Xa levels of 0.1 to 0.3units/ml. Young people of all ages with an acute SCI should receive mechanical prophylaxis with graduated compression stockings. For those too small to wear commercially available graduated compression stockings, use of custom-made lower extremity stockings should be considered. Elastic wraps should be avoided because unevenness of application may result in constrictions with venous obstruction, increasing the risk of DVT or compartment syndrome (Vogel and Lubicky 2001). Pneumatic compression sleeves should be utilized for older children and adolescents during the first 2 weeks after sustaining an SCI.

Management of DVT includes anticoagulation with LMWH or intravenous unfractionated heparin (Monagle et al 2012) (see Chapter 14). LMWH is the preferred treatment because it is associated with decreased risk of bleeding, osteoporosis, and heparin-induced thrombocytopenia. Anticoagulation with LMWH should be adjusted to maintain anti-factor Xa levels of 0.5 to 1.0units/ml. Unfractionated heparin is administered intravenously and is adjusted to maintain an activated partial thromboplastin time between 60 and 85 seconds or anti-Xa levels of 0.35 to 0.70. Oral anticoagulation with warfarin sodium is begun within 72 hours after LMWH or unfractionated heparin has been initiated, and warfarin treatment should overlap by at least 5 days with LMWH or unfractionated heparin. Dosage adjustments are made to maintain a target international normalized ratio of 2.5 (range 2.0–3.0) (Monagle et al 2012). Individuals with clot progression while on therapy, completely occlusive clots on presentation, or persistently high levels of inflammatory markers (e.g. C-reactive protein, platelet count, and white blood cell count), are at risk of treatment failure and may benefit from a longer duration of anticoagulation therapy or placement of a vena caval filter (Monagle et al 2008).

Bladder

The extent of urinary tract dysfunction is dependent upon the level and severity of SCI (see Chapter 11). As a result of spinal shock after sustaining an SCI, the young person presents with an areflexic and acontractile bladder with urinary retention. Initial bladder management during this acute period consists of an indwelling urethral catheter, which also assists in monitoring urine output. However, once the young person is stable, the indwelling catheter should be removed to reduce the risk of urinary tract infections, and intermittent catheterization should be initiated.

Gastrointestinal complications

During the acute phase after sustaining an SCI, there are various gastrointestinal manifestations and complications including swallowing dysfunction, gastritis and stress ulcers, superior mesenteric artery syndrome, decreased gastrointestinal motility (ileus and gastroparesis), pancreatitis, and gall bladder disorders (cholecystitis and cholelithiasis) (see Chapter 14). In addition, for those who had intra-abdominal injuries associated with their SCI, complications related to the original intra-abdominal injury or its surgical management, such as intra-abdominal sepsis or small bowel obstruction, may also occur. Young people with acute SCI should receive prophylactic histamine 2 receptor blockers or proton pump inhibitors to reduce the risk of stress ulceration and gastrointestinal bleeding, although the duration of this therapy is unknown (Kewalramani 1979). Enteral feeding should be started orally or via an enteral feeding tube as soon as the child is hemodynamically stable. Once the child begins receiving enteral nutrition, a bowel program should be initiated with a goal of one bowel movement per day or every other day to prevent constipation (Merenda and Hickey 2005) (see Chapter 11). This may require stool softeners, prokinetic agents, suppositories, and/or enemas.

Skin care

Skin care is an essential component in the care of young people with SCI, which must begin during the acute stage after sustaining an SCI (see Chapter 15). Pressure ulcers are a serious and, unfortunately, common complication in this population, even during the acute phase of caring for a young person with an SCI (Caliri 2005). During the acute phase of SCI, the most common sites of pressure ulcers are the occiput, scapula, sacrum, and heels, which are sites associated with being supine or related to immobilization such as halo traction or cervical orthoses. Pressure ulcers that develop during the acute phase after an SCI adversely impact the young person in a number of ways. Pressure ulcers create a catabolic state that negatively affects wound healing. Pressure ulcers may lead to permanent lifelong defects such as localized baldness owing to an occipital pressure ulcer. Pressure ulcers acquired during acute care may adversely affect the ability of the young person to benefit from rehabilitation because of sitting or positioning limitations. Pressure ulcers may also lead to additional complications such as sepsis, osteomyelitis, and malnutrition, and may further delay transfer to a rehabilitation center (Vogel 1996). Therefore, preventive measures must be established immediately upon arrival to the emergency department and include padding over at-risk areas and bony prominences, removal of the child from the backboard as soon as safely possible, close monitoring of the skin especially under cervical collars and other braces, and frequent positional changes at a minimum of every 2 hours. Thermal injuries may also occur to insensate areas with the use of warming blankets.

Fever

Fever is a common occurrence in young people with SCI during the acute phase and can be the result of infections or non-infectious processes (see Chapters 13 and 14). The more common infections include pneumonia and urinary (urinary tract infection or epididymitis), gastrointestinal (antibiotic-associated diarrhea or intra-abdominal infections), and surgical site and intravascular catheter-associated infections. Non-infectious etiologies of fever may include atelectasis, pathologic fractures, heterotopic ossification, and DVT. Not uncommonly, young people, especially those with cervical and high-thoracic SCI, have a fever known as 'quad fever', which is presumably a manifestation of autonomic dysfunction (Colachis and Otis 1995) (see Chapter 13). Evaluation of a febrile young person with an SCI must include a thorough history and physical examination, and appropriate laboratory and imaging studies guided by the clinical evaluation (see Chapter 14).

Neuroprotection

Although initial enthusiasm was high for the use of high-dose methylprednisolone within 8 hours of SCI in adults after the National Acute Spinal Cord Injury Study trials, more rigorous post-hoc analysis of the data has raised considerable doubt about, and in some cases convincing arguments against, the use of this therapy (Bracken et al 1997, Hall and Springer 2004). Only a small number of adolescents and no young people below the age of 12 years were included in these trials. There is no evidence of any clinical benefit of corticosteroids in young people with SCI. Given this complete lack of evidence and the reports of increased morbidity after the use of high-dose corticosteroids for adults with SCI, as well as those with traumatic brain injury, lung injury, or sepsis, there is no evidence to support using this therapy in young people with SCI (Coleman et al 2000). Similarly, therapeutic hypothermia after SCI has not been proven to improve outcome, although clinical trials are currently under way in adults. Given the recently reported hypotensive effects of systemic hypothermia in young people with traumatic brain injury, the use of hypothermia therapy in young people with SCI should be approached with caution owing to the potential for an additive effect of hypothermia to the cardiovascular instability seen with SCI (Hutchison et al 2008).

Acute rehabilitation

Young people who have sustained an SCI will require rehabilitative services to maximize recovery and minimize secondary complications. Early rehabilitation may be key in the prevention of many of the potential complications that occur. Early consultation by a rehabilitation medicine specialist can provide guidance in initiating therapeutic interventions in the acute setting and assist with plans for transition to an acute in-patient spinal cord rehabilitation unit. Occupational and physical therapists should be involved as soon as possible in the pediatric intensive care unit in order to prevent contractures, muscle atrophy, and skin breakdown through careful use of upper and lower extremity splinting. Recently, an effort has been made to initiate early mobilization of critically ill but stable adult patients, with noted benefits in the prevention of muscle loss and improvement in respiratory function (Truong et al 2009, Jia et al 2013).

Summary

From the pre-hospital setting to initial trauma resuscitation, intra-operative intervention (when indicated), intensive care, and preparation for transfer to a rehabilitation center, young people with acute SCI require an interprofessional team of physicians, nurses, psychologists, social workers, and therapists in order to achieve the best outcome from the life-threatening impact of SCI. In the absence of proven therapeutic interventions for SCI, the primary goal of acute care management is to maintain physiological homeostasis and prevent secondary spinal cord and systemic insults in order to provide the injured cord with the best chance for recovery. The most commonly and severely affected organ systems are the respiratory and cardiovascular systems, although multi-organ system dysfunction and failure may occur. The best outcome for the young person with SCI will be achieved when secondary complications are prevented or anticipated in advance, identified early, and rapidly managed.

REFERENCES

Anthes DL, Theriault E, Tator CH (1996) Ultrastructural evidence for arteriolar vasospasm after spinal cord trauma. *Neurosurgery* 39: 804–14. doi.org/10.1097/00006123-199610000-00032

Bascom AT, Lattin CD, Aboussouan LS, Goshgarian HG (2005) Effect of acute aminophylline administration on diaphragm function in high cervical tetraplegia: a case report. *Chest* 127: 658–61. doi.org/10.1378/chest.127.2.658

Bracken MB, Shepard MJ, Holford TR et al (1997) Administration of methylprednisolone for 24 or 48 hours or tirilazad mesylate for 48 hours in the treatment of acute spinal cord injury. Results of the Third National Acute Spinal Cord Injury Randomized Controlled Trial. National Acute Spinal Cord Injury Study. *JAMA* 277: 1597–604. http://dx.doi.org/10.1001/jama.1997.03540440031029

Caliri MH (2005) Spinal cord injury and pressure ulcers. *Nurs Clin North Am* 40: 337–47. doi:10.1016/j.cnur.2004.09.009

Chung S, Mikrogianakis A, Wales PW et al (2011) Trauma association of Canada Pediatric Subcommittee National Pediatric Cervical Spine Evaluation Pathway: consensus guidelines. *J Trauma* 70: 873–84. doi.org/10.1097/TA.0b013e3182108823

Colachis SC, Otis SM (1995) Occurrence of fever associated with thermoregulatory dysfunction after acute traumatic spinal-cord injury. *Am J Phys Med Rehabil* 74: 114–19. doi.org/10.1097/00002060-199503000-00005

Coleman WP, Benzel D, Cahill DW et al (2000) A critical appraisal of the reporting of the national acute spinal cord injury studies (I and II) of methylprednisolone in acute spinal cord injury. *J Spinal Disord* 13: 185–99. http://dx.doi.org/10.1097/00002517-200006000-00001

Congress of Neurological Surgeons (2002) Guidelines for the management of acute cervical spine and spinal cord injuries. *Neurosurgery* 50: S1. doi.org/10.1227/01.neu.0000430319.32247.7f.

Easter JS, Barkin R, Rosen CL, Ban K (2011) Cervical spine injuries in children, part I: mechanism of injury, clinical presentation, and imaging. *J Emerg Med* 41: 142–50. doi.org/10.1016/j.jemermed.2009.11.034

Frank JB, Lim CK, Flynn JM, Dormans JP (2002) The efficacy of magnetic resonance imaging in pediatric cervical spine clearance. *Spine (Phila Pa 1976)* 27: 1176.

Furlan JC, Fehlings MG (2008) Cardiovascular complications after acute spinal cord injury: pathophysiology, diagnosis, and management. *Neurosurg Focus* 25: E13. doi.org/10.3171/FOC.2008.25.11.E13

Garg BP, Ottinger CJ, Smith RR, Fishman MA (1993) Strokes in children due to vertebral artery trauma. *Neurology* 43: 2555–8. doi.org/10.1212/WNL.43.12.2555

Gebauer G, Osterman M, Harrop J, Vaccaro A (2012) Spinal cord injury resulting from injury missed on CT scan: the danger of relying on CT alone for collar removal. *Clin Orthop Relat Res* 470: 1652–7. doi.org/10.1007/s11999-012-2286-7

Hall ED, Springer JE (2004) Neuroprotection and acute spinal cord injury: a reappraisal. *NeuroRx* 1: 80–100. http://dx.doi.org/10.1602/neurorx.1.1.80

Hanson SJ, Punzalan RC, Greenup RA, Liu H, Sato TT, Havens PL (2010) Incidence and risk factors for venous thromboembolism in critically ill children after trauma. *J Trauma* 68: 52–6. doi.org/10.1007/s11999-012-2286-7

Haque I, Zaritsky A (2007) Analysis of the evidence for the lower limit of systolic and mean arterial pressure in children. *Pediatr Crit Care Med* 8: 138–44. doi.org/10.1097/01.PCC.0000257039.32593.DC

Heath KJ (1994) The effect of laryngoscopy of different cervical spine immobilisation techniques. *Anaesthesia* 49: 843–5. doi.org/10.1111/j.1365-2044.1994.tb04254.x

Herzenberg JE, Hensinger RN, Dedrick DK et al (1989). Emergency transport and positioning of young children who have an injury of the cervical spine. The standard backboard may be hazardous. *J Bone Joint Surg* 71A: 15–22.

Holtz A, Nyström B, Gerdin B (1988) Regulation of spinal cord blood flow in the rat as measured by quantitative autoradiography. *Acta Physiol Scand* 133: 485–93. doi.org/10.1111/j.1748-1716.1988.tb08432.x

Holtz A, Nyström B, Gerdin B (1989) Spinal cord blood flow measured by 14C-iodoantipyrine autoradiography during and after graded spinal cord compression in rats. *Surg Neurol* 31: 350–60. doi.org/10.1016/0090-3019(89)90066-9

Hutchings L, Willett K (2009) Cervical spine clearance in pediatric trauma: a review of current literature. *J Trauma* 67: 687–91. doi.org/10.1097/TA.0b013e3181b5ecae

Hutchison J, Ward R, Lacroix J et al; HyP-HIT Investigators and the Canadian Critical Care Trials Group (2008) Hypothermia therapy after traumatic brain injury in children. *N Engl J Med* 358: 2447–56. doi: 10.1056/NEJMoa0706930.

Ishikawa Y, Bach JR (2010) Physical medicine respiratory muscle aids to avert respiratory complications of pediatric chest wall and vertebral deformity and muscle dysfunction. *Eur J Phys Rehabil Med* 46: 581–97.

Jia X, Kowalski RG, Sciubba DM, Geocadin RG (2013) Critical care of traumatic spinal cord injury. *J Intensive Care Med* 28: 12–23. doi.org/10.1177/0885066611403270

Kewalramani LS (1979) Neurogenic gastroduodenal ulceration and bleeding associated with spinal cord injuries. *J Trauma* 19: 259–65. http://dx.doi.org/10.1097/00005373-197904000-00008

Krassioukov A, Claydon VE (2006) The clinical problems in cardiovascular control following spinal cord injury: an overview. *Prog Brain Res* 152: 223–9. doi.org/10.1016/S0079-6123(05)52014-4

Krassioukov A, Warburton DE, Teasell R, Eng JJ; Spinal Cord Injury Rehabilitation Evidence Research Team (2009) A systematic review of the management of autonomic dysreflexia after spinal cord injury. *Arch Phys Med Rehabil* 90: 682–95. doi.org/10.1016/j.apmr.2008.10.017

Lehmann KG, Lane LG, Piepmeier JM, Batsford WP (1987) Cardiovascular abnormalities accompanying acute spinal cord injury in humans: incidence, time course and severity. *J Am Coll Cardiol* 10. 46–52. doi.org/10.1016/S0735-1097(87)80158-4

Levi L, Wolf A, Belzberg H (1993) Hemodynamic parameters in patients with acute cervical cord trauma: description, intervention, and prediction of outcome. *Neurosurgery* 33: 1007–17. doi.org/10.1227/00006123-199312000-00008

Martyn JA, Richtsfeld M (2006) Succinylcholine-induced hyperkalemia in acquired pathologic states: etiologic factors and molecular mechanisms. *Anesthesiology* 104: 158–69. doi.org/10.1097/00000542-200601000-00022

Merenda LA, Hickey K (2005) Key elements of bladder and bowel management for children with spinal cord injuries. *SCI Nurs* 22: 8–14.

Miller PR, Fabian TC, Croce MA et al (2002) Prospective screening for blunt cerebrovascular injuries: analysis of diagnostic modalities and outcomes. *Ann Surg* 236: 386. doi.org/10.1097/00000658-200209000-00015

Monagle P, Chalmers E, Chan A, DeVeber G, Kirkham F, Massicotte P, Michelson AD (2008) Antithrombotic therapy in neonates and children: American College of Chest Physicians Evidence-Based Clinical Practice Guidelines (8th Edition). *Chest* 6: 887S–968S. doi: 10.1378/chest.08-0762

Monagle P, Chan AKC, Goldenberg NA et al (2012) Antithrombotic therapy in neonates and children. Antithrombotic therapy and prevention of thrombosis, 9th Ed: American College of Chest Physicians evidence-based clinical practice guidelines. *Chest* 141(Suppl): e737S–801S. doi: 10.1378/chest.

Nantwi KD, Goshgarian HG (2005) Adenosinergic mechanisms underlying recovery of diaphragm motor function following upper cervical spinal cord injury: potential therapeutic implications. *Neurol Res* 27: 195–205. doi.org/10.1179/016164105X21977

Nileshwar A, Garg V (2010) Comparison of Bullard laryngoscope and short-handled Macintosh laryngoscope for orotracheal intubation in pediatric patients with simulated restriction of cervical spine movements. *Paediatr Anaesth* 20: 1092–7. doi: 10.1111/j.1460-9592.2010.03439.x

Norwood S, Myers MB, Butler TJ (1994) The safety of emergency neuromuscular blockade and orotracheal intubation in the acutely injured trauma patient. *J Am Coll Surg* 179: 646–52.

Padman R, Alexander M, Thorogood C, Porth S (2003) Respiratory management of pediatric patients with spinal cord injuries: retrospective review of the duPont experience. *Neurorehabil Neural Repair* 17: 32–6. doi.org/10.1177/0888439003251751

Panczykowski DM, Tomycz ND, Okonkwo DO (2011) Comparative effectiveness of using computed tomography alone to exclude cervical spine injuries in obtunded or intubated patients: meta-analysis of 14 327 patients with blunt trauma. *J Neurosurg* 115: 541. doi.org/10.3171/2011.4.JNS101672

Qaiyum M, Tyrrell PN, McCall IW, Cassar-Pullicino VN (2001) MRI, detection of unsuspected vertebral injury in acute spinal trauma: incidence and significance. *Skeletal Radiol* 30: 299–304. doi.org/10.1007/s002560100329

Schottler J, Vogel LC, Sturm P (2012) Spinal cord injuries in young children: a review of children injured at five years of age and younger. *Dev Med Child Neurol* 54: 1138–43. doi: 10.1111/j.1469-8749.2012.04411.x

Seidl RO, Wolf D, Nusser-Müller-Busch R, Niedeggen A (2010) Airway management in acute tetraplegics: a retrospective study. *Eur Spine J* 19: 1073–8. doi.org/10.1007/s00586-010-1328-7

Silver JR (2000) Early autonomic dysreflexia. *Spinal Cord* 4: 229–33. http://dx.doi.org/10.1038/sj.sc.3100996

Tator CH (1995) Update on the pathophysiology and pathology of acute spinal cord injury. *Brain Pathol* 5: 407–13. doi.org/10.1111/j.1750-3639.1995.tb00619.x

Tator CH, Fehlings MG (1991) Review of the secondary injury theory of acute spinal cord trauma with emphasis on vascular mechanisms. *J Neurosurg* 75: 15–26. doi.org/10.3171/jns.1991.75.1.0015

Truong AD, Fan E, Brower RG, Needham DM (2009) Bench-to-bedside review: mobilizing patients in the intensive care unit--from pathophysiology to clinical trials. *Crit Care* 13: 216. doi.org/10.1186/cc7885

Vale FL, Burns J, Jackson AB, Hadley MN (1997) Combined medical and surgical treatment after acute spinal cord injury: results of a prospective pilot study to assess the merits of aggressive medical resuscitation and blood pressure management. *J Neurosurg* 87: 239–46. doi.org/10.3171/jns.1997.87.2.0239.

Viccellio P, Simon H, Pressman BD, Shah MN, Mower WR, Hoffman JR (2001) A prospective multicenter study of cervical spine injury in children. *Pediatrics* 108: e20. doi: 10.1542/peds.108.2.e20

Vogel LC (1996) Medical management of pressure ulcers. In: Betz RR, Mulcahey MJ (eds). *The Child with a Spinal Cord Injury*. Rosemont, IL: American Academy of Orthopaedic Surgeons, pp. 293–304.

Vogel LC, Lubicky JP (2001) Lower extremity compartment syndrome in an adolescent with a spinal cord injury. *J Spinal Cord Med* 24: 278–83.

Vogel L, Betz R, Mulcahey M (2011) Pediatric spinal cord disorders. In: Kirshblum S, Campagnolo DI (eds). *Spinal Cord Medicine*. 2nd Ed. Philadelphia, PA: Lippincott Williams & Wilkins, pp. 533–64.

Zahra M, Samdani A, Piggott K et al (2010) Acute changes in systemic hemodynamics and serum vasopressin after complete cervical spinal cord injury in piglets. *Neurocrit Care* 13: 132–40. doi.org/10.1007/s12028-010-9364-z

7
PRINCIPLES OF TREATMENT OF SPINE STABILITY IN CHILDREN WITH SPINAL CORD INJURY

Nigel Price

Introduction

Although many of the treatment principles of spine injuries associated with spinal cord injury (SCI) are similar to adults, the unique anatomical differences in children may alter the approach to the acute management of children's spinal injuries. The child's spine continues to grow until 14 years of age in females and 16 to 18 years in males. The enduring presence of a cartilaginous endplate and synchondroses can affect the injury patterns in children. Until complete ossification of the child's spine occurs, interpretation of radiographs can be challenging and may require an experienced pediatric specialist in radiology, neuroscience, or orthopedics. Children do have the advantage of better rates of healing and more predictable fusion. Non-operative techniques are generally better tolerated with fewer complications.

Acute management of the child with SCI must take into account the pediatric physiology, anatomy, behavioral differences, and mechanisms of injury. Once the patient has been triaged and resuscitated, the team involved with the assessment and treatment of the axial injury must determine the best treatment algorithm based on the bone age of the patient and the injury pattern. Other considerations in treating the child with an SCI include the neurologic classification utilizing the International Standards for the Neurological Classification of Spinal Cord Injury (injury level and severity on the American Spinal Injury Association Impairment Scale [AIS] [American Spinal Injury Association 2011]); the presence of other significant injuries to the limbs, abdomen, and chest; the presence of significant abrasions; and the presence of traumatic brain injury. The overall goal is to restore normal alignment and stability in order to prevent neurologic deterioration and improve neurologic status.

Acutely, children should be treated on a pediatric backboard or a board modified to accommodate the relatively larger head-to-trunk ratio in a child by supporting the upper trunk with a pad or blanket (see Chapter 7). Side bolsters or sand bags and a cervical collar are standard treatment. Once the patient is off the backboard, the collar should be maintained until clinical or radiographic analysis has been done and the spine has been cleared.

According to the National Emergency X-Radiography Utilization Study criteria, clinical examination alone can be used to clear a cervical spine (Viccellio et al 2001) (see Box 7.1). Although plain radiographs demonstrate most bony injuries in childhood cervical spine injuries, many pediatric spine clearance protocols recommend computed tomography (CT) of C1–C2 in place of the open-mouth odontoid view in all patients and CT of the head and

Box 7.1 National Emergency X-Radiography Utilization Study criteria for clinical clearance of the cervical spine

- No posterior midline cervical tenderness
- No evidence of intoxication
- A normal level of alertness
- No focal neurologic deficit
- No painful distracting injuries

C1–T1 in the unconscious patient immobilized in a cervical collar (Hoffman et al 1998). CT of the head, trunk, and abdomen in pediatric trauma activation scenarios with sagittal reconstructions of the axial skeleton is increasingly seen, particularly with reduced dosage pediatric CT protocols. Magnetic resonance imaging (MRI) can help in scenarios where plain radiographs and CT images are normal or equivocal and to clear a cervical spine in obtunded patients (Flynn et al 2002). Plain radiographs are useful to evaluate the spinal column and global alignment. Flexion and extension views are rarely used in the setting of an acute SCI and are more commonly used to assess stability after acute pain and spasm have abated (Kokoska et al 2001).

Spinal cord injury without radiographic abnormality

Spinal cord injury without radiographic abnormality (SCIWORA) was initially described as an SCI in the absence of radiographic or tomographic abnormality (Pang and Wilberger 1982). This occurs more frequently in children than adults and relates to the greater flexibility of the pediatric spine. The spinal column can stretch up to 7cm, but the cord is injured when stretched beyond 10mm (Pang and Wilberger 1982, Pang 2004). These authors note that up to 38% of pediatric SCIs are SCIWORAs.

In a meta-analysis of SCIWORAs, Launay et al (2005) noted that 90% of SCIWORAs are seen in persons less than 18 years old. The same authors noted a wide clinical spectrum in 133 children: 73 (55%) with partial cord syndrome, 36 (27%) with complete cord syndrome, 13 (10%) with central cord syndrome, 7 (5%) with Brown–Séquard syndrome, and 4 (3%) with anterior cord syndrome. In analyzing the subgroups, the authors recommended immobilization of patients with SCIWORA for 12 weeks. In the patients immobilized for 8 weeks, there was a recurrent SCIWORA after removal of the immobilization in 17%. No recurrence was seen in patients immobilized for 12 weeks.

Subaxial cervical injuries

Generally, pediatric fracture stability is determined based on adult criteria. There is no universally accepted adult or pediatric classification, but, as with adult fractures, there are several recognized injury patterns: compression, burst, facet dislocation, and traumatic spondylolysis/spondylolisthesis. Classification schemes of cervical trauma generally follow adult guidelines. Occipital cervical dissociations are often fatal. Survivors have unstable spines that can have occipital cervical wiring or more contemporary occipital plating systems that connect to cervical rods or plates. In very young patients, non-operative treatment may be attempted.

Subaxial cervical injuries in children can be classified according to several adult classification schemes including the subaxial injury classification and severity scale (Vaccaro et al 2009) and the cervical spine injury severity score (Anderson et al 2007). The two classification systems have good interobserver reliability compared with existing classifications (Stone et al 2010). Pediatric patients are generally faster healers and tolerate non-operative (i.e. cast and brace treatment) much better, and hence the frequent use of pinless and conventional halos.

Non-operative Management

Indications for non-operative treatment of subaxial cervical injuries include absence of spinal cord compression, stable neurologic examination, reduced unilateral or bilateral facet dislocations, and no radiographic instability.

Pinless halos were designed as an alternative to Minerva casts and have evolved from earlier designs of cervicothoracic orthoses (Fig. 7.1a). The indications for use include occipital-cervical injuries and upper C-spine injuries, and can include upper thoracic injuries in some cases. Halos can be used in children as young as 6 months of age, but because of the thinness of the skull, a pre-halo CT is recommended to assess skull osteology (Wong and Haynes 1994). The halo is applied with 10 to 12 halo pins, which are torqued to 11.2cm/kg (2in/lbs; i.e. finger tight) (Mubarak et al 1989). The number of pins decreases and torque increases with age. In a child between 2 and 6 years of age, 8 or 10 pins can be used at up to 22.4 to 33.6cm/kg (4–6in/lbs) (Fig. 7.1b). After 12 years of age, the adult four-pin configuration is typically used at 44.8cm/kg (8in/lbs). Frequent clinical check-ups for pin and skin integrity

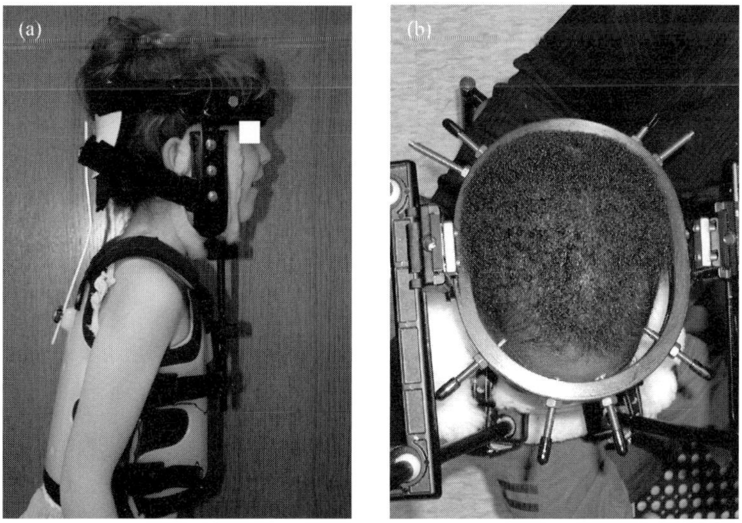

Fig. 7.1 (a) Pinless halo. (b) Halo for thin skull osteology using eight pins.

should be done. Complications of halo include inner table penetration, infection, and loosening (Dormans et al 1995).

In subaxial cervical SCI with the above indications, a rigid collar can be worn until fracture healing, usually 6 weeks in children and young adolescents. Older adolescents can heal in a period similar to that of an adult of 8 to 12 weeks.

Operative Treatment

Indications for surgical stabilization of subaxial cervical injuries include neurologic deterioration, spinal cord compression, irreducible unilateral or bilateral facet dislocations, and persisting instability. Children and adolescents are more likely to have endplate avulsions that can be compared to Salter–Harris 1 growth plate injuries. Displacement of the endplate into the canal with an injury to the pedicle, facets, or facet capsules represents a more significant injury (Hadley 2002). These represent unstable injuries that may require anterior decompression and plate stabilization. Anterior cervical plating systems may be too large for many children, so preoperative planning is necessary. Posterior ligamentous injuries of the subaxial cervical spine with associated instability generally require posterior instrumentation and fusion.

A variety of methodologies of fracture fixation is available, with anterior or posterior approaches used at the discretion of the surgeon. Stable fracture fixation with anterior plating in shown in Figure 7.2a–e. Sometimes, posterior wiring or screw and rod/plate techniques are used in very unstable fractures or where postoperative brace or collar use may not be complied with. Stable subaxial fractures can be treated in a collar for 6 to 8 weeks.

Thoracolumbar injuries

Classification

Currently, most classifications of spinal injury that are used as the basis of treatment of pediatric spine injuries are based on adult series. Until modified/unique trauma classifications are developed for children, this seems the most logical approach to the assessment of spine stability.

The AO spine injury classification (AOSpine TL Injury Classification) is a classification system based on morphologic classification of the fracture, a grading system for neurologic status, and a description of the relevant patient-specific modifiers (Vaccaro et al 2013).

The AOSpine TL classification system is based on the following three parameters:

1 morphologic classification of the fracture, which can be divided into:
  - i type A: compression injuries;
  - ii type B: failure of the posterior or anterior tension band with evidence of either gross translation or the potential for gross translation;
  - iii type C: failure of all elements leading to dislocation or displacement in any plane or complete disruption of a soft tissue hinge, even in the absence of translation;

2 neurologic status;

3 clinical modifiers.

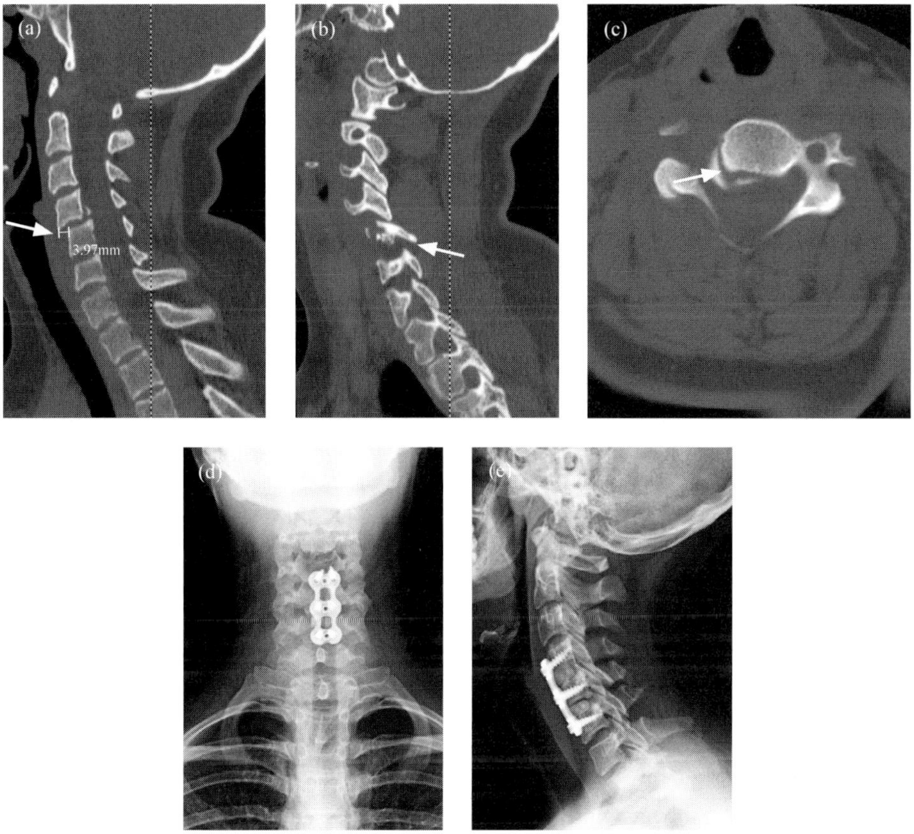

Fig. 7.2 (a) Lateral computed tomography image of a 15-year-old with C4–C5 fracture dislocation from a rollover motor vehicle crash. The fracture propagates through the apophysis of the vertebral body. The white arrow shows the subluxation of C4 on C5. The posterior elements of C5–C6 are unstable, as shown in (b). (b) Lateral computed tomography image of the patient in (a) showing unstable posterior elements of C5–C6. Open and disrupted facet is shown by the white arrow. (c) Axial computed tomography image of the patient shown in (a) showing displacement of the C4 apophysis. The apophysis, shown with a white arrow, was surgically decompressed. (d) Postoperative anteroposterior radiograph of the patient showing C4–C5–C6 anterior plating and bone grafting of disk space after decompression. (e) Postoperative lateral radiograph of the patient. This shows anterior plating with disk and apophysis decompression and autograft tricortical bone graft in disk space.

The injures can be subtyped according to severity and pattern. The following grading of neurologic deficits is used:

- N0 is used to designate patients who are neurologically intact.
- N1 means that a patient had a transient neurologic deficit, which is no longer present.
- N2 denotes patients with symptoms or signs of radiculopathy.
- N3 designates incomplete SCI or cauda equina injury.
- N4 is a complete SCI (AIS A).

- Nx is used to designate a patient who cannot be examined because of head injury or another condition which limits the ability to complete a neurologic examination, such as intoxication, multiple trauma, or intubation/sedation.

The clinician, on an as-needed basis, applies the following patient-specific modifiers to assist in deciding on a treatment:

- M1: designates fractures with an indeterminate injury to the tension band based on spinal imaging such as MRI or clinical examination. This helps to determine if ligamentous instability exists and whether operative stabilization is a consideration.
- M2: designates a patient-specific comorbidity, which contributes to decision making about the need for surgery for injuries and conditions such as burns over the spine, low bone density, and systemic illness such as rheumatologic or oncologic conditions.

Treatment planning is primarily based on the stability of the fracture. Using the AOSpine classification, the more severe patterns such as A4 and all of the B and C combinations of the letter system classifications would constitute potentially unstable fracture patterns, such as thoracolumbar burst pattern with neurologic injury and canal compromise, distraction and shear injuries with displacement, and soft tissue Chance injuries. These would generally be considered for surgical stabilization.

There is currently no universal agreement on thoracolumbar spinal injury classification. The AOSpine classification does allow further study using objective criteria. In a patient with SCI, one of the key principles of treatment is early mobilization and rehabilitation. External immobilization can effectively treat many compressions and burst fractures, but it can impede rehabilitation. Surgical treatment is indicated when there is an unstable fracture pattern and/or deterioration of neurologic status.

Immobilization

For stable fractures such as AOSpine types A1 and A2 with or without B1 bony injury, either an off-the-shelf or a custom brace can be used for 6 to 12 weeks. When possible, because of more prompt healing of pediatric fractures, non-operative techniques such as casting or bracing can be employed. Casting challenges the team to assess the skin and, in patients with SCI, increases the likelihood of skin breakdown, respiratory issues, feeding issues, and reduced hygiene levels. The application of body casts requires personnel trained in the technique to avoid skin complications.

Operative Fixation

The extent and level of instability dictate the operative fixation of a pediatric thoracolumbar spine fracture. Surgical stabilization is generally considered for significant bony compromise such as A4 injuries with greater than 20 degrees of kyphosis as well as canal compromise, distraction, and shear injuries (B and C types) with failure of anterior and posterior tension bands and displacement, particularly with neurologic compromise N3 and N4 and with significant M1 or M2 determinants. In older adolescents with unstable fracture patterns, concurrent non-spine injuries that preclude the use of external support (abdominal injury, or significant pelvic or limb injuries), worsening neurologic deficits, and/or desire for early rehabilitation, the indications for operative fixation are more compelling.

Management of specific injuries

Compression Fractures (A1, A2, and A3)

Compression fractures are common, often resulting from an axial load to the spine with an element of flexion such as a fall from height. As they are considered mainly as anterior column injuries, they are generally not associated with spinal cord dysfunction and can be treated in most cases with an 'off-the-shelf' extension brace (Jewitt, Florida Brace Corporation, Winter Park, FL, USA) or thoracolumbosacral orthosis for 6 to 8 weeks. In some cases, the age of the injury is not obvious, and clinical examination and advanced imaging such as MRI or a bone scan can help determine the acuity of the fracture. Occasionally, a patient will present with multiple compression fractures from either a more significant injury mechanism or a more fragile bone. The etiology of the reduced bone density should be determined in order to find a preventive strategy or treatment (Fig. 7.3a,b).

Unless the amount of compression is in excess of 40% or 50% with significant clinical deformity or sagittal imbalance, typically an extension brace can be fitted and worn for 4 to 6 weeks in younger children and 6 to 8 weeks in older patients. They may be weaned out over

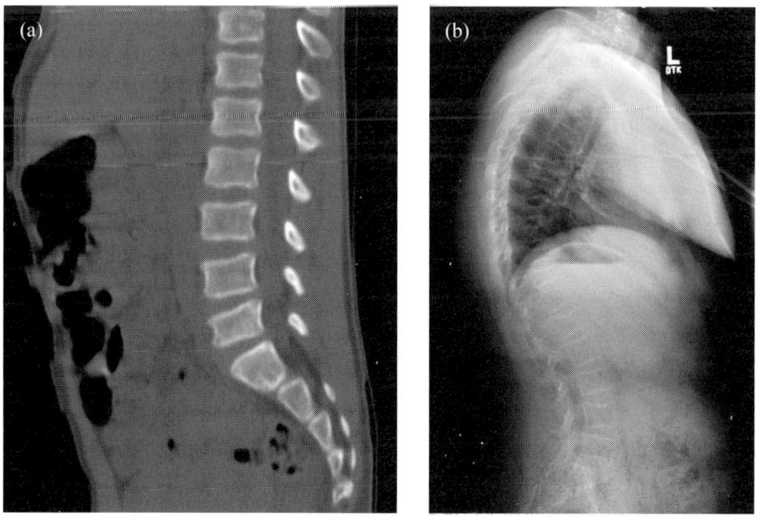

Fig. 7.3 (a) Fifth lumbar vertebra showing a moderate compression fracture in a 9-year-old male who had a fall from 3m. The patient had no neurologic symptoms. The patient was treated in a lumbar corset for 6 weeks. (b) Multiple compression fractures in an 11-year-old female patient with juvenile osteoporosis. She was treated medically and with a thoracic lumbar sacral orthosis for 1 year with good resolution of her symptoms.

several weeks as the patient regains trunk strength. Physical therapy can enhance this weaning process and return to normal activity as the neurologic status dictates.

Patients with multiple compression fractures, particularly if they have a systemic low bone density for their age verified by dual-energy X-ray absorptiometry, should have an endocrine and/or renal workup and treatment if necessary. More prolonged use of external brace support may be required as the vertebrae heal and remodel. The role of vertebroplasty/kyphoplasty in children has not been thoroughly investigated, although there has been significant experience in adult patients.

The surgical options include posterior instrumentation and fusion with screw or hook constructs into stable vertebrae, at least one above and one below the fracture. Adjunctive brace use can be tolerated in children but longer constructs and more stable fixation would diminish the need for external support and make rehabilitation easier. Anterior plating or rods are effective but are seldom needed with modern posterior implants that are available, even for small children.

Burst Fractures (A4)

Burst fractures are more significant injuries involving the middle column of the spine and may extend into the posterior column, creating a three-column and potentially more unstable spine. These are typically created by an axial loading mechanism such as a fall from height or high-speed motor vehicle crash injury (Lalonde et al 2001) (Fig. 7.4a–d). This injury is more likely to be associated with an SCI and dural tear and/or entrapment of nerve roots in the lumbar spine (Wang et al 2004).

Surgeon preference and experience often dictates the surgical approach. Posterior surgery is readily extended superiorly and inferiorly. Direct and indirect decompression can be done via this approach and alignment and height of the vertebra can be improved via ligamentotaxis. Retropulsed bone or disk and endplate fragments can be removed and reduced via a posterolateral or transpedicular approach, and bone grafting can also be added to the repair with this method.

The Chance Injury (Lap Belt)

Chance injuries, AOSpine B and C injuries, are secondary to a flexion/distraction mechanism of injury and involve the three columns of the spine. A soft-tissue Chance injury disrupts the disk or the vertebral body and continues through the ligamentum flavum or capsules posteriorly and is generally considered to lead to some persisting instability. The bony Chance injury, which involves bony posterior elements, may represent a scenario where closed treatment (extension cast or brace) may be adequate (Mulpuri et al 2007).

The constellation of findings resulting from wearing a two-point restraint (lap belt) include abdominal wall ecchymoses, intra-abdominal organ injuries (intra- and/or retroperitoneal), and vertebral fractures with SCI, and together they characterize seat belt or lap belt injuries. Hence, when evaluating children involved in motor vehicle crashes with any of the components of seat belt injury, a high index of suspicion must be maintained for associated injuries to avoid the devastating consequences of a delayed diagnosis. In a seat belt injury, the most common injury is intra-abdominal, which is thought to result from the compression of organs

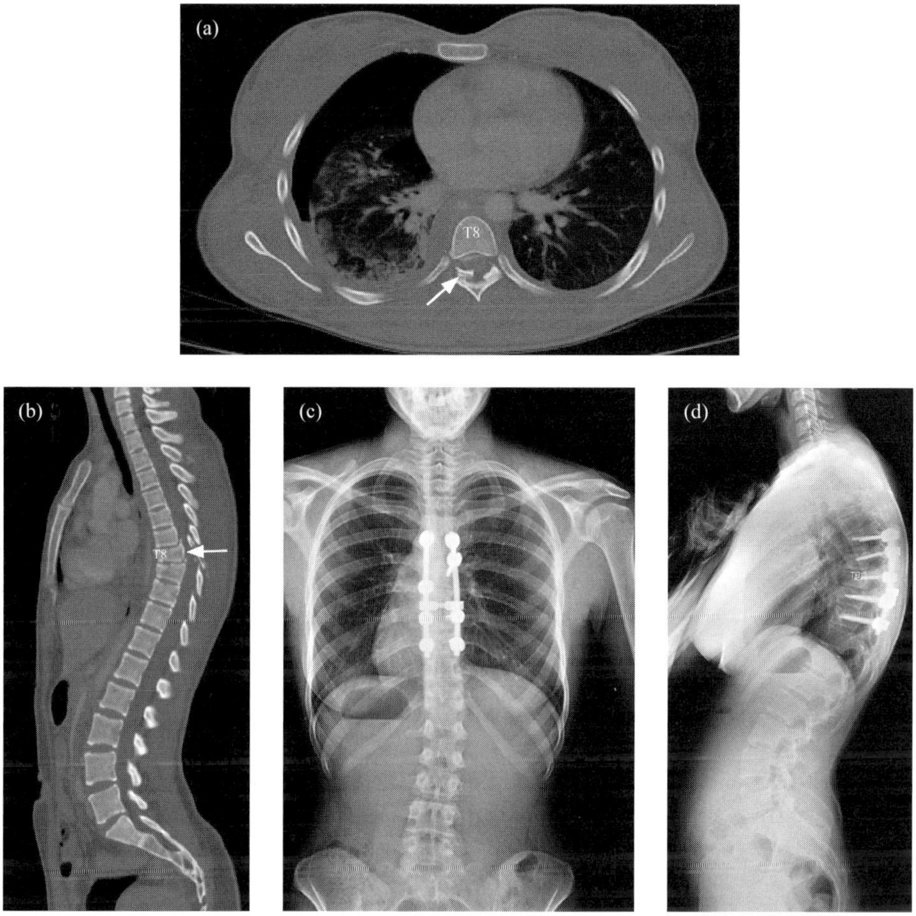

Fig. 7.4 (a) Lateral computed tomography image of a T8 burst fracture in a rollover motor vehicle crash victim. This 16-year-old patient had an incarcerated facet in canal (see white arrow) and a diagnosis of American Spinal Injury Association Impairment Scale (AIS) C. (b) Axial computed tomography image showing a T8 burst fracture with an incarcerated right inferior facet of T8 displacing the spinal cord (see white arrow). (c) Anteroposterior scoliosis view showing a patient after urgent decompression (within 8h) and posterior reconstruction. She had the facet removed and her spinal cord decompressed. A posterior construct was used and all levels were fused. The posterior ligamentous structures were disrupted from T6 to T10. (d) Lateral scoliosis view showing a posterior reconstruction of a T8 burst fracture. She had implants from T6 to T10. Within 4 months, she had no motor deficits and had a diagnosis of AIS E.

between the lap belt anteriorly and the bony vertebral column posteriorly, especially considering the small anteroposterior diameter of a child (Prince et al 2004). Moreover, the less muscular, thinner abdominal wall in children offers less protection against blunt trauma. The most common intra-abdominal injuries are hollow viscous injuries, with the small intestine most commonly involved (Bruny and Bensard 2004). The jejunum is the most common site of small intestine involvement, especially around the ligament of Treitz, since the fixation promotes shear stress tears; another vulnerable fixed site is the ileocecal valve (Bruny and Bensard 2004). Other commonly involved intra-abdominal or retroperitoneal organs are the mesentery; solid organs such as the liver, spleen, and kidneys; vascular structures; and the genitourinary system (ureters and bladder). Injuries to the vertebral column and spinal cord are the second most common seat belt injuries.

Appropriate surgical repair of any injuries to the hollow viscous and any other involved intra-abdominal organs should be undertaken; however, if the spine has not been cleared, spine precautions are essential during transfer to and from the operating room. Chance fractures are three-column injuries derived from flexion/distraction mechanisms. In the pediatric population, they are often associated with lap belt injuries in which the child is flexed over a fulcrum of the lap belt/lower abdomen. The ensuing injury pattern involves oblique injury through disk/endplate/vertebra, which continues posteriorly through pedicle and either facet capsules or interspinous ligaments or bony posterior elements.

The treatment choices are based on the spectrum of injury. In younger children with bony injuries, an extension body cast that reduces and holds the fracture in good alignment may be used for 6 to 8 weeks. Severe abdominal injuries would preclude this, and operative stabilization with or without a brace would be indicated.

When the posterior column injury involves more soft tissue elements such as capsule and ligaments, an operative technique with tension band wiring or rods and hooks or pedicle screws can be used (Fig. 7.5a–d).

The Fracture Dislocation

Fracture dislocation, AOSpine C injury, of the spine is caused by high-speed injuries, generally motor vehicle crashes or falls from significant heights. It is most often associated with SCI and is considered very unstable, as all three columns are involved, typically with significant displacement. These typically represent the most severe of injuries, often with complete SCI and very unstable spines.

Operative fixation is almost universally indicated, and the approach is generally at the surgeon's discretion. Surgical planning includes stable fixation at the fracture site to incorporate an additional level above and below the injury to allow early rehabilitation and less reliance on external bracing. Young patients with complete injuries at a high anatomical level have a high incidence of scoliosis. Some surgeons advocate longer instrumentations to counter the trend toward neurogenic scoliosis (Fig. 7.6a–h).

Timing of surgery

The timing of surgery, particularly when decompression of the spinal cord is involved, has been debated for decades. Fehlings et al (2012), in a study of patients older than 16 years, found in the Surgical Timing of Acute Spinal Cord Injury Study that early cervical decompression within 24 hours led to statistically improved neurologic outcomes of greater than or equal to two AIS grades. Papadopoulos et al (2002) also showed more improvement in neurologic outcome in half of the early decompression group than in the delayed decompression cohort. No known data exist for children.

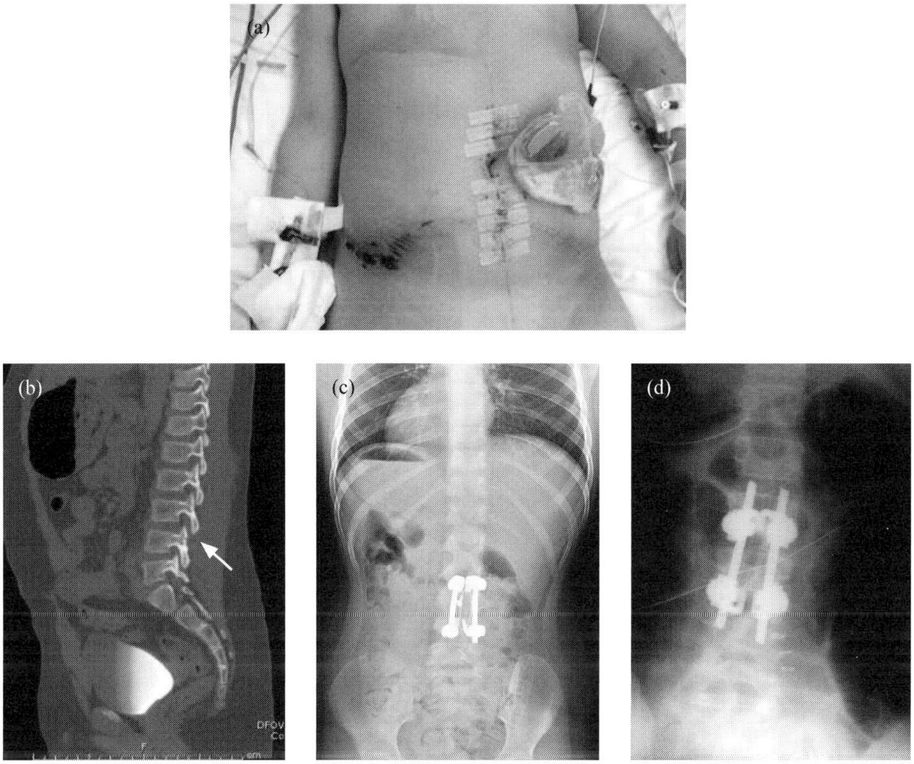

Fig. 7.5 (a) Photograph of a male child with lap belt injury requiring bowel resection and colostomy. He also had an operative Chance fracture, which was repaired on a delayed basis several days later. (b) Sagittal computed tomography reconstruction of an unstable L3–L4 Chance injury in a female patient, which propagated through disk and facet joint capsules (white arrow). (c) Anteroposterior radiograph of the same patient with internal fixation. She had a cast and then a brace to ensure healing. (d) Lateral radiograph of the same patient.

Summary

Young people with SCI and spine trauma generally have better outcomes than adults (Parent et al 2011). Currently the trend is toward early decompression and stabilization of unstable fractures. In most cases, classification systems that apply to adult fracture patterns are employed for analysis and decision making, although unique anatomical differences in children, such as the presence of endplates and synchondroses, also enter into decision making. Children and adolescents are more likely to have a SCIWORA. Now, in the era of MRI use, that term may be antiquated. Protection of the spine for 6 to 8 weeks seems prudent to reduce further injury. Children are also more likely to incur a Chance mechanism of injury, so thorough assessment of intra-abdominal injuries is important. There are more technical options for operative pediatric spine fixation of both spine injuries and limb injuries with the creation of pediatric-sized implants. This has allowed the surgeon to create stable constructs; this aids in early rehabilitation.

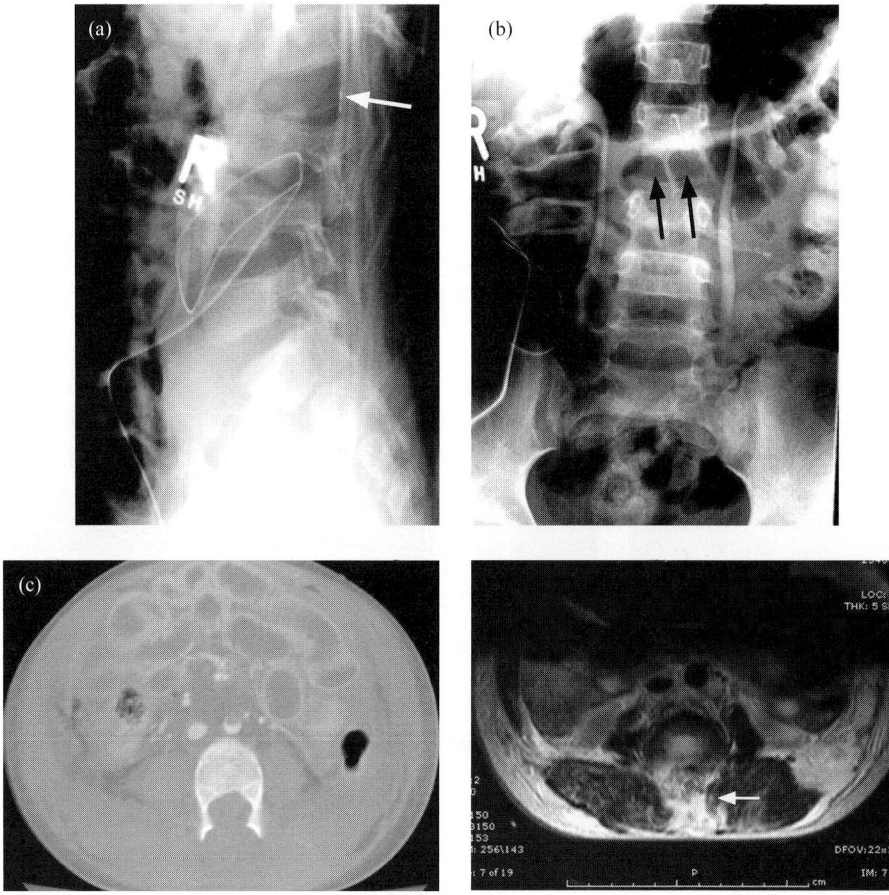

Fig. 7.6 (a) Lumbar plain lateral trauma radiograph of a L2–L3 spine dislocation in a 6-year-old female. She was a back-seat passenger, wearing a lap belt, in a head-on collision, sustaining a flexion and distraction injury to her spine. She had significant visceral injuries. She presented as a T6 American Spinal Injury Association Impairment Scale (AIS) grade A, even though her obvious injury was mid-lumbar. (b) Lumbar anteroposterior view of the same patient showing L2–L3 with a widened distance (white arrows) between vertebrae. (c) Axial computed tomography of the same patient showing the 'empty facet sign' indicating complete disruption of posterior elements. (d) Axial magnetic resonance image of the same patient showing severe spinal disruption with dural contents shifted posteriorly (white arrow). Her diagnosis was T6 AIS A from a second spinal cord injury without radiographic abnormality (SCIWORA) injury.

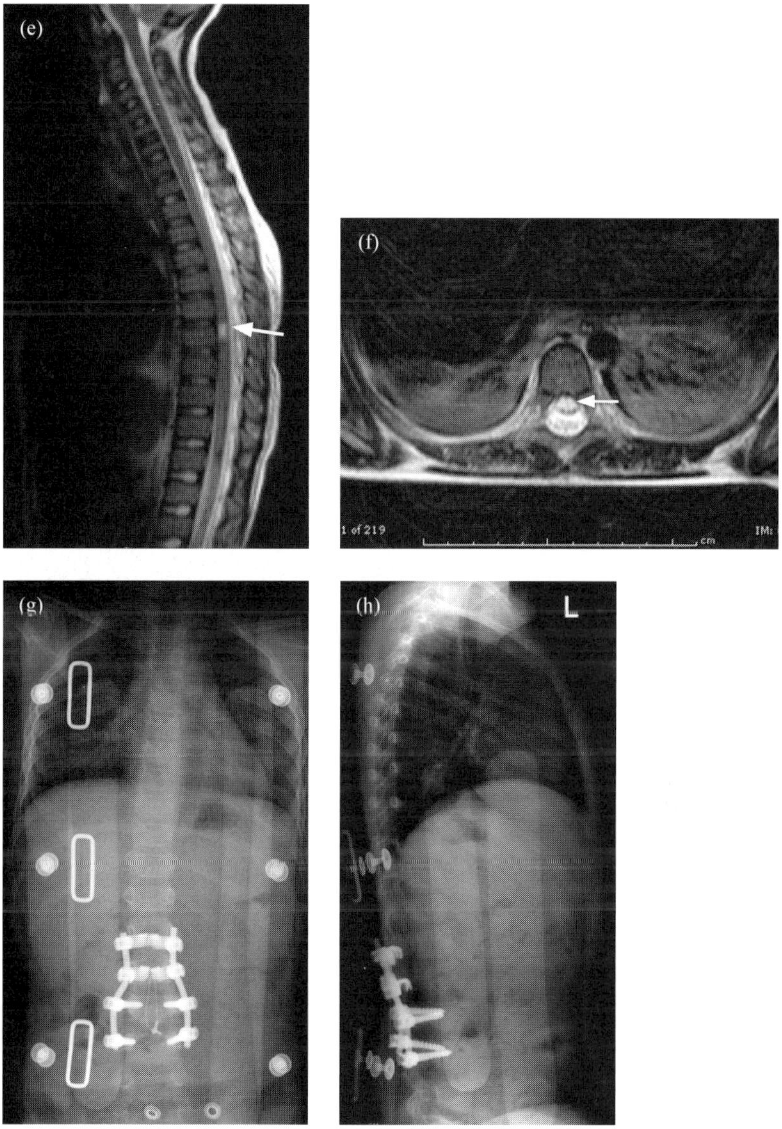

Fig. 7.6 (continued) Second lesion and treatment of the same female patient. (e) Lateral magnetic resonance image of the same patient showing a T6–T7 level of injury. This SCIWORA was the highest anatomic level of injury. The white arrow depicts the spinal cord injury. (f) Axial magnetic resonance image showing the extent of the T6–T7 spinal cord injury. The majority of the area of the cord was traumatized at this level (white arrow). (g) She underwent urgent decompression and posterior instrumentation and fusion. A brace was used for 3 months because of the SCIWORA in the mid-thoracic spine. This is an anteroposterior showing her instrumentation. She underwent extensive repair of the dural tear with a dural graft and the cauda equina was placed back into the spinal canal. She underwent a hybrid hook and screw construct at four levels and was also fused. (h) Lateral view of the same patient.

REFERENCES

American Spinal Injury Association (2011) *International Standards for the Neurologic Classification of Spinal Cord Injury Revised 2011* (booklet). Atlanta, GA: American Spinal Injury Association.

Anderson P, Moore T, Davis K, Molinari R, Resnick D, Vaccaro A; Spinal Trauma Study Group (2007) Cervical spine injury severity score. Assessment of reliability. *J Bone Joint Surg Am* 89: 1057–65. http://dx.doi.org/10.2106/JBJS.F.00684

Bruny JL, Bensard DD (2004) Hollow viscous injury in the pediatric patient. *Semin Pediatr Surg* 13: 112–18. http://dx.doi.org/10.1053/j.sempedsurg.2004.01.007

Dormans JP, Criscitiello AA, Drummond DS, Davidson RS (1995) Complications in children managed with immobilization in a halo vest. *J Bone Joint Surg* 77: 1370–3.

Fehlings MG, Vaccaro A, Wilson JR et al (2012) Early versus delayed decompression for traumatic cervical spinal cord injury: results of the Surgical Timing in Acute Spinal Cord Injury Study (STASCIS). *PLoS One* 7: e32037. doi: 10.1371/journal.pone.0032037

Flynn JM, Closkey RF, Mahboubi S, Dormans JP (2002) Role of magnetic resonance imaging in the assessment of pediatric cervical spine injuries. *J Pediatr Orthop* 22: 573–7. doi: 10.1097/01241398-200209000-00002

Hadley MN (2002) Management of pediatric cervical spine and spinal cord injuries. *Neurosurgery* 50: S85–S99. doi: 10.1097/00006123-200203001-00016

Hoffman JR, Wolfson AB, Todd K, Mower WR (1998) Selective cervical spine radiography in blunt trauma: methodology of the National Emergency X-Radiography Utilization Study (NEXUS). *Ann Emerg Med* 32: 461–9. doi: 10.1016/S0196-0644(98)70176-3

Kokoska ER, Keller MS, Rallo MC, Weber TR (2001) Characteristics of pediatric cervical spine injuries. *J Pediatr Surg* 36: 100–5. doi: 10.1053/jpsu.2001.20022

Lalonde F, Letts M, Yang JP, Thomas K (2001) An analysis of burst fractures of the spine in adolescents. *Am J Orthop* 30: 115–20.

Launay F, Leet AI, Sponseller PD (2005) Pediatric spinal cord injury without radiographic abnormality: a meta-analysis. *Clin Orthop Relat Res* 433: 166–70. doi: 10.1097/01.blo.0000151876.90256.bf PMid:15805953

Mubarak SJ, Camp JF, Vuletich W, Wenger DR, Garfin SR (1989) Halo application in the infant. *J Pediatr Orthop* 9: 612–14. doi: 10.1097/01241398-198909010-00021

Mulpuri K, Reilly CW, Perdios A, Tredwell SJ, Blair GK (2007) The spectrum of abdominal injuries associated with chance fractures in pediatric patients. *Eur J Pediatr Surg* 17: 322–7. doi: 10.1055/s-2007-965587

Pang D (2004) Spinal cord injury without radiographic abnormality in children, 2 decades later. *Neurosurgery* 55: 1325–43. http://dx.doi.org/10.3171/jns.1982.57.1.0114

Pang D, Wilberger J (1982) Spinal cord injury without radiographic abnormalities in children. *J Neurosurg* 57: 114–29. http://dx.doi.org/10.3171/jns.1982.57.1.0114

Papadopoulos SM, Selden NR, Quint DJ, Patel N, Gillespie B, Grube S (2002) Immediate spinal cord decompression for cervical spinal cord injury: feasibility and outcome. *J Trauma Acute Care Surg* 52: 323–32. doi: 10.1097/00005373-200202000-00019

Parent S, Mac-Thiong JM, Roy-Beaudry M, Sosa JF, Labelle H (2011) Spinal cord injury in the pediatric population: a systematic review of the literature. *J Neurotrauma* 28: 1515–24. doi: 10.1089/neu.2009.1153

Prince JS, LoSasso BE, Senac MO Jr (2004) Unusual seat-belt injuries in children. *J Trauma Acute Care Surg* 56: 420–7. doi: 10.1097/01.TA.0000113256.49300.2B

Stone A, Bransford R, Lee M et al (2010) Reliability of classification systems for subaxial cervical injuries. *Evid Based Spine Care J* 1: 19–26. doi: 10.1055/s-0030-1267064

Vaccaro AR, Rihn JA, Saravanja D et al (2009) Injury of the posterior ligamentous complex of the thoracolumbar spine: a prospective evaluation of the diagnostic accuracy of magnetic resonance imaging. *Spine* 34: E841–7. doi: 10.1097/BRS.0b013e3181bd11be

Vaccaro A, Oner C, Kepler C et al; AOSpine Spinal Cord Injury & Trauma Knowledge Forum (2013) AOSpine thoracolumbar spine injury classification system: fracture description, neurological status, and key modifies. *Spine* 38: 2028–37. doi: 10.1097/BRS.0b013e3182a8a381

Viccellio P, Simon H, Pressman BD, Shah MN, Mower WR, Hoffman JR (2001) A prospective multicenter study of cervical spine injury in children. *Pediatrics* 108: e20. doi: 10.1542/peds.108.2.e20

Wang MY, Hoh DJ, Leary SP, Griffith P, McComb JG (2004) High rates of neurological improvement following severe traumatic pediatric spinal cord injury. *Spine* 29: 1493–7; discussion E266. doi: 10.1097/01.BRS.0000129026.03194.0F

Wong W, Haynes R (1994) Osteology of the pediatric skull. Considerations of halo pin placement. *Spine* 19: 1451–4. http://dx.doi.org/10.1097/00007632-199407000-00005

Section 3 Unique Issues in Pediatric Spinal Cord Injury

8 NON-TRAUMATIC PEDIATRIC SPINAL CORD INJURY

David W Pruitt

Case vignette

A 14-year-old previously healthy female experienced sudden, severe cramping in her epigastric region during an intensive track practice. The pain became more severe, radiating to her back, followed by numbness and tingling in her back, abdomen, buttocks, and thighs. She was transported by ambulance to the local emergency room. Within 90 minutes, she was unable to move either leg and developed urinary retention and loss of rectal tone, with a sensory level at T6. She was treated acutely with high-dose intravenous corticosteroids and transferred to a higher level of care.

On initial examination, she was found to have flaccid paralysis bilaterally from T6. On the right, she demonstrated total anesthesia at a T6 level and her left lower extremity sensory examination demonstrated intact light touch and proprioception only. Patellar or ankle muscle stretch reflexes were absent, and Babinski examination was negative.

Spine magnetic resonance imaging (MRI) was conducted and the results demonstrated no evidence of cord compression or injury, no abnormal disk signal, and no Schmorl nodes. Brain MRI with and without contrast revealed no evidence of demyelinating disease or other abnormalities.

Computed tomography of the spine was conducted and revealed no abnormalities. Lumbar puncture was performed and the results revealed neither elevation in cerebrospinal fluid protein nor any white cell abnormalities. Coagulopathy evaluation revealed that factor V Leiden was normal. She tested negative for G20210A mutation (possibly an independent risk factor for spinal cord infarction). Protein S, protein C, cardiolipin antibodies, and homocysteine were all within normal limits. Echocardiogram was negative for valvular abnormalities. The patient is a non-smoker and has never used oral contraceptives.

A diagnosis of fibrocartilaginous embolus was made by exclusion, based on the facts that the patient exhibited paresthesias and paralysis within minutes to hours after sudden, severe back pain; had normal cerebrospinal fluid; and displayed no evidence of underlying disease or prodromal illness. Moreover, there was no evidence of forceful trauma, but the event was probably precipitated by physical exertion. However, collapsed disk space and associated acute cord swelling on MRI were not seen. Follow-up serial imaging with MRI would be suggested in the next week to assess for any progressive changes in her spinal cord.

Introduction

The great majority of studies reporting on the demographics, injury patterns, and functional outcomes in children and adolescents have focused on traumatic spinal cord injury (SCI), rather than non-traumatic etiology. Epidemiologic data from the National SCI Statistical Database reveal that in children less than 15 years of age, 7.7% of all etiologies are classified as 'other' causes, excluding vehicular crashes, violence, sports, and falls (National Spinal Cord Injury Statistical Center 2010). Incidence, demographics, and outcomes for the pediatric and adolescent non-traumatic SCI population have not been well studied. The pathogenesis of non-traumatic SCI in children includes such entities as craniovertebral junction abnormalities, spinal stenosis, vascular ischemia, tumorous compression, and infectious and inflammatory disorders (Box 8.1).

Box 8.1 Causes of non-traumatic spinal cord injury in infants and children

Craniovertebral junction anomalies

- Down syndrome
- Ehlers–Danlos syndrome
- Skeletal dysplasias
  - Achondroplasia
  - Mucopolysaccharidosis
  - Spondyloepiphyseal dysplasia
  - Kniest dysplasia
  - Chondrodysplasia punctata
  - Metatropic dysplasia
  - Metaphyseal chondrodysplasia
  - Larsen syndrome

Vertebral anomalies

- Os odontoideum
- Klippel–Feil syndrome
- Spinal stenosis

Vascular

- Arteriovenous malformation

Inflammatory/infectious etiologies

- Juvenile rheumatoid arthritis

- Inflammation after adenotonsillectomy
- Spinal cord abscess
- Transverse myelitis
- Acute disseminated encephalomyelitis
- Multiple sclerosis

Oncologic

- Intramedullary spinal cord tumors
- Spinal cord compression
  - Extramedullary spinal cord tumors
  - Metastasis
- Radiation fibrosis syndrome

Craniovertebral and cervicomedullary compression

Certain genetic and congenital conditions can predispose the infant or young child to spinal cord damage, from cord compression secondary to associated trauma from birth and delivery or minor trauma during growth and maturation of the spine. The craniovertebral junction (CVJ) has been identified as the most complex joint of the axial skeleton from an anatomical and kinetic point of view (Giussani et al 2009). CVJ instability of non-traumatic origin represents 27% of all of the CVJ instabilities in the pediatric age group (Rahimi et al 2003), and refers to the presence of different anatomical and motion abnormalities of the osteoligamentous elements with an increased risk of developing severe cervicomedullary compressions (Steinmetz et al 2003). Down syndrome, mucopolysaccharidosis, odontoid malformations, achondroplasia, and spondyloepiphyseal and metaphyseal dysplasia are some of the conditions commonly associated with pediatric symptomatic CVJ instability.

ACHONDROPLASIA

Achondroplasia is the most common form of human short-limbed dwarfism, occurring in 1 in 10 000 to 30 000 live births, and is one of a spectrum of diseases caused by mutations in the *FGFR3* gene (Orioli et al 1986, Okudera et al 1994, Deng et al 1996). The *FGFR* gene is a regulator of bone growth, inhibiting proliferation and differentiation of growth plate chondrocytes. Mutations resulting in achondroplasia exaggerate this inhibitory function, resulting in diminished growth of the skull base (Orioli et al 1986, Okudera et al 1994, King et al 2009). Children with achondroplasia are susceptible to hydrocephalus, cervicomedullary compression, spinal canal stenosis (both cervical and lumbar), syringomyelia, and spinal instability (King et al 2009). Defects in endochondral bone formation in the cranial base result in a shortened basicranium, shallow posterior fossa, shortened clivus, and abnormal cranium and spinal relationships (Moorthy and Rajshekhar 2011). Foramen magnum stenosis occurs commonly (Hecht et al 1989, Bagley et al 2006). The foramen magnum dimensions in children without achondroplasia and in symptomatic and asymptomatic children with achondroplasia have been studied and demonstrate that more than 70% of symptomatic children will have foramen magnum dimensions between the mean and two standard deviations below the mean for children with achondroplasia (Hecht et al 1985, 1989). Compression of the cervicomedullary region can result in tetraplegia with associated bladder dysfunction, lower cranial nerve dysfunction including dysphagia, apnea, and associated respiratory difficulties.

Surveillance for CVJ abnormalities and cervicomedullary compression in this population is essential. Initial evaluation is advocated for infants at 6 months of age, including both magnetic resonance imaging (MRI) and polysomnography (King et al 2009). Those children with radiographic abnormality alone, who are otherwise asymptomatic, should undergo re-imaging in 1 year. Indications for surgery include myelopathy with upper motor neuron signs, central apnea, or the presence of syrinx, with evidence of a narrow foramen magnum (King et al 2009). Decompression of the CVJ is the recommended treatment in symptomatic individuals and involves removal of the posterior rim of the foramen magnum up to the medial aspect of the occipital condyles bilaterally and excision of the posterior arch of the atlas (Moorthy and Rajshekhar 2011). Re-operation rates are reported from 9.3% to 11.1% (Bagley et al 2006, King et al 2009).

Individuals with achondroplasia also have short pedicles, small neural foramina, and reduced interpedicular distance and, with age, these individuals are prone to thickening of the ligamentum flavum and subsequent cervical, thoracic, and lumbar canal stenosis (Kopits 1988, Bagley et al 2006). Symptomatic canal stenosis requiring surgery in the pediatric population is thought to be relatively rare (King et al 2009).

Down Syndrome

Craniovertebral junction instability in Down syndrome is caused by laxity of the tectorial membrane and cruciate ligaments, by the presence of an os odontoideum or hypoplasia of various craniovertebral elements (Giussani et al 2009). Atlantoaxial subluxation associated with ligamentous laxity occurs in 14% to 24% of individuals with Down syndrome; however, symptomatic atlantoaxial subluxation is estimated to occur in only 1% of cases (Nader-Sepahi et al 2005). Symptoms associated with subluxation may include neck pain, cervical deformity, or cervicomedullary compression leading to neurologic deficit and even sudden death (Nader-Sepahi et al 2005).

Assessment and screening for atlantoaxial instability has been debated since the 1980s. In 1983, the Special Olympics mandated cervical spine screening with plain lateral and flexion–extension views in all athletes with Down syndrome participating in high-risk sports (Wills and Dormans 2006). However, the American Academy of Pediatrics Committee on Sports Medicine has concluded that 'lateral plain radiographs of the cervical spine are of potential but unproven value in detecting individuals at risk for developing spinal cord injury during sports participation' (American Academy of Pediatrics Committee on Sports Medicine and Fitness 1995). The committee felt a greater priority was identifying those individuals with signs or symptoms consistent with symptomatic SCI. Recommendations on the need and frequency of radiographic screening may vary from clinical sites, but examination of neurologic function should be performed at least annually.

Some controversy exists regarding the treatment of asymptomatic children with Down syndrome found to have atlantoaxial subluxation (Nader-Sepahi et al 2005). Some surgeons use the atlantodens interval as a criterion on which to base the decision to operate. The atlantodens interval is the space between the posterior aspect of the anterior ring of C1 and the anterior border of the odontoid and should be less than 4mm in children younger than 8 years of age and less than 3mm in children older than 8 years of age and throughout adulthood (Steel 1982, Eubanks et al 2006, Wills and Dormans 2006). The correlation between the atlantodens interval and the risk of developing a neurologic deficit, however, is unclear; furthermore, the measurements of the atlantodens interval have been shown to be inconsistent and can vary significantly on repeated radiographs on the same day (Selby et al 1991). The importance of individualized patient assessment in deciding whether to perform occipital cervical arthrodesis in young people with Down syndrome and who have significant asymptomatic upper cervical spine instability cannot be overemphasized (Wills and Dormans 2006). Initial external reduction of the dislocation followed by immediate stabilization with a halo orthosis is a common surgical pathway, particularly in younger children with Down syndrome.

Mucopolysaccharidoses

Mucopolysaccharidoses comprise a group of 11 genetic lysosomal storage disorders that result from the deficiency of one or more of the enzymes required for glycosaminoglycan catabolism (Horovitz et al 2011). Cervical myelopathy is a well-known long-term complication in children with mucopolysaccharidoses, which is usually caused by diffuse thickening of the dura and of the extradural soft tissues in the cervical region, especially the posterior longitudinal ligament, and by posterior indentation by the arch of the atlas (Kaufman et al 1982). Storage of glycosaminoglycans in the dura mater and supporting ligaments, kyphoscoliosis, odontoid hypoplasia, and cervical bony stenosis are thought to be the main causes of myelopathy in mucopolysaccharidoses. MRI is the method of choice to detect spinal cord compression and intramedullary signal abnormalities, but functional assessment may also be warranted, including somatosensory evoked potentials and motor evoked potential studies (Horovitz et al 2011). The C1–C2 instability is nearly universal in Morquio syndrome (mucopolysaccharidoses type IV), and can be effectively treated by posterior occipitocervical arthrodesis (Stevens et al 1991). Children with Morquio syndrome frequently have progressive instability and therefore preventive fusion is often recommended before neurologic symptoms develop (Stevens et al 1991).

Vertebral anomalies

Os Odontoideum

Os odontoideum is a radiographic diagnosis and is defined as an ossicle with smooth circumferential cortical margins and no osseous continuity with the body of C2 (Klimo et al 2008). The incidence of os odontoideum is higher in individuals with conditions characterized by instability at the CVJ, such as Down syndrome, Morquio syndrome, and spondyloepiphyseal dysplasia (Nader-Sepahi et al 2005). This abnormality seems to be related to a traumatic hypermobility of the CVJ that may result in abnormal shearing stresses at the cartilaginous stage of development with an abnormal ossification (Stevens et al 1991, 1994, Klimo et al 2008) (Fig. 8.1). Individuals with this abnormality may be asymptomatic or have neck pain, torticollis, or neurologic symptoms that may develop either acutely or chronically from repeated spinal cord trauma or vertebral artery compromise (Klimo et al 2008). Without a united odontoid

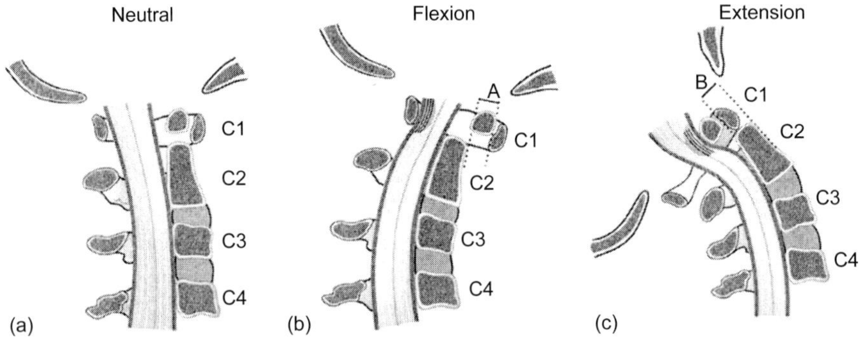

Fig. 8.1 Diagrams depicting an os odontoideum in neutral (a), flexed (b), and extended (c) positions. The ossicle and the ring of C1 move as a unit. The spinal cord may be injured anteriorly by the ossicle if there is excessive movement on extension or posteriorly by the posterior ring of C1 if there is too much movement on flexion. The amount of movement (C1 translation) was calculated as the distance between the posterior cortical margin of the anterior tubercle of C1 and the anterior margin of the C2 vertebral body as indicated by the dotted lines and 'A' or 'B' in panels (b) and (c). With either anterior or posterior instability, this distance increases. Reproduced with permission from Klimo et al (2008).

process, the atlantoaxial joint is supported only by ligamentous structures, which may not be able to tolerate minor stresses. Published reports provide only class III evidence, opinions of respected authorities based on clinical experience, descriptive studies, or reports of expert committees regarding this problem and much of the evidence that is available is contradictory (Klimo et al 2008, American Association of Neurological Surgeons/Congress of Neurological Surgeons Joint Section on Disorders of the Spine and Peripheral Nerves 2002).

Klippel–Feil Syndrome

Klippel–Feil syndrome refers to a spectrum of congenital osseous anomalies of the cervical spine, often with congenital fusion of two or more cervical vertebrae, and is believed to result from faulty segmentation along the embryo's developing axis during weeks 3 to 8 of gestation. The triad of short neck, low posterior hairline, and limitations in cervical motion with associated congenital cervical fusions is seen in less than half of the individuals with this disorder (Herman and Pizzutillo 1999). Decrease in cervical motion, especially lateral bend and rotation, is the most common physical finding (Herman and Pizzutillo 1999). Specific anomalous patterns are classified to identify risk of neurologic compromise. Type I is defined as C2–C3 fusion with occipitalization of the atlas. Type II is a long cervical fusion with an abnormal occipital junction and type III is defined as two blocked vertebral segments with a single open interspace (Hensinger and MacEwen 1982).

Individuals with Klippel–Feil syndrome and cervical stenosis may be at an increased risk of sustaining neurologic deficit after minor trauma. This is probably related to the fused segments and the resultant altered mechanical force transfer that makes the adjacent non-fused segments excessively mobile (Karasick et al 1998). Single-level Klippel–Feil deformity at the C3 level and below with no evidence of instability or stenosis noted on

MRI is a relative contraindication to sports participation (Ellis and Gottlieb 2007). Fusions above C3 and multiple-level Klippel–Feil deformity are absolute contraindications to sports participation (Vaccaro et al 2002, Eddy et al 2005). Surgical intervention is pursued for those individuals with progressive symptomatic segmental instability or the presence of neurologic compromise.

Vascular

Vascular Malformations

Vascular malformations of the spinal cord are a rare cause of spinal cord myelopathy (Madhugiri et al 2013). Most spinal aneurysms do not occur at vascular branching points because spinal vessels are low-flow arteries (Berlis et al 2005). Any process that increases flow through the spinal vessels would predispose the individual to the formation of a spinal aneurysm. In children and adolescents, these conditions include coarctation of the aorta, spinal arteriovenous malformation, and renal transplant, to name a few (Madhugiri et al 2013). Disease processes that cause weakening of the vessel wall (connective tissue disorders, infections, trauma, vasculitis) could also lead to the development of a spinal aneurysm (Madhugiri et al 2013). Spinal cord vascular myelopathies can be divided into intramedullary arteriovenous malformations, perimedullary arteriovenous malformations, spinal–dural arteriovenous fistulas, epidural arteriovenous malformations, paravertebral vascular malformations, vertebral hemangiomas, spinal cord hemangiomas, telangiectasias, venous angiomas, and complex angiomatosis including metameric angiomatosis (Cobb syndrome) and disseminated angiodysplasias (Osler–Weber–Rendu syndrome) (Caragine et al 2002).

Spinal aneurysms can present with a myriad of symptoms, most commonly resulting from hemorrhage. Children and adolescents typically present with backache (with or without radiculopathy, myelopathy, sensory loss, or bladder involvement) or headache (with or without vomiting) (Madhugiri et al 2013). For those who present without associated hemorrhage, children and adolescents can present with a host of different symptoms including scoliosis, patchy sensory loss, or compressive myelopathy-like features.

Selective spinal angiography is the 'criterion standard' for visualization of the intricate vascular anatomy (Caragine et al 2002). The ideal management technique (surgical clipping/excision or endovascular coiling) and the outcome with respect to clinical recovery and spinal aneurysm obliteration rates have not been established, as most descriptions of spinal aneurysms in the literature are reports of single cases and only a few case series have been published (Madhugiri et al 2013).

Infarction

Spinal cord infarction is a rare condition in children and can be caused by decreased blood flow owing to hypotension resulting from vascular injury, compression, thrombosis, or embolization to the spinal arteries. Systemic hypotension leading to spinal cord infarction in children can be caused by cardiac arrest or cardiac tamponade. Surgery on the aorta, particularly in children with congenital heart diseases such as coarctation of the aorta, can also risk subsequent spinal cord myelopathy. Several thrombotic disorders have been reported in cases of spinal cord infarction in children (Young et al 1999, Ramelli et al 2001, Hakimi and Massagli 2005). Diagnostic evaluation should include MRI with both axial and sagittal T1-, T2-, and diffusion-weighted imaging (Nance and Golomb 2007). Evaluating potential etiologies for the infarction will help to determine appropriate treatment.

Fibrocartilaginous Emboli

Spinal cord infarction secondary to fibrocartilaginous embolism (FCE) was once thought to be a rare and usually fatal event (Han et al 2004). FCE myelopathy may be more prevalent than commonly thought, may not typically be fatal, and may actually be the underlying cause in many cases of acute transverse myelitis and anterior spinal syndrome (Han et al 2004). In general, it is agreed that an acute vertical disk herniation can lead to spinal cord infarction via retrograde spread of FCE to the central artery (Han et al 2004). The nucleus pulposus is thought to be the origin of FCE. The nucleus pulposus is a semifluid, fibrocartilaginous cushion considered a remnant of the embryonic notochord (Toro et al 1994). Throughout childhood, the nucleus pulposus transitions from a mucoid, collagenous matrix to fibrocartilage. The pathophysiology of the embolism of this material is unclear, but a number of postulations exist to explain the eventual retrograde embolization of the nucleus pulposus material to the vasculature supplying the anterior spinal cord (Davis and Klug 2000).

Typical presentation of FCE includes rapid onset of weakness often after a sudden onset of severe pain (Toro et al 1994). In a review of most of the cases published thus far, the majority of cases occurred in females (69%) with an age range of 13 to 77 years (Toro et al 1994). Young people seem to be prone to FCE, as vessels can persist in intervertebral discs until adolescence, whereas vascularization is lost at a later age (Beer and Kesselring 2002). Many of the cases reported have no precipitating factor preceding the paralysis. Currently, there are no non-invasive tests to confirm the diagnosis, and the risk of histologic confirmation is too great (Han et al 2004). Imaging the spinal cord with MRI may or may not identify an area of cord ischemia at the time of presentation but should not rule out FCE myelopathy as a cause of symptoms. Short-term serial imaging with MRI has been demonstrated as helpful in assisting with eventual clinical diagnosis of FCE (Davis and Klug 2000, Han et al 2004). Findings including intervertebral disk disease, progressive cord edema, increased T2-weighted signal, and lack of contrast enhancement in the acute phase, and the clinical picture of an acute anterior spinal artery syndrome are suggestive of FCE myelopathy (Davis and Klug 2000). Because there are limited individuals reported in the literature who have been diagnosed ante mortem, there is limited information available as regards treatment recommendations and the spectrum of recovery reported following diagnosis in children (Davis and Klug 2000, Beer and Kesselring 2002, Han et al 2004).

Infectious/inflammatory

Infectious Myelopathies

Although infectious myelopathies in young people are rare, timely and accurate diagnosis is essential for improving outcomes. There is a broad spectrum of potential infectious etiologies of myelopathy, including human immunodeficiency virus, human T-cell lymphotropic virus type 1, herpes viruses (varicella-zoster, herpes simplex type 2, cytomegalovirus), enteroviruses, *Treponema pallidum*, *Mycobacterium tuberculosis*, fungi, and parasites (Berger and Sabet 2002). It is essential when evaluating an individual with myelopathy of unknown etiology to consider their premorbid medical history and to inquire about potential exposures that an individual may have had to organisms known to be associated with myelopathy. Inquiring about recent infections and symptomatology, history or risk of immunodeficiency, travel history, and sexual history are important features of the historical intake. Further diagnostic workup would include neuroimaging with MRI and cerebrospinal fluid studies. Antimicrobial treatment is initiated to treat presumed causes of myelitis, most often after specimens have been obtained for culture.

Spinal epidural abscess may result in myelopathy and is regarded as a surgical emergency. Although a variety of organisms may be etiologic agents, *Staphylococcus aureus* has been demonstrated to be the most likely etiology in over 50% of cases (Kaufman et al 1980). The spread of infection may be directly from a focus of osteomyelitis or hematogenously from a distant site, such as skin furuncles or pulmonary infections (Berger and Sabet 2002). Back pain and fever occur in 70% of individuals with spinal epidural abscess (Reihsaus et al 2000). Radicular involvement is followed by myelopathic symptoms including weakness, sensory loss, and sphincter incontinence (Berger and Sabet 2002). The diagnostic procedure of choice is MRI and treatment typically includes laminectomy and antibiotic therapy.

Acute Transverse Myelitis

Acute transverse myelitis is a rare disorder with about 1400 new cases diagnosed in the USA per year with approximately 20% occurring in individuals younger than 18 years of age (Berman et al 1981, Jeffery et al 1993, Kerr et al 2005). Utilizing criteria developed by the Transverse Myelitis Consortium Working Group, the diagnosis of acute transverse myelitis requires both the presence of spinal cord inflammation, as shown by cerebrospinal fluid pleocytosis, elevated cerebrospinal fluid immunoglobulin G index, or gadolinium enhancement on a spinal MRI, and the absence of an identified central nervous system infection (Therapeutics and Technology Assessment Subcommittee of the American Academy of Neurology 2002). The diagnosis also requires exclusion of acute myelopathy secondary to a known underlying disease and from compressive myelopathies.

The largest reported single case series of 47 individuals under 18 years of age diagnosed with acute transverse myelitis revealed a bimodal presentation of incidence with one peak occurring in toddlers less than 3 years of age and the other in individuals between the ages of 11 and 17 years with males and females being affected equally (Pidcock et al 2007). There was no significant relationship identified between onset of acute transverse myelitis and preceding illness, immunization, or trauma (Pidcock et al 2007). In total, 42 individuals had monophasic idiopathic transverse myelitis, two individuals had recurrent transverse myelitis, and three individuals had transverse myelitis that was later associated with another disease, specifically neuromyelitis optica, acute disseminated encephalomyelitis, and systemic lupus erythematosus (Pidcock et al 2007). Factors associated with a better functional outcome included older age at the time of diagnosis, shorter time to diagnosis, lower sensory and anatomic neurologic levels of SCI, absence of T1 hypointensity on spinal MRI during the acute period, lack of white blood cells in the cerebrospinal fluid, and fewer affected spinal cord segments (Pidcock et al 2007).

In regards to the level of injury, T2 signal abnormalities were identified predominantly in the cervicothoracic levels. Most of the 47 children were noted to have longitudinally extensive transverse myelitis, with an average of six segments affected. Another study of 27 individuals diagnosed with acute transverse myelitis before the age of 18 years demonstrated that 21 individuals had abnormal MRI results and 14 of these 21 had enhancement of three or more segments on spinal MRI (Alper et al 2011). Additionally, all lesions were shown to be centrally located with high signal intensity involving gray matter and occasionally surrounding white matter (Alper et al 2011). Longitudinally extensive transverse myelitis is also reported in association with acute disseminating encephalomyelitis; however, this condition is characterized by multifocal involvement (cerebral, cerebellar, optic nerve, and spinal cord), and therefore isolated spinal cord syndrome is not consistent with acute disseminating encephalomyelitis by definition (Krupp et al 2007).

Transverse myelitis is a result of inflammation in the spinal cord and presents clinically with neurologic dysfunction in motor, sensory, and autonomic nerves. Antecedent febrile illnesses as well as preceding infections have been reported to occur in a number of cases of acute transverse myelitis and it remains to be determined whether parainfectious transverse myelitis is the result of immune-cell targeting of pathogen-related proteins that bear molecular similarity to neural proteins, or whether the heightened immune state that follows recent infection simply increases the pool of circulating T- or B-cell clones that already possess the capacity to recognize neural proteins (Banwell 2007). Although a variety of conditions should be considered, studies reveal that the disease presenting with non-compressive acute spinal cord syndrome in children is most likely to be inflammatory in origin and not associated with another central nervous system or systemic disease (Alper et al 2011). Treatment options for acute transverse myelitis have included intravenous steroids, intravenous immunoglobulin, oral steroids, plasma exchange, and acyclovir with high-dose steroid treatment. Despite the lack of randomized controlled studies, administration of high-dose intravenous corticosteroids should be utilized in individuals with acute transverse myelitis in efforts to hasten recovery, reduce disease activity, and restore neurologic function (Defresne et al 2001, Therapeutics and Technology Assessment Subcommittee of the American Academy of Neurology 2011). Plasma exchange may be considered in individuals with acute transverse myelitis who fail to improve after corticosteroid treatment (Therapeutics and Technology Assessment Subcommittee of the American Academy of Neurology 2011).

The functional evolution of acute transverse myelitis after its nadir is roughly divided into three groups: one-third completely recovers, one-third has some improvement but has residual symptoms, and the remaining group has no improvement at all (Ropper and Poskanzer 1978). In Pidcock's case series of 33 individuals, at an average of 8 years' follow-up, 21 were independent with transfers, 22 were independent with mobility (either walking or with the propulsion of a manual wheelchair), 24 were independent with self-care skills, and 15 were independent with sphincter control. Impaired bladder control has been demonstrated to be the most common long-term neurologic deficit following acute transverse myelitis (Defresne et al 2003, Pidcock et al 2007).

Oncologic

Spinal Cord Tumors

Tumors of the central nervous system constitute the second most prevalent type of cancer in children and the most common solid tumor in children. Intrinsic tumors of the spinal cord make up 1% to 10% of pediatric central nervous system tumors (Allen et al 1998, Lonjon et al 1998, Nadkarni and Rekate 1999). These tumors occur throughout childhood, and the median age at diagnosis is 10 years (Blaney et al 2011). The gross classification of spinal tumors based on anatomic location can be divided into three discrete areas: extradural tumors and intradural tumors (which are then subdivided into extramedullary and intramedullary) (Wilson et al 2007). The most common spinal cord tumors are intramedullary (Wilson et al 2007). In children, 60% of intramedullary tumors are astrocytomas and 30% are ependymomas. Tumor anatomic location in the spinal cord appears to be random, with the incidence in each anatomic region (cervical, thoracic, lumbar) roughly proportional to the length of that region (Blaney et al 2011). The only exception is the myxopapillary ependymoma, which has a predilection for the conus medullaris and filum terminale (Blaney et al 2011).

The small number of participants and relative lack of inclusion in clinical trials with prescribed treatment approaches makes the identification of prognostic factors difficult (Blaney et al 2011). One study reviewed the experience of 13 French treatment centers with spinal cord astrocytoma and found high-grade histology and short duration of presenting symptoms to be associated with poorer prognosis (Bouffet et al 1998).

The spinal cord and cauda equina may be compressed by tumor in the epidural or subarachnoid space or, less commonly, by metastatic spread to the cord parenchyma (Fisher and Rheingold 2011). Metastatic involvement of the vertebral bodies and secondary compression of the spinal cord, common in adults with cancer, is rare in childhood (Boogerd and van der Sande 1993). Spinal cord compression resulting from epidural metastases can result in significant morbidity in children with advanced cancer.

Epidural compression may occur with a known malignancy or may be the presenting symptom of an undiagnosed malignancy. One study, documenting rates of spinal cord compression secondary to metastasis, found evidence of compression in 6% of all children treated for all types of cancer over a 17-year time period (Pollono et al 2003). Initial symptoms in this population resulting from compression were motor dysfunction with paresis, radicular or back pain, and alterations in sensation. The etiologic tumors responsible for metastatic spinal cord compression included extradural tumors, which were the most common primary tumor. Sarcomas account for the majority of spinal cord metastases (Ewing sarcoma 19.9%, osteosarcoma 6.5%, rhabdomyosarcoma, soft-tissue sarcoma 3.9%), with neuroblastoma (7.9%), germ cell tumors (3.8%), Hodgkin disease (2%), and dropped metastases from primary central nervous system tumors accounting for most of the remainder (Klein et al 1991).

Local or radicular back pain occurs in 80% of children with cord compression and is often worse at night and when the individual lies flat (Lewis et al 1986). Children with back pain and systemic cancer should be considered to have spinal cord compression until proven otherwise. Pain can start weeks to months before diagnosis of the primary cancer (Fisher and Rheingold 2011). Other symptoms of cord compression can include weakness, sensory impairment, and bowel and/or bladder incontinence. MRI is the criterion standard for diagnosis (Fisher and Rheingold 2011).

Early intervention can lead to improved functional outcomes. Corticosteroid therapy reduces cord edema and pain and may improve overall outcome after specific antineoplastic therapy (Sorensen et al 1994, Abrahm 1999). If the diagnosis is known and the tumor is radioresponsive, radiation therapy is often the treatment of choice. In addition, for children able to undergo surgery, laminectomy may also relieve the effects of spinal cord compression (Ullrich et al 2011). A clear indication for surgery is an unknown primary tumor, particularly in those without known dissemination, and it offers the dual benefit of decompression plus identification of the tumor type (Fisher and Rheingold 2011).

Radiation Myelopathy

Myelopathy is a potential complication following radiation to the spinal cord and individuals will present with progressive spastic paraplegia or tetraplegia depending on the level of the spinal cord irradiated. It usually has a subtle onset after a latency of more than 5 to 6 months but can occur up to several years after treatment (New 2001, Blaney et al 2011). Craniospinal irradiation is commonly used in children, although dose levels to the entire spine rarely approach or exceed the 44Gy level identified as 'safe' in the USA using conventional fractionation (Emami et al 1991, Schultheiss et al 1995). With contemporary three-dimensional image-guided irradiation for low-lying posterior fossa lesions, subacute white matter lesions can occur in the cervicomedullary or upper cervical cord regions (Fouladi et al 2004). Although most subacute effects are transitory, such changes can be associated with permanent neurologic signs and symptoms (Blaney et al 2011). Awareness of the long-term effects of radiation treatment is useful to consider in a differential diagnosis for progressive weakness, especially when evaluation of the spinal cord by imaging reveals no progressive compression or other changes to explain the deficits.

Damage to white matter (and sometimes dorsal root ganglion) is associated with diffuse demyelination, swollen axons, and vascular necrosis (McKinley 2009). The pathogenesis of radiation myelopathy involves postmitotic cell death of endothelial cells or oligodendrocytes, which subsequently induces a complex pathophysiological reaction in which the response of surviving cells may contribute to the impact of radiation on tissue integrity and functions (Blaney et al 2011). Owing to the resulting increased vascular permeability, this increased expression of tissue factors and increased thrombin formation occurs intravascularly, in the perivascular areas, and within the extracellular matrix (Stubblefield 2009). It is the abnormal accumulation of thrombin in both the intravascular and extravascular compartments that is responsible for the progressive fibrotic tissue sclerosis that characterizes radiation fibrosis and underlies the radiation fibrosis syndrome (Stubblefield 2009). There is no cure for the progressive fibrotic sclerosis that occurs as a result of radiation treatment and, thus, there is no cure for radiation fibrosis syndrome (Stubblefield 2009).

Summary

Etiologies of non-traumatic SCI in children are extensive with both congenital and acquired medical conditions. Assessment and medical management of spinal cord dysfunction as a result of all of these etiologies should mirror the care given to children with traumatic etiologies (see Chapter 21). Although developed for traumatic injuries and not well established for non-traumatic injuries, the International Standards for Neurological Classification of children with Spinal Cord Injury should be utilized for assessment of neurologic level of injury (see Chapter 4) as well as evaluation of autonomic function. With many of the etiologies having the potential for progressive disease, the standardized examination will allow the clinician to objectively assess for neurologic progression and be prepared for the possibility of medical complications associated with progression in spinal cord dysfunction.

REFERENCES

Abrahm JL (1999) Management of pain and spinal cord compression in patients with advanced cancer. ACP-ASIM End-of-life Care Consensus Panel. American College of Physicians – American Society of Internal Medicine. *Ann Intern Med* 131: 37–46. http://dx.doi.org/10.7326/0003-4819-131-1-199907060-00009

Allen JC, Aviner S, Yates A et al (1998) Treatment of high-grade spinal cord astrocytoma of childhood with '8-in-1' chemotherapy and radiotherapy: a pilot study of CCG-945. Children's Cancer Group. *J Neurosurg* 88: 215–20. http://dx.doi.org/10.3171/jns.1998.88.2.0215

Alper G, Petropoulou KA, Fitz CR, Kim Y (2011) Idiopathic acute transverse myelitis in children: an analysis and discussion of MRI findings. *Mult Scler* 17: 74–80. doi: 10.1177/1352458510381393.

American Academy of Pediatrics Committee on Sports Medicine and Fitness (1995) Atlantoaxial instability in Down syndrome: subject review. *Pediatrics* 96: 151–4.

American Association of Neurological Surgeons/Congress of Neurological Surgeons Joint Section on Disorders of the Spine and Peripheral Nerves (2002) Os odontoideum. *Neurosurgery* 50: S148–55.

Bagley CA, Pindrik JA, Bookland MJ, Camara-Quintana JQ, Carson BS (2006) Cervicomedullary decompression for foramen magnum stenosis in achondroplasia. *J Neurosurg* 104: 166–72.

Banwell BL (2007) The long (-itudinally extensive) and the short of it: transverse myelitis in children. *Neurology* 68: 1447–9. doi: 10.1212/01.wnl.0000264553.99997.45

Beer S, Kesselring J (2002) Fibrocartilaginous embolisation of the spinal cord in a 7-year-old girl. *J Neurol* 249: 936–7. http://dx.doi.org/10.1007/s00415-002-0713-5

Berger JR, Sabet A (2002) Infectious myelopathies. *Semin Neurol* 22: 133–42. http://dx.doi.org/10.1055/s-2002-36536

Berlis A, Scheufler KM, Schmahl C, Rauer S, Gotz F, Schumacher M (2005) Solitary spinal artery aneurysms as a rare source of spinal subarachnoid hemorrhage: potential etiology and treatment strategy. *AJNR Am J Neuroradiol* 26: 405–10.

Berman M, Feldman S, Alter M, Zilber N, Kahana E (1981) Acute transverse myelitis: incidence and etiologic considerations. *Neurology* 31: 966–71. http://dx.doi.org/10.1212/WNL31.8.966

Blaney S, Haas-Kogan D, Poussaint T et al (2011) Gliomas ependymomas and other nonembyonal tumors of the central nervous system. In: Pizzo P, Poplack D (eds). *Principles and Practice of Pediatric Oncology*. 6th Ed. Philadephia, PA: Lippincott Williams & Wilkins.

Boogerd W, van Der Sande JJ (1993) Diagnosis and treatment of spinal cord compression in malignant disease. *Cancer Treat Rev* 19: 129–50. doi: 10.1016/0305-7372(93)90031-L

Bouffet E, Pierre-Kahn A, Marchal JC et al (1998) Prognostic factors in pediatric spinal cord astrocytoma. *Cancer* 83: 2391–9. doi: 10.1002/(SICI)1097-0142(19981201)83: 11<2391::AID-CNCR20>3.0.CO;2-0

Caragine LP Jr, Halbach VV, Ng PP, Dowd CF (2002) Vascular myelopathies-vascular malformations of the spinal cord: presentation and endovascular surgical management. *Semin Neurol* 22: 123–32. http://dx.doi.org/10.1055/s-2002-36535

Davis G, Klug G (2000) Acute-onset nontraumatic paraplegia in childhood: fibrocartilagenous embolism or acute myelitis? *Childs Nerv Syst* 16: 551–4. http://dx.doi.org/10.1007/s003810000268

Defresne P, Meyer L, Tardieu M et al (2001) Efficacy of high dose steroid therapy in children with severe acute transverse myelitis. *J Neurol Neurosurg Psychiatry* 71: 272–4. doi: 10.1136/jnnp.71.2.272

Defresne P, Hollenberg H, Husson B et al (2003) Acute transverse myelitis in children: clinical course and prognostic factors. *J Child Neurol* 18: 401–6. http://dx.doi.org/10.1177/08830738030180060601

Deng C, Wynshaw-Boris A, Zhou F, Kuo A, Leder P (1996) Fibroblast growth factor receptor 3 is a negative regulator of bone growth. *Cell* 84: 911–21. http://dx.doi.org/10.1016/S0092-8674(00)81069-7

Eddy D, Congeni J, Loud K (2005) A review of spine injuries and return to play. *Clin J Sport Med* 15: 453–8. http://dx.doi.org/10.1097/01.jsm.0000186681.13416.0c

Ellis JL, Gottlieb JE (2007) Return-to-play decisions after cervical spine injuries. *Curr Sports Med Rep* 6: 56–61.

Emami B, Lyman J, Brown A et al (1991) Tolerance of normal tissue to therapeutic irradiation. *Int J Radiat Oncol Biol Phys* 21: 109–22. http://dx.doi.org/10.1016/0360-3016(91)90171-Y

Eubanks JD, Gilmore A, Bess S, Cooperman DR (2006) Clearing the pediatric cervical spine following injury. *J Am Acad Orthop Surg* 14: 552–64.

Fisher M, Rheingold S (2011) Oncologic emergencies. In: Pizzo P, Poplack D (eds). *Principles and Practice of Pediatric Oncology*. 6th Ed. Philadelphia, PA: Lippincott Williams & Wilkins.

Fouladi M, Chintagumpala M, Laningham FH et al (2004) White matter lesions detected by magnetic resonance imaging after radiotherapy and high-dose chemotherapy in children with medulloblastoma or primitive neuroectodermal tumor. *J Clin Oncol* 22: 4551–60. http://dx.doi.org/10.1200/JCO(2004)03.058

Giussani C, Roux FE, Guerra P et al (2009) Severely symptomatic craniovertebral junction abnormalities in children: long-term reliability of aggressive management. *Pediatr Neurosurg* 45: 29–36. doi: 10.1159/00020(2621)

Hakimi K, Massagli T (2005) Anterior spinal artery syndrome in two children with genetic thrombotic disorders. *J Spinal Cord Med* 28: 69–73.

Han J, Massagli T, Jaffe K (2004) Fibrocartilagenous embolism – an uncommon cause of spinal cord infarction: a case report and review of literature. *Arch Phys Med Rehabil* 85: 153–7. http://dx.doi.org/10.1016/S0003-9993(03)00289-2

Hecht JT, Nelson FW, Butler IJ et al (1985) Computerized tomography of the foramen magnum: achondroplastic values compared to normal standards. *Am J Med Genet* 20: 355–60. http://dx.doi.org/10.1002/ajmg.1320200219

Hecht JT, Horton WA, Reid CS, Pyeritz RE, Chakraborty R (1989) Growth of the foramen magnum in achondroplasia. *Am J Med Genet* 32: 528–35. http://dx.doi.org/10.1002/ajmg.1320320421

Hensinger R, MacEwen G (1982) Congenital anomalies of the spine. In: RH, R FA, S (eds). *The Spine*. Philadelphia, PA: WB Saunders.

Herman MJ, Pizzutillo PD (1999) Cervical spine disorders in children. *Orthop Clin North Am* 30: 457–66, ix. http://dx.doi.org/10.1016/S0030-5898(05)70098-5

Horovitz DD, Magalhaes Tde S, Pena e Costa A et al (2011) Spinal cord compression in young children with type VI, mucopolysaccharidosis. *Mol Genet Metab* 104: 295–300. doi: 10.1016/j.ymgme.(2011)07.019

Jeffery DR, Mandler RN, Davis LE (1993) Transverse myelitis. Retrospective analysis of 33 cases with differentiation of cases associated with multiple sclerosis and parainfectious events. *Arch Neurol* 50: 532–5. http://dx.doi.org/10.1001/archneur.(1993)00540050074019

Karasick D, Schweitzer ME, Vaccaro AR (1998) The traumatized cervical spine in Klippel–Feil syndrome: imaging features. *AJR Am J Roentgenol* 170: 85–8. http://dx.doi.org/10.2214/ajr.170.1.9423605

Kaufman DM, Kaplan JG, Litman N (1980) Infectious agents in spinal epidural abscesses. *Neurology* 30: 844–50. http://dx.doi.org/10.1212/WNL30.8.844

Kaufman HH, Rosenberg HS, Scott CI, Lee YY, Pruessner JL, Butler IJ (1982) Cervical myelopathy due to dural compression in mucopolysaccharidosis. *Surg Neurol* 17: 404–10. http://dx.doi.org/10.1016/S0090-3019(82)80004-9

Kerr D, Krishnan C, Pidcock F (2005) Acute transverse myelitis. In: Singer H, Kossoff E, Hartman A, Crawford T (eds). *Treatment of Pediatric Neurologic Disorders*. Boca Raton, FL: Taylor & Francis. http://dx.doi.org/10.1201/b14120-65

King JA, Vachhrajani S, Drake JM, Rutka JT (2009) Neurosurgical implications of achondroplasia. *J Neurosurg Pediatr* 4: 297–306. doi: 10.3171/(2009)3.PEDS08344.

Klein SL, Sanford RA, Muhlbauer MS (1991) Pediatric spinal epidural metastases. *J Neurosurg* 74: 70–5. http://dx.doi.org/10.3171/jns.(1991)74.1.0070

Klimo P Jr, Kan P, Rao G, Apfelbaum R, Brockmeyer D (2008) Os odontoideum: presentation diagnosis and treatment in a series of 78 patients. *J Neurosurg Spine* 9: 332–42. doi: 10.3171/SPI(2008)9.10.332.

Kopits SE (1988) Orthopedic aspects of achondroplasia in children. *Basic Life Sci* 48: 189–97.

Krupp LB, Banwell B, Tenembaum S (2007) Consensus definitions proposed for pediatric multiple sclerosis and related disorders. *Neurology* 68: S7–12. http://dx.doi.org/10.1212/01.wnl.0000259422.44235.a8

Lewis DW, Packer RJ, Raney B, Rak IW, Belasco J, Lange B (1986) Incidence presentation and outcome of spinal cord disease in children with systemic cancer. *Pediatrics* 78: 438–43.

Lonjon M, Goh KY, Epstein FJ (1998) Intramedullary spinal cord ependymomas in children: treatment results and follow-up. *Pediatr Neurosurg* 29: 178–83. http://dx.doi.org/10.1159/000028718

McKinley W (2009) Rehabilitation of patients with spinal cord dysfunction in the cancer setting. In: Stubblefield M, O'Dell M (eds). *Cancer Rehabilitation, Principles and Practice*. New York, NY: Demos Medical Publishing.

Madhugiri VS, Ambekar S, Roopesh Kumar VR, Sasidharan GM, Nanda A (2013) Spinal aneurysms: clinicoradiological features and management paradigms. *J Neurosurg Spine* 19: 34–48. doi: 10.3171/(2013)3. SPINE12(1026)

Moorthy R, Rajshekhar V (2011) Craniovertebral junction abnormalities associated with metabolic and genetic disorders. In: Goel A, Cacciola F (eds). *The Craniovertebral Junction: Diagnosis, Pathology, Surgical Techniques*. New York, NY: Georg Thieme Varlag.

Nader-Sepahi A, Casey AT, Hayward R, Crockard HA, Thompson D (2005) Symptomatic atlantoaxial instability in Down syndrome. *J Neurosurg* 103: 231–7.

Nadkarni TD, Rekate HL (1999) Pediatric intramedullary spinal cord tumors. Critical review of the literature. *Childs Nerv Syst* 15: 17–28. http://dx.doi.org/10.1007/s003810050321

Nance JR, Golomb M (2007) Ischemic spinal cord infarction in children without vertebral fracture. *Pediatr Neurol* 36: 209–16. doi: 10.1016/j.pediatrneurol.(2007)01.006

National Spinal Cord Injury Statistical Center (2010) The 2010 Annual Statistical Report for the Spinal Cord Injury Model Systems. Birmingham, AL: National Spinal Cord Injury Statistical Center.

New P (2001) Radiation injury to the nervous system. *Curr Opin Neurol* 14: 725–34. http://dx.doi.org/10.1097/00019052-200112000-00008

Okudera T, Huang Y, Ohta T et al (1994) Development of posterior fossa dural sinuses emissary veins and jugular bulb: morphological and radiologic study. *Am J Neuroradiol* 15: 1871–83.

Oriolli M, Castilla F, Barbosa-Neto J (1986) The birth prevalence rates for the skeletal dysplasias. *J Med Genet* 23: 328–32. http://dx.doi.org/10.1136/jmg.23.4.328

Pidcock F, Krishnan C, Crawford T, Salorio C, Trovato M, Kerr D (2007) Acute transverse myelitis in childhood: center-based analysis of 47 cases. *Neurology* 68: 1474–80. http://dx.doi.org/10.1212/01.wnl.0000260609.1(1357)6f

Pollono D, Tomarchia S, Drut R, Ibanez O, Ferreyra M, Cedola J (2003) Spinal cord compression: a review of 70 pediatric patients. *Pediatr Hematol Oncol* 20: 457–66. http://dx.doi.org/10.1080/08880010390220126

Rahimi S, Stevens E, Yeh D, Flannery A, Choudhri H, Lee M (2003) Treatment of atlantoaxial instability in pediatric patients. *Neurosurg Focus* 15: ECP1. http://dx.doi.org/10.3171/foc.(2003)15.6.7

Ramelli G, Wyttenbach R, Cvon der Weid N, Ozdoba C (2001) Anterior spinal artery syndrome in an adolescent with protein S, deficiency. *J Child Neurol* 16: 134–5. http://dx.doi.org/10.1177/088307380101600213

Reihsaus E, Waldbaur H, Seeling W (2000) Spinal epidural abscess: a meta-analysis of 915 patients. *Neurosurg Rev* 23: 175–204; discussion 205. http://dx.doi.org/10.1007/PL00011954

Ropper A, Poskanzer D (1978) The prognosis of acute and subacute transverse myelopathy based on early signs and symptoms. *Ann Neurol* 4: 51–9. http://dx.doi.org/10.1002/ana.410040110

Schultheiss TE, Kun LE, Ang KK, Stephens LC (1995) Radiation response of the central nervous system. *Int J Radiat Oncol Biol Phys* 31: 1093–112. http://dx.doi.org/10.1016/0360-3016(94)00655-5

Selby KA, Newton RW, Gupta S, Hunt L (1991) Clinical predictors and radiological reliability in atlantoaxial subluxation in Down's syndrome. *Arch Dis Child* 66: 876–8. http://dx.doi.org/10.1136/adc.66.7.876

Sorensen S, Helweg-Larsen S, Mouridsen H, Hansen HH (1994) Effect of high-dose dexamethasone in carcinomatous metastatic spinal cord compression treated with radiotherapy: a randomised trial. *Eur J Cancer* 30A: 22–7. http://dx.doi.org/10.1016/S0959-8049(05)80011-5

Steel H (1982) Anatomical and mechanical considerations of the atlanto-axial articulation. *J Bone Joint Surg Br* 64: 422–8.

Steinmetz MP, Lechner RM, Anderson JS (2003) Atlantooccipital dislocation in children: presentation diagnosis and management. *Neurosurg Focus* 14: ecp1. http://dx.doi.org/10.3171/foc.(2003)14.2.11

Stevens JM, Kendall BE, Crockard HA, Ransford A (1991) The odontoid process in Morquio-Brailsford's disease. The effects of occipitocervical fusion. *J Bone Joint Surg Br* 73: 851–8.

Stevens JM, Chong WK, Barber C, Kendall BE, Crockard HA (1994) A new appraisal of abnormalities of the odontoid process associated with atlanto-axial subluxation and neurological disability. *Brain* 117: 133–48. http://dx.doi.org/10.1093/brain/117.1.133

Stubblefield M (2009) Radiation fibrosis syndrome. In: Stubblefield M, O'Dell M (eds). *Cancer Rehabilitation, Principles and Practice*. New York, NY: Demos Medical Publishing.

Therapeutics and Technology Assessment Subcommittee of the American Academy of Neurology (2002) Proposed diagnostic criteria and nosology of acute transverse myelitis. *Neurology* 59: 499–505. http://dx.doi.org/10.1212/WNL59.4.499

Therapeutics and Technology Assessment Subcommittee of the American Academy of Neurology (2011) Evidence-based guideline: clinical evaluation and treatment of transverse myelitis. *Neurology* 77: 2128–34. doi: 10.1212/WNL0b013e31823dc535

Toro G, Roman GC, Navarro-Roman L, Cantillo J, Serrano B, Vergara I (1994) Natural history of spinal cord infarction caused by nucleus pulposus embolism. *Spine (Phila Pa 1976)* 19: 360–6.

Ullrich C, Sourkes B, Wolfe J (2011) Palliative care for the child with cancer. In: Pizzo P, Poplack D (eds). *Principles and Practice of Pediatric Oncology*. 6th Ed. Philadelphia, PA: Lippincott Williams & Wilkins.

Vaccaro AR, Klein GR, Ciccoti M et al (2002) Return to play criteria for the athlete with cervical spine injuries resulting in stinger and transient quadriplegia/paresis. *Spine J* 2: 351–6. http://dx.doi.org/10.1016/S1529-9430(02)00202-4

Wills BP, Dormans JP (2006) Nontraumatic upper cervical spine instability in children. *J Am Acad Orthop Surg* 14: 233–45.

Wilson PE, Oleszek JL, Clayton GH (2007) Pediatric spinal cord tumors and masses. *J Spinal Cord Med* 30(Suppl 1): S15–20.

Young G, Krohn K, Packer R (1999) Prothrombin g20210a mutation in a child with spinal cord infarction. *J Pediatr* 134: 777–9. http://dx.doi.org/10.1016/S0022-3476(99)70298-2

9
MANAGEMENT OF HIGH TETRAPLEGIA

Virginia Simson Nelson

Case vignette

Rachel is a 3-year-old female who sustained a C2 complete spinal cord injury in a motor vehicle crash in which her mother died. For the first 2 months after her injury, she was critically ill and was cared for in the pediatric intensive care unit during which time she required continuous mechanical ventilation, underwent tracheostomy and gastrostomy tube placements, and experienced several bouts of pneumonia. During this time, the focus of the healthcare providers and her father was survival. It was not until she was transferred to the in-patient rehabilitation floor 2 months after the injury that the father asked the question out loud: 'Now what?'.

Introduction

Children with high spinal cord injury (SCI) (C4 and higher) present unique problems, both at the time of the initial injury and during rehabilitation and follow-up. These children will have respiratory problems because innervation of the diaphragm and intercostal muscles is either absent or decreased, depending on the level and completeness of the injury. There are various opinions in the medical and rehabilitation communities about whether or not long-term mechanical ventilation should be offered and whether parents should be given a choice of long-term ventilation or withdrawing support. These children often require resuscitation at the scene of the accident, before details of the extent of the injury are known. Once the complete situation is known, should the parents (and children if they are old enough) be given a choice about long-term mechanical ventilation or should the medical team make such a choice? Ultimately, a shared decision-making approach is prudent. This discussion must take place before further medical treatment and rehabilitation can proceed. Information that must be provided within the discussion includes:

- the extent of the injury and prognosis for recovery and life;
- what home management will entail, including knowledge that caregivers must learn, equipment that will be necessary, and resources that will be available to the child and family;

- the schedule to be followed in training the caregivers before they can take their child home.

Issues unique to children with high tetraplegia are airway management, ventilator management, the developmental impact of being dependent on a machine for life support, and the impact of a tracheostomy on swallowing and communication. Since these children will be completely dependent on caregivers and equipment, they will also have the psychological impact of never being alone or without a trained adult present. Children with motor complete high tetraplegia will also have minimal to no arm function, and thus will be dependent on technology or others to manipulate their environment.

Mechanical ventilation

Complete details of mechanical ventilation are beyond the scope of this chapter. Rehabilitation professionals must understand the mechanics of respiration, the equipment available, the procedures necessary to keep the child healthy, and what must be done to optimize the child's quality of life as a person with both high tetraplegia and ventilator dependence. The goals of respiratory management both during in-patient rehabilitation and when the child is at home are to prevent complications such as pneumonia and atelectasis and to maximize respiratory function for well-being and communication.

Respiratory Mechanics

Quiet respiration is primarily accomplished by the diaphragm, which is innervated by C3, C4, and C5 spinal nerves. When the diaphragm contracts, air is drawn in. Exhalation is primarily passive. During exercise, intercostal and neck muscles (primarily the sternocleidomastoid and scalene muscles) move the ribs outward during inspiration. The abdominal muscles assist expiration. Coughing is also assisted by contraction of the abdominal muscles. A child with complete tetraplegia at C2 or higher will have no function of the diaphragm, or intercostal or abdominal muscles of respiration. Neck muscles may be weak or non-functional. Thus, respiration will need to be supported 24 hours a day. Children with injuries at C3–C4 may have partial function of these muscles, which may mean that they can sustain unsupported respiration while awake but not when asleep. There are two basic types of respiratory problems: intrinsic lung disease (obstructive lung disease) and restrictive lung disease ('bellows failure'), which is caused by muscular or skeletal problems such as neuromuscular scoliosis or weak chest muscles. Restrictive lung disease caused by weak intercostal muscles reduces functional lung volume, causing shallow breathing or reduced tidal volume.

Types of Respiratory Support

Respiratory support can be either non-invasive (delivered via a face or nasal mask or mouthpiece) or invasive (delivered via a tracheostomy). Phrenic or diaphragm pacers may also be used, but are still not widely available for those children requiring full-time ventilation. The first article on the use of diaphragm pacing in children with SCI was published in 2011 (Onders et al 2011), the results of which suggest that these systems show promise for the future. Earlier articles have been published about the use of diaphragm or phrenic pacing in adults with childhood-onset SCI (Onders et al 2007). Table 9.1 provides some information about each of these types of support.

There are several types of tracheostomy tubes, including cuffed and uncuffed. A cuffed tube is designed to seal the tracheostomy so that all air delivered by the ventilator goes to the lungs and none escapes around the tube, over the larynx, and through the mouth and nose. This type of tube makes phonation difficult or impossible. If the child can be adequately ventilated with either an uncuffed tube or the cuff deflated, this is preferable so the child can phonate.

There are several types of portable ventilators that can be used in the community setting, such as the LTV ventilator (Care Fusion/Pulmonetics, San Diego, CA; http://www.carefusion.com/medical-products/respiratory/ventilation/) and Trilogy ventilator (Phillips/respironics, Murraysville, PA; http://trilogy100.respironics.com/). There are other, older, brands of mechanical ventilators, which are no longer used in the USA but are still in use in developing countries. As with most technologies, advancements are made and newer types of ventilators are seen every few years. Ventilators may support respiration via volume or pressure or both. These ventilators may be used via tracheostomy (invasive ventilation), face mask, or mouthpiece (non-invasive).

Continuous positive airway pressure or bilevel positive airway pressure devices are designed to support respiration by continuous pressure, thus keeping the airways open. Continuous positive airway pressure devices provide one level of continuous positive airway pressure; BiPap devices provide both inspiratory and expiratory positive airway pressure and may provide a breath rate. They are typically used in obstructive sleep apnea or to rest weakened muscles during sleep in those with muscle disorders. They do not have internal batteries, which limits their use to times when the person using them is near an electrical outlet.

TABLE 9.1
Types of ventilation

Type	Indications	Limitations	Advantages
Mask: positive pressure (may be nasal mask, nasal–mouth mask, or full-face mask). May be done with ventilator, or continuous positive airway pressure or bilevel positive airway pressure unit	Support for child with weak respiratory muscles who needs part-time support (e.g. at night)	Not applicable for child with no respiratory effort or who needs 24h ventilation	No tracheostomy Better humidification than through tracheostomy
Tracheostomy: positive pressure	Airway problems Need for full ventilator support	Tracheostomy imposes changes in lifestyle (e.g. no swimming)	Direct access to trachea for suctioning
Phrenic or diaphragm pacers	Ability to ventilate with electrical stimulation of phrenic nerves or diaphragm	Not widely available Usually does not eliminate need for tracheostomy	May not adequately ventilate child with scoliosis or who requires full ventilator support

The type of ventilation will be decided upon by the intensive care physician or pulmonologist before the child's transfer to the rehabilitation service. The device that is chosen will impact the design of the child's wheelchair, since his or her wheelchair will become a 'traveling intensive care unit', supporting the child, ventilator, suction machine, and any ancillary equipment (see Chapter 22). For children who are dependent on mechanical ventilation all of the time, there must be a back-up ventilator in the home for emergency use. Typically, one of these ventilators is used during the day on the wheelchair and the other at night at the bedside. There must also be a back-up suction machine for emergency use. A care plan must be made for those times when power is lost, which typically will be some type of generator. Portable ventilators have internal batteries that power the ventilator from 1 to 5 hours. An auto battery can be added to the set-up to extend the power time to approximately 12 hours. Humidifier units used with bedside ventilators do not typically have any internal battery and must be plugged in for use.

Management of Children who use Ventilation During Rehabilitation

Respiratory management during the stay in the intensive care unit will be aimed at getting the child healthy and medically stable (see Chapter 6). Once the child is able to begin intensive rehabilitation, attention needs to be paid daily to the pulmonary status. This includes physical examination, monitoring of oxygen saturation (Spo_2), and transcutaneous ($Ptcco_2$) or end-tidal carbon dioxide ($ETco_2$). Radiographs lag behind clinical symptoms of pneumonia, so careful monitoring of clinical status is more important than 'routine' chest radiographs. Daily pulmonary management may include airway clearance techniques (percussion and drainage or high-frequency chest wall oscillation, commonly called a therapy vest), mechanical insufflator/exsufflator, and possibly bronchodilators, inhaled steroids, and dornase alfa. Percussion and drainage or the therapy vest are used to loosen secretions that can then be either coughed up or suctioned out. The mechanical insufflator/exsufflator provides a breath then sucks it out, pulling out secretions at the same time. This is useful in the child who cannot effectively cough out secretions because of weakened or paralyzed muscles. For most children with SCI in the cervical or high thoracic areas, use of one or more of these techniques, at least during times of respiratory illness, is necessary to maintain pulmonary health.

Weaning from the ventilator may be possible for some children with high tetraplegia, especially those who have a C4 level of motor function or those with American Spinal Injury Association Impairment Scale (AIS) grade D classification. Weaning should not start until the child is medically stable and can tolerate a full rehabilitation program (or full community activity if the child is at home). Weaning may be accomplished either with 'sprinting' off the ventilator or by changing the child to pressure support (which increases the work of breathing the child must do). Because weaning is a form of muscle strengthening, it must follow general principles of exercise to gradually build up strength. The child must be monitored closely, following vital signs, Spo_2, $ETco_2$, activity level, and the child's appearance. Initial weaning should not occur during therapies that require more energy and endurance than resting in bed or in the wheelchair. Weans should begin at 5 to 10 minutes several times a day and should be stopped if the child is tired or develops atelectasis or cannot participate in therapies. Weaning should initially be done with one-to-one attention from a trained staff member, such as a respiratory therapist or nurse.

Policies and practices vary regarding whether children who use invasive mechanical ventilation must be accommodated on the rehabilitation unit. One model is that a pulmonologist and a physiatrist concurrently care for these children. All staff members must be fully trained in tracheostomy and ventilator management before working with these patients, with training updated annually. Training includes suctioning, bagging, changing the tracheostomy, basic operation of the ventilator, and trouble-shooting problems. Staff members who are not trained must have a trained staff member or trained parent present for the therapy session. Children who are ventilated non-invasively may be cared for on the rehabilitation unit, and, if they use a full-face mask, they must be able to remove it independently. Non-invasive ventilation is used for a child who can breathe independently, and is thus 'safe' should the ventilator fail to function. A child who uses a full-face mask covering the nose and mouth and who cannot independently remove the mask because of age, cognitive, or physical status is at risk of aspiration should he or she vomit. In that situation, the child would need immediate attention, which is not typically available around the clock on rehabilitation units. Non-invasive ventilation should never be used in a child who cannot breathe on his or her own. A rate added to BiPap ventilation may assist with supporting ventilation, but this does not substitute for full ventilator support in a child unable to breathe at all.

Part of the rehabilitation process includes parent and caregiver training in all aspects of care that SCI requires (see Chapter 21) as well as ventilator management. Every family is required to have two fully trained caregivers, even if it is anticipated that they will have nursing care 24 hours/day (which few patients have). Details of this education and training can be found in Ramsey et al (2006). Family education begins when the child is still in the pediatric intensive care unit, starting with tracheostomy training. Details of this training can be found in Vander Hyde (2012).

Once caregivers have read the tracheostomy training book and have been taught by trained staff members (generally nurses or respiratory therapists), they practice tracheostomy management skills until they have mastered all skills and demonstrated three successful tracheostomy changes. Concurrent with the final stages of practice, parents/caregivers are educated on the ventilator and its management by a respiratory therapist. Tracheostomy cardiopulmonary resuscitation is also taught by the respiratory therapist. This is pediatric cardiopulmonary resuscitation as performed on a child with a tracheostomy. Parents then practice their skills by taking 'road trips' off the rehabilitation unit to various places in the hospital. Once the child is stable and has nearly completed in-patient rehabilitation, parents are then scheduled to care for their child for 12 hours in the hospital without assistance from hospital staff. Upon completion, they are scheduled for a pass to the hotel attached to the hospital where they practice their skills for 24 hours. The goal of progressive care is to make sure parents/caregivers can do all of the necessary care (including usual care needed by children with SCI as well as ventilator management) and to have them practice initially in an environment where help is near if they need to request it. Other centers have different discharge criteria for children with high ventilator dependence. One example in the UK is noted in the article by Jardine and Wallis (1998).

Communication

Oral communication is a complex process that requires intact respiratory, vocal cord, and oral motor function. If any of these functions is impaired, normal oral communication is affected. Children with high tetraplegia typically experience difficulty with oral communication. For those utilizing invasive ventilation, they must learn to speak on inhalation rather than exhalation, since expiration while on a ventilator is a slow passive process, which rarely produces enough airflow for phonation. The tracheostomy tube must be small enough to permit a 'leak' of air around it to flow up through the larynx. Vocal cords may be abnormal either because of the initial injury or because of prolonged intubation before tracheotomy. Because of the complexity of the situation, a team approach is needed, with the team comprising the patient and family, a speech pathologist, an otolaryngologist, a physiatrist, a pulmonologist, a nurse, and a respiratory therapist. Manipulating ventilator settings to optimize oral communication should be done jointly with the respiratory therapist and speech pathologist. For children who are invasively ventilated only part of the time, the use of a one-way speaking valve may help to improve oral communication (Hull et al 2005). Evaluation for this requires clearance from the otolaryngologist and evaluation by the speech pathologist. The speaking valve should only be used when the child is awake and being closely observed, since it forces exhaled air up the airway and over the larynx instead of out of the tracheostomy.

Feeding and nutrition

Although nutrition is important for all children with SCI, this may be more complicated in children who are invasively ventilated. Coordinating breathing and swallowing with a tracheostomy and ventilator requires a learning curve. For most of these children, they will require nutrition via either a nasogastric or a gastrostomy tube, at least until they have learned to coordinate swallowing with the ventilator and are willing to eat. Close attention must be paid to caloric need. One study by Patt et al (2007) looked at resting energy expenditure in children with SCIs without mechanical ventilation and found that traditional methods of predicting resting energy expenditure overestimated needs. This is particularly the case in children on full-time mechanical ventilation, because these children use almost no calories when breathing. These children should be followed closely, monitoring their resting energy expenditure and/or by a dietitian familiar with the nutrient needs of children with high tetraplegia. More details about spinal cord nutrition can be found in Chapter 16.

Assistive technology

To gain any control over their environment, children with high tetraplegia need to be given access to and learn how to use assistive technology. New technologies emerge continuously and a dedicated person or persons is required to keep abreast of those that emerge that may be most relevant for children with high-level tetraplegia. Children should be introduced to assistive technology early in the rehabilitation process. The role that assistive technology will play in a child's life depends on physical, cognitive, and emotional needs, as well as parental wishes and skills and financial resources. Types of assistive technology include augmentative communication, computer access, environmental control, power mobility, and robotic arms and implantable functional electrical stimulation systems (see Chapter 20). To become and remain a successful user of assistive technology, a child must have an adult who can set up the equipment and assist with its use. Although therapists can help with the initial set-up, daily use will require the assistance of a caregiver and/or teacher. As assistive technology changes, types that will prove useful to children with high tetraplegia will also change. Robots of various types are currently being used experimentally and, in some cases, clinically to enhance function (Siedziewski et al 2012, Yozbatiran et al 2012).

Initial evaluation, and continuing re-evaluation and updating of assistive technology equipment, should be a team effort. Members should include the patient and family, speech pathologist, rehabilitation engineer (or another team member who is an expert in technology), physical and occupational therapists, and a rehabilitation technology supplier who assists with mounting assistive technology equipment on the wheelchair and bed. Some equipment will require an upright position for use and not be readily useable in bed.

Assistive technology evaluation and provision of equipment may be available through the public school system and/or dedicated assistive technology centers run by various disability-related groups. The Assistive Technology Industry Association publishes a funding resources guide for assistive technology (see http://www.atia.org/i4a/pages/index.cfm?pageid=4219#Federal Programs).

Communication

Various devices are readily available, with new applications, 'apps', being developed daily. These include smartphones and tablet computers, which have several voice-output apps currently available. These devices can be accessed via touch using fingers or a mouth stick. Dedicated communication devices include those that use eye gaze (such as the Tobii products; see http://www.tobii.com/), scanning, or direct select (which can be activated using a mouth stick). The power of newer tablet computers lowers the cost of these products to make them more affordable, since many health insurance policies do not cover the cost of speech-generating devices. A knowledgeable speech pathologist should evaluate the child with high tetraplegia, trying a variety of devices to see which one best suits the child's abilities and needs.

Computer Access

There are many ways to access computers for those with high tetraplegia: a keyboard using fingers or a mouth stick; a touch screen using a stylus, mouth stick, or finger; voice-activated software such as Dragon Naturally Speaking by Nuance Software (Burlington, MA, USA, http://nuance.software.net); and Headmaster by Prentke-Romich (Wooster, OH, USA, http://www.prentrom.com/), which allows head movements to act like a mouse. Tablet and laptop computers can be mounted on a wheelchair, as can smartphones that have some of the functions of computers. Some of these devices can also be used from bed. An experienced assistive technology provider can assist with determining how to use assistive technology devices in bed.

Other Assistive Technology Equipment

Mouth sticks play a vital role in allowing a child with high tetraplegia to access his environment. These are lightweight sticks with specifically designed distal ends for various activities. The mouth end may be a custom-fabricated or prefabricated 'Y' design and may be fitted with tongue-activated plungers that operate the distal end. Custom fabrication is typically done by a dentist and is not commonly used because of cost and the fact that stock mouth sticks work well. Training in the use of mouth sticks starts as soon as the child is able to be upright in his wheelchair and is able to participate in therapy. Activities with mouth sticks may include a variety of craft projects and games so that the child associates mouth sticks with fun activities. Mouth stick activities may be used clinically to improve neck strength, range of motion, and endurance.

Balanced forearm orthoses (BFOs) or mobile arm supports are devices that assist in balancing gravity forces while permitting motion at the shoulder and elbow. These are fastened to the wheelchair or table top and are used for table-top activities. BFOs are commercially available in custom sizes to fit the child (http://jaecoorthopedic.com/products/). Parts of the BFO include the positioning bracket plus the proximal arm, distal arm, and arm trough. Movement of the arm is made possible by gross shoulder movements in the horizontal plane. To use a BFO, a child must have some shoulder movement, a nearly full passive range of motion at the shoulder and elbow, and minimal spasticity. The BFO must be properly sized and set up correctly.

Financial Considerations

Unfortunately, most US health insurance does not cover assistive technology completely, and often does not cover it at all. In the USA, public schools must provide the necessary equipment to enable a child to attend school, under the auspice of the Individuals with Disability Education Act, specifically the 1990 amendment (Public Law 101-476) and 1997 amendment (Public Law 105-17) (see Chapter 23). Although this may include assistive technology, devices that are more complex are rarely provided because of the costs and lack of expertise in the evaluation and use of such devices. When devices are provided by the school, they may only allow the child to use it in the school setting and not at home, even if the device is to be used for homework. Rehabilitation team members will need to spend a lot of time documenting the need of the child, writing letters of medical necessity, and filling out the myriad forms required by third-party payers. Parents will also need to learn to advocate for their children by pushing their insurance companies for coverage, and perhaps even doing fundraisers and/or working with their legislators and schools. In the USA, rehabilitation centers can assist their patients by raising funds to assist with coverage of assistive technology. Funding in other countries varies. Information about funding for assistive technology in the UK is available from the following website: http://techdis.palepurple.co.uk/sites/techdis/funding.

Therapy and equipment needs unique to children with high tetraplegia

In addition to typical therapy for children with SCI (as described in Chapter 21), there are special considerations for children with high tetraplegia. Typically, neck strength is weak, either because of the level of injury or, with lower levels of injury, because of immobilization in the period after injury. Thus, neck strengthening is often one of the first therapeutic activities that must be done when the child begins to sit up. Isometric, active, and resistive exercises may be done when medically approved. Isometric exercises can be done while a child is immobilized in a cervical immobilizing device such as a halo vest or cervical collar if permitted by the treating surgeon. More functional ways of working on neck strengthening are with mouth sticks and driving a power wheelchair. For a child with high tetraplegia, access to drive a power wheelchair is by a chin-controlled joystick, a pneumatic switch activated with breath control, or a head array system (see also Chapter 22). The joystick requires small head and chin movements to drive the chair. The chin must be in a consistent position, which requires enough muscle strength to hold the head upright, even with the provision of a headrest. Pneumatic control of the wheelchair requires precision with breath control and less head control to drive the chair.

Abdominal support is often necessary to maintain blood pressure and assist with ventilation. This may be accomplished utilizing an elastic abdominal binder or thoracolumbosacral orthosis. If a thoracolumbosacral orthosis is to be used, it should be casted with the child upright at approximately 40 degrees, since the shape of the body is different in supine and upright positions and much of the time spent wearing the thoracolumbosacral orthosis will be in the upright position.

Mobility devices for children with high tetraplegia often include power wheelchairs. In addition to other seating needs, the wheelchair must accommodate the ventilator, suction machine, and other necessary supplies such as ambu bag, feeding supplies, extra tracheostomy, and suction supplies. It is possible to run the ventilator off the wheelchair battery using a unit such as the PowerTech Vent Power Center by Richardson Products (Frankfort, IL, USA).

School and community

Once children are discharged home, most will return to school. For this to be successful, the school must be wheelchair accessible for all school activities. Caregivers may be a nurse or paraprofessional, depending on the stability and age of the child, school rules, and governmental regulations. The caregiver must have the same training as parents had before the child's discharge, including practicing tracheostomy changes. Although routine tracheostomy changes will not be done at school, the school caregiver must be prepared for emergency tracheostomy changes. For children who use non-invasive ventilation at night, school caregivers only need to be trained in all other care, which may be done during the school day (bladder management, positioning, range of motion activities if these are to be done at school, feeding, medications, etc.). For children who use invasive ventilation only during non-school hours, the caregiver needs to be trained in tracheostomy management and all other management that is to be done during the school day. For adolescents who will be entering college, the college or university is not required by law to provide caregivers, and the student will be responsible for arranging his or her own caregivers.

Recreation

Recreation is a big part of every child's life, and the exact form it takes varies between ages and different geographic regions. Once a child has had an SCI, especially high tetraplegia, it is difficult to take part in many activities. In addition, before 1990, summer camp for children who are ventilator dependent was almost non-existent. In 1990, we started the University of

Michigan Trails Edge Camp for Ventilator-dependent Children. This camp now accommodates 32 children who use any form of home mechanical ventilation, whether non-invasive, invasive, or pacers. Children have a variety of disabilities, but many of them have high tetraplegia SCI. Children stay for 5 days without their families or usual caregivers. For many campers, this is the first time they have been away from their families other than when they are hospitalized. All staff are volunteers and the staffing ratio is approximately 3.5 staff to 1 camper. About 50% to 60% of staff are medical professionals (physicians, nurses, respiratory therapists, and therapists), with the remaining staff having non-medical backgrounds. Volunteers come from all over the USA and from the UK. Staff positions include the director, people in charge of all supplies, the camp physician and nurse, partners (direct caregivers for the campers during the day), cabin leaders (senior staff who provide care at night and assist partners during the daytime), cabin respiratory therapists and nurses, activity staff, kitchen staff, a handyman, and a rehabilitation technology specialist (who keeps the wheelchairs running).

Planning the camp required a number of steps that are detailed in Dekeon and Howell (1997). These include, at a minimum, the following:

- securing the campsite;
- finding financial support;
- securing a license;
- obtaining liability coverage;
- securing supplies;
- recruitment and training of volunteer staff;
- planning activities;
- logistics (meal planning, safety, laundry, etc.).

The mission of the camp is to provide a respite for families and caregivers and to provide a camp experience for children who otherwise would not have the opportunity. Some other camps that currently operate include the Ventilation-assisted Children's Center (http://www.vacccamp.com/about/index.asp) from Miami Children's Hospital, and a ventilator camp started in 2013 by Pittsburgh Children's Hospital.

Summary

The management of children with high tetraplegia is a complex and dynamic process. Successful management requires close attention to all body systems and the close coordination among all members of the team, including physiatrists, pulmonologists, therapists, nurses, social workers, psychologists, and, most of all, the child and his or her family. As one of our adolescents with high tetraplegia stated (Juntunen 1997), 'There are many hardships in life, but there is also happiness, and without both, neither is meaningful. I hope to express the outlook of people in situations similar to mine, and I hope my experiences can provide commentary on the personal experiences of other disabled persons and on the field of health care'.

REFERENCES

Dekeon M, Howell B (1997) Establishing a recreational camp for ventilator-assisted children. In: Driver LE, Nelson VS, Warschausky SA (eds). *The Ventilator-Assisted Child: A Practical Resource Guide*. San Antonio, TX: Communication Skill Builders, pp. 143–50.

Hull EM, Dumas HM, Crowley RA, Kharasch VS (2005) Tracheostomy speaking valves for children: tolerance and clinical benefits. *Pediatr Rehab* 8: 214–19.

Juntunen D (1997) Transitions: a personal perspective. In: Driver LE, Nelson VS, Warschausky SA (eds). *The Ventilator-Assisted Child: A Practical Resource Guide*. San Antonio, TX: Communication Skill Builders, pp. 171–9.

Onders RP, Elmo MJ, Ignagni AR (2007) Diaphragm pacing stimulation system for tetraplegia in individuals injured during childhood or adolescence. *J Spinal Cord Med* 30(Suppl 1): S25–9.

Onders RP, Ponsky TA, Elmo M, Lidsky K, Barksdale E (2011) First reported experience with intramuscular diaphragm pacing in replacing positive pressure mechanical ventilators in children. *J Pediatr Surg* 46: 72–6. doi: 10.1016/j.jpedsurg.2010.09.071

Patt PL, Agena SM, Vogel LC, Foley S, Anderson CJ (2007) Estimation of resting energy expenditure in children with SCI. *J Spinal Cord Med* 30(Suppl 1): S83–7. http://dx.doi.org/10.2165/11531960-000000000-00000

Ramsey AM, Tsai WC, Nelson VS (eds) (2006) *Growing and Thriving with Respiratory Support: A Family Education Manual*. Ann Arbor, MI: University of Michigan Hospitals.

Siedziewski L, Schaaf RC, Mount J (2012) Use of robotics in spinal cord injury: a case report. *Am J Occup Ther* 66: 51–8. http://dx.doi.org/10.5014/ajot.2012.000943

Vander Hyde K (2012) *Growing and Thriving with a Tracheostomy*. Ann Arbor, MI: University of Michigan Health System. Available at: http://issuu.com/kiimmmmmyy/docs/trach_book_2012_update_v3_web

Yozbatiran N, Berliner J, O'Malley MK et al (2012) Robotic training and clinical assessment of upper extremity movements after spinal cord injury: a single case report. *J Rehabil Med* 44: 186–8. http://dx.doi.org/10.2340/16501977-0924

10
DUAL DIAGNOSIS: CONCOMITANT TRAUMATIC BRAIN INJURY IN SPINAL CORD INJURY

Miriam Hwang

Case vignette

Jason, 11 years old, was a happy, healthy male in the fourth grade when he sustained a C5 American Spinal Injury Association Impairment Scale C spinal cord injury at 9 years of age following a diving accident. He experienced loss of consciousness at the time of injury which lasted for 2 days, after which he spontaneously regained consciousness and memory. Jason had previously achieved high academic marks before the injury, but is currently repeating the fourth grade and experiences difficulty keeping up his grades. Additionally, his dad states that Jason often forgets to catheterize his bladder at designated times and has episodes of irritability that occasionally alarm his friends. Although Jason's motor recovery allows him to have modified independence in the community, Jason and his family would like further evaluation and management of his cognitive and emotional status.

Introduction

Spinal cord injury (SCI) rehabilitation requires the patient to have insight into the life changes resulting from SCI, have an understanding of the extent of their functional capabilities, cope with the psychological issues of a disability, acquire new information and skills, and have the ability to instruct caregivers regarding required assistance. The presence of a concomitant traumatic brain injury (TBI) in an individual with an SCI, that is dual diagnosis, presents an additional challenge as the physical, cognitive, psychological, and behavioral complications associated with a TBI can hinder the learning and executive functioning skills needed for effective rehabilitation (Watanabe et al 1999, Bowman and Macciocchi 2004, Sommer and Witkiewicz 2004). TBI in children adds additional complexity to the rehabilitative efforts, as the injury may disrupt the developing neural connections in the immature brain which support acquisition of cognitive and psychological development, subsequently leading to persistent disorders of learning and behavior (Chapman and McKinnon 2000, Anderson et al 2005). This chapter will discuss the epidemiology of SCI/TBI dual diagnosis, neurocognitive and behavioral aspects of TBI, medical complications, and rehabilitation of children with dual diagnosis.

Epidemiology

The Centers for Disease Control and Prevention (CDC) report an estimated 1.7 million people in the USA sustain a TBI annually (Faul et al 2010). In the pediatric population, children aged 0 to 4 years and adolescents aged 15 to 19 years were most likely to sustain a TBI, with more than 630 000 emergency department visits made annually by children 19 years and younger (Faul et al 2010). The etiologies of TBI in children vary according to age, with infants and toddlers sustaining the majority of their injuries through falls or inflicted trauma, whereas school-aged children and older adolescents sustain injuries through sports or motor vehicle crashes (Faul et al 2010, Li and Liu 2013). As falls, sports injuries, and motor vehicle crashes, all involving high-velocity forceful impact to the body, are etiologies common to both SCI and TBI, it is intuitive that the diagnosis of one condition should add suspicion of the presence of the other. Immediately following a traumatic incident, however, loss of consciousness can preclude determination of any motor deficit of either TBI or SCI, whereas when the motor deficit is the predominant feature, mild or subtle changes in mental status can be missed, thus rendering the simultaneous detection of both conditions difficult. In the adult SCI population, the incidence of dual diagnosis ranges from 28% to 74% depending on the criteria used to establish a diagnosis of TBI (Wilmot et al 1985, Davidoff et al 1988, Tolonen et al 2007, Hagen et al 2010). Dual diagnosis in the pediatric SCI population is rarely reported. One case series from a rehabilitation unit of a tertiary children's hospital found that 3 out of 21 children with SCI demonstrated cognitive impairments which were attributed to the SCI-inducing incident (Miles and Cawley 1996). The paucity of literature on dual diagnosis in the pediatric population is likely to be the result of insufficient assessment in the acute care setting (especially when the TBI is mild or not apparent), the absence of standardized diagnostic criteria of dual diagnosis in children, and the lack of population-based epidemiologic data.

Diagnosis and classification of SCI is relatively straightforward and is based on the International Standards of Neurological Classification of Spinal Cord Injury (see Chapter 4). On the other hand, TBI diagnosis and severity classification involve a combination of loss of consciousness, duration of post-traumatic amnesia, Glasgow Coma Scale score, and neuroimaging results (Teasdale and Jennett 1974, Tolonen et al 2007, Macciocchi et al 2008). The diagnostic value of loss of consciousness is somewhat debatable in pediatric dual diagnosis, as the traumatic events leading to the SCI can cause a loss of consciousness, irrespective of brain injury, especially in younger children under the age of 5 years (Ricker and Regan 1999, Palchak et al 2004). The Children's Orientation and Amnesia Test was developed to assess cognition in the early stages of recovery after the occurrence of TBI in children and adolescents, and was found to adequately measure the duration of post-traumatic amnesia in children (Ewing-Cobbs et al 1990). Neuroimaging studies, such as computed tomography (CT) or magnetic resonance imaging (MRI), provide objective evidence of brain injury; however, mild TBI, diffuse axonal injury, or post-concussion syndrome may present with non-specific or no abnormalities on conventional CT or MRI. In these cases, neuropsychological tests can provide sensitive diagnostic and objective assessment of cognitive or psychological changes of brain injury (Wilmot et al 1985, Bowman and Macciocchi 2004, Tolonen et al 2007), but must be age appropriate for the developing child as well as 'motor free', such that the impaired upper extremity function of either SCI or TBI does not influence the results of the tests. The most challenging aspect of determining dual diagnosis in children is when the TBI is mild or not immediately apparent, leading to subsequent difficulties in the rehabilitation setting. Thus, a high degree of suspicion of concomitant TBI in children with SCI is warranted with administration of neuropsychological tests when deemed necessary.

Risk factors associated with concomitant TBI in SCI include motor vehicle crashes (Davidoff et al 1988, Macciocchi et al 2008), alcohol use at the time of injury (Watanabe et al 1999, Hagen et al 2010), completeness of SCI (Hagen et al 2010), and cervical-level SCI (Iida et al 1999, Macciocchi et al 2008). The literature on the association between cervical-level SCI and dual diagnosis is conflicting. A number of studies report no significant relationship between cervical SCI and concomitant TBI, indicating that the concomitant TBI may be more likely owing to the acceleration/deceleration mechanism of injury rather than from direct impact to the head (Davidoff et al 1988, Watanabe et al 1999, Bowman and Macciocchi 2004). However, the possible association between concomitant TBI and cervical-level injury can be of concern in the pediatric population. The prevalence of cervical-level injury is approximately one-third of school-aged children with SCI (DeVivo and Vogel 2004; see also Chapter 3), and the anatomic features of a proportionately large head supported by underdeveloped neck musculature in younger children (Vogel et al 2011) can potentially lead to direct impact to the head as well as acceleration/deceleration injuries to the spinal cord at the time of injury.

Neurocognitive and behavioral aspects of pediatric traumatic brain injury

The neurocognitive and behavioral changes that occur after TBI can impede rehabilitation in children with dual diagnosis. Arousal and attention, memory, new skill acquisition, communication, visuoperception, and executive functioning are all cognitive functions required for effective rehabilitation, but are impaired to varying degrees depending on the type and severity of TBI (Davidoff et al 1992, Ricker and Regan 1999). Rehabilitative efforts may be negatively impacted by psychological and behavioral sequelae, such as depression, apathy, agitation, aggression, and impulsivity as well as by the potential side effects of the medications used to control such problems (Ricker and Regan 1999, Sommer and Witkiewicz 2004). Furthermore, these problems can lead to difficulties in academic performance and socialization with peers in children with dual diagnosis (Arroyos-Jurado et al 2000, Ginstfeldt and Emanuelson 2010).

The impact of injury to the developing brain can vary depending on the age at injury as well as injury severity. Research indicates that children sustaining severe injury in early childhood may be vulnerable to residual cognitive impairment, which is attributed to the disruption of the neural connective pathways in the early stages of brain development (Chapman and McKinnon 2000, Anderson et al 2005). Children with less severe injuries were found to recover to a healthy level of function and to make age-appropriate progress up to 10 years after injury (Anderson et al 2012). The physical and neurocognitive manifestations of brain injury can also vary as development progresses over time. For example, a TBI in younger children may not be apparent because they are in the earlier stages of development and are not expected to perform at higher levels of cognitive functioning. Upon reaching school age, however, the effects of the brain injury may present as low academic performance or behavioral problems, which were previously unrecognized.

Of particular concern in children with TBI is impaired attention. The ability to select, maintain, and divide attention appropriately is required for communication, following instructions, setting goals, and performing tasks, all of which are integral components of daily life, learning, and social participation. Attention deficit in children has been associated with incomplete myelination and interrupted frontal lobe maturation after injury, with a reported incidence of 30% to 50% in pediatric TBI (Ginstfeldt and Emanuelson 2010, Li and Liu 2013). Many studies have investigated the efficacy of methylphenidate and other psychostimulants for the treatment of attention deficits in pediatric TBI, but they report conflicting results, probably owing to differences in study design and variability in TBI severity, such as structural damage within the neural connections (Mahalick et al 1998, Williams et al 1998, Chapman and McKinnon 2000).

Given the importance of cognitive impairment and behavioral problems associated with TBI, identification of these changes should be an integral part of the comprehensive assessment of children with dual diagnosis. Equally important is the selection of instruments which can adequately assess children with limited use of the upper extremities or who are ventilator dependent with reduced verbal responsiveness. Although many tests of cognitive assessment can be performed 'motor free' or adjusted to accommodate children with motor impairment, assessment of attention and concentration in children with dual diagnosis is particularly difficult because such tests often require motor responses (Miles and Cawley 1996). As it is beyond the scope of this chapter to discuss in detail the available neuropsychological assessment instruments, the most commonly used measures are presented with their applications in Table 10.1. If available, the pre-injury status, including any learning disorders, cognitive issues, psychological disturbances, and substance-use problems, must also be considered in order to fully assess the child's current level of functioning. Findings from these assessments will provide the foundation for an individualized approach to optimize rehabilitation in children with dual diagnosis.

Medical complications

As complications of SCI are discussed in other chapters of this book, this section will present common complications associated with TBI and their impact on pediatric dual diagnosis.

Seizures

Post-traumatic seizure in the pediatric TBI population has an overall incidence of 5.5% to 40%, with the majority occurring within the first 24 hours after injury (Statler 2006, Arango et al 2012, Matsumoto et al 2013). Risk factors for post-traumatic seizure include younger age, subdural hematoma, contusion, severe cerebral edema, and severity of injury (Chiaretti et al 2000, Statler 2006). The occurrence of post-traumatic seizure is significant, as it can adversely affect long-term outcomes by worsening secondary brain damage and interrupting rehabilitative management. Post-traumatic epilepsy is a condition of recurrent, chronic seizures, intractable to medical management occurring in 10% to 20% of children with severe TBI. Risk factors for post-traumatic epilepsy include severe TBI and occurrence of early post-traumatic seizure (Statler 2006). In light of the negative consequences of post-traumatic seizure, prophylactic anticonvulsant therapy is recommended in the first 7 days after injury;

TABLE 10.1
Neuropsychological assessment instruments for children

Domain/function	Ages (y:mo)	Considerations
General intelligence		
Bayley Scales of Infant and Toddler Development – III	0:1–3:6	Performance and perceptual reasoning domains of intelligence can be highly dependent on motor ability. Consider use of tasks that require only verbal responses for children with physical limitations and high injury level
Differential Ability Scales – II (DAS-II)	2:6–17:11	
Kaufman Assessment Battery for Children – II (KABC-II)	3:0–18:11	
Mullen Scales of Early Learning	0:0–5:8	
Stanford–Binet Intelligence Scales, 5 (SB5)	2:0–89+	
Wechsler Intelligence Scale for Children – IV (WISC-IV)	6:0–16:11	
Wechsler Preschool and Primary Scale of Intelligence – IV (WPPSI-IV)	2:6–7:7	
Non-verbal Intelligence		
Leiter International Performance Scale – Revised (Leiter-R)	2:0–20:11	Non-verbal measures of intelligence may be an alternative for assessment of cognitive functioning in children with significant motor or language deficits
Raven Progressive Matrices (RPM)	6:0+	
Test of Nonverbal Intelligence – 3 (TONI-3)	6:0–89:11	
Academic achievement		
Peabody Individual Achievement Test – Revised (PIAT-R)	5:0–22:11	Achievement subtests that require written responses may need to be modified so that responses are dictated and recorded to the evaluator
Wechsler Individual Achievement Test – III (WIAT-III)	4:0–50:11	
Wide Range Achievement Test – 4 (WRAT4)	5:0–94:11	
Woodcock–Johnson III – Tests of Achievement (WJ-III)	2:0–90:11	
Executive functioning/attention		
Behavioral Rating Inventory of Executive Function (BRIEF)	5:0–18:11	Many of the subtests in the comprehensive batteries for executive functioning may not be appropriate for children with physical impairment. Use of single subtests that are not dependent on motor responses should be considered
Conners Continuous Performance Test (CPT-II)	6:0–55+	
Delis–Kaplan Executive Functions System (D-KEFS)	8:0–89:11	
Tests of Everyday Attention for Children (TEA-Ch)	6:0–15:11	
NEPSY-II – Attention and Executive Functioning Domain	3:0–16:11	
Wisconsin Card Sorting Test (WCST)	7:0–89:11	

TABLE 10.1
(Continued)

Domain/function	Ages (y:mo)	Considerations
Language		
Clinical Evaluation of Language Fundamentals – 4 (CELF-4)	5:0–21:11	The task demands of language assessments tend to depend on verbal responses rather than motor skills or speed. For tasks involving a muscle response, the format can be modified to allow for verbal indicators of choice or use of adaptive equipment
Expressive One Word Picture Vocabulary Test – 4 (EOWPVT-4)	2:0–80+	
Expressive Vocabulary Test – 2 (EVT-2)	2:6–90+	
NEPSY-II – Language Domain	3:0–16:11	
Peabody Picture Vocabulary Test – IV (PPVT-IV)	2:6–90+	
Receptive One Word Picture Vocabulary Test – 4 (ROWPVT-4)	2:0–80+	
Visual–motor and motor functioning		
Beery–Buktenica Developmental Test of Visual–Motor Integration – 6 (VMI)	2:0–100	If spinal cord injury has resulted in impairment or complete loss of motor function in the upper extremities, assessment of fine motor control may not be appropriate unless the purpose of the assessment is to evaluate the extent of the injury on motor functions or monitor progress in adaptive motor skills. In this event, modifications, including use of adaptive equipment, may be necessary to facilitate motor responding or compensate for lost motor skills
Bender Visual Motor Gestalt Test – II (Bender-II)	4:0–85+	
Grooved Pegboard Test (GPT)	5:0+	
Halstead–Reitan Neuropsychological Batteries	5:0+	
Finger Tapping Test (FFT)		
Grip Strength Test (GST)		
Motor-Free Visual Perception Test – 3 (MVPT-3)	4:0–70:11	
NEPSY-II – Sensorimotor and Visuospatial Processing Domains	3:0–16:11	
Rey–Osterrieth Complex Figure Test (CFT)	5:0–85:0	
Test of Visual Perceptual Skills – 3 (TVPS-3)	4:0–18:11	
Memory and learning		
California Verbal Learning Test – Children (CVLT-C)	5:0–16:11	For children with tracheostomy or ventilator dependency, verbal tasks that require immediate response may be inappropriate; however, memory subtests that do not require rapid, sequential, verbatim recall will allow children who are ventilator or tracheostomy dependent to better consolidate answers
Children's Memory Scale (CMS)	5:0–16:11	
NEPSY-II – Memory and Learning Domain	3:0–16:11	
Test of Memory and Learning – 2 (TOMAL-2)	5:0–59:11	
Rey Auditory Verbal Learning Test (AVLT)	7:0–89:11	
Wide Range Assessment of Memory and Learning – 2 (WRAML-2)	5:0–90:11	

however, routine seizure prophylaxis is not effective and thus not recommended later than 1 week after the TBI (Adelson et al 2003). Anticonvulsant medications approved for use in the pediatric population include valproic acid, carbamazepine, and lamotrigine, and are preferred over traditional medications such as phenytoin and phenobarbital, which have adverse cognitive side effects (Bowman and Macciocchi 2004, Pangilinan et al 2010). Potential side effects such as hepatotoxicity (valproic acid) and bone marrow suppression (carbamazepine) must be considered before administration, and children should be monitored closely with appropriate clinical examinations and laboratory tests.

Agitation

Agitation is a common symptom following TBI. It can manifest as physical or verbal aggression, explosive anger, restlessness, or inappropriate sexual behavior (Pangilinan et al 2010). Such behavior may be harmful not only to the patient but also to the rehabilitation staff, and can be disruptive to the rehabilitative environment. Before treatment initiation, it is important to rule out organic causes of agitation such as seizures, hypoxia, electrolyte imbalance, medications, or substance withdrawal. Modification to the patient's environment and behavior should be the first line of treatment of agitation; pharmacotherapy is indicated when such modifications alone are insufficient. Modifications include providing a quiet, stable, and consistent environment with minimal external stimuli; avoidance of activities which precipitate outbursts of agitation; and instantaneous and firm reprimand of inappropriate behaviors (Whyte et al 2002, Sommer and Witkiewicz 2004). Pharmacotherapy to control agitation must be selected based on the individual patient. Benzodiazepines, traditionally used to treat anxiety and agitation, are avoided after TBI, as they can cause sedation, memory loss, and potentially paradoxical increases in agitation. In recent years, atypical antipsychotic agents such as risperidone, quetiapine, clozapine, and olanzapine have been used for agitation management, as they have fewer cognitive side effects (Bowman and Macciocchi 2004, Pangilinan 2010). Their safety and efficacy in the pediatric population have not been established, however, and use of such agents should be carried out at the minimal effective dosage with close monitoring of adverse effects. Anticonvulsants such as valproic acid and carbamazepine can be used for management of agitation in children, but these also warrant close monitoring for side effects.

Hydrocephalus

Post-traumatic hydrocephalus is a late complication usually occurring weeks to months after the initial injury in approximately 40% of individuals with severe TBI. The hydrocephalus is usually of the communicating or normal-pressure type and is a treatable complication so recognition of its symptoms is important (Bowman and Macciocchi 2004). It classically presents as gait disturbance, incontinence, and dementia. These signs, however, can be easily overlooked in children with dual diagnosis because SCI precludes observing changes in gait, and the neurogenic bladder and bowel of SCI will mask any signs of new-onset incontinence. Furthermore, the clinical presentation of hydrocephalus can be variable or absent in children (Cantore et al 2012). Certainly, a high index of suspicion is necessary in children with dual diagnosis. Accompanying signs such as functional decline, increased spasticity, new-onset weakness, headache, or changes in mental status and behavior should alert the clinician to the possible presence of hydrocephalus. CT or MRI of the brain are used to detect ventricular dilation. In cases where brain imaging studies are equivocal, radionuclide cisternogram can be used to assess cerebrospinal fluid flow within the ventricular system, and lumbar puncture can also assist in the diagnosis with observable changes in behavior in response to withdrawal of cerebrospinal fluid (Whyte et al 2005). Treatment usually entails surgical placement of a ventriculoperitoneal shunt and the patient should be closely monitored thereafter, with awareness for the possibility of shunt obstruction.

Autonomic Dysfunction

Both SCI and TBI can lead to autonomic abnormalities, namely orthostatic hypotension and autonomic dysreflexia in SCI and dysautonomia in TBI. Orthostatic hypotension and autonomic dysreflexia (discussed in Chapter 14) are common and serious complications of SCI, which require immediate care; the presence of a concomitant TBI in SCI can make the detection of orthostatic hypotension and autonomic dysreflexia difficult if the child has cognitive deficits which preclude recognition of symptoms and communication of physical discomfort. Thus, both the child with dual diagnosis and the caregivers must be well educated on autonomic dysreflexia and orthostatic hypotension, and vigilant in recognizing their occurrences.

Dysautonomia, also known as paroxysmal sympathetic hyperactivity, is a sequela of acquired brain injury presenting with disturbances in temperature and hemodynamic homeostasis and dystonic muscle contractions (Kirk et al 2012). Dysautonomia usually manifests in the first few weeks after injury and continues for several months thereafter, presenting with fever, tachycardia, tachypnea, hypertension, diaphoresis, and dystonia. The incidence in children ranges from 10% to 14%, with the combination of hypertension, diaphoresis, and dystonia being the best predictor of dysautonomia in pediatric TBI (Krach et al 1997, Kirk et al 2012). Dysautonomia is associated with prolonged rehabilitation and less improvement in motor function and independence at discharge than pediatric TBI patients without dysautonomia (Kirk et al 2012). Therapeutic options include symptomatic pharmacotherapy and environmental modification, such as maintaining a cooler room temperature or reducing external stimuli that can induce autonomic hyperactivity (Baguley et al 2009). Pharmacologic agents are aimed at decreasing sympathetic hyperactivity with beta-blockers (atenolol) or centrally acting alpha-agonists (clonidine), increasing inhibitory neurotransmitter activity with GABAergic agents (gabapentin, baclofen, benzodiazepines), or modulating dopamine activity (chlorpromazine, bromocriptine). Beta-blockers should be used with caution in children who experience orthostatic hypotension, as it can worsen hypotension and impede compensatory increases in heart rate. The sedative and cognitive side effects of baclofen and benzodiazepines must also be considered before use in children with dual diagnosis.

Endocrine Dysfunction

Neuroendocrine changes have been well documented in the adult TBI population, with the syndrome of inappropriate antidiuretic hormone and central diabetes insipidus among the most common. The prevalence of endocrine changes following TBI in children ranges from 10% to 75% depending on the time since injury, and have been associated with loss of consciousness, subdural hematoma, or skull fracture (Acerini and Tasker 2007, Kaulfers et al 2010).

Most common in pediatric TBI is anterior pituitary dysfunction, especially deficiencies in growth hormone and gonadotrophic-releasing hormone, leading to disturbances in physical growth and pubertal development. Growth hormone deficiency has also been associated with decreased cognition and lower quality of life, further emphasizing its impact on the developing child (Ghigo et al 2005). Deficiency in thyroid-stimulating hormone can also cause developmental delay; adrenocorticotrophic hormone deficiency, although relatively rare, has been reported to persist following TBI (Rose and Auble 2012). Hyperprolactinemia has been reported in the first 1 to 2 years after injury, with resolution thereafter (Niederland et al 2007, Kaulfers et al 2010). Precocious puberty is a well-recognized condition in pediatric TBI with rapid progression of puberty within the first year after injury, and is thought to be caused by the brain's inability to inhibit gonadotropin release (Rose and Auble 2012). Disorders of water imbalance such as the syndrome of inappropriate antidiuretic hormone and diabetes insipidus have also been reported in the pediatric population but are transient, with resolution by 6 months (Kaulfers et al 2010). Although endocrine changes of TBI in children generally occur within the first year after injury, endocrine dysfunction is often overlooked during this period, especially in the prepubertal child. Therefore, serial assessment of endocrine function should be performed in children with dual diagnosis, especially during the early stages of recovery, in order to prevent delayed diagnosis and to ensure optimal growth and development.

Other Considerations

Speech, language, and swallowing function can be altered in children with dual diagnosis, as a result of both TBI and high cervical SCI. Moreover, the presence of a tracheostomy or ventilator dependency can lead to further difficulties in communication, inadequate nutrition, and increased risk of aspiration. Appropriate evaluation of speech and swallowing function as well as nutritional assessment is warranted for effective rehabilitation. Sleep disturbances, common in TBI, can negatively impact cognition, physical endurance, and functional outcomes, and have been reported to persist for more than 2 years after injury in children (Tham et al 2012). Strategies to maintain daytime wakefulness and improve sleep hygiene should be attempted before the use of medications. Melatonin can be used to adjust circadian rhythm (Cantore et al 2012). Benzodiazepines are avoided in TBI owing to its adverse effect on sleep architecture; the GABAergic agent zolpidem and antihistamines such as diphenhydramine can be administered for sleep onset, and the serotonergic agent trazodone is used for both sleep maintenance and agitation symptoms (Bowan and Macciocchi 2004, Cantore et al 2012). The side effect profiles of pharmacologic agents and interactions with other medications should be thoroughly assessed for each child.

Pressure ulcers, neurogenic bladder and bowel, pain, heterotopic ossification, and increased muscle tone are conditions that are common to both SCI and TBI and are discussed in other chapters of this book. Heterotopic ossification is notable in that the location of new bone formation commonly occurs around the shoulder and hip joints in the hemiplegic side in TBI, and below the neurologic level of injury in SCI, most commonly around the hip and knees. It is associated with immobility and spasticity, and thus range-of-motion exercises of the joints and spasticity management, in addition to indomethacin administration, can be helpful in preventing or minimizing its occurrence (Black and DeSantis 1999, Cipriano et al 2009,

Ayyoub and Aragaki 2010). Increased muscle tone commonly manifests as spasticity in both SCI and TBI. Dystonia, involuntary sustained muscle contractions causing abnormal posturing or repetitive movements, and extrapyramidal syndromes such as akathisia and muscle stiffness are abnormalities of muscle tone frequently observed in TBI, and should be differentiated from spasticity for appropriate management in children with dual diagnosis. Strategies to treat the common conditions are generally identical for both SCI and TBI. Medications, however, should be used with caution in the child with dual diagnosis being mindful of any sedative effects. For example, pharmacologic management for general spasticity usually involves oral administration of baclofen, tizanidine, or clonidine, all of which have sedative side effects; dantrolene sodium, on the other hand, is a peripherally acting muscle relaxant with fewer sedating effects, and thus can be used as an alternative agent, but regular monitoring of liver function is required.

Rehabilitation of spinal cord injury/traumatic brain injury dual diagnosis

Rehabilitation efforts in children with dual diagnosis should begin with measures to address cognitive and behavioral issues because these may interfere with new learning and problem solving (see also Chapter 21). When the child demonstrates the ability to retain learned information, more active rehabilitative measures can gradually be introduced. All members of the rehabilitation team must be cognizant of the problems associated with the TBI and provide a structured and consistent approach to therapy in order to keep the child focused and minimize confusion. The therapy environment should be controlled to minimize external stimuli. Therapeutic tasks are best started with short sessions consisting of simple one-step actions and frequent repetition, with sufficient time allotted for completion of tasks and rest periods. Provision of positive feedback is beneficial in controlling behavioral problems as well as in encouraging progress in rehabilitation (Sommer and Witkiewicz 2004). Attention should be given to any assistive devices or equipment as children can quickly outgrow them. The clinician should be diligent in checking for skin breakdown or neurovascular compression caused by any device or brace, especially in children with deficits in sensation or communication.

Reintegration into school and social participation with peers are important aspects of rehabilitation in children with dual diagnosis (see also Chapter 23). Although the majority of children with SCI are able to attend regular education classes, this may not be possible for children with a concomitant TBI. Cognitive and behavioral problems may hinder the child's ability to learn in a regular classroom setting, which in turn can limit socializing with peers. From an academic standpoint, it is imperative that teachers are aware of the child's cognitive and behavioral status and an individualized education plan is developed (Arroyos-Jurago et al 2000).

Research reports better quality of life and positive long-term outcomes in children with disabilities when they are able to actively participate in social settings (Bedell and Dumas 2004, Kelly et al 2012). The degree of participation in children with disabilities, however, is relatively lower than in those without a disability (Bedell et al 2013). In pediatric SCI, obstacles to community participation include living in a small town, younger age at injury, incomplete injury, and experiencing recent medical complications (Gorzowski et al 2011). The child with TBI is restricted in areas of managing daily routines, play with peers, unstructured physical activities, and structured community activities (van Tol et al 2011, Bedell et al 2013). Factors related to participation in pediatric TBI include pre-injury cognitive and behavioral status, severity of the injury, and functional performance at discharge from acute rehabilitation (Arroyos-Jurado et al 2000, Bedell and Dumas 2004). For the child with dual diagnosis, factors influencing social participation in both pediatric SCI and TBI should be considered throughout rehabilitation in order to better prepare the child for return to school and reintegration into peer relationships. Additionally, greater efforts are needed to advocate and enhance participation of children with dual diagnosis in the community to prepare for their transition to adulthood and assimilation into society.

Family participation is essential not only for successful functional rehabilitation and transition to home, but also for more positive long-term outcomes. Numerous studies have shown better functional, cognitive, and psychosocial outcomes in children with TBI when family members actively participate in the rehabilitation process (Chapman and McKinnon 2000, Sommer and Witkiewicz 2004, Anderson et al 2012, Li and Liu 2013). Family members and caregivers should be educated about changes in medical, cognitive, psychological, and rehabilitative management as the child develops, and should also be able to communicate the child's needs to healthcare providers as well as to teachers and peers in the community.

Summary

Developmental changes in brain function, physical and cognitive development, and social relationships are important aspects to be considered in working toward functional improvement in children with dual diagnosis. Therapy should be individualized for each child with the family as active participants in medical management and rehabilitation, with the ultimate goal of achieving reintegration into society. Future research should include the development of accurate assessment tools for early diagnosis and effective rehabilitation methods, as well as investigations of long-term neuropsychological and functional outcomes in children with dual diagnosis.

REFERENCES

Acerini CL, Tasker RC (2007) Traumatic brain injury induced hypothalamic–pituitary dysfunction: a paediatric perspective. *Pituitary* 10: 373–80. doi: 10.1007/s11102-007-0052-8

Adelson PD, Bratton SL, Carney NA et al (2003) Guidelines for the acute medical management of severe traumatic brain injury in infants, children, and adolescents. Chapter 19. The role of anti-seizure prophylaxis following severe pediatric traumatic brain injury. *Pediatr Crit Care Med* 4: S72–5. doi: 10.1097/00130478-200307001-00020

Anderson V, Catroppa C, Morse S, Haritou F, Rosenfeld J (2005) Functional plasticity or vulnerability after early brain injury? *Pediatrics* 116: 1374–82. doi: 10.1542/peds.2004-1728

Anderson V, Godfrey C, Rosenfeld JV, Catroppa C (2012) Predictors of cognitive function and recovery 10 years after traumatic brain injury in young children. *Pediatrics* 129: e254–61. doi: 10.1542/peds.2011-0311

Arango JI, Deibery CP, Brown D, Bell M, Dvorchik I, Adelson PD (2012) Posttraumatic seizures in children with severe traumatic brain injury. *Childs Nerv Syst* 28: 1925–9. http://dx.doi.org/10.1007/s00381-012-1863-0

Arroyos-Jurado E, Paulsen JS, Merrell KW, Lindgren SD (2000) Traumatic brain injury in school-age children: academic and social outcome. *J Sch Psychol* 38: 571–87. doi: 10.1016/S0022-4405(00)00053-4

Ayyoub Z, Aragaki DLR (2010) Dual diagnosis: spinal cord injury and brain injury. In: Lin VW (ed.). *Spinal Cord Medicine: Principles and Practice*. 2nd Ed. New York, NY: Demos Medical Publishing, pp. 580–94.

Baguley IJ, Nott MT, Slewa-Younan S, Heriseanu RE, Perkes IE (2009) Diagnosing dysautonomia after acute traumatic brain injury: evidence for overresponsiveness to afferent stimuli. *Arch Phys Med Rehabil* 90: 580–6. doi: 10.1016/j.apmr.2008.10.020

Bedell GM, Dumas HM (2004) Social participation of children and youth with acquired brain injuries discharged from inpatient rehabilitation: a follow-up study. *Brain Inj* 18: 65–82. doi: 10.1080/0269905031000110517

Bedell G, Coster W, Law M et al (2013) Community participation, supports, and barriers of school-age children with and without disabilities. *Arch Phys Med Rehabil* 94: 315–23. doi: 10.1016/j.apmr.2012.09.024

Black KB, DeSantis N (1999) Medical complications common to spinal-cord-injured and brain-injured patients. *Top Spinal Cord Inj Rehabil* 5: 47–75. http://dx.doi.org/10.1310/7NV4-249J-AVPB-5XH4

Bowman BK, Macciocchi S (2004) Dual diagnosis: diagnosis, management, and future trends. *Top Spinal Cord Inj Rehabil* 10: 58–68. doi: 10.1310/VFHG-F2HU-PYKX-T85H

Cantore L, Norwood K, Patrick P (2012) Medical aspects of pediatric rehabilitation after moderate to severe traumatic brain injury. *NeuroRehabilitation* 30: 225–34. doi: 10.3233/NRE-2012-0749

Chapman SB, McKinnon L (2000) Discussion of developmental plasticity: factors affecting cognitive outcome after pediatric traumatic brain injury. *J Commun Disord* 33: 333–44. doi: 10.1016/S0021-9924(00)00029-0

Chiaretti A, De Benedictis R, Polidori G, Piastra M, Iannelli A, Di Rocco C (2000) Early post-traumatic seizures in children with head injury. *Childs Nerv Syst* 16: 862–6. doi: 10.1007/s003810000368

Cipriano CA, Pill SG, Keenan MA (2009) Heterotopic ossification following traumatic brain injury and spinal cord injury. *J Am Acad Orthop Surg* 17: 689–97.

Davidoff G, Thomas P, Johnson M, Berent S, Dijkers M, Doljanac R (1988) Closed head injury in acute traumatic spinal cord injury: incidence and risk factors. *Arch Phys Med Rehabil* 69: 869–72.

Davidoff GN, Roth EJ, Richards JS (1992) Cognitive deficits in spinal cord injury: epidemiology and outcome. *Arch Phys Med Rehabil* 73: 275–84.

DeVivo MJ, Vogel LC (2004) Epidemiology of spinal cord injury in children and adolescents. *J Spinal Cord Med* 27: S4–10.

Ewing Cobbs L, Levin HS, Fletcher JM, Miner MF, Eisenberg HM (1990) The Children's Orientation and Amnesia Test: relationship to severity of acute head injury and to recovery of memory. *Neurosurgery* 25: 683–91. doi: 10.1227/00006123-199011000-00003

Faul M, Xu L, Wald MM, Coronado VG (2010) *Traumatic Brain Injury in the United States: Emergency Department Visits, Hospitalizations and Deaths 2002–2006*. Atlanta, GA: Centers for Disease Control and Prevention, National Center for Injury Prevention and Control.

Ghigo E, Masel B, Aimaretti G et al (2005) Consensus guidelines on screening for hypopituitarism following traumatic brain injury. *Brain Inj* 19: 711–24. doi: 10.1080/02699050400025315

Ginstfeldt T, Emanuelson I (2010) An overview of attention deficits after paediatric traumatic brain injury. *Brain Inj* 24: 1123–34. doi: 10.3109/02699052.2010.506853

Gorzowski J, Kelly EH, Klaas SJ, Vogel LC (2011) Obstacles to community participation among youth with spinal cord injury. *J Spinal Cord Med* 34: 576–85. doi: 10.1179/2045772311Y.0000000037

Hagen EM, Eide GE, Rekand T, Gilhus NE, Gronning M (2010) Traumatic spinal cord injury and concomitant brain injury: a cohort study. *Acta Neurol Scand Suppl* 122: 51–7. doi: 10.1111/j.1600-0404.2010.01376.x

Iida H, Tachibana S, Kitahara T, Horiike S, Ohwada T, Fujii K (1999) Association of head trauma with cervical spine injury, spinal cord injury, or both. *J Trauma* 46: 450–2. doi: 10.1097/00005373-199903000-00018

Kaulfers AM, Backeljauw PF, Reifschneider K et al (2010) Endocrine dysfunction following traumatic brain injury in children. *J Pediatr* 157: 894–9. doi: 10.1016/j.jpeds.2010.07.004

Kelly EH, Klass SJ, Garma S, Russell HF, Vogel LC (2012) Participation and quality of life among youth with spinal cord injury. *J Pediatr Rehabil Med* 5: 315–25. doi: 10.3233/PRM-2012-00223

Kirk KA, Shoykhet M, Jeong JH et al (2012) Dysautonomia after pediatric brain injury. *Dev Med Child Neurol* 54: 759–64. doi: 10.1111/j.1469-8749.2012.04322.x

Krach LE, Kriel RL, Morris WF, Warhol BL, Luxenberg MG (1997) Central autonomic dysfunction following acquired brain injury in children. *J Neuro Rehab* 11: 41–5. doi: 10.1177/154596839701100107

Li L, Liu J (2013) The effect of pediatric traumatic brain injury on behavioral outcomes: a systematic review. *Dev Med Child Neurol* 55: 37–45. doi: 10.1111/j.1469-8749.2012.04414.x

Macciocchi S, Seel RT, Thompson N, Byams R, Bowman B (2008) Spinal cord injury and co-occurring traumatic brain injury: assessment and incidence. *Arch Phys Med Rehabil* 89: 1350–7. doi: 10.1016/j.apmr.2007.11.055

Mahalick DM, Carmel PW, Greenberg JP et al (1998) Psychopharmacologic treatment of acquired attention disorders in children with brain injury. *Pediatr Neurosurg* 29: 121–6. doi: 10.1159/000028705

Matsumoto JH, Caplan R, McArthur DL, Forgey MJ, Yudovin S, Giza CC (2013) Prevalence of epileptic and nonepileptic events after pediatric traumatic brain injury. *Epilepsy Behav* 27: 233–7. http://dx.doi.org/10.1016/j.yebeh.2013.01.024

Miles MA, Cawley MF (1996) Dual diagnosis: spinal cord injury and traumatic brain injury. In: Betz RR, Mulcahey MJ (eds). *The Child with a Spinal Cord Injury*. Rosemont, IL: American Academy of Orthopedic Surgeons, pp. 761–71.

Niederland T, Makovi H, Gal V, Andreka B, Abraham CS, Kovacs J (2007) Abnormalities of pituitary function after traumatic brain injury in children. *J Neurotrauma* 24: 119–27. 10.1089/neu.2005.369ER

Palchak MJ, Holmes JF, Vance CW et al (2004) Does an isolated history of loss of consciousness or amnesia predict brain injuries in children after blunt head trauma? *Pediatrics* 113: e507. doi: 10.1542/peds.113.6.e507

Pangilinan PH, Giacoletti-Argento A, Shellhaas R, Hurvitz EA, Hornyak JE (2010) Neuropharmacology of pediatric brain injury: a review. *PM R* 2: 1127–40. doi: 10.1016/j.pmrj.2010.07.007

Ricker JH, Regan T (1999) Neuropsychological and psychological factors in acute rehabilitation of individuals with both spinal cord injury and traumatic brain injury. *Top Spinal Cord Inj Rehabil* 5: 76–82. doi: 10.1310/0YJX-2KYE-VY3Q-9D5V

Rose SR, Auble B (2012) Endocrine changes after pediatric traumatic brain injury. *Pituitary* 15: 267–75. doi: 10.1007/s11102-011-0360-x

Sommer JL, Witkiewicz PM (2004) The therapeutic challenges of dual diagnosis: TBI/SCI. *Brain Inj* 18: 1297–308. doi: 10.1080/02699050410001672288

Statler KD (2006) Pediatric posttraumatic seizures: epidemiology, putative mechanisms of epileptogenesis and promising investigations progress. *Dev Neurosci* 28: 354–63. doi: 10.1159/000094162

Teasdale G, Jennett B (1974) Assessment of coma and impaired consciousness: a practical scale. *Lancet* 2: 81–4. doi: 10.1016/S0140-6736(74)91639-0

Tham SW, Palermo TM, Vavilala MS et al (2012) The longitudinal course, risk factors, and impact of sleep disturbances in children with traumatic brain injury. *J Neurotrauma* 29: 154–61. doi: 10.1089/neu.2011.2126

Tolonen A, Turkka J, Salonen O, Ahoniemi E, Alaranta H (2007) Traumatic brain injury is under-diagnosed in patients with spinal cord injury. *J Rehabil Med* 39: 622–6. doi: 10.2340/16501977-0101

van Tol E, Gorter JW, DeMatteo C, Meester-Delver A (2011) Participation outcomes for children with acquired brain injury: a narrative review. *Brain Inj* 25: 1279–87. doi: 10.3109/02699052.2011.613089

Vogel LC, Betz RR, Mulcahey MJ (2011) Pediatric spinal cord disorders. In: Kirshblum S, Campagnolo DI (eds). *Spinal Cord Medicine*. 2nd Ed. Philadelphia, PA: Lippincott Williams & Wilkins, pp. 533–64.

Watanabe TK, Zafonte RD, Lairson EJ (1999) Traumatic brain injury associated with acute spinal cord injury: risk factors, evaluation, and outcomes. *Top Spinal Cord Inj Rehabil* 5: 83–90. doi: 10.1310/JDDU-W8FQ-8XQQ-LNT7

Whyte J, Hart T, Laborde A, Rosenthal M (2002) Rehabilitation issues in traumatic brain injury. In: DeLisa JA (ed.). *Physical Medicine and Rehabilitation: Principles and Practice*. Philadelphia, PA: Lippincott Williams & Wilkins, pp. 1677–713.

Williams SE, Ris MD, Ayyangar R, Schefft BK, Berch D (1998) Recovery in pediatric brain injury: is psychostimulant medication beneficial? *J Head Trauma Rehabil* 13: 73–81. doi: 10.1097/00001199-199806000-00007

Wilmot CB, Cope DN, Hall KM, Acker M (1985) Occult head injury: its incidence in spinal cord injury. *Arch Phys Med Rehabil* 66: 227–31. doi: 10.1016/0003-9993(85)90148-0

Section 4 Medical Management

11
NEUROGENIC BLADDER AND BOWEL: ASSESSMENT, MANAGEMENT, AND OUTCOMES

Lisa Merenda and Gregory Dean

Case vignette

Kara is a 10-year-old female who sustained a T7 American Spinal Injury Association Impairment Scale A spinal cord injury at the age of 5 years in a motor vehicle crash. Kara's mother performs intermittent bladder catheterization every 6 hours; however, Kara wears diapers owing to urinary incontinence between catheterizations. For bowel management, her mother performs a manual evacuation every 2 days. Lately, Kara has been experiencing bowel accidents, sometimes at school, which has led to teasing by classmates and feelings of embarrassment. Kara lives in a very rural community and, owing to the extreme distance from the nearest medical center, she has not followed up with her urologist and rehabilitation team since she was injured 5 years ago.

Introduction

Bladder and bowel management after spinal cord injury (SCI) can be one of the most challenging aspects of life for children and adults alike. Impaired bladder and bowel functioning can lead to decreases in self-esteem and life satisfaction. Essential goals of bladder management include preservation of renal function and bladder health, social continence, and fostering independence. Essential goals of a bowel program are to control constipation, achieve elimination at socially convenient times, and foster age-appropriate independence.

Pathophysiology of the neurogenic bladder

The extent of urinary tract dysfunction is dependent upon the level and severity of SCI (Consortium for Spinal Cord Medicine 2006). Initially after SCI, there is a period of spinal shock manifested by an areflexic, acontractile bladder and urinary retention. Initial bladder management during this acute period is an indwelling urethral catheter; this also helps to monitor urine output. However, once the patient is stabilized, intermittent urethral catheterization should begin. After spinal shock resolution, there are generally two types of neurogenic bladder presentations. A reflexic or upper motor neuron (UMN) bladder, also known as a spastic bladder, is present in children who sustain supraconal SCI. The sacral reflex arc remains intact as demonstrated by the bulbocavernosus reflex. Detrusor overactivity is typically present, which results in incontinence, and the child is at risk of detrusor sphincter dyssynergia in which the detrusor contracts at the same time as the urethral sphincter. The lack of coordination between the detrusor and sphincter can lead to poor bladder compliance, high storage pressures, vesicoureteral reflux, and hydronephrosis. Classic urodynamic findings for an UMN lesion include uninhibited bladder contractions, detrusor sphincter dyssynergia, and high intravesical pressures. In contrast, children who sustain injuries of the cauda equina or conus will present with a lower motor neuron (LMN) bladder, also known as a flaccid bladder. Sacral reflex pathways have been disrupted. There is an absence of the bulbocavernosus reflex, and continuous voiding owing to an open bladder neck impairs bladder storage. Classic urodynamic findings for a lesion at or below the conus will reveal an areflexic, low-pressure detrusor, absent electromyography activity, and an incompetent bladder outlet.

Urologic assessment

A baseline urologic evaluation should be completed within 3 to 6 months of injury. A comprehensive history should be obtained, including presence of congenital genitourinary anomalies, previous surgeries, past and present medications, history of urinary tract infections, past and present bladder emptying methods, and frequency of urinary incontinence. Bowel function is also a necessary component of evaluation because retained stool can mechanically impair bladder filling, increase detrusor irritability leading to incontinence, and contribute to urinary retention.

Essential elements of a physical examination of the child should include physical palpation of the abdomen for a full bladder, genital examination, assessment of deep tendon reflexes including anal wink and bulbocavernosus reflex, and rectal examination with attention to anal tone and presence of stool. The presence of visual impairments, postural control, and upper extremity motor function will be important factors when considering bladder management options. A urinalysis is routinely performed; urine cultures are only indicated when the child exhibits symptoms of urinary tract infection (e.g. fever, foul odor, incontinence). Blood urea nitrogen and creatinine should be obtained at baseline, but additional blood tests are generally not necessary.

Imaging studies such as renal bladder ultrasound assess renal size, the presence of renal scarring or hydronephrosis, bladder or renal calculi, and bladder wall thickening. A portable hand-held bladder scanner can be used to determine post-void residuals. Cystography, either as a separate study or as part of a video urodynamic study, can give important baseline information including the presence of bladder trabeculation, bladder diverticula, vesicoureteral reflux, the status of the bladder neck (intact or open), and the overall configuration of the bladder. Baseline urodynamic testing should be performed once spinal shock resolves to evaluate bladder function, and is a valuable tool for identifying early signs of pathology. A catheter is placed into the bladder, which permits the measurement of bladder or detrusor pressures. Bladder filling should be performed at a rate of 5% of the expected bladder capacity per minute with sterile saline or water (Schafer et al 2002). The expected bladder capacity can be derived from the formula of Koff: age in years + 2=capacity in ounces (Koff 1983). As the bladder is filled, pressure–volume relationships are determined. Bladder filling should continue until patient discomfort occurs, volitional micturition or leakage occurs, or detrusor storage pressures exceed 40cm H_2O. A second catheter can be placed in the rectum to measure intra-abdominal pressure during the bladder filling and emptying. True bladder pressure is determined by subtracting intra-abdominal pressure from the measured bladder pressure. Electromyography is often performed simultaneously to measure external urethral sphincter activity and pelvic floor musculature during bladder filling and emptying. This measurement permits the determination of the presence or absence of detrusor sphincter dyssynergia. A critical portion of the urodynamic evaluation is to determine whether the child is storing urine at safe pressures. If the bladder stores at less than 40cm of water pressure, the risk of upper tract deterioration is unlikely (Lapides et al 1972). The upper limit of daily catheterized volumes should be determined and then correlated to the corresponding urodynamic pressure. Should the child not be storing at a safe pressure, measures need to be taken to alleviate high-pressure storage.

After children undergo the initial urologic evaluation and are on an established and appropriate method of bladder management, they should be followed up annually at a minimum. Urologic status may deteriorate over time, often without overt clinical signs and symptoms. Children may also need to be monitored more frequently if clinically indicated, for example in instances of medication changes, alterations in bladder management methods, changes in continence, recurring infection, presence of calculi, or traumatic catheterization. The annual evaluation should include an updated urologic history (type of bladder management program, medications, urinary tract infections, frequency of bladder emptying, episodes of urinary incontinence), bowel program history, and level of satisfaction with both the bladder and bowel methods. A physical examination should assess the genitalia, bladder fullness, and constipation status. A urinalysis and urine culture are indicated only with the new onset of urinary incontinence or in the presence of foul-smelling or cloudy urine. Renal bladder ultrasounds should be performed annually for ongoing surveillance of the urinary tract. Urodynamics can be useful in predicting upper tract deterioration and can permit the clinician to modulate therapy and the patient's catheterization regimen in response to this information, and should be performed whenever the patient's clinical status changes. This would include deterioration of the patient's continence status or the development of hydronephrosis. Some clinicians prefer to take a more proactive approach and perform annual urodynamics in order to modulate therapy in order to avoid clinical deterioration.

Urinary tract infections and antibiotic prophylaxis

Asymptomatic bacteriuria is common and can often be found regardless of the type of bladder method utilized in individuals with SCI. Intermittent catheterization can facilitate the introduction of enteric organisms into the bladder, which are typically colonized at the periurethral area (Lapides et al 1973). Treatment of asymptomatic bacteriuria or antibiotic prophylaxis is typically not recommended because it may result in the selection of resistant organisms. Cultures and antibiotic treatment are reserved for children who present with symptoms such as fever, chills, foul-smelling urine or pyuria. Vesicoureteral reflux may be present in some of these children as an incidental finding or as the result of a high-pressure bladder. In those children who have reflux secondary to high bladder pressures, the underlying detrusor instability and poor compliance should be addressed. The treatment of reflux in children is evolving with some recent studies questioning the role of antibiotic prophylaxis (Finnell et al 2011). In children with vesicoureteral reflux on intermittent catheterization, observation of prophylaxis is advocated by some because of the concerns over antibiotic-resistant strains of bacteria. In patients with recurrent symptomatic pyelonephritis, antibiotic prophylaxis can be considered as well as mechanical management of the reflux. Mechanical management of the reflux can be accomplished by endoscopic correction with dextranomer hyaluronic acid copolymer/dextranomer, which has been combined with simultaneous detrusor botulinum neurotoxin A injection, recognizing the importance of good bladder compliance (Dean and Doumanian 2006). An alternative approach is ureteral re-implantation. While effective, this is associated with the risk of obstruction after re-implantation as the result of bladder wall thickening.

Bladder management methods for enhanced storage

Pharmacologic Intervention

Anticholinergic therapy

Anticholinergic therapy may be useful in maintaining safe storage pressures and adequate storage volumes, limiting bladder wall hypertrophy and promoting urinary continence. The timing of initiating this therapy should be guided by the patient's course but is commonly started at the first sign of bladder instability. In patients with UMN lesions, this is at the time that spinal shock begins to recede.

Anticholinergic therapy may have troublesome side effects including facial flushing, dry mouth, dry eyes, tachycardia, constipation, and blurred vision. There is evidence that it also may have a reversible impact on cognitive ability and concentration, although some have suggested that this may not be the case (Sommer et al 2005). Hallucinations can occur, although rarely, in some patients. Although these side effects can be troublesome in some patients, they are usually dose dependent and can be managed by changing the drug formulation or dosage. Anticholinergics include:

- oxybutynin (Food and Drug Administration [FDA] approved for use in children 6 years and older);
- tolterodine (FDA approved for use in children 12 years and older);
- trospium (not FDA approved in children);
- hyoscyamine (not FDA approved in children);
- darifenacin (not FDA approved in children);
- solifenacin (not FDA approved in children); and
- fesoterodine (not FDA approved in children).

Oxybutynin is widely use as both an oral preparation and a skin patch. Because the dermal patch bypasses gastrointestinal absorption, it is believed to result in less *N*-desethyloxybutynin, a hepatic metabolite produced from oral ingestion which may be responsible for some adverse side effects of anticholinergic therapy (Staskin and Salvatore 2010). Oxybutynin can also be directly instilled into the bladder via a urethral catheter with the potential advantage of limiting systemic side effects (Lazarus 2009); however, there remains some systemic absorption through the bladder wall. This approach is limited because of its relative inconvenience. Oxybutynin has both a short-acting preparation used as often as *quater in die* (q.i.d.) and a long-acting preparation that can be administered one or two times a day. Care must be taken not to crush the long-acting preparation before oral administration to prevent an unwanted rapid delivery to the patient. The oral form of oxybutynin is usually administered to older children as a 5mg tablet twice a day and can be increased to three times per day. Oxybutynin is also available in a liquid form (1mg/1ml) and can be given at 0.3 to 0.6mg/kg per day in three divided doses. Dose adjustments are made based on clinical response as well as the presence of anticholinergic side effects.

Other anticholinergic options are available, but many can be used only off label in children. Some of them, including tolterodine, have a larger molecular weight than oxybutynin, which may have the advantage of limiting transmission across the blood–brain barrier, limiting central nervous system side effects.

Botulinum neurotoxin therapy

Botulinum neurotoxin therapy is a useful adjunct to anticholinergic therapy in improving bladder capacity and compliance. It can replace or decrease the dose of anticholinergics for many patients, and can be very useful in children who are having difficulty tolerating the side effects of anticholinergics. In some instances, it may delay or prevent the need for surgical bladder augmentation. Its use has been demonstrated in children with non-neurogenic overactive bladder (Hoebeke et al 2006), as well as in children with neurogenic bladders (Game et al 2009). Various botulinum neurotoxin A brands are available. Its effects generally wear off over a 4- to 9-month period, requiring repeat therapy. Some have demonstrated that, with repeat injections, antibodies may develop, limiting the efficacy of this approach (Schulte-Baukloh et al 2011). Patients and their families need to be alerted to the potential side effects of botulinum neurotoxin, particularly respiratory depression. Although deaths from urologic uses of botulinum neurotoxin A have not been reported, it has been seen in other clinical situations, such as injections of botulinum neurotoxin into large lower extremity muscle groups. Also of note is that systemic effects can be quite delayed before developing, in some cases days or weeks after the injection (Allergan 2011).

Intravesical botulinum neurotoxin is administered via cystoscopy while the patient is under general anesthesia. This procedure should not be performed in the face of an active bladder infection. In this procedure, 4IU botulinum neurotoxin A/kg can be utilized with up to a maximum of 300IU. Injection sites should be dispersed throughout the bladder. The trigone has been traditionally avoided because of concerns that this might induce reflux; however, there has been a report suggesting that injection into the trigone may enhance response of this therapy (Abdel-Meguid 2010). Future development includes the potential for an electromotive delivery system eliminating the need for cystoscopy (Kajbafzadeh et al 2011). This method employs an electrical current to permit migration of botulinum neurotoxin directly into the bladder wall.

Bladder Augmentation

In some patients, bladder compliance and capacity remain inadequate, despite conservative measures. When this is encountered, the clinician may consider the option of bladder augmentation. Evidence that the patient may benefit from this procedure is based on the combined clinical, radiologic, and urodynamic picture. Clinical signs of concern include persistent urinary incontinence. Radiographic signs include sonographic evidence of new hydronephrosis and bladder wall thickening or cystographic findings of bladder wall thickening or trabeculation. In the presence of these signs, urodynamics should be performed to confirm inadequate compliance manifested by elevated storage pressures (>40cm H_2O) at normal catheterized volumes or diminished volumes.

Auto-augmentation is a technique whereby the detrusor is surgically incised, thereby permitting the mucosa to expand. This has the theoretical benefit of increasing the compliance of the bladder rather than increasing the capacity. The popularity of this approach has waned over time, in part because of the lack of favorable outcome data (MacNeily et al 2003). When it is employed, it is in those instances where the bladder volume is normal but the bladder compliance is impaired.

Intestinal augmentation

This approach involves harvesting a segment of large or small bowel, reconfiguring it as a patch, and then anastomosing it to the bladder in order to increase bladder compliance and capacity. Ileum is the most commonly used segment of bowel for bladder augmentation. Large bowel, usually sigmoid colon, is relatively simple to harvest but often results in large volumes of mucus within the urine, necessitating bladder irrigation. Although ileum has the advantage of exuding less mucus, it is more likely to result in vitamin B_{12} deficiency. Care must be taken to ensure that the segment used is completely detubularized to prevent spontaneous contractions, which can elevate bladder pressures.

Complications of intestinal augmentation include spontaneous perforation of the augmented segment with a mortality rate as high as 10% (Metcalfe et al 2006). Perforation may be associated with poor compliance with intermittent catheterization but can also occur sporadically. Should a patient with a bladder augmentation develop abdominal pain, computed tomography cystography or standard cystography should be performed. For patients who have undergone bladder augmentation, annual cystoscopy is recommended to begin 3 to 10 years after the initial procedure to monitor for the risk of carcinoma (Metcalfe and Rink 2007); vitamin B_{12} levels should also be evaluated for any patients having undergone ileal bladder augmentation (Metcalfe and Rink 2007).

Bladder Outlet Management

In patients with LMN disease, the presence of an open bladder neck can result in urinary incontinence, which may be continuous or exacerbated with movement or valsalva maneuvers. Radiographic evidence of this is usually demonstrated on the cystogram. Video urodynamics demonstrate a low leak point pressure with an open bladder neck. Potential treatment options for this group of patients ranges from surgical urethral closures, artificial sphincters, sling procedures, and bladder neck bulking.

Bladder neck reconstruction, such as the Kropp procedure through open surgery, is a reasonable consideration but can be associated with difficult catheterization and the loss of the bladder neck pop-off valve, which protects against excessive intravesical pressure (Kropp and Angwafo 1986). The artificial urinary sphincter is another consideration (Scott 1985). Although this device can render some patients dry, the potential for urethral erosion, need for revision, and difficulty with manipulating the sphincteric mechanism have limited wide adoption.

Sling procedures provide an alternative to the artificial sphincter and perform by providing constant passive urethral compression. In males, sling procedures can be performed either in an open abdominal fashion or through a perineal approach, but both have a moderate failure rate (Dean and Kunkle 2009). The pubovaginal sling has good success in females but can be difficult to perform in the prepubertal female because of space constraints within the introitus.

Because of these shortcomings, endoscopic bulking procedures have been explored. The application of polytetrafluoroethylene as a bladder neck-bulking agent spurred initial interest in this approach but was discarded because of evidence of distal migration (Malizia et al 1984). Other materials have been utilized and, most recently, dextranomer hyaluronic acid copolymer/dextranomer bladder bulking has become an option, which is a copolymer with many advantages over other substances, including ease of injection through a thin needle and good tissue tolerance. Although it has been FDA approved in the treatment of vesicoureteral reflux, its use as a bladder neck-bulking agent remains off label. Although initial studies demonstrated success (Caione and Capozza 2002), the need for ongoing retreatment is a limiting factor (Dean et al 2007).

Bladder management methods for enhanced emptying

Intermittent Catheterization

Clean intermittent catheterization (CIC) (Lapides et al 1972) is the preferred treatment for children with a neurogenic bladder owing to its relatively low complication rate. CIC prevents overdistension of the bladder, reduces the risk of urinary infection, and decreases episodes of urinary incontinence. Complications associated with this technique include urethral trauma, false passages, and urethral strictures. The frequency of catheterization can be based on timed hourly intervals or can be volume dependent. Most children catheterize four to six times a day. In children with SCI, catheterized volumes should not exceed those that elevate bladder pressures over 40cm of water pressure. Early intervention with CIC may begin as early as infancy if there is evidence of a poorly emptying high-pressure bladder. More commonly, it is initiated at the age of 2 to 3 years, when their peers are becoming toilet trained. Parents initially perform CIC and gradually transfer the process to the child upon school age. For those who are able to perform CIC, independence should be expected between 7 and 8 years of age. Independently performed CIC should not be expected in children whose developmental level is less than 5 years of age. Depending on the level of injury, a child may not be able to independently perform catheterization. Children with tetraplegia, particularly C5 injuries or above, are typically not able to perform a self-CIC program owing to limitations in hand function. Importantly, children with tetraplegia should be able to describe and appropriately direct catheterization to another person in the event of an emergency. Adaptive equipment is available, as well as upper extremity reconstructive procedures, to enhance independence and improve hand function in children with tetraplegia (see Chapter 20). Children with paraplegia can usually become quite proficient in self-CIC. Factors that inhibit independence include cognition and body habitus. Because young people with SCI are at risk of latex allergy, catheters should be non-latex. Longer catheters are used by males, whereas females usually prefer shorter ones. The size of the catheter should be increased as the child grows, with the following suggested sizes: infants, 5 French; toddlers and preschool children, 6 to 8 French; school-aged children, 8 to 12 French; and adolescents, 12 to 16 French.

The use of chronic indwelling urethral or suprapubic catheters is not recommended for children with SCI because of the risk of bladder malignancy associated with this approach (Gormley 2010) and the development of bladder calculi. Additional risks associated with indwelling catheters include urethral erosion and recurrent urinary tract infections.

It is important to note that other options sometimes utilized by adults with SCI are not routinely recommended for children with SCI. Crede and valsalva techniques, once thought to be harmless, are not recommended owing to risks of increased intravesical pressure, vesicoureteral reflux, and hydronephrosis. Reflex voiding with or without external collection devices should not be used because of poor bladder emptying, urinary tract infections, and risk of autonomic dysreflexia and vesicoureteral reflux in the presence of detrusor sphincter dyssynergia (Consortium for Spinal Cord Medicine 2006). Although not available in all countries, electrical stimulation and posterior sacral rhizotomy can be applied to sacral nerve roots innervating the bladder to produce urination on demand without the use of catheters. This technique has been predominantly applied to adults with SCI; however, its use in skeletally mature children and adolescents with SCI has been explored (Merenda et al 2000). Owing to the irreversibility of this procedure, it has not been widely accepted as a form of bladder management for children with SCI.

Continent Catheterizeable Stoma

The continent catheterizeable stoma is a reconstructive procedure that permits enhanced ease of emptying by either the patient or their caregiver. It is particularly useful for those who have difficulty performing CIC owing to diminished hand function, body habitus, or difficulty with hand–eye coordination. Continent catheterizeable stomas are especially appealing in females because of the difficulty in accessing their urethra, along with clothing issues and the necessity for physical transfer from the wheelchair to the toilet.

Mitrofanoff

In the Mitrofanoff procedure (Mitrofanoff 1980), a native tissue tube is used to construct a channel into the bladder with continence achieved by compression of the tube by the bladder wall. Although the tissue of choice is the appendix, an alternative is a small segment of ileum (Monti technique; Monti et al 1997). Other less common alternatives to the appendix include the fallopian tube or native ureter. The stoma that is created at the skin level can be located anywhere on the abdominal wall with the umbilicus being the most common site because of its favorable ergonomic and cosmetic location. Although the Mitrofanoff technique is associated with high levels of patient satisfaction, full disclosure of the potential complications should be reviewed, including stomal stenosis, which occurs in approximately 15% of individuals (Thomas et al 2006). Other complications include urinary leakage and small bowel obstruction. A relatively non-invasive treatment for stomal incontinence is endoscopic bulking with dextranomer hyaluronic acid copolymer/dextranomer.

An option for use of the appendix for both urinary bladder emptying and fecal washout (antegrade continence enema procedure) has been described and is known as the split appendix technique (VanderBrink et al 2011). This is commonly performed with one stoma situated within the umbilicus and the other in a nearby but separate abdominal location. Recently, a variant of this has been described using the umbilicus for both stomas. In this approach, the appendix is split and both stomas are created within the umbilicus yielding a cosmetically appealing appearance.

Incontinence stomas

Incontinence stomas may be considered for children with severe cognitive deficits who would obtain no significant social or emotional benefit from urinary continence or in children with recurrent ruptures of an augmented bladder. This can be particularly useful if the family or caregivers are unable to perform intermittent catheterization. Caution must be exercised in this situation to ensure that aggressive skin care precautions are practiced and, if a collection device is used, it should be emptied routinely. Options for incontinence stomas include vesicostomy and an ileal chimney. A vesicostomy is an excellent option for bladder drainage, particularly in children who are not yet toilet trained. As the child becomes older, vesicostomies are not easily managed with a urinary collection device. Furthermore, attempts at constructing vesicostomies in older children can be difficult because of trouble bringing the bladder out to the level of the abdominal wall. An ileal chimney is a technique whereby a short segment of ileum is isolated and used to bridge the bladder with the abdominal wall. It has the advantage of simplifying the fitment of a urinary collection device. It obviates the difficulty of bringing the bladder to skin level in older patients and it avoids the need for ureteral implantation as is required with an ileal conduit.

Pathophysiology of the neurogenic bowel

The mechanisms behind neurogenic bowel dysfunction are in many ways similar to those underlying the neurogenic bladder. There are two clinical presentations of bowel dysfunction after SCI. Supraconal lesions result in an UMN bowel or hyper-reflexic bowel, manifested by increased colonic and anal tone. Disruption of voluntary control of the external anal sphincter causes it to tighten and retain stool. Reflexive coordination and stool propulsion are preserved owing to intact nerve connections between the sacral spinal cord and colon. Patients with a hyper-reflexic bowel typically exhibit constipation and fecal retention. Stool evacuation in these patients occurs owing to reflexive activity in response to some type of stimulus introduced into the rectum (suppositories or digital stimulation) (Krassioukov et al 2010).

Injuries at the conus or cauda equina result in a LMN bowel, often referred to as areflexic bowel, manifested by decreased peristalsis and slower stool propulsion. Constipation and incontinence are associated with a hyporeflexic bowel owing to an atonic external anal sphincter and a lack of control of the levator ani muscle, which causes the rectal lumen to open (Krassioukov et al 2010).

Assessment

Clinical assessment should include a detailed history of defecation patterns including the time of day, stool consistency, frequency, medications, diet, and fluid intake. Stool consistency is affected by dietary fiber and fluid intake. Foods high in fiber contribute to softer stool, whereas flours, breads, cereals, and dairy products tend to make the stool firmer. Hard and dry stools can lead to impaction and trauma to the rectum or bowel. Ideally, stool should be soft and formed. Cognitive level, postural control, joint contractures, and upper extremity function may present a challenge in establishing a bowel program. Evaluating both the pre-injury bowel patterns and any previously attempted bowel management methods can be particularly useful when selecting a bowel program. The child's daily routines and family schedules should also be assessed. Bowel programs are more likely to be carried out if they are reasonable and acceptable to both the child and family. Bowel programs should not cause major interruptions to the child's schedule (meals, school, bedtime) and lifestyle (recreational and community activities).

Management

Goals of a successful bowel program are to control constipation, achieve elimination at socially convenient times, obtain an absence of fecal incontinence, and gain independence (Merenda and Brown 2004). Bowel regimens will differ based upon the level of the lesion and whether it is an upper or lower neuron lesion. Bowel programs are typically initiated when children are 2 to 4 years of age; this is consistent with typical age-appropriate development of continence. Bowel programs can be instituted earlier if the child is experiencing difficulties with diarrhea or constipation. Although the parents will primarily be providing the direct care for the toddler/preschool-aged child, the child should still be involved in his or her care early on. By the time the child reaches school age, he or she should be gaining more independence in his or her bowel care. Total independence with performing bowel routines is typically expected by the time the child reaches 10 to 12 years of age. Similar to bladder management, independence levels depend upon level of injury. Children with high tetraplegia will have limitations in upper extremity function that affect their ability to perform bowel management. Children with tetraplegia may undergo upper extremity reconstructive procedures, which can enhance their ability to perform bowel management (see Chapter 20). Children with paraplegia should be able to perform all aspects of bowel care. Factors that may inhibit independence in the child with paraplegia include cognitive maturity and body habitus. In addition, consultation with occupational therapy is beneficial, as the use of adaptive equipment can afford greater independence with bowel management. As the child enters adolescence, compliance with care may become a factor; the need to be accepted by peers may conflict with the need for carrying out physical care tasks. Regardless of the child's age, bowel programs must be carried out consistently at the same time of day (every day or every other day), even if incontinence occurs. Whatever bowel program is used, it should be carried out on the toilet or commode chair so that gravity can aid in stool passage, and privacy should be afforded to young people of all ages.

Conservative Measures

Manual evacuation involves the insertion of one or two gloved, lubricated fingers into the rectum to break up or grab the stool and remove it from the rectum. Children with LMN injuries typically utilize manual evacuation as their primary means for bowel management. Manual evacuation may yield only limited amounts of stool and can produce irritation to the anus and rectal vault.

Digital stimulation is the direct stimulation of the anal sphincter to elicit evacuation. It can increase motility in the left colon by activating preserved anorectal colonic reflexes. A gloved, lubricated finger is gently inserted into the anal canal and small circular motions are performed to stimulate the external and internal anal sphincters. The sphincters relax and the smooth muscles of the lower colon contract to expel stool. Digital stimulation can be repeated every 10 minutes as necessary until stool evacuation is complete. Digital stimulation is more effective in patients with a UMN lesion as they have anal tone and can reflexively empty their bowel. Digital stimulation is less useful for those with LMN lesions, but can be trialed to see if it assists in bowel evacuation during manual stool removal.

Suppositories and small-volume enemas stimulate complete emptying of stool from the lower colon and are generally most effective in those with UMN lesions. These options can provide predictability, as evacuation is closer to the time of administration. Glycerin and bisacodyl are common active ingredients in suppositories utilized for children and adults. Polyethylene glycol-based suppositories containing bisacodyl, better known as the magic bullet, are also available and have grown in popularity. They have been shown to stimulate reflex defecation sooner and significantly shorten the total bowel care time compared with traditional hydrogenated vegetable oil-based bisacodyl suppositories (Stiens et al 1998). Docusate sodium (5ml) or liquid glycerin (5–10ml) are the most common mini enemas (or liquid suppositories) used, whereas bisacodyl and sodium phosphate are the most common small enemas used. The suppositories and mini enemas are administered rectally to stimulate evacuation. Response times vary with the products but the stimulant should ideally work within 15 to 30 minutes (Merenda and Brown 2004). Manual stool removal is necessary before administration of any suppositories or mini enemas so that the medication makes contact directly with the rectal wall. Large-volume enemas are not preferred for daily management as retaining fluid, premature expulsion of fluid, and independent administration can be challenging for children with SCI. More recently, a transanal irrigation system, known as Peristeen (Coloplast, Denmark), has been utilized to assist with emptying the lower part of the bowel (Pacilli et al 2014). This system uses tap water that is introduced into the rectum via a precoated rectal catheter that contains a soft inflatable balloon to help anchor it in place during irrigation. This system offers rectal catheters in pediatric and adult sizes.

Oral medications used in bowel management for children include stool softeners (with or without stimulants), bulk laxatives, and osmotic agents. Stool softeners, such as docusate sodium, may be used on a daily basis; they assist with drawing water into the stool making it softer for passage. Stimulant laxatives, such as senna and bisacodyl, can induce defecation by stimulating peristaltic activity in the intestine; they can be administered approximately 4 to 6 hours before the desired bowel evacuation. Osmotic agents such as polyethylene glycol cause water to be retained within the small intestine and colon, aiding in softer stool.

Surgical Measures

When conservative measures fail with bowel management, either through difficulty with chronic constipation or incontinence, or through failure to simplify bowel management and enhance independence, surgical options should be considered. A basic requirement is that a patient needs to be able to be positioned over a commode on a regular basis for periods up to 60 minutes in duration. These techniques promote bowel management by permitting the passage of fluid within the colon thereby performing an antegrade enema. These approaches are distinct from a colostomy in that they promote fecal continence rather than the use of an external appliance.

Malone procedure

The Malone technique brings the tip of the appendix out to the skin level. A catheter can then periodically be placed into the stoma to permit antegrade washouts of stool. This is also referred to as the antegrade continence enema procedure or Malone Antegrade Continence Enema (MACE) procedure. This procedure can be performed in conjunction with other reconstructive procedures including the Mitrofanoff procedure and bladder augmentation. During surgical planning for these other procedures, consideration for construction of an antegrade continence enema should be made because of the added complexity and risk of asynchronous reconstruction.

Cecostomy button

A cecostomy button can be accomplished through open surgery or by utilizing interventional radiology. These buttons are small silastic appliances with a trap door that can be connected to permit irrigation. They are easily placed and can be used as a temporary means to determine if this approach will be effective before creating a MACE or a permanent device. Compared with a MACE, the disadvantages of a cecostomy include the difficulty to manipulate, limited speed of irrigation depending on sizing, and cosmetics.

Summary

Bladder and bowel management for children with SCI can be one of the most difficult aspects of their disability. In addition, bladder and bowel issues can affect long-term health and well-being. It is essential that children are placed on bladder and bowel regimens that foster independence and promote continence. Methods should be realistic and acceptable to both the child and family. Satisfaction with daily methods ultimately affects long-term compliance and health. Medical monitoring of children is critical; subtle changes can occur over time, often without overt clinical signs and symptoms. Today's surgical methods for enhanced bladder and bowel emptying continue to improve and evolve. These methods can afford children with high-level injuries greater independence and function.

REFERENCES

Abdel-Meguid TA (2010) Botulinum toxin-A injections into neurogenic overactive bladder--to include or exclude the trigone? A prospective, randomized, controlled trial. *J Urol* 184: 2423–28. doi: 10.1016/j.juro.2010.08.028

Allergan (2013) *Highlights of Prescribing Information: Botox* [online]. Available at: www.allergan.com/assets/PDF/botox_pi.pdf

Caione P, Capozza N (2002) Endoscopic treatment of urinary incontinence in pediatric patients: 2-year experience with dextranomer/hyaluronic acid copolymer. *J Urol* 168: 1868–71. doi: 10.1016/S0022-5347(05)64432-1

Consortium for Spinal Cord Medicine (2006) Bladder management for adults with spinal cord injury: a clinical practice guideline for health care providers. Washington, DC: Paralyzed Veterans of America.

Dean GE, Doumanian LR (2006) The extended use of deflux (dextranomer/hyaluronic acid) in pediatric urology. *Curr Urol Rep* 7: 143–8. http://dx.doi.org/10.1007/s11934-006-0074-1

Dean GE, Kunkle DA (2009) Outpatient perineal sling in adolescent boys with neurogenic incontinence. *J Urol* 182: 1792–6. doi:10.1016/j.juro.200904.082

Dean GE, Kirsch AJ, Packer MG, Scherz HC, Zaontz MR (2007) Antegrade and retrograde endoscopic dextranomer/hyaluronic Acid bladder neck bulking for pediatric incontinence. *J Urol* 178: 652–5. doi:10.1016/j.juro.200704.005

Finnell SM, Carroll AE, Downs SM (2011) Technical report-diagnosis and management of an initial UTI, in febrile infants and young children. *Pediatrics* 128: e749–70. doi: 10.1542/peds.2011-1332

Game X, Mouracade P, Chartier-Kastler E et al (2009) Botulinum toxin-A (Botox) intradetrusor injections in children with neurogenic detrusor overactivity/neurogenic overactive bladder: a systematic literature review. *J Pediatr Urol* 5: 156–64. doi: 10.1016/j.jpurol.2009.01.005

Gormley EA (2010) Urologic complications of the neurogenic bladder. *Urol Clin North Am* 37: 601–7. doi: 10.1016/j.ucl.201007.002

Hoebeke P, De CK, Vande WJ et al (2006) The effect of botulinum A toxin in incontinent children with therapy resistant overactive detrusor. *J Urol* 176: 328–30. doi:10.1016/S0022-5347(06)00301-6

Kajbafzadeh AM, Ahmadi H, Montaser-Kouhsari L, Sharifi-Rad L, Nejat F, Bazargan-Hejazi S (2011) Intravesical electromotive botulinum toxin type A administration--part II: clinical application. *Urology* 77: 439–45. doi: 10.1016/j.urology.201006.003

Koff SA (1983) Estimating bladder capacity in children. *Urology* 21: 248. doi: 10.1016/0090-4295(83)90079-1

Krassioukov A, Eng JJ, Claxton G, Sakakibara BM, Shum S (2010) Neurogenic bowel management after spinal cord injury: a systematic review of the evidence. *Spinal Cord* 48: 718–33. doi: 10.1038/sc.201014

Kropp KA, Angwafo FF (1986) Urethral lengthening and reimplantation for neurogenic incontinence in children. *J Urol* 135: 533–6.

Lapides J, Diokno AC, Silber SJ, Lowe BS (1972) Clean intermittent self-catheterization in the treatment of urinary tract disease. *J Urol* 107: 458–61.

Lapides J, Diokno AC, Lowe BS, Kalish MD (1973) Followup on unsterile intermittent self-catheterization. *Trans Am Assoc Genitourin Surg* 65: 44–50.

Lazarus J (2009) Intravesical oxybutynin in the pediatric neurogenic bladder. *Nat Rev Urol* 6: 671–4. doi: 10.1038/nrurol.2009214

MacNeily AE, Afshar K, Coleman GU, Johnson HW (2003) Autoaugmentation by detrusor myotomy: its lack of effectiveness in the management of congenital neuropathic bladder. *J Urol* 170: 1643–6. doi:10.1097/01.ju.0000083800.25112.22

Malizia AA Jr, Reiman HM, Myers RP et al (1984) Migration and granulomatous reaction after periurethral injection of polytef (Teflon). *JAMA* 251: 3277–81. doi:10.1001/jama.1984.03340480059030

Merenda L, Brown JP (2004) Bladder and bowel management for the child with spinal cord dysfunction. *J Spinal Cord Med* 27(Suppl 1): S16–23.

Merenda LA, Spoltore TA, Betz RR (2000) Progressive treatment options for children with spinal cord injury. *SCI Nurs* 17: 102–9.

Metcalfe PD, Rink RC (2007) Bladder augmentation: complications in the pediatric population. *Curr Urol Rep* 8: 152–6. http://dx.doi.org/10.1007/s11934-007-0065-x

Metcalfe PD, Casale AJ, Kaefer MA et al (2006) Spontaneous bladder perforations: a report of 500 augmentations in children and analysis of risk. *J Urol* 175: 1466–70. doi:10.1016/S0022-5347(05)00672-5

Mitrofanoff P (1980) Trans-appendix continent vesicostomy in treatment of neurogenic bladder in children [in French]. *Chir Pediatr* 21: 297–305.

Monti PR, Lara RC, Dutra MA, de Carvalho JR (1997) New techniques for construction of efferent conduits based on the Mitrofanoff principle. *Urology* 49: 112–5. doi:10.1016/S0090-4295(96)00503-1

Pacilli M, Pallot D, Andrews A, Downer A, Dale L, Willetts I (2014) Use of Peristeen transanal irrigation for bowel management in children: a single-center experience. *J Ped Surgery* 49: 269–72. doi:10.1016/j.jpedsurg.201311.036

Schafer W, Abrams P, Liao L et al (2002) Good urodynamic practices: uroflowmetry filling cystometry and pressure-flow studies. 21: 261–74.

Schulte-Baukloh H, Herholz J, Bigalke H, Miller K, Knispel HH (2011) Results of a BoNT/A, antibody study in children and adolescents after onabotulinumtoxin A (Botox(R)) detrusor injection. *Urol Int* 87: 434–8. doi: 10.1159/000331726

Scott FB (1985) Use of the artificial sphincter in the treatment of urinary incontinence. *Clin Obstet Gynaecol* 12: 415–29.

Sommer BR, O'Hara R, Askari N, Kraemer HC, Kennedy WA (2005) The effect of oxybutynin treatment on cognition in children with diurnal incontinence. *J Urol* 173: 2125–7. doi:10.1097/01.ju.0000157685.83573.79

Staskin DR, Salvatore S (2010) Oxybutynin topical and transdermal formulations: an update. *Drugs Today (Barc)* 46: 417–25. http://dx.doi.org/10.1358/dot.2010.46.6.1487750

Stiens SA, Luttrel W, Binard JE (1998) Polyethylene glycol versus vegetable oil based bisacodyl suppositories to initiate side-lying bowel care: a clinical trial in persons with spinal cord injury. *Spinal Cord* 36: 777–81. http://dx.doi.org/10.1038/sj.sc.3100702

Thomas JC, Dietrich MS, Trusler L et al (2006) Continent catheterizable channels and the timing of their complications. *J Urol* 176: 1816–20. doi:10.1016/S0022-5347(06)00610-0

VanderBrink BA, Cain MP, Kaefer M, Meldrum KK, Misseri R, Rink RC (2011) Split-appendix technique for simultaneous appendicovesicostomy and appendicocecostomy. *J Pediatr Surg* 46: 259–62. doi: 10.1016/j.jpedsurg.2010.08.001

12
SPASTICITY

Loren T Davidson, James W Middleton and Joyce Oleszek

Case vignette

Jason is a 17-year-old male with a C5 American Spinal Injury Association Impairment Scale A spinal cord injury who attends the clinic for spasticity management. Physical examination reveals Modified Ashworth Scale (MAS) 3 tone in the lower extremities with easily triggered flexion withdrawal response to tactile stimulation. Skin examination reveals stage 2 wounds of the bilateral posterior heels owing to friction against the bed surface when spasticity is triggered. Relieving and exacerbating factors were enquired about and no contributing factors to exacerbate spasticity were identified; the current degree of tone has been present for more than 6 months. Jason has tried conservative treatment with regular stretching, therapy, and a functional electrical stimulation cycle with little alleviation of spasticity. A trial of oral baclofen in combination with oral diazepam and dantrolene sodium was initiated; however, sedative side effects and the risk of hepatic toxicity have limited effective dosing. After a successful intrathecal baclofen bolus trial, Jason elected to have an intrathecal baclofen pump implanted. Once the spasticity and flexion withdrawal response were controlled via the pump, Jason was finally able to heal the open sores and discontinue the previous oral antispasticity medications.

Introduction

Spasticity is a component of upper motor neuron syndrome characterized by velocity-dependent resistance to passive range of motion resulting from an increase in tonic stretch reflexes and accompanied by exaggerated tendon jerks (Sanger et al 2003). Spasticity is a form of hypertonia, although the terms are not synonymous, as hypertonia is a descriptive term intended to describe only the increase in resistance to passive motion. Hypertonia encompasses a broader category of motor disorders associated with upper motor neuron syndrome including disorders that arise from brain pathology, specifically dystonia, rigidity, and hyperkinetic movement disorders (tremor, athetosis, chorea, and ballismus), which are not present in spinal cord injury (SCI). It is often difficult to clinically differentiate the component of hypertonia that is attributable to spasticity rather than soft tissue stiffness or shortening (rheologic changes) (Sheean and McGuire 2009). Spasticity is not immediately apparent after complete SCI during the period of spinal shock. Spinal shock is a temporary loss of spinal reflex activity occurring below the zone of injury and is associated with flaccid paralysis and absent muscle stretch reflexes (MSRs) (Kirshblum and Campagnolo 2011: p. 107). The duration of spinal shock is variable but generally resolves within weeks of injury. Spasticity generally follows spinal shock but may be delayed for up to 2 months or more in some circumstances. Of note is that an SCI characterized by concomitant damage to the anterior horn cell, nerve root, or distal lower motor neuron including cauda equina is characterized by flaccid paralysis and may mitigate the development of spasticity.

Pathophysiology

In the setting of SCI, the complex interplay of regulatory feedback loops that modulate MSRs is disrupted (Fig. 12.1). The precise mechanism of spasticity is not known and is probably multifactorial. Although a number of mechanisms have been proposed, most attribute spasticity to a disruption of normal descending control of spinal segmental reflexes which serve to modulate α-motor neuron firing and the associated muscle contraction in response to an afferent stimulus. The purpose of spinal reflexes is to allow rapid motor responses to external stimuli without requiring the additional time needed for central processing by the brain. The response to a stimulus or reflex may be excitatory, inhibitory, or both. The following section will serve as a brief overview of spinal reflexes, their role in daily activities, and how dysregulation of these complex feedback loops leads to spasticity. A basic understanding of spinal reflex physiology is helpful in understanding the treatment options for spasticity and their mechanisms of action.

Muscle stretch reflexes

Muscle stretch reflexes or deep tendon reflexes are normal physiological responses to changes in muscle length, tension, and velocity of stretch with MSR being the preferred terminology, as

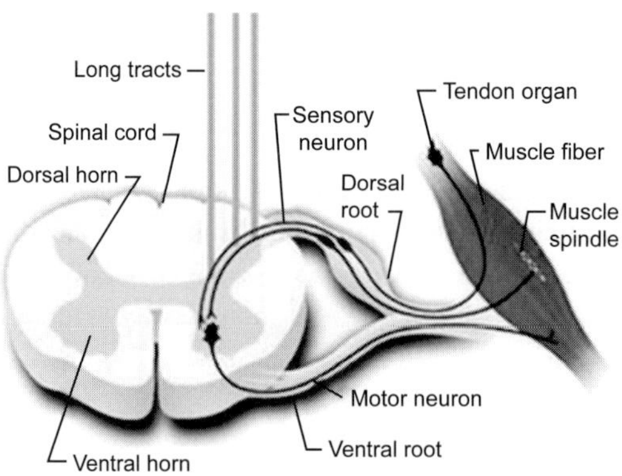

Fig. 12.1 Reflex arc.

the receptor to the external stimulus or stretch is located in the muscle rather than the tendon. The MSR has both phasic and tonic components. The phasic component is a response to a change in muscle length and is a short-acting monosynaptic reflex. An example of a phasic MSR response is the patellar tendon reflex that results in a rapid non-sustained contraction of the quadriceps muscle. In contrast, the tonic component of a MSR is a long-acting polysynaptic reflex that functions to maintain postural reflexes in response to changes in muscle stretch. Specialized receptors for muscle length and tension are known as muscle spindles and Golgi tendon organs, respectively. Muscle spindles are activated by muscle stretch and lengthening but are silent during active muscle contraction and shortening of the muscle. Golgi tendon organs are activated by lengthening of the muscle during stretch or shortening of the muscle during contraction. Thus, passive stretching of a muscle causes afferents from both Golgi tendon organs and muscle spindles to fire, but active muscle contraction silences input from muscle spindles, while causing Golgi tendon organs to fire at a faster rate (Kirshblum and Campagnolo 2011: p. 265).

Physiological modulation of the stretch reflex is facilitated by a number of different pathways both at the muscle level and from brain centers via inhibitory interneurons. Examples of normal spinal reflex modulation include reciprocal inhibition, presynaptic Ia inhibition, recurrent inhibition, and non-reciprocal inhibition. Each of these mechanisms has been implicated in the pathophysiology of spasticity. Reciprocal inhibition is mediated by afferent feedback from the muscle spindle via group Ia and group II fibers to excite both the agonist muscle and its synergists while simultaneously inhibiting the antagonist muscle. The purpose of reciprocal inhibition is to prevent co-contraction of both the agonist and antagonist muscles. Presynaptic Ia inhibition is facilitated by modulation of the excitatory signal traveling from the α-motor neuron to the muscle via axo-axonal connections. Presynaptic inhibition serves to modify the monosynaptic stretch reflex and its disruption is believed to cause hyper-reflexia. Recurrent inhibition is a mechanism of negative feedback on the α- and γ-motor neuron that involves a specialized type of interneuron called the Renshaw cell. Finally, non-reciprocal inhibition involves Ib fibers from Golgi tendon organs, which synapse on interneurons to cause inhibition of the α-motor neuron.

Assessment and pharmacologic treatment of spasticity in children

Assessment

Comprehensive clinical evaluation by an experienced interprofessional team is the foundation for treatment planning and decision making. This involves not only careful assessment of various aspects of spasticity (e.g. tonic stretch reflexes; clonus, flexor, or extensor reflexes; muscle co-contraction, weakness, contracture), but, more importantly, their overall functional impact on the child. Spasticity is not always undesirable and the rehabilitation approach to its treatment must consider both the positive and the negative effects. The art of spasticity management is determining the degree of spasticity that may be tolerable and whether there may be a functional benefit or if it is just counterproductive and potentially injurious. Evaluation begins by eliciting a thorough history, establishing the type, frequency, severity, distribution (i.e. generalized versus localized), chronicity, and diurnal variation of spasms; the impact of spasms on sleep and positioning; the exacerbating and relieving factors; and any recent changes. It is also important to evaluate age-appropriate motor development and self-care, mobility, and health-related issues (e.g. contractures, deformities, pain, hip subluxation, or skin breakdown). Evaluation of function will entail reviewing activities of daily living and enquiring about negative effects of spasticity such as interference with positioning, transfers, dressing, bathing, toileting, sitting balance, wheelchair propulsion, or ambulation. For example, extensor spasms of the trunk and lower limbs may interfere with safe and independent transfer board-assisted or hoist transfers. Severe hip adductor spasticity may lead to difficulties in self care including perineal hygiene, bladder catheterization, dressing, and bed positioning. It may also impact sexuality and sexual function and impair ambulation. Spasticity in the elbow, wrist, and finger flexors may interfere with upper limb and hand function.

Physical examination includes the assessment of joint range of motion; measurement of resistance to passive range of motion, which will vary by body position; MSRs; reflex spread; cutaneomuscular reflexes (e.g. flexion withdrawal response); and clonus. Voluntary muscle strength is graded on the Medical Research Council scale from 0 to 5. However, given that static strength may be strong (recruitment facilitated by hyperactive stretch reflexes), it is critical to evaluate selective motor control. It is important to observe the quality and ease of movements, posture, and voluntary control, and how spontaneous spasms and muscle overactivity interfere with the child's age-appropriate motor tasks and functional activities. The ultimate aim is to correlate findings from the assessment of body system/structure impairments (e.g. spasticity, hypertonia, hyperactive reflexes, muscle weakness, altered balance, impaired motor control, joint contracture) with activity limitations and participation restrictions to determine their relative contributions.

A sudden increase in spasticity or progressive deterioration of function owing to spasticity may signify secondary complications. Potential etiologies of the exacerbation are numerous and may include urinary tract infections, urinary calculi, epididymo-orchitis, constipation, hemorrhoids, fissures, cholecystitis, pressure sores, burns, ingrown toenails, heterotopic ossification, hip subluxation, fracture, or post-traumatic syringomyelia.

A variety of clinical and research tools exist to assess spasticity both quantitatively and qualitatively. Unfortunately, many of these do not provide a practical or reliable way to assess spasticity in a clinic setting, and they have not been validated for use with children (Platz et al 2005, Biering-Sorensen et al 2006). Special consideration must also be given to the environment in which testing occurs in order to minimize confounding factors such as fear, anxiety, ambient temperature, and discomfort. For young children, it is often helpful to examine them in their parent's lap and incorporate play in the clinical assessment. The Ashworth scale (Ashworth 1964) and its subsequent modified version (Bohannon and Smith 1987) are used most commonly to assess resistance to passive movement through a range on a five-point (or modified six-point) ordinal scale at an unspecified velocity without standardization of testing posture (e.g. sitting or supine position). Despite simplicity and wide use, the Ashworth scale and its modified version lack content validity to distinguish the velocity-dependent nature of spasticity from hypertonia (Fleuren et al 2010), with reliability of testing possibly depending on the examiner's experience and varying depending on the limb/joint being tested (Platz et al 2005, Biering-Sorensen et al 2006). Of all the available scales, only the Tardieu scale (Gracies et al 2010) conforms to the definition of spasticity, passively moving the joint at three specified velocities (slow, under gravity, and fast) and rating intensity, duration of muscle response to stretch, and the joint angle where tone first increases; however, it is time consuming (Scholtes et al 2006). The modified Tardieu scale (Boyd and Graham 1999) is simpler in that it records joint angle at the moment of 'catch' (increase in tone) with a fast stretching movement and can be used to calculate the 'dynamic component' by subtraction from the angle reached with slow passive movement.

In addition, a range of other scales may be applied to measure indirect effects of spasticity on daily functioning (activity limitation) and the level of assistance required, such as the pediatric version of the FIM[a] (WeeFIM®, Amherst, NY, USA) (Ottenbacher et al 2000) or the Pediatric Evaluation of Disability Inventory (PEDI™, San Antonio, TX, USA) (Feldman et al 1990), which is a more comprehensive clinical assessment of key functional capabilities and performance in children between the ages of 6 months and 7 years. For children, particularly those under the age of 5 years, unlike adolescents and adults, several developmental scales are commonly used for assessing gross and fine motor performance (e.g. Bayley Scales of Infant Development, Peabody Developmental Motor Scales) (Bayley 1993, Fewell and Folio 2000). However, the developmental scales are not validated for children with SCI and do not assess the quality or ease of movement and, thus, are often not sensitive to changes with treatment of spasticity. For an in-depth review of the available measures of spasticity and outcome with SCI, readers could refer to the SCI Rehabilitation Evidence website (http://www.scireproject.com). It should be noted that few measures are established for use in children and this should be a research priority.

Assessment of gait may take different forms, including observational gait analysis; spatiotemporal measurement of characteristics such as gait speed, cadence, step length, and stride length on an electronic walkway (Thorpe et al 2005); and full kinematic/kinetic motion analysis. Motion analysis cannot directly measure spasticity but may demonstrate the effect of spasticity reduction on mobility by comparing before and after treatment.

Treatment

Non-operative management

Management of spasticity must be individually tailored to specific goals based on factors already discussed. Taking an incremental approach with a treatment hierarchy has traditionally been recommended (Merritt 1981). For example, after excluding potential nociceptive factors exacerbating spasticity, physical therapy and modalities are introduced before consideration of oral medications or injections. If less invasive options are insufficient, more invasive

a FIM is a trademark of Uniform Data System for Medical Rehabilitation (UDSMR), a division of UB Foundation Activities, Inc. The use of the FIM instrument to collect data for this research study was authorized and conducted in accordance with the terms of a special purpose license granted to the licensee by UDSMR. The patient data collected in the course of this research study have not been processed by UDSMR and there is no implication that such data have been or will be subjected to UDSMR's standard data processing procedures or that they are otherwise comparable to data processed by UDSMR.

orthopedic and neurosurgical treatments such as tendon lengthening surgery or intrathecal baclofen (ITB) pump implantation should be considered.

Therapy plays a critical role in the management of spasticity. Interventions employed often include range of motion, prolonged passive muscle stretching via splinting, and education in a home program (Hsieh et al 2010). Evidence for long-term efficacy of passive physical treatments such as stretching is lacking (Hsieh et al 2010), although regular standing on a tilt table or standing frame is frequently encouraged to stretch hip, knee, and ankle flexors. Passive stretching may be more effective when combined with other modalities, such as the application of heat (Lee and Ng 2008), cooling (Abd El-Maksouda et al 2011), neuromuscular electrical stimulation (Hsieh et al 2010), or selective nerve blocks (Kwon and Kim 2009). The addition of neuromuscular electrical stimulation of antagonist muscles may improve the efficacy of lower limb stretching (Khalili and Hajihassanie 2008). Functional electrical stimulation using a cycle has also been shown to reduce spasticity and preserve range of motion. In addition, hydrotherapy has been shown to help reduce spasticity and the amount of antispasmodic medication needed (Kesiktas et al 2004).

Oral antispasmodic medications used for systemic treatment of generalized spasticity commonly include baclofen, diazepam, dantrolene sodium, tizanidine, and clonidine (Table 12.1). These medications differ in their mechanism of action and little is known about the pharmacokinetics/dynamics in children. There is limited evidence of efficacy and considerable potential for adverse effects (Gracies et al 1997, Tilton et al 2010). A review of 100 randomized controlled trials, systematic reviews, and meta-analyses of comparative efficacy and safety of various antispasmodic agents reported that most studies were not of a high quality and had methodologic flaws (Chou et al 2004). In general, baclofen, tizanidine, and dantrolene appear reasonably effective compared with placebo for treating spasticity, with baclofen and tizanidine having similar efficacy in adults (Chou et al 2004). The choice of medication is often based on clinical experience, commencing at a low dose with careful titration to optimal dose (Kopec 2008), and monitoring for adverse effects or detrimental changes in function such as increased muscle weakness. Medications may be used in combination to achieve complementary or synergistic effects. Baclofen is usually the first choice (Tilton et al 2010), with diazepam often added as an adjunct to baclofen initially at night to assist with sleep and reduce night-time spasms (Mathew and Mathew 2005). Clonidine or tizanidine may also be useful adjuncts to baclofen and are initiated as a single night-time dose owing to sedative side effects. Dantrolene may be preferred in spasticity related to supraspinal injury, such as traumatic brain injury, to avoid sedation caused by baclofen and diazepam, although concerns about liver toxicity limit its use and necessitate monitoring of hepatic function (Gracies et al 1997, Kopec 2008). Dantrolene may be useful in the treatment of hyperthermia after abrupt baclofen withdrawal (Mandac et al 1993). Dosing guidelines, precautions, and adverse effects (Gracies et al 1997, Kopec 2008) are summarized for each medication in Table 12.1.

Surgical management

Surgical management should be considered when spasticity causes significant functional impairments that are refractory to more conservative management. The majority of research

TABLE 12.1
Dosing guidelines, pharmacologic actions, and side-effect profile of commonly prescribed oral antispasmodic medications for children

Oral medication (dosing guideline)	Mode of action	Side effects/precautions
Baclofen (0.125–1mg/kg/d)		
2–7y: 2.5–10mg q.i.d. (10–40mg/d) 8–12y: 5mg t.i.d.–15mg q.i.d. (15–60mg/d) 12–16y: 5–20mg q.i.d. (20–80mg/d) Note: adult doses may reach up to 150–200mg/d. Caution advised with renal impairment; consider reducing dose	Centrally acting structural analog of GABA Binds to $GABA_B$ receptors of presynaptic excitatory interneurons (and postsynaptic primary afferents) causing presynaptic inhibition of mono/polysynaptic spinal reflexes Rapid absorption Blood-level peaks in 1h Half-life of 3–4h Renal and hepatic (15%) excretion	CNS depression (sedation, drowsiness, fatigue), nausea, headache, dizziness, confusion, euphoria, hallucinations, hypotonia, ataxia, paraesthesiae Note: abrupt withdrawal may cause seizures, hallucinations, rebound muscle spasms, and hyperpyrexia
Diazepam (0.12–0.8mg/kg/d)		
0.5–10mg t.i.d. Note: prescription of a bedtime dose only, or proportionately larger dose at bedtime, may help to limit problems owing to sedation	Centrally acting Binds to $GABA_A$ receptors mediating presynaptic inhibition in brain stem reticular formation and spinal polysynaptic pathways Rapid absorption Blood-level peaks in 1h Half-life of 20–80h Metabolized in the liver, producing pharmacologically active metabolites with a long duration of action Increased potential for side effects with low albumin levels, as it is 98% protein bound	CNS depression (sedation, impaired memory, and attention), ataxia Dependence/potential for substance abuse/overdose Withdrawal syndrome (including anxiety, agitation, irritability, tremor, muscle twitching, nausea, insomnia, seizures, hyperpyrexia)
Dantrolene sodium (3–12mg/kg/d)		
Children >5y: commence at 0.5mg/kg b.i.d. for 7d, then 0.5mg/kg t.i.d. for 7d, then 1mg/kg t.i.d. for 7d, then 2mg/kg t.i.d. to a maximum of 3mg/kg q.i.d. or 400mg/d	Peripheral action, blocking release of calcium from sarcoplasmic reticulum with uncoupling of nerve excitation and skeletal muscle contraction Blood-level peaks in 3–6h (active metabolite 4–8h) Half-life of approximately 15h Metabolized largely in the liver, with 15–25% of non-metabolized drug excreted in urine	Malaise, fatigue, nausea, vomiting, diarrhea, muscle weakness with high dose Note: hepatotoxicity (baseline liver function tests *must* be checked before starting dantrolene and tested weekly during dose titration and regularly every 1–2mo thereafter). Drug *should be discontinued* promptly if liver enzymes become elevated

TABLE 12.1
(Continued)

Oral medication (dosing guideline)	Mode of action	Side effects/precautions
Tizanidine		
Children <10y: commence 1mg orally at bedtime initially, increasing to 0.3–0.5mg/kg in four divided doses Children ≥10y: commence 2mg orally at bedtime initially, increased according to response, to a maximum of 24mg/d in three to four divided doses	Centrally acting α-2 adrenoceptor agonist with activity at both spinal and supraspinal sites. Prevents release of excitatory amino acids, facilitating presynaptic inhibition Good oral absorption Blood-level peaks in 1–2h Half-life of 2.5h Extensive first pass hepatic metabolism with urinary excretion of inactive metabolites	Dry mouth, drowsiness, tiredness, headache, dizziness, insomnia, anxiety, aggression, mood swings, visual hallucinations, risk of hypotension (although 10 times less antihypertensive potency than clonidine), nausea, vomiting, and constipation Liver function tests should be monitored for elevation in enzymes in view of possible hepatotoxicity
Clonidine		
0.025–0.1mg in two or three divided doses Note: a retrospective chart review of literature about clonidine in children reported an average dosage based on weight was 0.02–0.03mg/kg/d (0.4–0.5mg/d), with a range of 0.0014 to 0.15mg/kg/d	Centrally acting mixed alpha adrenoceptor agonist with predominant α-2 activity causing membrane hyperpolarization at multiple sites in the brain, brainstem, and dorsal horns of spinal cord. Inhibition of substance P may also contribute to tone reduction via an antinociceptive effect Rapidly absorbed orally Blood-level peaks in 1–1.5h Half-life of 2.5h	Drowsiness, dry mouth, bradycardia, orthostatic hypotension Abrupt cessation may result in rebound hypertension

q.i.d., *quater in die*; GABA, γ-aminobutyric acid; CNS, central nervous system; t.i.d., *ter in die*; b.i.d., *bis in die*.

on pediatric surgical spasticity management involves children with cerebral palsy. These procedures are also very effective and widely used in spasticity of spinal origin (Elbasiouny et al 2010).

Chemical denervation and neurolysis

Focal hypertonicity can be managed with intramuscular botulinum neurotoxin (BoNT) injections and phenol/alcohol neurolysis. Injections are most effective in children with dynamic muscle shortening caused by spasticity or dystonia that is localized to specific muscles, and those without significant contracture (Graham et al 2000).

Children undergoing injection with BoNT may require sedation for comfort if multiple muscles are injected. In contrast, neurolysis with phenol is a technically more difficult procedure requiring precision to avoid sclerosis of surrounding structures and is more likely to require sedation. Electrical stimulation or ultrasound guidance can be used for muscle localization when injecting BoNT into muscles that are not easily palpated. Phenol requires electrical stimulation for nerve identification and avoidance of iatrogenic injury.

Botulinum neurotoxin

Botulinum neurotoxin blocks signal transmission at the neuromuscular junction by preventing the release of acetylcholine from the presynaptic axon at the motor endplate (Koman et al 2001). Treatment with BoNT-A is most common but BoNT-B is also used. The choice of toxin subtype is a matter of physician preference and experience.

Extensive literature exists on the use of BoNT in children with cerebral palsy, and long-term use of BoNT-A with repeated rounds of injection in children with cerebral palsy has been found to be safe and efficacious (Naumann et al 2006). A practice parameter published in 2010 originating from a multidisciplinary panel systematically reviewing relevant literature of pharmacologic treatment of spasticity in children and adolescents with cerebral palsy found that BoNT-A is an effective and generally safe treatment to reduce spasticity in the upper and lower extremities. There was conflicting evidence regarding functional improvement, and data on BoNT-B or phenol were inconclusive (Delgado et al 2010).

In adults with SCI, BoNT has been shown to be effective; however, there are no published reports regarding children with SCI (Marciniak et al 2008, Elbasiouny et al 2010). In a review of 28 adults with SCI receiving BoNT-A, patients were asked to identify goals for the injection, and success was reported in 5 out of 9 patients for ambulation, in 5 out of 7 for positioning, in 5 out of 7 for upper extremity function, in 2 out of 3 for hygiene, and in 5 out of 6 for pain (Marciniak et al 2008). Effectiveness was not influenced whether BoNT injections were used less than 1 year after SCI or later (Marciniak et al 2008). BoNT-A use in small muscles may be an important adjunctive therapy to increase the therapeutic effect of antispasticity medications and ITB, which would result in a more focal effect, and to improve the use of orthoses and the effectiveness of rehabilitation programs in patients with SCI (Santamato et al 2010).

Dosing and dilution guidelines in children have not been established but consensus statements, systematic reviews, and randomized controlled trials provide recommendations (Graham et al 2000, Kawamura et al 2007). Considerations used in dosing include the child's weight, muscle size, location of muscle, and degree of spasticity. The period of clinically useful relaxation is typically 12 to 16 weeks, and it is recommended that injections are spaced at a minimum of 3-month intervals owing to concern for neutralizing antibody formation (Graham et al 2000). Adverse events related to BoNT are rare but include injection-site pain and focal muscle weakness (Graham et al 2000, Delgado et al 2010). Since 2009, the Food and Drug Administration has required black box labeling on BoNT products cautioning that the effects of BoNT may spread from the area of injection to other areas of the body, causing symptoms similar to those of botulism. Co-administration of BoNT and aminoglycosides or other agents interfering with neuromuscular transmission is contraindicated. Further research on the use of BoNT in children with SCI is needed to determine efficacy, dosing, and functional outcomes in this population.

Phenol

Phenol perineural injections or motor point blocks have been used for many years to reduce focal spasticity. The low cost of phenol is a significant advantage over BoNT, but the need for electrical stimulation guidance and general anesthesia in children may offset any cost savings. Duration of clinical effect varies between 3 and 18 months (Kwon and Kim 2009). Phenol neurolysis is typically used for large proximal muscles such as the biceps brachii, hip adductors, and hamstrings (Fig. 12.2). Phenol motor point blocks can also be performed in the posterior tibialis and gastrocnemius muscles with minimal risk of sensory dysesthesia. Since the 1960s, phenol has also been used to treat spasticity and, more recently, has been used for patients with SCI (Gunduz et al 1992). In adults with SCI, phenol neurolysis of the obturator nerve using fluoroscopy and nerve stimulator guidance has been shown to decrease spasticity and pain, increase hip range of motion, and improve hygiene with an efficacy lasting for approximately 3 months (Akkaya et al 2010). Another study showed that buttock–seat interface pressure (a factor in the development of pressure ulcers) was reduced after phenol neurolysis of the obturator nerve in adults with SCI (Yasar et al 2010). Phenol injections have been combined safely with BoNT in children, and this combination allows an increased number of injections at the maximal recommended dose during one procedure (Gooch and Patton 2004, Kolaski et al 2008). Phenol has been shown to be safe in children, but transient sensory dysesthesias occur rarely and were reported at a level of 0.4% in one study (Gooch and Patton 2004, Kolaski et al 2008).

Intrathecal baclofen

Intrathecal baclofen is highly effective in treating generalized spasticity in both children and adults. ITB is delivered to the intrathecal space via a catheter connected to an implanted pump

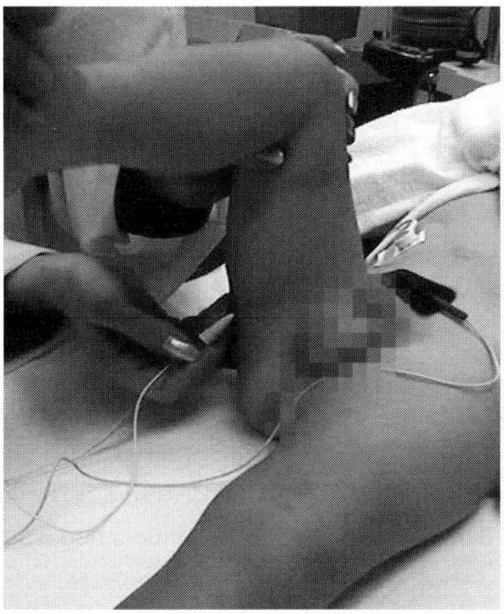

Fig. 12.2 Phenol neurolysis.

in the abdomen. This method of delivery confers an advantage over oral baclofen in that central nervous system depressive effects are minimized and dosages can be titrated to functional effect. A thorough assessment of the patient and careful selection are crucial for a successful outcome. Goals of treatment – whether they are to improve function, comfort, or care – need to be firmly established (Albright 2007). Patient and family education and close follow-up are essential. Cost and maintenance can be prohibitive for some families. The battery life of the newer pumps is approximately 7 years. A screening lumbar intrathecal bolus dose of baclofen is recommended to evaluate responsiveness and the impact on abilities, as well as adverse effects, but these trials are not performed universally (Albright 2007, Dan et al 2010). Catheter tips are typically positioned at C5–T2 in patients with spastic tetraplegia and T10–T12 in those with paraplegia. Both the 20- and 40-ml pumps are 8.75cm in diameter; however, the 20-ml pump is 19.5mm thick, whereas the 40-ml pump is 26mm thick. Depending on the reservoir size and the patient's dosing regimen, the refill interval is between 2 and 6 months. The surgical technique of placing pumps subfascially (Fig. 12.3) rather than subcutaneously (Fig. 12.4) in children may result in better esthetics and lower incidence of wound erosion.

Several studies demonstrate the effectiveness of ITB in children (Albright et al 2003). A consensus statement on the use of ITB in children with spasticity was published in 2010 and provides recommendations on treatment guidelines (Dan et al 2010). Numerous studies have shown efficacy and safety in adults with SCI. Only a small amount of research has been performed in children with SCI, but one study in two ventilator-dependent children showed efficacy with ITB (Armstrong et al 1992). A long-term multicenter study of 93 adults with SCI and multiple sclerosis showed ITB to be safe and effective for the long-term treatment of intractable spasticity (Coffey et al 1993), and another study in adults with SCI showed improvement in pain and functional abilities (Jagatsinh 2009). It has been shown that control of spasticity can be achieved without detrimental effects on strength in incomplete SCI, which suggests there is a need to include strength testing in comprehensive clinical assessments of spasticity (Bowden and Stokic 2009). ITB may help stabilize autonomic dysreflexia and orthostatic hypotension in patients with SCI, but more research is needed (Kofler et al 2009).

Potential complications of ITB include infections, respiratory depression, cerebrospinal fluid leaks, and catheter problems such as disconnection, migration, or kinking. Pump malfunction is less common. In one study, the most common complications of surgery

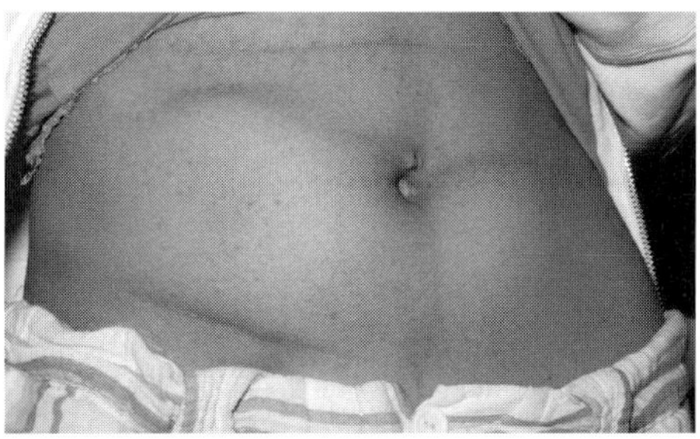

Fig. 12.3 Subfascial implantation of intrathecal baclofen.

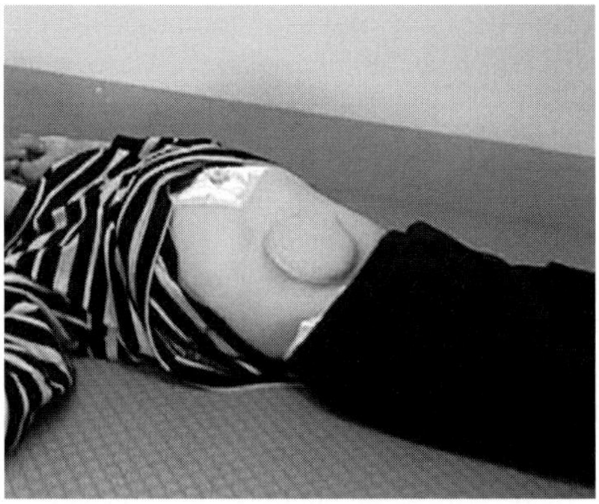

Fig. 12.4 Subcutaneous implantation of intrathecal baclofen.

were catheter-related problems (31%), seromas (24%), and cerebrospinal fluid leaks (15%) (Albright et al 2003). An analysis of 200 consecutive children (with cerebral palsy, hereditary spastic paraparesis, multiple sclerosis, or traumatic brain injury) who received ITB pumps showed that 11% had cerebrospinal fluid leaks, 7% had catheter-related problems, 7.5% had infections, and 5.5% had more than one complication (Motta et al 2007). The results corresponded to one complication for every 11 years 4 months of treatment, and the onset of at least one complication was statistically more likely in patients with a greater degree of spasticity and in those aged 10 years or younger. The incidence of infection was found to be lower with subfascial pump placement. Another study reported a 31% rate of complications requiring surgical management over a 3-year period (Borowski et al 2010). ITB has not been found to significantly impact the rate of progression of scoliosis in children with cerebral palsy (Shilt et al 2008), but no such studies exist in children with SCI. ITB withdrawal is a medical emergency and needs to be identified early and managed aggressively. Caregivers should have a home supply of oral baclofen and be instructed to administer it at the first signs of baclofen withdrawal. Causes can include a catheter problem, human programming error, failure to refill the pump, or medication error.

Selective dorsal rhizotomy

Selective dorsal rhizotomies (SDRs) involve single- or multilevel osteoplastic laminectomies that expose the L2–S1 nerve roots, and typically 25% to 70% of dorsal rootlets are selectively cut with the aid of electrophysiologic monitoring (Hays et al 1998, Steinbok 2007). SDR is most often performed in children with spastic diplegic cerebral palsy, and little research is available to evaluate the potential benefit of SDR in children with SCI whose spasticity is severe and causing functional limitations, positioning challenges, or pain. The primary disadvantage of a SDR is its permanence. Although studies in children with cerebral palsy have shown long-term improvement in spasticity and function after SDR (Nordmark et al 2008), minimal research exists in patients with SCI. SDR can reduce the need for orthopedic surgeries in children with cerebral palsy, with 35% of patients avoiding surgery (Steinbok 2007).

One concern with multilevel laminectomies is the potential for an increased risk of spinal deformities, but there is no clear evidence to support this.

Percutaneous thermal rhizotomy was first described in 1977 for the treatment of pain and spasticity (Turnbull 1983). It is a procedure that involves radiofrequency electrocoagulation and selective destruction of the sensory portion of the nerve, while preserving motor, proprioceptive, and touch sensation. It is thought to be less destructive than a traditional rhizotomy, but the reduction in spasticity is temporary. A few studies have reported improvement in painful spasms without significant adverse effects in patients with paraplegia (Turnbull 1983, Herz et al 1990). The procedure is recommended primarily for those with complete injuries. Spasticity may recur to some degree, but the procedure can be repeated. Further research on these spinal procedures is needed.

Summary

The art of spasticity management is determining the degree of spasticity that may be tolerable and whether there may be a functional benefit or if it is just counterproductive and potentially injurious. When devising a treatment plan, it is imperative to consider both the positive and the negative effects of spasticity on function. Ideally, treatment should maximize function while minimizing sedation and adverse effects. A barrier to spasticity management has been the sedative potential of various treatments; thus, a goal of future research should be to achieve effective tone reduction without sedation.

REFERENCES

Abd El-Maksouda G, Sharafb MA, Rezz-Allahc SS (2011) Efficacy of cold therapy on spasticity and hand function in children with cerebral palsy. *J Adv Res* 2: 319–25. doi: 10.1016/j.jare.2011.02.003

Akkaya T, Unlu E, Alptekin A, Gumus HI, Umay E, Cakci A (2010) Neurolytic phenol blockade of the obturator nerve for severe adductor spasticity. *Acta Anaesthesiol Scand* 54: 79–85. doi: 10.4103/1658-354X.101223

Albright AL (2007) Intrathecal baclofen for childhood hypertonia. *Childs Nerv Syst* 23: 971–9. doi 10.1007/s00381-007-0397-3

Albright AL, Gilmartin R, Swift D, Krach LE, Ivanhoe CB, Mclaughlin JF (2003) Long-term intrathecal baclofen therapy for severe spasticity of cerebral origin. *J Neurosurg* 98: 291–5. doi: 10.1111/j.1469-8749.200803034.x

Armstrong RW, Steinbok P, Farrell K, Cochrane D, Norman MG, Kube S (1992) Continuous intrathecal baclofen treatment of severe spasms in two children with spinal-cord injury. *Dev Med Child Neurol* 34: 731–8. doi: 10.1111/j.1469-8749.1992tb11509x

Ashworth B (1964) Preliminary trial of carisoprodol in multiple sclerosis. *Practitioner* 192: 540–2.

Bayley N (1993) *Bayley Scales of Infant Development*. San Antonio, TX: The Psychological Corporation.

Biering-Sorensen F, Nielsen JB, Klinge K (2006) Spasticity-assessment: a review. *Spinal Cord* 44: 708–22. doi:10.1038/sj.sc.3101928

Bohannon RW, Smith MB (1987) Interrater reliability of a modified Ashworth scale of muscle spasticity. *Phys Ther* 67: 206–7.

Borowski A, Littleton AG, Borkhuu B et al (2010) Complications of intrathecal baclofen pump therapy in pediatric patients. *J Pediatr Orthop* 30: 76–81. doi: 10.1097/BPO0b013e3181c6b257

Bowden M, Stokic S (2009) Clinical and neurophysiologic assessment of strength and spasticity during intrathecal baclofen titration in incomplete spinal cord injury: single-subject design. *J Spinal Cord Med* 32: 183–90.

Boyd R, Graham H (1999) Objective measurement of clinical findings in the use of botulinum toxin type A for the management of children with cerebral palsy. *Eur J Neurol* S23–35. doi: 10.1111/j.1468-13311999tb00031.x

Chou R, Peterson K, Helfand M (2004) Comparative efficacy and safety of skeletal muscle relaxants for spasticity and musculoskeletal conditions: a systematic review. *J Pain Symptom Manage* 28: 140–75. doi: 10.1016/j.jpainsymman.200405.002

Coffey JR, Cahill D, Steers W et al (1993) Intrathecal baclofen for intractable spasticity of spinal origin: results of a long-term multicenter study. *J Neurosurg* 78: 226–32. doi: 10.3171/jns.199378.2.0226

Dan B, Motta F, Vles JS et al (2010) Consensus on the appropriate use of intrathecal baclofen (ITB) therapy in paediatric spasticity. *Eur J Paediatr Neurol* 14: 19–28. doi: 10.1016/j.ejpn.2009.05.002

Delgado MR, Hirtz D, Aisen M et al (2010) Practice parameter: pharmacologic treatment of spasticity in children and adolescents with cerebral palsy (an evidence-based review): report of the Quality Standards Subcommittee of the American Academy of Neurology and the Practice Committee of the Child Neurology Society. *Neurology* 74: 336–43. doi: 10.1212/WNL.0b013e3181cbcd2f

Elbasiouny SM, Moroz D, Bakr MM, Mushahwar VK (2010) Management of spasticity after spinal cord injury: current techniques and future directions. *Neurorehabil Neural Repair* 24: 23–33. doi: 10.1177/1545968309343213

Feldman AB, Haley SM, Coryell J (1990) Concurrent and construct validity of the Pediatric Evaluation of Disability Inventory. *Phys Ther* 70: 602–10.

Fewell R, Folio M (2000) *Peabody Developmental Motor Scales*. Austin, TX: Pro-Ed.

Fleuren JF, Voerman GE, Erren-Wolters CV et al (2010) Stop using the Ashworth Scale for the assessment of spasticity. *J Neurol Neurosurg Psychiatry* 81: 46–52. doi: 10.1136/jnnp.2009.177071

Gooch JL, Patton CP (2004) Combining botulinum toxin and phenol to manage spasticity in children. *Arch Phys Med Rehabil* 85: 1121–4. doi:10.1016/j.apmr.200309.032

Gracies JM, Nance P, Elovic E, Mcguire J, Simpson DM (1997) Traditional pharmacological treatments for spasticity. Part II: General and regional treatments. *Muscle Nerve Suppl* 6: S92–120. doi: 10.1002/(SICI)1097-4598(1997)6+<92::AID-MUS7>3.3.CO;2-E

Gracies JM, Burke K, Clegg NJ et al (2010) Reliability of the Tardieu Scale for assessing spasticity in children with cerebral palsy. *Arch Phys Med Rehabil* 91: 421–8. doi: 10.1016/j.apmr.200911.017

Graham HK, Aoki KR, Autti-Ramo I et al (2000) Recommendations for the use of botulinum toxin type A in the management of cerebral palsy. *Gait Posture* 11: 67–79. doi: 10.1016/S0966-6362(99)00054-5

Gunduz S, Kalyon TA, Dursun H, Mohur H, Bilgic F (1992) Peripheral nerve block with phenol to treat spasticity in spinal cord injured patients. *Paraplegia* 30: 808–11. doi: 10.1038/sc.1992156

Hays RM, Mclaughlin JF, Bjornson KF, Stephens K, Roberts TS, Price R (1998) Electrophysiological monitoring during selective dorsal rhizotomy and spasticity and GMFM performance. *Dev Med Child Neurol* 40: 233–8. doi: 10.1111/j.1469-8749.1998b15455.x

Herz DA, Looman JE, Tiberio A et al (1990) The management of paralytic spasticity. *Neurosurgery* 26: 300–6. doi: 10.1097/00006123-199002000-00018

Hsieh JTC, Wolfe DL, Townson AF et al (2010). Spasticity following spinal cord injury. In: Eng JJ, Teasell RW, Miller WC et al (eds). *Spinal Cord Injury Rehabilitation Evidence. Version 3.0.* Vancouver, BC, Canada: SCIRE.

Jagatsinh Y (2009) Intrathecal baclofen: its effect on symptoms and activities of daily living in severe spasticity due to spinal cord injuries: a pilot study. *Indian J Orthop* 43: 46–9. doi: 10.4103/0019-5413.45323

Kawamura A, Campbell K, Lam-Damji S, Fehlings D (2007) A randomized controlled trial comparing botulinum toxin A dosage in the upper extremity of children with spasticity. *Dev Med Child Neurol* 49: 331–7. doi: 10.1111/j.1469-8749.200700331.x

Kesiktas N, Paker N, Erdogan N, Gulsen G, Bicki D, Yilmaz H (2004) The use of hydrotherapy for the management of spasticity. *Neurorehabil Neural Repair* 18: 268–73. doi: 10.1177/1545968304270002

Khalili MA, Hajihassanie A (2008) Electrical simulation in addition to passive stretch has a small effect on spasticity and contracture in children with cerebral palsy: a randomised within-participant controlled trial. *Aust J Physiother* 54: 185–9. doi: 10.1016/S0004-9514(08)70025-4

Kirshblum S, Campagnolo DI (eds) (2011) *Spinal Cord Medicine*. 2nd Ed. New York, NY: Wolters Kluwer; Lippincott Williams & Wilkins.

Kofler M, Poustka K, Saltuari L (2009) Intrathecal baclofen for autonomic instability due to spinal cord injury. *Auton Neurosci* 146: 106–10. doi: 10.1016/j.autneu.200812.003

Kolaski K, Ajizian SJ, Passmore L, Pasutharnchat N, Koman LA, Smith BP (2008) Safety profile of multilevel chemical denervation procedures using phenol or botulinum toxin or both in a pediatric population. *Am J Phys Med Rehabil* 87: 556–66. doi: 10.1097/PHM0b013e31817c115b

Koman LA, Brashear A, Rosenfeld S et al (2001) Botulinum toxin type A neuromuscular blockade in the treatment of equinus foot deformity in cerebral palsy: a multicenter open-label clinical trial. *Pediatrics* 108: 1062–71. doi: 10.1542/peds.108.5.1062

Kopec K (2008) Cerebral palsy: pharmacologic treatment of spasticity. *US Pharm* 33: 22–6.

Kwon JY, Kim JS (2009) Selective blocking of the anterior branch of the obturator nerve in children with cerebral palsy. *Am J Phys Med Rehabil* 88: 7–13. doi: 10.1097/PHM0b013e31815b6381

Lee GP, Ng GY (2008) Effects of stretching and heat treatment on hamstring extensibility in children with severe mental retardation and hypertonia. *Clin Rehabil* 22: 771–9. doi: 10.1177/0269215508090067

Mandac BR, Hurvitz EA, Nelson VS (1993) Hyperthermia associated with baclofen withdrawal and increased spasticity. *Arch Phys Med Rehabil* 74: 96–7.

Marciniak C, Rader L, Gagnon C (2008) The use of botulinum toxin for spasticity after spinal cord injury. *Am J Phys Med Rehabil* 87: 312–17. doi: 10.1097/PHM0b013e318168ceaf

Mathew A, Mathew MC (2005) Bedtime diazepam enhances well-being in children with spastic cerebral palsy. *Pediatr Rehabil* 8: 63–6. doi:10.1080/13638490410001731180

Merritt JL (1981) Management of spasticity in spinal cord injury. *Mayo Clin Proc* 56: 614–22.

Motta F, Buonaguro V, Stignani C (2007) The use of intrathecal baclofen pump implants in children and adolescents: safety and complications in 200 consecutive cases. *J Neurosurg* 107: 32–5.

Naumann M, Albanese A, Heinen F, Molenaers G, Relja M (2006) Safety and efficacy of botulinum toxin type A following long-term use. *Eur J Neurol* 13(Suppl 4): 35–40. doi: 10.1111/j.1468-1331.2006.01652.x

Nordmark E, Josenby AL, Lagergren J et al (2008) Long-term outcomes five years after selective dorsal rhizotomy. *BMC Pediatr* 8: 54. doi: 10.1186/1471-2431-8-54

Ottenbacher KJ, Msall ME, Lyon N et al (2000) The WeeFIM instrument: its utility in detecting change in children with developmental disabilities. *Arch Phys Med Rehabil* 81: 1317–26. doi:10.1053/apmr.2000.9387

Platz T, Eickhof C, Nuyens G, Vuadens P (2005) Clinical scales for the assessment of spasticity, associated phenomena, and function: a systematic review of the literature. *Disabil Rehabil* 27: 7–18. doi:10.1080/09638280400014634

Sanger TD, Delgado MR, Gaebler-Spira D, Hallett M, Mink JW (2003) Classification and definition of disorders causing hypertonia in childhood. *Pediatrics* 111: e89–97. doi: 10.1542/peds.111.1.e89

Santamato A, Panza F, Ranieri M et al (2010) Effect of intrathecal baclofen, botulinum toxin type A and a rehabilitation programme on locomotor function after spinal cord injury: a case report. *J Rehabil Med* 42: 891–4. doi: 10.2340/16501977-0596

Scholtes VA, Becher JG, Beelen A, Lankhorst GJ (2006) Clinical assessment of spasticity in children with cerebral palsy: a critical review of available instruments. *Dev Med Child Neurol* 48: 64–73. doi: 10.1017/S0012162206000132

Sheean G, McGuire JR (2009) Spastic hypertonia and movement disorders: pathophysiology, clinical presentation, and quantification. *PM R* 1: 827–33. doi: 10.1016/j.pmrj.2009.08.002

Shilt JS, Lai LP, Cabrera MN, Frino, J, Smith BP (2008) The impact of intrathecal baclofen on the natural history of scoliosis in cerebral palsy. *J Pediatr Orthop* 28: 684–7. doi: 10.1097/BPO.0b013e318183d591

Steinbok P (2007) Selective dorsal rhizotomy for spastic cerebral palsy: a review. *Childs Nerv Syst* 23: 981–90. doi: 10.1007/s00381-007-0379-5

Thorpe DE, Dusing SC, Moore CG (2005) Repeatability of temporospatial gait measures in children using the GAITRite electronic walkway. *Arch Phys Med Rehabil* 86: 2342–6. doi:10.1016/j.apmr.2005.07.301

Tilton A, Vargus-Adams J, Delgado MR (2010) Pharmacologic treatment of spasticity in children. *Semin Pediatr Neurol* 17: 261–7. doi: 10.1016/j.spen.2010.10.009

Turnbull IM (1983) Percutaneous lumbar rhizotomy for spasms in paraplegia. *Paraplegia* 21: 131–6. doi: 10.1038/sc.1983.21

Yasar E, Tok F, Taskaynatan MA, Yilmaz B, Balaban B, Alaca R (2010) The effects of phenol neurolysis of the obturator nerve on the distribution of buttock–seat interface pressure in spinal cord injury patients with hip adductor spasticity. *Spinal Cord* 48: 828–31. doi: 10.1038/sc.2010.34

13
AUTONOMIC DYSFUNCTION AFTER SPINAL CORD INJURY

Andrei Krassioukov

Introduction

Paralysis is a devastating consequence of spinal cord injury (SCI) that predominantly affects young and healthy adults (Ackery et al 2004). However, SCIs in young children are relatively rare (see Chapter 2). The literature on pediatric SCI gives some evidence on unique features associated with SCI in children, specifically regarding the use of neurologic classification and some rehabilitation strategies (Vogel et al 2009). Little is known about autonomic dysfunction after pediatric SCI. This chapter will provide an overview of some autonomic dysfunctions after SCI, predominantly based on our present understanding of clinical data available from adults and the limited pediatric data.

Injury to the fragile neuronal structures in the spinal cord results in significant functional alterations of the autonomic nervous system. Although the injury itself generally affects only a small area of the neuronal tissue and pathways of the spinal cord, the effect of this local disruption can commonly be seen in all spinal autonomic functions controlled by both sympathetic and parasympathetic components of the autonomic nervous system. Despite these widespread effects, the clinical presentation of these individuals is dominated by the effects of the initial alteration of spinal sympathetic control, as the most devastating effect of the SCI on autonomic control is the disruption of the descending sympathetic tonic pathways (Krassioukov 2009). For example, on a daily basis, individuals with SCI face the challenge of managing their unstable blood pressure, which frequently results in persistent hypotension and/or episodes of uncontrolled hypertension. These cardiovascular abnormalities have been well documented in human studies, as well as in animal models (Krassioukov and Fehlings 1999, Mathias and Frankel 2002, Claydon and Krassioukov 2006). The recognition and management of these cardiovascular dysfunctions after SCI represent challenging clinical issues. Moreover, cardiovascular disorders in the acute and chronic stages of SCI are among the most common causes of death in individuals with SCI (Garshick et al 2005). Until recently, the majority of basic science and clinical investigations were focused on finding a cure for paralysis and re-establishing motor function. Unfortunately, little attention has been paid to the function of the autonomic nervous system after SCI (Krassioukov et al 2007). However, a recent survey that evaluated the functional priorities for individuals with SCI revealed that sexual function and other autonomic-related functions (including abnormal blood pressure control) were the main areas that were important to individuals with SCI (Anderson 2004); these findings are articulated by the child profiled in Chapter 1 of this book.

This chapter will focus on the range of clinical issues associated with abnormal autonomic control after SCI, including various cardiovascular disorders, abnormal temperature, and sweating control.

Autonomic dysfunctions following spinal cord injury: anatomical and physiological correlates

After SCI, supraspinal autonomic control to the spinal autonomic circuits is disrupted. Autonomic circuits in the spinal cord include sympathetic preganglionic neurons (SPNs), whose cell bodies are located in the lateral horns of the spinal gray matter of the thoracic and upper lumbar spinal segments (T1–L2, Fig. 13.1), and parasympathetic preganglionic neurons, whose cell bodies lie within the sacral spinal segments (S2–S4). Both types of spinal preganglionic neurons receive supraspinal tonic and inhibitory nervous system control (Calaresu and Yardley 1988) via spinal autonomic pathways, which are pathways commonly disrupted after SCI (Furlan et al 2003). Conversely, vagal parasympathetic pathways, which exit supraspinally, are generally intact in individuals with SCI. As a result of the anatomical structure of the autonomic nervous system, the level of SCI has important consequences for the autonomic dysfunctions observed after injury. Cardiac function, for example, is under dual control of sympathetic (T1–T5) and parasympathetic (vagus, cranial nerve X) nervous systems. After high cervical SCI, parasympathetic (vagal) control will remain intact, whereas the sympathetic nervous system will lose its tonic autonomic control. On the other hand, in individuals with an injury below the sixth thoracic segment, both the sympathetic and the parasympathetic control of the heart is intact. Because of their injury level, individuals with tetraplegia will have very different cardiovascular responses to injury than those with paraplegia (Sheel et al 2005, Claydon et al 2006a). It is important to appreciate that similar relationships can exist between the level of SCI and the functioning of organs that are under autonomic control (urinary bladder, bowel, sweat gland, etc.).

Since the early 2000s, clinical observations and experimental animal studies have significantly contributed to our understanding of the pathophysiology of autonomic dysfunctions after SCI (Teasell et al 2000, Krassioukov et al 2002, Mathias and Frankel 2002). Changes have been identified in numerous components of autonomic circuits that could contribute to abnormal cardiovascular control after SCI (Krassioukov and Claydon 2006). For example, it has been shown that SCI disrupts the descending sympatho-excitatory pathways from neurons in the rostral ventrolateral medulla (Krassioukov and Fehlings 1999, Furlan et al 2003), which usually provides tonic input to spinal SPNs. Disruption of these descending cardiovascular pathways results in at least four phenomena: initial sympathetic hypoactivity (Maiorov et al 2000), alterations in the morphology of SPNs (Krassioukov and Weaver 1995, Krassioukov et al 1999), plastic changes within the spinal circuits (including dorsal root afferents sprouting and the potential formation of inappropriate synaptic connections) (Krenz et al 1999), and the development of changes in peripheral sympathetic neurovascular responsiveness (Alan et al 2010, Ramer et al 2012).

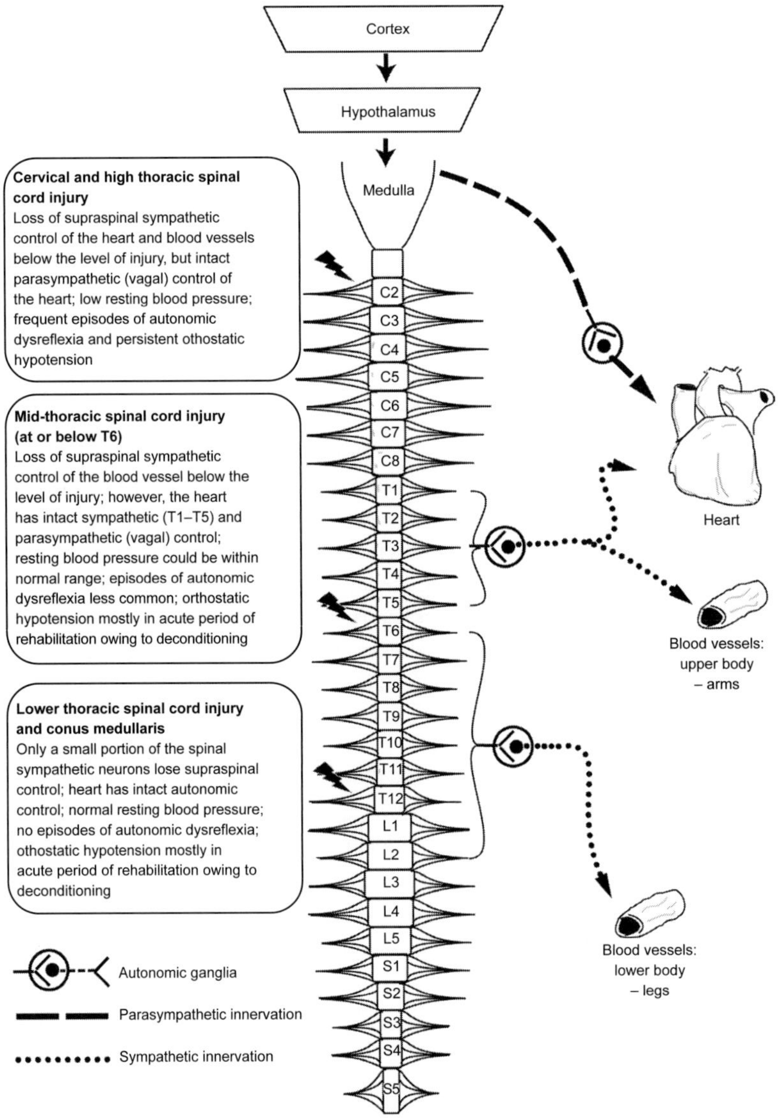

Fig. 13.1 Schematic diagram of autonomic cardiovascular control. The cerebral cortex and hypothalamus project to the various nuclei within the medulla oblongata, where cardiovascular autonomic control is coordinated. The parasympathetic control of the cardiovascular system exits at the level of the brainstem via the vagus nerve. The preganglionic fibers of the vagus nerve then synapse with postganglionic parasympathetic neurons in ganglia on or near the target organ. Descending sympathetic pathways provide tonic control to sympathetic preganglionic neurons involved in cardiovascular control. Sympathetic preganglionic neurons are found within the lateral horn of the spinal cord in segments T1–L2 and exit the spinal cord via the ventral root. They then synapse with postganglionic neurons located in the sympathetic chain (paravertebral ganglia). Finally, the sympathetic postganglionic neurons synapse with the target organs, the heart, and blood vessels. The different levels of spinal cord injury commonly present with various degrees of cardiovascular dysfunctions (see boxed text).

The initial sympathetic hypoactivity results in low resting blood pressure, loss of blood pressure homeostasis, and disturbed blood pressure reflex control (Mathias and Frankel 2002). In addition, over time after SCI, the loss of descending inhibitory pathways, coupled with plastic changes within the spinal cord and peripheral neurovascular changes, are likely to predispose individuals with SCI to episodes of extreme hypertension associated with autonomic dysreflexia. Indeed, autonomic dysreflexia frequently develops in both acute and chronic stages of spinal injury.

It is only recently that the morphologic changes within spinal autonomic circuits responsible for the variety of autonomic dysfunctions after SCI have begun to be identified. Evaluation of SPN morphology in animals and in humans (Krassioukov et al 1999) has demonstrated that in the acute stage after spinal cord transection, these neurons show signs of atrophy. With time, however, these SPNs regain their normal morphology (Krassioukov and Weaver 1996). The initial morphologic changes within the SPNs probably occur as a consequence of partial deafferentation from the loss of descending projections from medullary neurons, a proportion of which are thought to synapse directly on SPNs. In addition to the immediate depression of autonomic functions resulting from a loss of important excitatory input from the brainstem, the atrophy of SPNs also probably contributes to the initial sympathetic atonia. Conversely, over time after SCI, sustained excitatory responses develop that manifest as autonomic dysreflexia (Mathias and Frankel 2002, Krassioukov and Claydon 2006). Autonomic dysreflexia is generally seen during the subacute and chronic stages of human SCI, becoming obvious within the first few months after SCI in individuals with cervical or high- to mid-thoracic SCI (Krassioukov 2004). In the chronic stage of SCI, additional mechanisms may contribute to impaired cardiovascular control. For example, in animals, after an SCI, dorsal root afferents have been shown to sprout (Krenz et al 1999) and spinal neurons that initially lose synaptic inputs appear to have them replaced with synapses from a different source (Beattie et al 1990). Therefore, new inappropriate afferent inputs from different afferent sources could contribute to the eventual development of autonomic dysreflexia after SCI in humans (Ackery et al 2007).

Finally, in addition to plastic changes within the central nervous system, changes within the periphery could also contribute to unstable autonomic control after SCI. In recent studies, we demonstrated aberrant sprouting of the sympathetic fibers within the dorsal root ganglions in animals with chronic SCI. This aberrant sprouting could contribute to the vicious cycle of the sensory–autonomic interactions that previously were identified as a possible underlying mechanism for the development of autonomic dysreflexia (Ramer et al 2007). Furthermore, there is evidence from both animal and human studies that changes within the peripheral blood vessel could also contribute to the development of autonomic dysfunctions after SCI. Hypersensitivity of peripheral vascular α-adrenoceptors also could contribute to the development of autonomic dysreflexia (Alan et al 2010).

Baseline cardiovascular parameters in children and adolescents

Before we can understand autonomic dysfunctions after SCI, we first have to be familiar with normal/baseline cardiovascular parameters for the pediatric population. According to the National Heart, Lung, and Blood Institute, there are three factors that determine blood pressure in children and adolescents: height, sex, and age (National High Blood Pressure

Education Program Working Group on High Blood Pressure in Children and Adolescents 2007). Presently, numerous tables are available for clinicians to estimate normative blood pressure parameters in children, accounting for height, sex, and age. For example, the upper limit for normal systolic pressure in children aged 3 to 5 years will range from 104 to 116mmHg, depending on height and sex, whereas diastolic blood pressure will range from 63 to 74mmHg. For example, for a 10-year-old female who is about 1.4m tall, systolic blood pressure of less than 114mmHg would be considered healthy and normal. For a 10-year-old male of about the same height, the number is very similar: 115mmHg for systolic blood pressure is normal. As children get older and taller, normal readings are closer to adult standards. In a child with normal blood pressure, the recommendation by the National Heart, Lung, and Blood Institute is to recheck the blood pressure in 1 year. A retrospective study of resting blood pressure and heart rates in young people with SCI aged under 19 years demonstrated that systolic and diastolic blood pressure increased and heart rate decreased with increasing age. Systolic blood pressure was higher in males, in those with incomplete injury, and in those with paraplegia, whereas heart rate was higher in females. There was no association between cardiovascular measures and injury duration (Hwang et al 2013, Zebracki et al 2013).

Abnormal cardiovascular control

Acute Post-injury Period and Neurogenic Shock

Cardiovascular control is severely compromised in the majority of individuals with SCI (Hadley et al 2002). In the acute period, especially when the injury is at the cervical level, patients present clinically with severe hypotension and persistent bradycardia, which are common components of the phenomenon known as neurogenic shock (Krassioukov et al 2007). Clinical observations strongly suggest that the extent to which prolonged and severe hypotension requires vasopressive therapy correlates well with the severity of cervical or high-thoracic SCI, and can last up to 5 weeks after the injury (Hadley 2002, Mathias and Frankel 2002). Glenn and colleagues, when studying adults with SCI, reported that severe hypotension was present in all of the 31 adults with tetraplegia assessed with severe SCI, half of whom required vasopressor therapy in order to maintain adequate arterial blood pressure (Glenn and Bergman 1997). In addition to this pronounced hypotension, many patients with acute SCI experience severe abnormalities in heart rate. In the acute post-injury stage, bradycardia was reported in 64% of patients with cervical SCI, with the most severe and frequent episodes occurring within the first 5 weeks after SCI (Piepmeier et al 1985, Winslow et al 1986). Bradycardia is a less severe problem when the injury is below the upper-thoracic spinal cord, as cardiac sympathetic neurons remain under brainstem control, leaving vagal and sympathetic influences more in balance. Both the level and the completeness of injury are important determinants of the severity of bradycardia. Indeed, we have also shown that the initial hypotension and bradycardia observed after injury persisted in the individuals with more severe injury of the descending cardiovascular autonomic pathways (Furlan et al 2003). Moreover, all individuals in this group required vasopressor therapy in order to maintain systolic arterial blood pressure above 90mmHg (Furlan et al 2003). In contrast, individuals with less severe injury to the descending cardiovascular pathways tended to have higher blood pressure and heart rate, although minor and short-term hypotension and low heart rates were occasionally observed.

In addition to neurogenic shock, the acute phase of SCI is also associated with 'spinal shock' (Ditunno et al 2004). Although some authors use these terms interchangeably, it is important to recognize that these are two clinically important and distinct conditions. Neurogenic shock is characterized by changes in autonomic blood pressure control after SCI, whereas spinal shock is characterized by a marked reduction or abolition of sensory, motor, and reflex function of the spinal cord below the level of injury (Ditunno et al 2004). Clinically, spinal shock is characterized by flaccid paralysis and areflexia.

Autonomic Dysreflexia

The mechanisms underlying the development of autonomic dysreflexia are still poorly understood. However, there are some experimental animal and clinical data suggesting that a loss of descending sympathetic inhibitory influences (Krassioukov and Fehlings 1999), plastic changes within the spinal and peripheral autonomic circuits (Krassioukov and Weaver 1995, 1996), and changes within the peripheral vasculature (Alan et al 2010) are the main contributing factors in the development of autonomic dysreflexia. As described earlier in this chapter, changes occurring within the spinal autonomic circuits in both the acute and the chronic stages after SCI have been identified among the possible causes of autonomic dysreflexia (Teasell et al 2000, Mathias and Frankel 2002). This condition is characterized by episodes of extreme hypertension after SCI and is well documented in the adult SCI population (Krassioukov et al 2009, Kirshblum et al 2002). However, there are only two studies that describe this condition in a pediatric population (Hickey et al 2004, Schottler et al 2012). Schottler and colleagues reported that up to 34% of children injured at 5 years of age or younger with injuries at or above T6 experienced episodes of autonomic dysreflexia (Schottler et al 2012). Typically, arterial blood pressure is low in individuals with high-level SCI and could range from 90 to 110mmHg (West et al 2012). In adults with SCI, an elevation of systolic blood pressure by 20 to 40mmHg above baseline can be a sign of autonomic dysreflexia in the proper clinical context. Autonomic dysreflexia is characterized by extreme hypertension (Fig. 13.2), with systolic blood pressure reaching up to 300mmHg, and usually accompanied by a pounding headache, slow heart rate, and upper-body flushing in adults (Mathias and Frankel 2002). However, in the pediatric population, the most common symptoms were facial flushing (43%), headaches (24%), sweating (15%), and piloerection (14%) (Hickey et al 2004).

In adults, untreated episodes of autonomic dysreflexia may have serious consequences, including intracranial hemorrhage, retinal detachments, seizures, cardiac arrhythmias, and even death (Yarkony et al 1986, Eltorai et al 1992). These sudden increases in arterial blood pressure can be provoked by a range of different noxious and non-noxious stimuli, including bladder and bowel distension, muscle spasms, and pressure sores (Teasell et al 2000). Similar to the adult population, in a pediatric population the most common causes of dysreflexia were urologic issues (75%) and bowel impaction (18%) (Hickey et al 2004).

In the adult SCI population, it is well documented that routine procedures, such as catheterization and manipulation of an indwelling catheter, as well as urinary tract infection, detrusor sphincter dyssynergia, and bladder percussion, are the most common precipitating

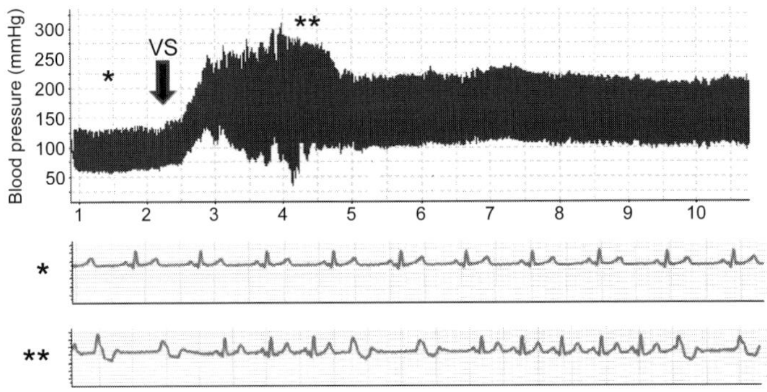

Fig. 13.2 Autonomic dysreflexia in a male with cervical spinal cord injury (C7 American Spinal Injury Association Impairment Scale [AIS] B, motor complete, sensory incomplete) during the vibrostimulation (VS) procedure for sperm retrieval. Blood pressure (using a finger cuff; Finapres, Arnhem, the Netherlands) and one-lead electrocardiography were recorded continuously during the procedure. Blood pressure during the procedure (top diagram); representative 10-second samples of the electrocardiography recorded at rest (before the vibrostimulation; middle recording); and electrocardiography results at the time of ejaculation (bottom recording) are shown. Before vibrostimulation there was relative hypotension (100/65mmHg) with a regular heart rate of 78bpm. With initiation of vibrostimulation there was a sharp increase in arterial blood pressure suggestive of a typical episode of autonomic dysreflexia. Finally, at the time of ejaculation, arterial blood pressure surged to 305/120mmHg accompanied by bradyarrhythmia (38bpm) with a short run of premature ventricular contractions observed in the 3 minutes after ejaculation (electrocardiography recording at the bottom). Time of recorded premature ventricular contractions is indicated by an asterisk. At 15 minutes after ejaculation, arterial blood pressure was still slightly elevated (130mmHg; heart rate 66bpm). During the next 30–35min, arterial blood pressure and heart rate gradually returned to resting values. This episode of autonomic dysreflexia was accompanied by significant spasms in the upper and lower extremities, profuse sweating on the forehead and neck, and piloerection on the forearms. Interestingly, during this episode of autonomic dysreflexia, the patient reported only a mild headache. (Personal observations.) A color version of this figure is available in the color plate section.

factors of autonomic dysreflexia (Teasell et al 2000). There are also numerous reports of iatrogenic triggering factors such as cystoscopy, cystometry, vibration, or functional electrostimulation for ejaculation, and electrical stimulation of muscles (Giannantoni et al 1998, Sheel et al 2005). Autonomic dysreflexia may also present with minimal symptoms, such as sweating and piloerection, or it may be asymptomatic, even in individuals with tetraplegia (Kirshblum et al 2002). Finally, the level and completeness of injury are also important in the prevalence of autonomic dysreflexia, with dysreflexia being three times more common in those with tetraplegia with complete injury than those with an incomplete injury (Curt et al 1997). Among young people with T6 and higher level SCI and who were injured at 5 years of age and younger, those with complete lesions were three times more likely to experience autonomic dysreflexia than those with incomplete lesions (Schottler et al 2012). There is limited information with respect to a correlation between the severity of injury and presentation of autonomic dysreflexia in the pediatric population. However, Hickey and colleagues noted that there were some age differences relative to certain symptoms of autonomic dysreflexia. For example, headaches (5%) and piloerection (0%) were seen uncommonly in children 5 years of age and younger (Hickey et al 2004).

It is, however, important to note that, although autonomic dysreflexia occurs more often in the chronic stage of SCI at or above the sixth thoracic segment, there is clinical evidence of episodes of autonomic dysreflexia during the acute phase of the SCI within the first days or weeks after the injury (Krassioukov et al 2003). In fact, it seems likely that the presence of autonomic dysreflexia is simply under-recognized in the acute phase of SCI (Krassioukov et al 2003).

Although autonomic dysreflexia is unpleasant and life threatening (Eltorai et al 1992, Ho and Krassioukov 2010), some wheelchair athletes with SCI voluntarily induce it before the competition in order to enhance their performance (Harris 1994). Self-induced autonomic dysreflexia is commonly referred to as 'boosting' (Bhambhani et al 2010) and is considered unethical and illegal by the International Paralympic Committee Medical Commissions.

Orthostatic Hypotension

Although orthostatic intolerance and orthostatic hypotension are well documented in the pediatric population without SCI (Stewart 2002), there are no data available on the frequency or severity of orthostatic hypotension in the pediatric SCI population. In adults, it is well recognized that, for individuals with an SCI, in addition to low resting arterial blood pressure, many also experience a further drop in arterial blood pressure when they assume an upright position (Fig. 13.3). This is particularly common in the acute phase of injury (Mathias 1995, Cariga et al 2002). Orthostatic hypotension is defined as a decrease in systolic blood pressure of 20mmHg or more, or a decrease in diastolic blood pressure of 10mmHg or more, upon the assumption of an upright posture from a supine position, regardless of whether symptoms occur (Consensus Committee of the American Autonomic Society and the American Academy of Neurology 1996). The symptoms of orthostatic hypotension in individuals with SCI are similar to those in able-bodied individuals (Cleophas et al 1986) and include fatigue or weakness, light headedness, dizziness, blurred vision, dyspnea, restlessness, or even loss of consciousness in severe cases (Frisbie and Steele 1997, Sclater and Alagiakrishnan 2004). However, orthostatic hypotension can also be asymptomatic; Illman and colleagues reported that 41.1% of individuals with SCI who developed orthostatic hypotension were asymptomatic, despite significant blood pressure decline (Illman et al 2000). In a more recent study, we also found that orthostatic hypotension could persist asymptomatically in the chronic stage of SCI, despite a marked decrease in arterial blood pressure (Claydon and Krassioukov 2006). In this study, blood pressure decreases indicative of orthostatic hypotension were observed in 7 out of 14 participants with cervical SCI, and in 2 out of 11 participants with thoracic SCI. Symptomatic orthostatic hypotension was present in 5 out of 14 participants with cervical SCI and 2 out of 11 participants with thoracic SCI, and required early termination of the test in two symptomatic participants with cervical SCI (Claydon and Krassioukov 2006).

Concerning the incidence and prevalence of orthostatic hypotension in the adult population, orthostatic maneuvers performed during physiotherapy and mobilization are reported to induce blood pressure changes at levels indicative of orthostatic hypotension in 74% of individuals with SCI, suggesting that orthostatic hypotension is a common phenomenon in this population (Illman et al 2000).

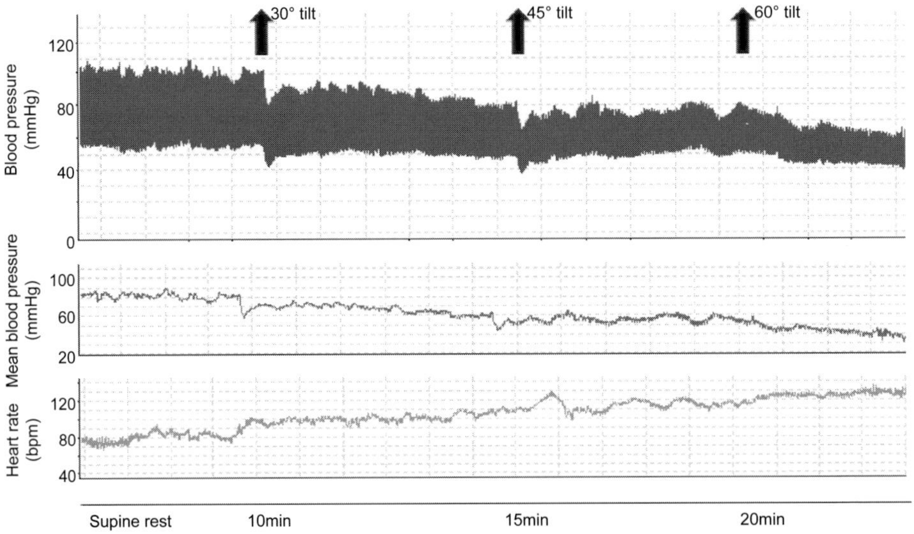

Fig. 13.3 A 16-year-old male with C5 American Spinal Injury Association Impairment Scale (AIS) A was examined for his blood pressure instability using a progressive tilt table test 2 months after the initial onset of a traumatic spinal cord injury. His main complaints were ongoing episodes of dizziness, light headedness, and periods of blurred vision that he experienced with transfer to his wheelchair or with the initiation of sessions of physical therapy. On numerous occasions during the previous few weeks he also had a few episodes of passing out while seated in his wheelchair. He was positioned on a tilt table in a supine position and was instrumented with a one-lead electrocardiography (lead II). Beat-to-beat arterial blood pressure was recorded continuously from the left hand using a Finometer (Finapres, Arnhem, the Netherlands). The upper panel shows the beat-by-beat blood pressure, the middle panel shows the arterial pressure, and the lower panel shows the heart rate during the progressive tilt test (30, 45, and 60 degrees, as indicated by arrows). His supine resting arterial blood pressure was measured as 100/60mmHg with a heart rate of 79bpm. There was a gradual decline in arterial blood pressure with reflex tachycardia with each progressive tilt up in this case. After 4min on the tilt table at 60 degrees, his arterial blood pressure declined to the level of 60/40mmHg and he became light headed, dizzy, and nauseous. The test was interrupted and he was returned to a supine position. Within 2 minutes of returning to the supine position, his cardiovascular parameters returned to the baseline level and his symptoms dissipated. The changes in his cardiovascular parameters were consistent with symptomatic orthostatic hypotension that had also interfered with his rehabilitation. Recommendations on non-pharmacologic and pharmacologic measures were made and the patient was followed until his discharge from acute rehabilitation. His orthostatic hypotension required prolonged management during his rehabilitation. (Personal observations.) A color version of this figure is available in the color plate section.

Several mechanisms have been proposed for the development of orthostatic hypotension in the population with SCI. Interruption of sympatho-excitatory efferent pathways from the brainstem to the spinal SPNs involved in vasoconstriction causes failure of short-term reflex blood pressure regulation (Claydon et al 2006a). This leads to pooling of blood in the viscera and dependent vasculature below the level of injury. Resting catecholamine levels are also lower in individuals with cervical SCI than in those with paraplegia and able-bodied individuals, and there is no significant increase in epinephrine or norepinephrine levels when individuals with tetraplegia undergo a head-up tilt (Claydon and Krassioukov 2006, Claydon et al 2006b, Mathias et al 1980). Individuals with SCI are also reported to have impaired baroreflex function (Wecht et al 2003), smaller plasma volumes owing to hyponatremia (Frisbie and Steele 1997), and possible cardiovascular deconditioning, at least in the early period after SCI, owing to prolonged periods of bed rest (Vaziri 2003). Any combination of these factors can further increase the likelihood and severity of orthostatic hypotension. On the other hand, there are a number of changes that occur after SCI that can mitigate the severity of orthostatic hypotension, including the recovery of spinal sympathetic reflexes, development of spasticity, increased muscle tone, and changes in the renin–angiotensin system (Teasell et al 2000). Although these changes have the potential to reduce the severity of orthostatic hypotension, the reality is that orthostatic hypotension remains a significant problem for the majority of the population with SCI.

Temperature Dysregulation after Spinal Cord Injury

Abnormal temperature control is another well-recognized clinical phenomenon that occurs after SCI (Colachis and Otis 1995). Although it often occurs in the acute period, it can potentially be a lifelong complication (McLean et al 1999). A combination of factors probably contribute to the temperature dysregulation seen after an SCI, including reduction of sensory input to the thermoregulatory center of the brain and loss of both vasomotor and sudomotor sympathetic control below the level of injury (Freund et al 1984). A high-level SCI leaves a large area of skin disconnected from the supraspinal sympathetic control, including the sweat glands and blood vessels crucial for thermoregulation (Lee et al 2002). Consequently, patients with cervical and high-thoracic injuries are predisposed to a greater degree of temperature dysregulation (Boot et al 2006).

A variety of thermodysregulations have been described in individuals with SCI. First, there is a poikilothermia, that is the inability to maintain a constant core temperature independent of ambient temperature. This dysregulation has also been termed 'environmental fever'; in a high ambient temperature, the individual with SCI can develop hyperthermia, while exposure to cold temperatures can induce hypothermia (McLean et al 1999, Khan et al 2007). Fever in individuals with SCI is commonly associated with urinary tract or other infections. However, fever without an infectious source occurring within the first several weeks to months after an SCI has also been reported in individuals with cervical and high-thoracic SCI (known as 'quad fever') (Colachis and Otis 1995). Finally, the inability to maintain a body temperature during exercise is another phenomenon commonly seen in this population (Price 2006). Numerous studies have demonstrated that individuals with cervical or high-thoracic SCI are predisposed to developing hyperthermia during exercise (Nash 2005). In order to prevent or reduce the development of this high core temperature, these individuals can engage in either pre-exercise cooling (Webborn et al 2005) or cooling during exercise (Hagobian et al 2004). For example, Hagobian and colleagues demonstrated that extraction of heat through the foot (cooling of the foot) attenuated the rise in tympanic temperature (Hagobian et al 2004).

As individuals with SCI, particularly those with high lesion levels, lose the ability to maintain their body temperature, prevention of hyper- or hypothermia is an important component in the management of their temperature dysregulation. Therefore, the first and most important approach to management of the condition is to keep them either cool or warm in response to their environment or circumstance, including maintaining sufficient hydration and appropriate clothing. The second is to avoid or minimize drugs that compromise thermoregulation. For example, it is known that alcohol consumption results in vasodilatation and predisposes an individual to heat loss. Thus, this activity should be avoided when cold conditions are anticipated (Teresinski et al 2005).

Little is known about temperature dysregulation among children with SCI. However, considering our clinical experience and knowledge from adults with SCI, it is crucial to consider that infants and young children with SCI are particularly vulnerable to the extremes of environmental temperatures owing to their relatively large surface area and their variable communication, cognitive and problem-solving abilities. At the other extreme are adolescents with SCI, who may be susceptible to hypothermia or hyperthermia because of erratic judgment.

Sweating Disturbances after Spinal Cord Injury

Two types of sweat glands are present in the human skin: eccrine glands (present over the entire skin surface, but more numerous on the palms, soles, face, and axillae) and apocrine glands (confined to the axillae, genitals, and the areola of the nipple) (Leung et al 1999). Only eccrine glands receive direct sympathetic (cholinergic) innervation (Phillips 1985). However, apocrine glands do respond to locally or systemically released catecholamines. After SCI, a variety of sweating dysfunctions can be observed: excess sweating (hyperhidrosis), absence of sweating (anhidrosis), or decreased sweating (hypohidrosis). Excessive sweating is an especially common complaint among individuals with SCI. In the majority of individuals with SCI, episodic hyperhidrosis is usually associated with other autonomic dysfunctions or conditions, such as autonomic dysreflexia, orthostatic hypotension, or post-traumatic syringomyelia (Khurana 1987, Kramer and Levine 1997, Glasauer and Czyrny 1994, Nicotra et al 2005). The most common pattern of sweating after SCI is profuse sweating above the level of the lesion with minimal or no sweating below the level of the lesion. However, sweating exclusively below the level of the lesion can also occur. This type of sweating is reflexive and is usually a manifestation of mass reflex or autonomic crisis, occurring particularly in individuals with cervical or high-thoracic lesions. Individuals with an injury below T8–T10 usually do not present with reflex sweating (Fast 1977). There is some evidence that sweat glands below the level of SCI are less sensitive to cholinergic activation, regardless of central or exogenous stimulation. However, glands above the level of the lesion may exhibit increased productivity when individuals with SCI are exposed to physical training and physiological stress (Yaggie et al 2002).

Both temperature and sweating abnormalities are commonly observed in individuals with SCI. Temperature dysregulation can markedly influence both the mental and the physical function of individuals with SCI and can lead to numerous complications. For example, it has been shown that elevated sacral skin temperature in individuals with SCI could be among the risk factors predisposing the individual to the development of pressure ulcers (Sae-Sia et al 2005). The presence of moisture on the skin owing to excessive sweating could compromise the skin's natural barrier to injury and infection (Knight et al 2001). In addition, impaired sweating in individuals with SCI could contribute to thermoregulatory problems (Sawka et al 1989). Careful monitoring of the core temperature and adequate measures to maintain normothermia are of great importance in this population.

Summary

In addition to motor and sensory deficits, individuals with SCI face lifelong abnormalities of the autonomic system. However, until 2009, the impact of an SCI on a person's neurologic function was evaluated only by motor and sensory assessment, in line with the International Standards for the Neurological Classification of Spinal Cord Injury (Kirshblum et al 2011). These assessments do not examine the status of a person's autonomic function. In order to address this deficiency, the American Spinal Injury Association and the International Spinal Cord Society commissioned a group of international experts to develop a common strategy for documenting any remaining autonomic function after SCI (Krassioukov 2012).

REFERENCE

Ackery A, Tator C, Krassioukov A (2004) A global perspective on spinal cord injury epidemiology. *J Neurotrauma* 21: 1355–70. doi.org/10.1089%2Fneu.2004.21.1355

Ackery A, Norenberg M, Krassioukov A (2007) Calcitonin gene-related peptide immunoreactivity in chronic human spinal cord injury. *Spinal Cord* 45: 678–86. doi.org/10.1038%2Fsj.sc.3102020

Alan N, Ramer LM, Inskip JA et al (2010) Recurrent autonomic dysreflexia exacerbates vascular dysfunction after spinal cord injury. *Spine J* 10: 1108–17. doi.org/10.1016%2Fj.spinee.201009.018

Anderson KD (2004) Targeting recovery: priorities of the spinal cord-injured population. *J Neurotrauma* 21: 1371–83. doi.org/10.1089%2Fneu.200421.1371

Beattie MS, Bresnahan JC, Leedy MG (1990) Synaptic plasticity in the adult sacral spinal cord: effects of lesions and hormones. In: *Trophic Factors and the Nervous System*. New York, NY: Raven Press Ltd. pp. 263–76.

Bhambhani Y, Mactavish J, Warren S et al (2010) Boosting in athletes with high-level spinal cord injury: knowledge, incidence and attitudes of athletes in paralympic sport. *Disabil Rehabil* 32: 2172–90. doi: 10.3109/09638288.2010.505678

Boot CR, Binkhorst RA, Hopman MT (2006) Body temperature responses in spinal cord injured individuals during exercise in the cold and heat. *Int J Sports Med* 27: 599–604. doi.org/10.1055/s-2005-865955

Calaresu FR, Yardley CP (1988) Medullary basal sympathetic tone. *Ann Rev Physiol* 50: 511–24. doi.org/10.1146%2Fannurev.ph.50.030188.002455

Cariga P, Ahmed S, Mathias CJ, Gardner BP (2002) The prevalence and association of neck (coat-hanger) pain and orthostatic (postural) hypotension in human spinal cord injury. *Spinal Cord* 40: 77–82. doi.org/10.1038/sj.sc.3101259

Claydon VE, Krassioukov A (2006) Orthostatic hypotension and autonomic pathways following spinal cord injury. *J Neurotrauma* 23: 1713–25. http://dx.doi.org/10.1089/neu.2006.23.1713

Claydon VE, Hol AT, Eng JJ, Krassioukov AV (2006a) Cardiovascular responses and postexercise hypotension after arm cycling exercise in subjects with spinal cord injury. *Arch Phys Med Rehabil* 87: 1106–14. doi.org/10.1016%2Fj.apmr.200605.011

Claydon VE, Steeves JD, Krassioukov A (2006b) Orthostatic hypotension following spinal cord injury: understanding clinical pathophysiology. *Spinal Cord* 44: 341–51. doi.org/10.1038/sj.sc.3101855

Cleophas TJM, Kauw FHW, Bijl C, Meijers J, Stapper G (1986) Effects of beta adrenergic receptor agonists and antagonists in diabetics with symptoms of postural hypotension – a double-blind placebo-controlled study. *Angiology* 37: 855–62. doi.org/10.1177/000331978603701110

Colachis SC, Otis SM (1995) Occurrence of fever associated with thermoregulatory dysfunction after acute traumatic spinal-cord injury. *Am J Phys Med Rehabil* 74: 114–19. doi.org/10.1097/00002060-199503000-00005

Consensus Committee of the American Autonomic Society and the American Academy of Neurology (1996) Consensus statement on the definition of orthostatic hypotension, pure autonomic failure, and multiple system atrophy. *Neurology* 46: 1470. http://dx.doi.org/10.1212/WNL.46.5.1470

Curt A, Nitsche B, Rodic B, Schurch B, Dietz V (1997) Assessment of autonomic dysreflexia in patients with spinal cord injury. *J Neurol Neurosurg and Psychiatry* 62: 473–7. doi.org/10.1136%2Fjnnp.62.5.473

Ditunno JF, Little JW, Tessler A, Burns AS (2004) Spinal shock revisited: a four-phase model. *Spinal Cord* 42: 383–95. doi.org/10.1038%2Fsj.sc.3101603

Eltorai I, Kim R, Vulpe M, Kasravi H, Ho W (1992) Fatal cerebral hemorrhage due to autonomic dysreflexia in a tetraplegic patient: case report and review. *Paraplegia* 30: 355–60. doi.org/10.1038%2Fsc.199282

Fast A (1977) Reflex sweating in patients with spinal cord injury: a review. *Arch Phys Med Rehabil* 58: 435–7.

Freund PR, Brengelmann GL, Rowell LB, Halar E (1984) Attenuated skin blood flow response to hyperthermia in paraplegic men. *J Appl Physiol* 56: 1104–9.

Frisbie JH, Steele DJR (1997) Postural hypotension and abnormalities of salt and water metabolism in myelopathy patients. *Spinal Cord* 35: 303–7. doi.org/10.1038/sj.sc.3100436

Furlan JC, Fehlings MG, Shannon P, Norenberg MD, Krassioukov AV (2003) Descending vasomotor pathways in humans: correlation between axonal preservation and cardiovascular dysfunction after spinal cord injury. *J Neurotrauma* 20: 1351–63. doi.org/10.1089%2F089771503322686148

Garshick E, Kelley A, Cohen SA et al (2005) A prospective assessment of mortality in chronic spinal cord injury. *Spinal Cord* 43: 408–16. doi.org/10.1038%2Fsj.sc.3101729

Giannantoni A, Di Stasi SM, Scivoletto G et al (1998) Autonomic dysreflexia during urodynamics. *Spinal Cord* 36: 756–60. doi.org/10.1038%2Fsj.sc.3100684

Glasauer FE, Czyrny JJ (1994) Hyperhidrosis as the presenting symptom in post-traumatic syringomyelia. *Paraplegia* 32: 423–9. doi.org/10.1038/sc.199469

Glenn MB, Bergman SB (1997) Cardiovascular changes following spinal cord injury. *Top Spinal Cord Inj Rehabil* 2: 47–53.

Hadley M (2002) Blood pressure management after acute spinal cord injury. *Neurosurgery* 50: S58–62. http://dx.doi.org/10.1097/00006123-200203001-00012

Hadley MN, Walters BC, Grabb PA et al (2002) Guidelines for the management of acute cervical spine and spinal cord injuries. *Neurosurgery* 50: S1–199. doi.org/10.1227%2FNEU.0b013e3182773549

Hagobian TA, Jacobs KA, Kiratli BJ, Friedlander AL (2004) Foot cooling reduces exercise-induced hyperthermia in men with spinal cord injury. *Med Sci Sports Exercise* 36: 411–17. doi.org/10.1249/01.MSS0000117133.75146.66

Harris P (1994) Self-induced autonomic dysreflexia ('boosting') practised by some tetraplegic athletes to enhance their athletic performance. *Paraplegia* 2: 289–91. doi.org/10.1038%2Fsc.199450

Hickey KJ, Vogel LC, Willis KM, Anderson CJ (2004) Prevalence and etiology of autonomic dysreflexia in children with spinal cord injuries. *J Spinal Cord Med* 27: S54–60.

Ho CP, Krassioukov AV (2010) Autonomic dysreflexia and myocardial ischemia. *Spinal Cord* 48: 714–15. doi:10.1038/sc.2010.2

Hwang M, Zebracki K, Betz RR, Mulcahey MJ, Vogel LC (2013) Normative blood pressure and heart rate in pediatric spinal cord injury. *Top Spinal Cord Inj Rehabil* 19: 87–95. doi: 10.1310/sci1902-87

Illman A, Stiller K, Williams M (2000) The prevalence of orthostatic hypotension during physiotherapy treatment in patients with an acute spinal cord injury. *Spinal Cord* 38: 741–7. doi.org/10.1038/sj.sc.3101089

Khan S, Plummer M, Martinez-Arizala A, Banovac K (2007) Hypothermia in patients with chronic spinal cord injury. *J Spinal Cord Med* 30: 27–30.

Khurana RK (1987) Orthostatic hypotension – induced autonomic dysreflexia. *Neurology* 37: 1221–24. doi.org/10.1212/WNL37.7.1221

Kirshblum SC, House JG, O'Connor KC (2002) Silent autonomic dysreflexia during a routine bowel program in persons with traumatic spinal cord injury: a preliminary study. *Arch Phys Med Rehabil* 83: 1774–6. doi.org/10.1053%2Fapmr.200236070

Kirshblum SC, Burns SP, Biering-Sørensen F et al (2011) International standards for neurological classification of spinal cord injury (revised 2011). *J Spinal Cord Med* 34: 535–46. doi: 10.1179/204577211X13207446293695

Knight SL, Taylor RP, Polliack AA, Bader DL (2001) Establishing predictive indicators for the status of loaded soft tissues. *J Appl Physiol* 90: 2231–7.

Kramer KM, Levine AM (1997) Posttraumatic syringomyelia: a review of 21 cases. *Clin Orthop Relat Res* 334: 190–9. doi.org/10.1097/00003086-199701000-00025

Krassioukov A (2004) Autonomic dysreflexia in acute spinal cord injury: incidence, mechanisms and management. *SCI Nurs* 21: 215–16. doi: 10.1089/089771503767869944

Krassioukov A (2009) Autonomic function following cervical spinal cord injury. *Respir Physiol Neurobiol* 169: 157–64. doi.org/10.1016%2Fj.resp.2009.08.003

Krassioukov A (2012) Introducing the revised International Standards on documentation of remaining Autonomic Function after SCI (ISAFSCI). *J Spinal Cord Med* 35: 201. doi: 10.1179/1079026812Z.00000000054

Krassioukov A, Claydon VE (2006) The clinical problems in cardiovascular control following spinal cord injury: an overview. *Prog Brain Res* 152: 223–9. doi.org/10.1016%2FS0079-6123%2805%2952014-4

Krassioukov AV, Fehlings MG (1999) Effect of graded spinal cord compression on cardiovascular neurons in the rostroventrolateral medulla. *Neuroscience* 88: 959–73. http://dx.doi.org/10.1016/S0306-4522(98)00267-X

Krassioukov AV, Weaver LC (1995) Reflex and morphological changes in spinal preganglionic neurons after cord injury in rats. *Clin Exp Hypertens* 17: 361–73. doi.org/10.3109%2F10641969509087077

Krassioukov AV, Weaver LC (1996) Morphological changes in sympathetic preganglionic neurons after spinal cord injury in rats. *Neuroscience* 70: 211–26. doi.org/10.1016%2F0306-4522%2895%2900294-S,

Krassioukov AV, Bunge RP, Puckett WR, Bygrave MA (1999) The changes in human spinal cord sympathetic preganglionic neurons after spinal cord injury. *Spinal Cord* 37: 6–13. doi.org/10.1038%2Fsj.sc.3100718

Krassioukov AV, Johns DG, Schramm LP (2002) Sensitivity of sympathetically correlated spinal interneurons renal sympathetic nerve activity and arterial pressure to somatic and visceral stimuli after chronic spinal injury. *J Neurotrauma* 19: 1521–9. doi.org/10.1089%2F089771502762300193

Krassioukov AV, Furlan JC, Fehlings MG (2003) Autonomic dysreflexia in acute spinal cord injury: an under-recognized clinical entity. *J Neurotrauma* 20: 707–16. doi.org/10.1089%2F089771503767869944

Krassioukov AV, Karlsson AK, Wecht JM, Wuermser LA, Mathias C, Marino RJ (2007) Assessment of autonomic dysfunction following spinal cord injury: rationale for additions to the International Standards for Neurological Assessment. *J Rehabil Res Dev* 44: 103–12. doi.org/10.1682%2FJRRD.2005.10.0159

Krassioukov A, Warburton DE, Teasell R, Eng JJ (2009) A systematic review of the management of autonomic dysreflexia after spinal cord injury. *Arch Phys Med Rehabil* 90: 682–95. doi.org/10.1016%2Fj.apmr.200810.017

Krenz NR, Meakin SO, Krassioukov AV, Weaver LC (1999) Neutralizing intraspinal nerve growth factor blocks autonomic dysreflexia caused by spinal cord injury. *J Neurosci* 19: 7405–14.

Lee SM, Williams WJ, Schneider SM (2002) Role of skin blood flow and sweating rate in exercise thermoregulation after bed rest. *J Appl Physiol* 92: 2026–34. doi: 10.1152/japplphysiol.00105.2001

Leung AK, Cho HY, Choi MC, Chan PY (1999) Hypohidrosis in children. *J R Soc Health* 119: 101–7. doi.org/10.1177/146642409911900208

McLean DE, Kearney J, Cawley MF (1999) Environmentally responsive temperature instability in pediatric spinal cord injury. *Spinal Cord* 37: 705–9. doi.org/10.1038/sj.sc.3100888

Maiorov DN, Adams MA, Krassioukov AV (2000) Telemetric blood pressure monitoring in conscious rats before and after compression injury of the spinal cord. *J Neurotrauma* 18: 727–36. doi.org/10.1089%2F089771501750357663

Mathias CJ (1995) Orthostatic hypotension: causes, mechanisms, and influencing factors. *Neurology* 45: S6–11.

Mathias CJ, Frankel HL (2002) Autonomic disturbances in spinal cord lesions. In: Bannister R, Mathias CJ (eds). *Autonomic Failure: A Textbook of Clinical Disorders of the Autonomic Nervous System*. 4th Ed. Oxford, UK: Oxford University Press. pp. 839–81.

Mathias CJ, Christensen NJ, Frankel HL, Peart WS (1980) Renin release during head-up tilt occurs independently of sympathetic nervous activity in tetraplegic man. *Clin Sci* 59: 251–6.

Nash MS (2005) Exercise as a health-promoting activity following spinal cord injury. *J Neurol Phys Ther* 29: 87–103, 106. doi.org/10.1097/01.NPT000028251494093.c6

National High Blood Pressure Education Program Working Group on High Blood Pressure in Children and Adolescents (2007) *A Pocket Guide to Blood Pressure Measurement in Children*. Washington DC: National Heart, Lung, and Blood Institute.

Nicotra A, Young TM, Asahina M, Mathias CJ (2005) The effect of different physiological stimuli on skin vasomotor reflexes above and below the lesion in human chronic spinal cord injury. *Neurorehabil Neural Repair* 19: 325–31. doi.org/10.1177/1545968305281210

Phillips DM (1985) Hypohidrosis. In: Taylor RB (ed.). *Difficult Diagnosis*. Philadelphia, PA: W.B. Sounders Company. pp. 252–6.

Piepmeier JM, Lehmann KB, Lane JG (1985) Cardiovascular instability following acute cervical spinal cord trauma. *Cent Nerv Syst Trauma* 2: 153–60. doi: 10.1089/cns.1985.2.153

Price MJ (2006) Thermoregulation during exercise in individuals with spinal cord injuries. *Sports Med* 36: 863–79. doi.org/10.2165/00007256-200636100-00005

Ramer LM, Ramer MS, Steeves JD, Krassioukov AV (2007) Sympathetic-sensory coupling in the peripheral nervous system may contribute to autonomic dysreflexia following spinal cord injury. *J Spinal Cord Med* 30: 177.

Ramer LM, van Stolk AP, Inskip JA, Ramer MS, Krassioukov AV (2012) Plasticity of TRPV1-expressing sensory neurons mediating autonomic dysreflexia following spinal cord injury. *Front Physiol* 3: 257. doi: 10.3389/fphys.2012.00257

Sae-Sia W, Wipke-Tevis DD, Williams DA (2005) Elevated sacral skin temperature (Ts): a risk factor for pressure ulcer development in hospitalized neurologically impaired Thai patients. *Appl Nurs Res* 18: 29–35. doi.org/10.1016/j.apnr.2004.03.005

Sawka MN, Latzka WA, Pandolf KB (1989) Temperature regulation during upper body exercise: able-bodied and spinal cord injured. *Med Sci Sports Exercise* 21: S132–40. doi.org/10.1249/00005768-198910001-00004

Schottler J, Vogel LC, Sturm P (2012) Spinal cord injuries in young children: a review of children injured at five years of age and younger. *Dev Med Child Neurol* 54: 1138–43. doi: 10.1111/j.1469-8749.2012.04411.x

Sclater A, Alagiakrishnan K (2004) Orthostatic hypotension – a primary care primer for assessment and treatment. *Geriatrics* 59: 22–7.

Sheel AW, Krassioukov AV, Inglis JT, Elliott SL (2005) Autonomic dysreflexia during sperm retrieval in spinal cord injury: influence of lesion level and sildenafil citrate. *J Appl Physiol* 99: 53–8. doi.org/10.1152%2Fj applphysiol.00154.2005

Stewart JM (2002) Orthostatic hypotension in pediatrics. *Heart Dis* 4: 33–9. doi.org/10.1097 %2F00132580-200201000-00006

Teasell R, Arnold AP, Krassioukov AV, Delaney GA (2000) Cardiovascular consequences of loss of supraspinal control of the sympathetic nervous system following spinal cord injuries. *Arch Phys Med Rehabil* 81: 506–16. http://dx.doi.org/10.1053/mr.2000.3848

Teresinski G, Buszewicz G, Madro R (2005) Biochemical background of ethanol-induced cold susceptibility. *Leg Med (Tokyo)* 7: 15–23. doi:10.1016/j.legalmed.2004.07.002

Vaziri ND (2003) Nitric oxide in microgravity-induced orthostatic intolerance: relevance to spinal cord injury. *J Spinal Cord Med* 26: 5–11.

Vogel L, Samdani A, Chafetz R, Gaughan J, Betz R, Mulcahey MJ (2009) Intra-rater agreement of the anorectal exam and classification of injury severity in children with spinal cord injury. *Spinal Cord* 47: 687–91. doi.org/10.1038%2Fsc.2008.180

Webborn N, Price MJ, Castle PC, Goosey-Tolfrey VL (2005) Effects of two cooling strategies on thermoregulatory responses of tetraplegic athletes during repeated intermittent exercise in the heat. *J Appl Physiol* 98: 2101–7. doi.org/10.1152/japplphysiol.00784.2004

Wecht JM, De Meersman RE, Weir JP, Spungen AM, Bauman WA (2003) Cardiac autonomic responses to progressive head-up tilt in individuals with paraplegia. *Clin Auton Res* 13: 433–8. doi: 10.1007/ s10286-003-0115-5

West CR, Mills P, Krassioukov AV (2012) Influence of the neurological level of spinal cord injury on cardiovascular outcomes in humans: a meta-analysis. *Spinal Cord* 50: 484–92. http://dx.doi.org/10.1038/sc.2012.17

Winslow EB, Lesch M, Talano JV, Meyer PR Jr (1986) Spinal cord injuries associated with cardiopulmonary complications. *Spine* 11: 809–12. doi.org/10.1097%2F00007632-198610000-00014

Yaggie JA, Niemi TJ, Buono MJ (2002) Adaptive sweat gland response after spinal cord injury. *Arch Phys Med Rehabil* 83: 802–5. doi.org/10.1053/apmr.200232670

Yarkony GM, Katz RT, Wu Y (1986) Seizures secondary to autonomic dysreflexia. *Arch Phys Med Rehabil* 67: 834–5.

Zebracki K, Hwang M, Patt PL, Vogel LC (2013) Autonomic cardiovascular dysfunction and vitamin D deficiency in pediatric spinal cord injury. *J Pediatr Rehabil Med* 6: 45–52. doi: 10.3233/PRM-130236

14
MEDICAL COMPLICATIONS AND MANAGEMENT

Glendaliz Bosques and Lawrence C Vogel

> **Case vignette**
> Taylor is a 5-year-old male who sustained a complete T6 spinal cord injury in a motor vehicle crash as a rear-seated passenger restrained with a lap belt and shoulder harness (three-point restraint). In addition to a Chance fracture of L3 requiring a posterior spine fusion, he had multiple small bowel perforations requiring surgical repair. Three weeks after his injury during intensive in-patient rehabilitation, he complained of not feeling well and of being nauseated and he vomited several times. He was afebrile and his abdominal examination demonstrated a non-distended abdomen with some diffuse tenderness and slightly diminished bowel sounds. While awaiting results of laboratory tests (serum calcium, amylase, and lipase; comprehensive chemistry panel; complete blood count; and urine analysis), he underwent an upper gastrointestinal study, which ruled out intestinal obstruction including superior mesenteric syndrome. When he returned from radiology, the diagnosis was established as hypercalcemia. He was managed with intravenous normal saline and one infusion of intravenous pamidronate with a resolution of the symptoms within 24 hours.

The approach to the diagnosis, treatment, and prevention of secondary health conditions that affect young people with spinal cord injuries (SCIs) must be developmentally based. Differences between the pediatric- and adult-onset SCI populations in the incidence and manifestations of secondary health conditions reflect a variety of factors that differ between these two groups. These factors include neurologic level and injury severity, age, growth and development, and subtle clinical manifestations in children, which may be the result of developmentally related communication skills. Hypercalcemia is an example of a medical complication that most commonly occurs in adolescent and young adult males because of their age-related active bone turnover. Another example is that infants and toddlers have limited abilities to articulate dysesthetic pain or the symptoms associated with autonomic dysreflexia because of their limited verbal abilities.

In addition to the medical complications described in this chapter, other chapters of this book cover additional secondary health conditions with unique features in children and young adults, including ventilator dependency (Chapter 9), neurogenic bladder and bowel (Chapter 11), spasticity (Chapter 12), autonomic dysfunctions (Chapter 13), pressure ulcers (Chapter 15), pain (Chapter 17), and musculoskeletal complications (Chapters 18 and 19).

Venous thromboembolism

Venous thromboembolism (VTE), which includes deep venous thrombosis (DVT) and pulmonary embolism, is a common complication after an SCI, and is a major cause of morbidity and mortality after an SCI. The Virchow triad, consisting of circulatory stasis, hypercoagulable state, and endothelial injury, predisposes individuals with SCI to VTE. Venous stasis results from the lack of both muscle tone and the pumping action of the leg muscles owing to paralysis. Endothelial damage may be a result of extrinsic pressure on the neurologically impaired leg or from free oxygen radicals or endotoxins generated by associated infections that individuals with SCI frequently experience. A transient hypercoagulable state occurs because of increased levels and activity of clotting factors, reduced fibrinolytic activity, and increased platelet aggregation.

There is limited literature available about the incidence, prevention, and treatment of VTE in pediatric SCI. Therefore, recommendations for the management of VTE in young people with SCI is extrapolated primarily from the adult SCI literature and, to a lesser degree, from studies on the general pediatric population, mainly critically ill young people (Kearon 2012).

Incidence

Data from the Shriners Hospitals for Children SCI program and the Model Systems SCI program databases reveal that DVT is extremely rare in children injured between birth and 5 years of age (0%) and in those injured between 6 and 12 years of age (2%) (Vogel et al 2011, Schottler et al 2012). In contrast, DVT was identified in 8% of those injured between 13 and 15 years of age and 9% of those injured between 16 and 21 years of age. In a retrospective cohort analysis of VTE in all SCI cases in California from 1991 to 2001, VTE was identified in only 1.1% of those aged 8 to 13 years and 4.8% of those aged 14 to 19 years (Jones et al 2005). In a retrospective study limited to one rehabilitation hospital, VTE was identified in 10% of those with SCI aged 15 to 18 years and in 5% of those under 15 years of age (Radecki and Gaebler-Spira 1994). Post-thrombotic syndrome develops in approximately 25% of young people with SCI who have developed DVT (David and Andrew 1993). Post-thrombotic syndrome is a manifestation of chronic venous insufficiency related to the preceding DVT and may present with chronic edema, varicosities, venous ulcers, and pain. Children who develop a thromboembolism may warrant further hematologic evaluation owing to the higher risk of pediatric patients having congenital or acquired anticoagulant deficiencies (Athale et al 2008).

Diagnosis

Although a classic presentation of an acute DVT is a warm, painful, and swollen extremity, individuals with SCI may be asymptomatic or exhibit non-specific signs and symptoms. In addition, other conditions, such as heterotopic ossification or a long-bone fracture, may present with signs and symptoms similar to a DVT, namely a warm and swollen leg. Pulmonary embolism may present with the acute onset of shortness of breath and tachycardia or sudden death. Therefore, a high degree of suspicion is required for the early diagnosis and timely management of VTE.

Clinical suspicion should be confirmed with diagnostic testing (Bates et al 2012). D-dimer levels may be used as a screening test for DVT in those individuals who are thought to be at a low to moderate risk of DVT. In the presence of elevated D-dimer levels, a duplex scan should be performed in order to make the definitive diagnosis of DVT. The duplex study consists of a Doppler component that measures venous flow and an ultrasound component that can identify the presence of a thrombus. One limitation of the duplex study is the inability to diagnose DVT in the iliac veins; magnetic resonance venography may be used for proximal and intrapelvic thrombosis (Macartney and Chan 2011). Although venography remains the criterion standard for diagnosing DVT, it is an invasive procedure that carries the risk of hypersensitivity reactions to the contrast material in addition to producing DVT itself. The diagnosis of a pulmonary embolism should be confirmed with spiral computed tomography rather than ventilation perfusion scans.

Prevention of Venous Thromboembolism

Because of the increased incidence of VTE and its associated high mortality in the general pediatric population since the early 2000s, guidelines have been established for risk stratification, assessment, and provision of thromboprophylaxis for at-risk pediatric populations (Raffini et al 2011, Sharthkumar et al 2012). Some authors suggest using Tanner stage II (presence of sparse pubic hair, and breast budding in females or testicular growth with texture changes in males) as the start of adolescence, instead of a specific onset age, as a cut-off for the provision of both mechanical and pharmacologic prophylaxis (Jackson and Morgan 2008).

There are no standard published guidelines for VTE prophylaxis in young people with an acute SCI. Early mobilization and passive movement should be instituted as soon as the patient is medically stable. Young people of all ages with acute SCI should receive mechanical prophylaxis with graduated compression stockings. For children who are too small to wear commercially available graduated compression stockings, use of custom-made lower extremity stockings may be a consideration. Using elastic wraps to wrap the legs is limited because unevenness of wrapping may result in constrictions with venous obstruction, increasing the risk of DVT or compartment syndrome (Vogel and Lubicky 2001). Additionally, some elastic wraps contain latex, which is contraindicated because of the risk of latex allergy in this patient population. Pneumatic compression sleeves can be utilized for older children and adolescents during the first 2 weeks after sustaining an SCI.

Because of the low incidence of DVT in children injured before adolescence, it may be reasonable to limit the use of anticoagulants to those young people with other factors that may increase the risk of DVT, such as lower extremity or pelvic trauma and fractures. Prophylactic anticoagulation should start within 24 to 72 hours after injury, if no active bleeding, other evidence of coagulopathy, or additional contraindications are present. Low-molecular-weight heparin (LMWH) can be administered subcutaneously; 0.75mg/kg of enoxaparin every 12 hours for infants younger than 2 months of age and 0.5mg/kg every 12 hours or 1mg/kg daily in those older than 2 months (Dix et al 2000). The target for prophylaxis with LMWH is 0.1 to 0.3units/ml of anti-factor Xa. Duration of prophylactic anticoagulation is generally 8 weeks or until discharge from rehabilitation; however, anticoagulation should be continued for 12 weeks or until discharge for those with motor complete lesions and who have additional risk factors such as lower extremity fractures, obesity, or history of previous VTE.

Thromboprophylaxis, both mechanical and anticoagulation, should be considered for children and young adults with chronic SCI who are hospitalized or who are restricted to bed rest for prolonged periods of time, such as those with pressure ulcers, as well as in the case of orthopedic interventions or other surgical procedures that may elevate the risk of developing VTE.

Treatment of Venous Thromboembolism

Management of DVT includes anticoagulation with LMWH or intravenous unfractionated heparin (UFH) (Monagle et al 2012). LMWH is the preferred treatment because it is associated with a decreased risk of bleeding, osteoporosis, and heparin-induced thrombocytopenia. LMWH is administered subcutaneously every 12 hours at 1.5mg/kg of enoxaparin for infants less than 2 months of age and at 1mg/kg for those more than 2 months of age. In individuals under 18 years of age, anticoagulation with LMWH should be monitored with anti-factor Xa levels (Monagle et al 2012) (see Table 14.1). Blood should be drawn 4 hours after the subcutaneous administration of LMWH with a target of 0.5 to 1.0units/ml of anti-factor Xa. UFH is administered intravenously with an initial bolus of 75 to 100units/kg followed by continuous infusion of 25 to 30units/kg/hour for infants or 18 to 20units/kg/hour for children over 1 year of age. The UFH infusion is adjusted to maintain the activated partial thromboplastin time between 60 and 85 seconds or an anti-Xa level of 0.35 to 0.70units/ml (Table 14.1). Oral anticoagulation with 0.2mg/kg of warfarin sodium is begun within 72 hours after LMWH or UFH has been initiated, and warfarin treatment should overlap by at least 5 days with LMWH or UFH. Dosage adjustments are made to maintain a target international normalized ratio of 2.5 (range 2.0–3.0) (Table 14.2) (Monagle et al 2012). The duration of anticoagulation is generally 3 to 6 months. In addition, graduated compression stockings should be worn for 2

TABLE 14.1

Monitoring low-molecular-weight heparin dose for venous thromboembolism treatment in children

Anti-factor Xa level	Dose titration	Next level check
≤0.35units/ml	Increase dose by 25%	4h after next dose
0.36–0.49units/ml	Increase dose by 10%	4h after next dose
0.5–1units/ml	Keep same dose	Next day, then 1wk later, then monthly
1.1–1.5units/ml	Decrease dose by 20%	Before next dose
1.6–2units/ml	Hold one dose for 3h and decrease next dose by 30%	Before next dose, then 4h after next dose
>2units/ml	Hold until anti-Xa level ≤0.5units/ml, then decrease previous dose by 40%	Before next dose, and every 12h until anti-Xa <0.5units/ml

Reproduced with permission from the American College of Chest Physicians and Monagle et al (2001).

TABLE 14.2
Protocol for oral anticoagulation therapy to maintain an international normalized ratio between 2 and 3 for pediatric patients

I	Day 1: if the baseline INR is 1.0–1.3, dose=0.2mg/kg orally	
II	Loading dose days 2–4: if the INR is	
	INR	*Action*
	1.1–1.3	Repeat initial loading dose
	1.4–1.9	50% of initial loading dose
	2.0–3.0	50% of initial loading dose
	3.1–3.5	25% of initial loading dose
	>3.5	Hold until INR <3.5 then restart at 50% decreased dose
III	Maintenance oral anticoagulation dose guidelines	
	1.1–1.4	Increase by 20% of dose
	1.5–1.9	Increase by 10% of dose
	2.0–3.0	No change
	3.1–3.5	Decrease by 10% of dose
	>3.5	Hold until INR <3.5 then restart at 20% decreased dose

Reproduced with permission from the American College of Chest Physicians and Monagle et al (2012). INR, international normalized ratio.

years after the onset of a VTE in order to decrease the incidence or severity of post-thrombotic syndrome (Kahn 2009).

Newer anticoagulant agents have been developed with the goal of more predictable and stable pharmacokinetics and pharmacodynamics (Kerlin 2012). Fondaparinux is a synthetic pentasaccharide that selectively inhibits factor Xa and is approved by the Food and Drug Administration (FDA) for use in the treatment and prophylaxis for VTE in adults. Compared with LMWH, its advantages include daily dosing, and reduced incidence of osteoporosis and heparin-induced thrombocytopenia. In a trial of 24 children, aged 1 to 18 years, with DVT or heparin-induced thrombocytopenia, fondaparinux was found to be safe, and pharmacokinetic modeling demonstrated that a once-daily dose at 0.1mg/kg resulted in similar concentrations known to be efficacious in adults (Young et al 2011a).

Argatroban is a small molecule that directly inhibits thrombin, is administered by continuous intravenous infusion, and is indicated as an anticoagulant for prophylaxis or the treatment of thrombosis in patients with heparin-induced thrombocytopenia. Argatroban has been studied in the pediatric population with pediatric dosage information being added to the FDA-approved labeling (Young et al 2011b). Similar to argatroban, bivalirudin is a direct thrombin inhibitor requiring continuous intravenous infusion. Although bivalirudin has been studied in children, pediatric-specific dosing has not been added to its labeling in the USA (Forbes et al 2011). Dabigatran is an orally administered drug that is a direct inhibitor of thrombin and is FDA approved for non-valvular atrial fibrillation (Kearon et al 2012). It is currently undergoing phase II trials in the pediatric population. It has the potential to replace warfarin as an orally administered anticoagulant. Rivaroxaban and apixaban are two orally administered drugs that are direct factor Xa inhibitors that are in various phases of study (Kearon et al 2012). Potential concerns with these agents are the lack of validated monitoring assays, which are particularly important for the pediatric population, and the lack of effective antidotes.

Hypercalcemia

Hypercalcemia affects 10% to 23% of individuals with SCI, and most commonly involves adolescent and young adult males during the first 3 months after injury (Tori and Hill 1978, Maynard 1986). Hypercalcemia results from increased bone resorption as a result of the immobilization associated with an SCI. The increased bone turnover characteristic of growing children and adolescents and the large and active bone mass that is characteristic of adolescent and young adult males in particular is the basis for the increased incidence of hypercalcemia. The excessive calcium load is not adequately excreted by the kidneys, because hypercalcemia depresses renal function, resulting in decreased calcium excretion and impairment in renal concentrating ability. Parathyroid hormone is usually depressed because of hypercalcemia.

Patients with hypercalcemia typically present with an insidious onset of abdominal pain, nausea, vomiting, lethargy, malaise, polydipsia, polyuria, and dehydration. Affected patients may exhibit behavioral changes or acute psychosis. In a series of 87 individuals younger than 16 years old, 18 (24%) experienced hypercalcemia (Tori and Hill 1978). Five of the patients with hypercalcemia had a clinical presentation consistent with an acute abdomen, and two of them underwent exploratory laparotomies. Patients with hypercalcemia can also be asymptomatic. Serum calcium and ionized calcium are higher than age-appropriate norms. Serum phosphorus is normal, and alkaline phosphatase is either normal or slightly higher than age-appropriate norms.

The mainstays of managing hypercalcemia are bisphosphonates and hydration with intravenous normal saline. Pamidronate is very effective in managing hypercalcemia and is administered intravenously at a dose of 1mg/kg (maximum dose of 60mg) over 4 hours (Kedlaya et al 1998). Generally, a single administration of pamidronate is sufficient to resolve an episode of hypercalcemia. Early mobilization and a weight-bearing program should also be instituted to assist in its management.

Complications of hypercalcemia can include urolithiasis, nephrocalcinosis, and renal failure. Tori and Kewalramani found that 11 of their 21 pediatric patients with hypercalcemia experienced urinary stones compared with 22% (17 out of 64) incidence of stones in patients without hypercalcemia (Tori and Kewalramani 1979). In an earlier report, 2 of the 18 patients with SCI developed renal failure and nephrocalcinosis (Tori and Hill 1978).

Latex hypersensitivity

Young people with SCI are susceptible to immediate-type, immunoglobulin E-mediated allergic reactions to latex with approximately 18% showing evidence of latex allergies (Vogel et al 1995). Among adults with SCI who had chronic indwelling catheters, 7 out of 15 had evidence of a latex allergy (Monasterio et al 2000). In addition, approximately 50% of young people with spina bifida are allergic to latex (Kwittken et al 1995).

An allergy to latex results from frequent and extensive contact with latex-containing materials. Other risk factors include young age of initial exposure and longer duration of exposure to latex-containing materials. Because children have a relatively immature immune system, they may be more prone to sensitization leading to immunoglobulin E-mediated reactions when exposures occur during infancy (Landwehr and Boguniewicz 1996). Atopy and exposure to latex-containing materials may act synergistically to increase the risk of developing a latex allergy (Moneret-Vautrin et al 1993). Reactions can be elicited by direct contact with latex via cutaneous, mucosal, intravenous, or serosal routes or by airborne dissemination of latex antigens that have adhered to glove powder.

Allergic reactions to latex may manifest as localized or generalized urticaria, wheezing, angioedema, or anaphylaxis. Intra-operative allergic reactions to latex may be life threatening, and they may be difficult to diagnose because of surgical drapes covering the patient's skin, which may be exhibiting urticaria.

The diagnosis of a latex allergy is established by a consistent history or utilizing in vitro assays or skin testing. Clinical manifestations may be subtle; for example, a child develops a blotchy facial rash when he blows up a latex-containing balloon. Latex allergy should be assumed in those who experience unexplained intra-operative allergic reactions, or in individuals who have allergic reactions to avocados, bananas, chestnuts, or kiwi. There is also a moderate degree of association between the following foods and latex: apples, carrots, celery, papaya, potato, tomato, and melon. Although skin tests are the most sensitive technique of identifying latex allergy, skin testing is limited by the lack of availability of skin-testing material and the potential for precipitating a severe allergic reaction (Landwehr and Boguniewicz 1996).

Because of the potential severity of latex allergy, individuals at risk, such as those with SCI or spina bifida, should be cared for in a latex-free environment, which should reduce the risk of sensitization and prevent allergic reactions in those with latex allergies. Young people with SCI, their families and caregivers, and other significant community personnel, such as teachers and school nurses, must be educated about latex allergy and the importance of avoiding latex-containing products. Individuals allergic to latex should wear a medical alert identification and carry auto-injectable epinephrine.

Respiratory insufficiency

Respiratory problems may affect young people with any level of an SCI with the possible exception of lumbar injuries. The extent of respiratory impairment is a function of the neurologic level of the SCI. Individuals with injuries at C2–C4 have varying degrees of significant respiratory compromise because of impairment of the diaphragm, intercostal muscles, and abdominal muscles. Those with C2–C3 injuries generally require chronic ventilatory support and are discussed in Chapter 9. Respiratory compromise in those with lower cervical and high-thoracic injuries (C5–T4) is a result of intercostal weakness and absence of abdominal musculature. Young people who have mid- to lower thoracic injuries (T5–T12) may still experience some degree of respiratory dysfunction, such as a weak cough, owing to abdominal musculature involvement.

In addition to the inherent respiratory impairments from neurologic involvement, children with an acute SCI may have concomitant complications, such as pneumothorax, hemothorax, or pulmonary contusions. As a result, young people with an acute SCI may experience respiratory insufficiency or failure, atelectasis, pulmonary edema, pneumonia, and acute respiratory distress syndrome (see Chapter 6).

Owing to intercostal muscle weakness, patients with cervical and high-thoracic injuries may experience restrictive lung dysfunction, with an associated decrease in vital capacity of 20% to 30% (Alvisi et al 2012). These young people may have ventilatory difficulty owing to diaphragmatic dysfunction in the seated position, which is most likely to be a result of the diaphragm collapsing into the abdominal cavity from abdominal muscle weakness compromising maximal diaphragmatic excursion. As a result, ventilation may be easier when the patient is in the supine position. An abdominal binder may provide enough support to improve diaphragmatic function when the young person is sitting. In addition, core muscle strengthening, including paraspinal muscles, aid respiration by strengthening accessory muscles.

Similar to adults, young people with tetraplegia are at risk of sleep-disordered breathing manifested as sleep problems, restlessness, confusion, cognitive changes, daytime sleepiness, or weight loss (Bach 1993). Therefore, healthcare providers must have a high index of suspicion for chronic alveolar hypoventilation, particularly in younger children with tetraplegia (Porth 2004). Young people should be assessed with a sleep study, and those with sleep-disordered breathing may benefit from continuous positive airway pressure or bilevel positive airway pressure (Tollefsen and Fondenes 2012).

Pneumonia is one of the most common causes of morbidity and mortality in patients with acute or chronic SCIs, regardless of age (DeVivo et al 1999). All individuals with SCI, regardless of neurologic level, should receive pneumococcal and annual influenza vaccinations. Young people with ineffective cough may benefit from cough assistance. This may be accomplished using manual cough assistance (quad cough), a mechanical device such as the mechanical insufflator/exsufflator (Tollefsen and Fondenes 2012), or lower thoracic spinal cord stimulation to activate the expiratory muscles (DiMarco et al 2009a,b).

Fever

Fever is a common presenting problem for young people with SCI, beginning during acute care and initial rehabilitation and extending throughout their lives. Developmental characteristics of the pediatric SCI population may impact the diagnostic evaluation of fever; for example, an infant or toddler may not be able to articulate a symptom such as a sore throat. In addition, although fever is not unique to children with SCI, children tend to become febrile more readily and experience higher temperature elevations than adults.

Acute infections are the most common cause of fevers in children with SCI, with the respiratory and genitourinary systems being the most frequently involved (McKinley et al 2006, Unsal-Delialioglu et al 2010). Other causes may include VTE, heterotopic ossification, pathologic fractures, surgical site infections, drug-related fever, or pressure ulcers. Fever related to an infectious cause is usually associated with higher maximal temperature elevations (>38.6ºC) and longer durations (>3d) (McKinley et al 2006).

Febrile episodes may be the result of non-infectious processes and may reflect autonomic dysfunction with associated thermoregulatory abnormalities (Unsal-Delialioglu et al 2010). Young people at greater risk of these non-infectious febrile episodes include those who are acutely injured, have tetraplegic injuries, or are ventilator dependent (McLean et al 1999). A temperature regulation protocol designed for children with injuries higher than T6 includes maintaining the room temperature at between 22.2ºC and 23.3ºC, maintaining ventilator temperature at between 30ºC and 32ºC, clothing adjustments for symptomatic episodes, and positioning thermostats above the head of the patient's bed (McLean et al 1999).

Evaluation of a young person with an SCI who is febrile must include a thorough history and physical examination, and appropriate laboratory and imaging studies guided by the clinical evaluation. The history should include recent blood transfusions and surgical procedures. The physical examination must encompass a general evaluation to identify problems such as otitis media or pneumonia. The evaluation must also be directed at SCI-specific problems, such as identifying a swollen extremity with limited range consistent with a fracture or heterotopic ossification or a swollen scrotum owing to epididymitis. Because of absent or altered pain sensation, an acute abdomen may present with fever and non-specific symptoms (see 'Gastrointestinal problems' section).

The choice of laboratory and imaging studies must be based on clinical findings, but usually includes a urine analysis and culture, a complete blood count with differential, erythrocyte sedimentation rate, and C-reactive protein. Liver function tests, serum amylase and lipase, plain abdominal radiographs, abdominal and pelvic ultrasound, and computed tomography may be helpful in evaluating the patient for potential intra-abdominal disorders (see 'Gastrointestinal problems' section below).

Gastrointestinal problems

Gastritis and stress ulcers are uncommon in the pediatric patient with acute SCI (Vogel 1996). Most patients benefit from a proton pump inhibitor or H2-blocker to provide protection to the gastrointestinal tract after the acute stress associated with an acute SCI. It is especially important if the patient has received steroids or is receiving thromboprophylaxis, since they are at a higher risk of developing complications such as gastrointestinal bleeds.

Superior mesenteric artery (SMA) syndrome, most commonly involving older adolescents or young adults (16–29y of age), may occur during acute care or initial rehabilitation (Laffont et al 2002). Factors contributing to the development of SMA syndrome include weight loss, paralysis with limited bed mobility, and spine fusions. SMA syndrome is probably caused by the loss of the retroperitoneal fat, which decreases the angle between the SMA and aorta resulting in compression of the third portion of the duodenum (Gore et al 1981). Patients typically present with persistent nausea, vomiting, and abdominal distention (Gore et al 1981, Laffont et al 2002). Differential diagnosis should include hypercalcemia, pancreatitis, cholecystitis, and intestinal obstruction related to intra-abdominal injuries incurred during the initial trauma. The diagnosis of SMA syndrome is usually confirmed by an upper gastrointestinal series, which demonstrates dilation of the stomach and first two segments of the duodenum and compression of the third portion of the duodenum (Laffont et al 2002). The finding of compression of the third portion of the duodenum can be intermittent in nature, similar to the clinical presentation. The diagnosis of SMA syndrome may also be accomplished utilizing endoscopy, abdominal computed tomography, or arteriography. Management should include nasogastric decompression and aggressive nutritional supplementation achieved by nasojejunal feedings, parenteral hyperalimentation, or a combination of both (Ramos 1975). For patients with milder forms of SMA syndrome and those in the recovery phase small frequent meals beginning with a mechanical soft diet should be provided. If medically and surgically permitted, positional changes such as lying on their side or lying knee to chest after meals may also be beneficial. For those with persistence of symptoms, despite conservative management, surgical intervention may be needed (Ylinen et al 1989).

Adynamic ileus is not an uncommon complication, which usually presents during the acute phase of spinal shock. Although the ileus usually resolves within a week of sustaining an SCI, the ileus may persist beyond the period of spinal shock and may be accompanied by gastric dilation and delayed gastric emptying. Management of ileus with or without gastroparesis includes nasogastric decompression, maintaining a nil-by-mouth status, and providing appropriate nutritional support, which may require parenteral hyperalimentation. Treatment may also include medications such as metoclopramide, erythromycin, or neostigmine.

Patients with tetraplegia or thoracic-level paraplegia may have a clinically silent acute abdomen owing to their neurologic impairments with absent or altered pain sensation and an inability to localize pain. These patients may present with persistent fevers or autonomic dysreflexia and subtle signs and symptoms, such as anorexia, abdominal distension, nausea, and vomiting. Therefore, the diagnosis of pancreatitis, appendicitis, and cholecystitis, among others, may require a high level of suspicion for prompt and adequate treatment (Zaremski et al 2010). Young people with SCI are at a greater risk of both pancreatitis and gall bladder disorders, which may coexist. Cholelithiasis and pancreatitis may be more common in individuals with tetraplegia and upper thoracic paraplegia because of impaired sympathetic innervation. The diagnosis of pancreatitis is established by an elevated serum lipase level, and management includes maintaining a nothing-by-mouth status of the young person, hydration with intravenous fluids, and central hyperalimentation. The diagnosis of cholelithiasis or cholecystitis is generally established utilizing ultrasound, whereas the diagnosis of choledocholithiasis is established by magnetic resonance cholangiopancreatography or endoscopic retrograde cholangiopancreatography. Treatment of cholelithiasis is usually accomplished by laparoscopic cholecystectomy.

Succinylcholine sensitivity

Individuals with neurologic injuries, such as SCI, may experience a massive release of intracellular potassium and consequent cardiac arrest after administration of succinylcholine. Therefore, succinylcholine should not be utilized in individuals with an SCI beyond 48 to 72 hours after injury. In addition, because the duration of sensitivity to succinylcholine is not known, it may be wise to avoid its use in those with neurologic impairments throughout their life (Martyn and Richtsfeld 2006).

REFERENCES

Alvisi V, Marangoni E, Zannoli S et al (2012) Pulmonary function and expiratory flow limitation in acute cervical spinal cord injury. *Arch Phys Med Rehabil* 93: 1950–6. http://dx.doi.org/10.1016/j.apmr.2012.04.015

Athale U, Siciliano S, Thabane L et al (2008) Epidemiology and clinical risk factors predisposing to thromboembolism in children with cancer. *Pediatr Blood Cancer* 51: 792–7. http://dx.doi.org/10.1002/pbc.21734

Bach JR (1993) Inappropriate weaning and late onset ventilatory failure of individuals with traumatic spinal cord injury. *Paraplegia* 31: 430–8. http://dx.doi.org/10.1038/sc.1993.72

Bates SM, Jaeschke R, Stevens SM et al (2012) Diagnosis of DVT: Antithrombotic therapy and prevention of thrombosis, 9th Ed: American College of Chest Physicians evidence-based clinical practice guidelines. *Chest* 141(Suppl 2): e351S–418S. doi:10.1378/chest.11-2299.

David M, Andrew M (1993) Venous thromboembolic complications in children. *J Pediatr* 123: 337–46. http://dx.doi.org/10.1016/S0022-3476(05)81730-5

DeVivo MJ, Krause JS, Lammertse DP (1999) Recent trends in mortality and causes of death among persons with spinal cord injury. *Arch Phys Med Rehabil* 80: 1411–19. http://dx.doi.org/10.1016/S0003-9993(99)90252-6

DiMarco AF, Kowalski KE, Geertman RT, Hromyak DR (2009a) Lower thoracic spinal cord stimulation to restore cough in patients with spinal cord injury: results of a National Institutes of Health-sponsored clinical trial. Part I: methodology and effectiveness of expiratory muscle activation. *Arch Phys Med Rehabil* 90: 717–25. doi: 10.1016/j.apmr.2008.11.013

DiMarco AF, Kowalski KE, Geertman RT et al (2009b) Lower thoracic spinal cord stimulation to restore cough in patients with spinal cord injury: results of a National Institutes of Health-sponsored clinical trial. Part II: clinical outcomes. *Arch Phys Med Rehabil* 90: 726–32. doi: 10.1016/j.apmr.2008.11.014

Dix D, Andrew M, Marzinotti V et al (2000) The use of low molecular weight heparin in pediatric patients: a prospective cohort study. *J Pediatr* 136: 439–45. http://dx.doi.org/10.1016/S0022-3476(00)90005-2

Forbes TJ, Hijazi ZM, Young G et al (2011) Pediatric catheterization laboratory anticoagulation with bivalirudin. *Catheter Cardiovasc Interv* 77: 671–9. doi: 10.1002/ccd.22817

Gore RM, Mintzer RA, Calenoff L (1981) Gastrointestinal complications of spinal cord injury. *Spine (Phila Pa 1976)* 6: 538–44.

Jackson PC, Morgan JM (2008) Perioperative thromboprophylaxis in children: development of a guideline for management. *Paediatr Anaesth* 18: 478–87. http://dx.doi.org/10.1111/j.1460-9592.2008.02597.x

Jones T, Ugalde V, Franks P, Zhou H, White RH (2005) Venous thromboembolism after spinal cord injury: incidence, time course, and associated risk factors in 16,240 adults and children. *Arch Phys Med Rehabil* 86: 2240–7. http://dx.doi.org/10.1016/j.apmr.2005.07.286

Kahn SR (2009) How I treat postthrombotic syndrome. *Blood* 114: 4624–31. doi: 10.1182/blood-2009-07-199174

Kearon C, Akl EA, Comerota AJ et al (2012) Antithrombotic therapy for VTE disease: Antithrombotic therapy and prevention of thrombosis, 9th Ed: American College of Chest Physicians evidence-based clinical practice guidelines. *Chest* 141(Suppl 2): e419S–4. doi:10.1378/chest.11-2301

Kedlaya D, Branstater ME, Lee JK (1998) Immobilization hypercalcemia in incomplete paraplegia: successful treatment with pamidronate. *Arch Phys Med Rehabil* 79: 222–5. http://dx.doi.org/10.1016/S0003-9993(98)90304-5

Kerlin BA (2012) Current and future management of pediatric venous thromboembolism. *Am J Hematol* 87(Suppl 1): S68–74. http://dx.doi.org/10.1002/ajh.23131

Kwittken PL, Sweinberg SK, Campbell DE, Pawlowski NA (1995) Latex hypersensitivity in children: clinical presentation and detection of latex-specific immunoglobulin E. *Pediatrics* 95: 693–9.

Laffont I, Bensmail D, Rech C, Prigent G, Loubert G, Dizien O (2002) Late superior mesenteric artery syndrome in paraplegia: case report and review. *Spinal Cord* 40: 88–91. http://dx.doi.org/10.1038/sj.sc.3101255

Landwehr LP, Boguniewicz M (1996) Current perspectives on latex allergy. *J Pediatr* 128: 305–12. http://dx.doi.org/10.1016/S0022-3476(96)70272-X

Macartney CA, Chan AK (2011) Thrombosis in children. *Semin Thromb Hemost* 37: 763–71. http://dx.doi.org/10.1055/s-0031-1297167

McKinley W, McNamee S, Meade M, Kandra K, Abdul N (2006) Incidence, etiology, and risk factors for fever following acute spinal cord injury. *J Spinal Cord Med* 29: 501–6.

McLean DE, Kearney J, Cawley MF (1999) Environmentally responsive temperature instability in pediatric spinal cord injury. *Spinal Cord* 37: 705–9. http://dx.doi.org/10.1038/sj.sc.3100888

Martyn JA, Richtsfeld M (2006) Succinylcholine-induced hyperkalemia in acquired pathologic states: etiologic factors and molecular mechanisms. *Anesthesiology* 104: 158–69. http://dx.doi.org/10.1097/00000542-200601000-00022

Monagle P, Michelson AD, Bovill E et al (2001) Antithrombotic therapy in children. *Chest* 119: 344–70S. http://dx.doi.org/10.1378/chest.119.1_suppl.344S

Monagle P, Chan AKC, Goldenberg NA et al (2012) Antithrombotic therapy in neonates and children: Antithrombotic therapy and prevention of thrombosis, 9th Ed: American College of Chest Physicians evidence-based clinical practice guidelines. *Chest* 141(Suppl 2): e737S–801S. doi: 10.1378/chest.11-2308

Monasterio EA, Barber DB, Rogers SJ et al (2000) Latex allergy in adults with spinal cord injury: a pilot investigation. *J Spinal Cord Med* 23: 6–9.

Moneret-Vautrin DA, Beaudouin E, Widmer S et al (1993) Prospective study of risk factors in natural rubber latex hypersensitivity. *J Allergy Clin Immunol* 92: 668–77. http://dx.doi.org/10.1016/0091-6749(93)90009-5

Porth SC (2004) Recognition and management of respiratory dysfunction in children with tetraplegia. *J Spinal Cord Med* 27(Suppl): S75–9.

Radecki RT, Gaebler-Spira D (1994) Deep vein thrombosis in the disabled pediatric population. *Arch Phys Med Rehabil* 75: 248–50. http://dx.doi.org/10.1016/0003-9993(94)90023-X

Raffini L, Trimarchi T, Beliveau J, Davis D (2011) Thromboprophylaxis in a pediatric hospital: a patient-safety and quality-improvement initiative. *Pediatrics* 127: e1326–32. doi: 10.1542/peds.2010-3282

Ramos M (1975) Recurrent superior mesenteric artery syndrome in a quadriplegic patient. *Arch Phys Med Rehabil* 56: 86–8.

Schottler J, Vogel LC, Sturm P (2012) Spinal Cord injuries in young children: a review of children injured at five years of age and younger. *Dev Med Child Neurol* 54: 1138–43. http://dx.doi.org/10.1111/j.1469-8749.2012.04411.x

Sharathkumar AA, Mahajerin A, Heidt L et al (2012) Risk-prediction tool for identifying hospitalized children with a predisposition for development of venous thromboembolism: Peds-Clot clinical Decision Rule. *J Thromb Haemost* 10: 1326–34. http://dx.doi.org/10.1111/j.1538-7836.2012.04779.x

Tollefsen E, Fondenes O (2012) Respiratory complications associated with spinal cord injury. *Tidsskr Nor Laegeforen* 132: 1111–14. http://dx.doi.org/10.4045/tidsskr.10.0922

Tori JA, Hill LL (1978) Hypercalcemia in children with spinal cord injury. *Arch Phys Med Rehabil* 59: 443–6.

Tori JA, Kewalramani LS (1979) Urolithiasis in children with spinal cord injury. *Paraplegia* 16: 357–65. http://dx.doi.org/10.1038/sc.1978.68

Unsal-Delialioglu S, Kaya K, Sahin-Onat S, Kulakli F, Culha C, Ozel S (2010) Fever during rehabilitation in patients with traumatic spinal cord injury: analysis of 392 cases from a national rehabilitation hospital in Turkey. *J Spinal Cord Med* 33: 243–8.

Vogel L (1996) Management of medical issues. In: Betz R (ed.). *The Child with a Spinal Cord Injury*. Rosemont, IL: American Academy of Orthopedic Surgeons. pp. 189–212.

Vogel LC, Lubicky JP (2001) Lower extremity compartment syndrome in an adolescent with a spinal cord injury. *J Spinal Cord Med* 24: 278–83.

Vogel LC, Schrader T, Lubicky JP (1995) Latex allergy in children and adolescents with spinal cord injuries. *J Pediatr Orthop* 15: 517–20. http://dx.doi.org/10.1097/01241398-199507000-00021

Vogel L, Betz R, Mulcahey M (2011) Pediatric spinal cord disorders. In: Kirshblum S, Campagnolo DI (eds). *Spinal Cord Medicine*. 2nd Ed. Philadelphia, PA: Lippincott Williams & Wilkins. pp. 533–64.

Ylinen P, Kinnunen J, Höckerstedt K (1989) Superior mesenteric artery syndrome. A follow-up study of 16 operated patients. *J Clin Gastroenterol* 11: 386–91. http://dx.doi.org/10.1097/00004836-198908000-00007

Young G, Yee DL, O'Brien SH, Khanna R, Barnbour A, Nugent DJ (2011a) FondaKIDS: a prospective pharmacokinetic and safety study of fondaparinux in children between 1 and 18 years of age. *Pediatr Blood Cancer* 57: 1049–54. doi: 10.1002/pbc.23011

Young G, Boshkov LK, Sullivan JE et al (2011b) Argatroban therapy in pediatric patients requiring nonheparin anticoagulation: an open-label, safety, efficacy, and pharmacokinetic study. *Pediatr Blood Cancer* 56: 1103–9. doi: 10.1002/pbc.22852

Zaremski JL, Jayawardena V, Lew HL (2010) An occult presentation of appendicitis in a patient with tetraplegia. *Am J Phys Med Rehabil* 89: 156–9. http://dx.doi.org/10.1097/PHM.0b013e3181c1ed30

15
SKIN INTEGRITY

Kelly M Johnson, Michelle Kauffman-Lawson and Kerry A Lavan

Case vignette

Adam is a 16-year-old male with a complex medical history, including inoperable spinal lymphangiomatosis resulting in complete T4 paraplegia and severe scoliosis. Adam required a custom-molded seating system in his wheelchair for stability and an air mattress for his bed. He was on an intermittent self-catheterization program. The wheelchair felt confining to Adam and he struggled with body image and the desire to 'fit in' with his friends. He frequently allowed classmates to sit on his lap for extended periods and he would sit on hard surfaces, such as unpadded classroom chairs and hard football bleachers. Adam stated the air mattress made him 'feel like an old man' so he frequently slept on the couch or other surfaces without the air mattress. Adam inconsistently adhered to his catheterization schedule resulting in urine incontinence, and his diet consisted primarily of canned soft drinks, energy drinks, and fast food.

Adam developed pressure ulcers on his sacrum and left ischial tuberosity that he did not disclose to his parents until they developed into stage 4 pressure injuries Adam was referred to a wound clinic where he was diagnosed with osteomyelitis; he was treated with long-term systemic antibiotics, negative pressure wound therapy for initial wound treatment, and eventually was referred to a plastic surgeon for surgical repair. Adam was referred to a dietitian who developed a nutritional plan with Adam and his family. Physical therapy evaluated his wheelchair and seating system, and modifications were made to provide him with more movement and flexibility. The modifications also addressed the look and feel of the wheelchair and seating system to help with body image. An assessment was also completed to provide a more acceptable option for a sleep surface.

Psychosocial assessment and support was provided to Adam, including access to a peer support group. Areas that were addressed included adherence to practices for prevention of pressure ulcers, nutrition, and self-catheterization.

Adam ultimately assumed ownership of his self care and acknowledged the importance of a preventive approach to his overall health and specifically skin health. Adam began to do skin checks routinely, independently manage safe skin practices, follow nutritional recommendations, and mange his neurogenic bladder.

Introduction

Children with spinal cord injury (SCI) are at risk of alterations in skin integrity including burns, maceration, scrapes, and pressure injuries. Pressure injuries can be devastating and are a common secondary complication in children with SCI (Hickey et al 2000). 'The misconception that children are not at risk for pressure injuries becomes a major risk factor in itself because their skin may not be thoroughly assessed and appropriate preventative measures may not be instituted' (Baharestani and Ratliff 2007). Early prevention and intervention through the pre-hospital, trauma, and critical care phases of recovery are important and are the responsibility of the healthcare team. Prevention remains vital throughout the lifetime of the individual with SCI, and responsibility transitions during rehabilitation and beyond from the healthcare team to the patient and their family/caregivers. The pediatric population may be dependent upon their caregivers, teachers, and parents to assist with optimizing skin integrity. This dependency can be due to age at the time of injury, level of injury, developmental and cognitive abilities, socio-economic status, and support systems. Prevention of pressure injuries requires active participation by the patient and their family/caregivers and consistency is key for maintaining skin. The goal is for children to increasingly assume responsibility for their personal care and the prevention of secondary conditions such as pressure injuries, while parents/caregivers serve as a safety net.

The goal of this chapter is to provide an overview of the prevention and management of pressure injuries in young people with SCI. For further information, the readers of this book are encouraged to read current clinical practice guidelines, best practice guidelines, and reviews on this topic (Houghton et al 2013, Smith et al 2013, Consortium for Spinal Cord Medicine 2014).

Effects of spinal cord injury on the skin

Many changes occur to the skin after an SCI. These occur because of sensory and motor impairments and alterations of the autonomic nervous system, which lead to changes in regulation of body temperature and reflex sweating. Biochemical changes to the skin after SCI include an increase in collagen catabolism and a decrease in collagen biosynthesis, resulting in more fragile skin below the level of injury (Consortium for Spinal Cord Medicine 2000). Changes in oxygen tension and vascular reaction, and reductions in blood supply and blood flow to the skin below the level of injury increase the risk of development of pressure injuries and impair wound healing (Consortium for Spinal Cord Medicine 2000).

Causes of alteration in skin integrity

Unrelieved pressure or pressure in combination with shear is the primary cause of pressure injuries. Other contributing factors include moisture, friction, and nutritional status. As many as 50% of pressure injuries reported in children with SCI are device and equipment related (Schluer et al 2009). Devices such as endotracheal or tracheotomy tubes, mechanical ventilators with associated tubing and circuits, orthotics, monitor leads, intravenous hubs, and pulse oximeters can contribute to skin breakdown owing to pressure, moisture, friction, and shearing in areas underneath these medical devices. Alterations in skin integrity may also be caused by exposure to extreme cold temperatures, or from scooting or bumping to get around on the floors or stairs.

Young people with SCI are also susceptible to burns that may be caused by scalding or exposure to hot surfaces such as exposed plumbing fixtures, playground equipment, exposed metal on adaptive equipment, hairdryers, or curling irons and other heated hair styling tools. Burns can occur from using the lap as a carrying surface for items such as hot plates, food items, or laptop computers or by exposure to the sun.

Risk, incidence, and prevalence

A retrospective analysis of Pediatric Health Information Systems (PHIS)[a] in-patient data from 38 US children's hospitals was conducted between 1 January 2007 and 31 December 2011. During this time, there were 858 pediatric patients (aged 18y or younger) with SCI diagnosis codes admitted to these 38 children's hospitals. Of the 858 pediatric patients with SCI, 41 were coded with a pressure injury with an incidence rate of 4.78 patients with pressure injuries per 100 patients with SCI or 4.78% (Children's Hospital Association, Pediatric Health Information Systems 2012). In 2003, a multisite pressure injury prevalence survey of 1064 children (aged <10d–17y) in nine US children's hospitals found the prevalence rate to be 4% (McLane et al 2004). The majority of pressure injuries identified were stage 1 (61%) and stage 2 (13%), and were most commonly located in the occiput (31%), followed by the sacrum (20%) and foot areas (19%) (McLane et al 2004).

Prevention

All children with SCI, no matter what age they are or level of injury they have, are at risk of pressure injuries. Accurate assessment and documentation of the skin are the foundations for prevention and treatment of alterations in skin integrity. It is important to note that skin assessment and pressure injury assessment are not the same but are two separate assessments. These assessments should begin during the acute admission, continue daily, and include the family/caregiver as integral parts of monitoring and education. Early and continued skin assessment for skin injury and pressure ulcers is more likely to discover alteration in the earliest stages when they are easier and quicker to heal.

Risk Assessment

The assessment of pressure injuries has two important components: (1) proper evaluation of the risk of ulceration in preparation for instituting the right preventive measures, and (2) accurate staging and documentation for appropriate management (Wu et al 2009). It is important

a Disclosure: data for this study were obtained from the Pediatric Health Information System (PHIS), an administrative database that contains in-patient, emergency department, ambulatory surgery, and observation data from 43 not-for-profit, tertiary-care pediatric hospitals in the USA. These hospitals are affiliated with the Child Health Corporation of America (Shawnee Mission, KS, USA), a business alliance of children's hospitals. Data quality and reliability are assured through a joint effort between the Child Health Corporation of America and participating hospitals. The data warehouse function for the PHIS database is managed by Thomson Reuters (Ann Arbor, MI, USA). For the purposes of external benchmarking, participating hospitals provide discharge/encounter data including demographics, diagnoses, and procedures. Of these hospitals, 42 also submit resource utilization data (e.g. pharmaceuticals, imaging, and laboratory) into PHIS. Data are de-identified at the time of data submission, and are subjected to a number of reliability and validity checks before being included in the database. For this study, in-patient data from 38 hospitals were included.

to note that risk assessment tools should be used in tandem with clinical judgment. Although risk assessment tools are a combination of measurable intrinsic and extrinsic factors, clinical judgments rely on visual inspection and individual experience and expertise. Both have their limitations and strengths; therefore, it is important to use a valid and reliable tool coupled with regular education of those conducting assessments for pressure injury.

Recommendations for risk assessment from the National Pressure Ulcer Advisory Panel (2007a) include the recommendation that all patients with impaired mobility be assessed utilizing a valid and reliable tool on in-patient admission and at least every 24 hours, and that out-patients and home-care patients are assessed on every visit.

Two risk assessment tools have been found valid and reliable in the pediatric population. The Braden Q scale was adapted for the pediatric population and is based on the Braden scale, which predicts the risk of pressure ulcers in adults (Wu et al 2009). The Neonatal Skin Risk Assessment Scale was also derived from the Braden scale. Reliability and validity testing was completed on a small sample of 32 patients in a neonatal intensive care unit and is therefore used sparingly (Wu et al 2009).

From 2009 to 2010, the Child Health Corporation of America (now the Children's Hospital Association) conducted a pediatric pressure injury prevention collaborative with 14 US children's hospitals participating. Each facility implemented a set of changes over 10 months, which consisted of (1) routine skin assessment, (2) routine risk assessment, (3) minimization of pressure, (4) management of clinical risk factors (moisture, nutrition, and hydration), and (5) maximization of team function (education, leadership, and family engagement). Consistent application of basic prevention practices achieved remarkable results with a 65% reduction in the prevalence of pressure injuries in intensive care units and major improvements in process compliance. The Child Health Corporation of America pediatric pressure injury prevention collaborative recommended and implemented a set of prevention interventions, referred to as a change package (daily skin care bundle). Children's Hospital Colorado, one of the participating hospitals, developed a bundle to facilitate implementation. A basic model of this bundle is displayed in Table 15.1.

Skin Assessment

The principal method of prevention is to complete skin checks on a regular basis. During the acute phase of hospitalization, skin checks should be completed on admission, at least every shift, and with every patient hand-off. Once skin tolerance has been established – which means skin does not exhibit non-blanchable red areas with times between turns or during wheelchair sitting – assessment should be performed, head to toe, at least daily. Special attention should be paid to pressure points including the sacrum, ischial tuberosities, trochanters, heels, elbows, and occiput, as well as skin around any medical devices. Visual and tactile assessment should be employed. The patient may need assistance from adaptive devices such as a hand mirror to assist in checking his or her skin as they gain independence. A parent or caregiver may be necessary to assist or supplement skin checks. As the young person with an SCI begins to transition into various positions to develop skin tolerance, it is vital to complete skin checks after the allotted time frame to assess skin tolerance for various surfaces and progression of sitting or position times. For example, as a patient is transitioned into a seated position in

TABLE 15.1
Daily skin care bundle: comprehensive assessment

Assessments	
Risk assessment	Outside of the NICU, use modified Braden Q upon admission and every shift
	All NICU patients are considered high risk
Skin assessment	Outside of the NICU, do a daily head-to-toe skin assessment
	All NICU patients require Neonatal Skin Condition Score every shift and daily head-to-toe skin assessment
Device protection assessment	Assess skin under medical devices each shift (i.e. splints, cervical collars, boots, intravenous lines, drains, restraints)
	Change pulse oximeter position and assess skin under devices each shift
Interventions	
Positioning	Based on modified Braden Q; reposition patients who are at moderate to high risk a minimum of every 2h. Reposition NICU patients with care
	Float/offload heels:
	Heel-protector boots if patient is agitated
	Pillows for sedated patient
	If on continuous lateral rotation therapy:
	Rotation 18h/d
	Manual turn every 2h: stop rotation, reposition right or left for 30min, place supine, resume rotation
Moisture/friction	Use barrier creams, moisturizers, and, as needed, incontinence cream
	Manage and minimize moisture by checking common moisture sites every 2–4h, intervening as appropriate
	Consider need for sacral dressing (see sacral dressing procedure)
	Use appropriate skin-care protective devices
Surface	Use pressure reduction surfaces for:
	Beds (refer to bed algorithm)
	Chairs
	Wheelchairs
	Use lift sheet/turn sheets and other transfer devices
Nutrition	Good nutrition is the first line of defense for prevention of pressure injuries
	Implement registered dietitian's nutrition care plan
	Promote adequate intake of calories, protein, fluid, vitamins, and minerals
	Encourage water and hydration
Family	Involve and educate families about:
	Basic skin care
	Prevention of pressure injuries
	Treatment of pressure injuries
	Provide pressure ulcer prevention family pamphlet

NICU, neonatal intensive care unit.

a wheelchair for a time allotment of 15 minutes, upon being transferred back to bed, a skin assessment should be completed. During the next scheduled seating time, the patient increases his or her sitting interval to 30 minutes with another skin check being completed after being transferred back to bed. Redness over a bony prominence suggests that the patient's skin is not tolerant of pressure for that amount of time, so that the next sitting time would be reduced back to 15 minutes. This process continues until time between turns can be increased without continued redness, or a specialty surface may need to be considered.

Prevention Interventions

The National Pressure Ulcer Advisory Panel (2007a) provided recommendations on the prevention of pressure injuries. The evidence on the prevention of pressure injuries largely pertains to adult populations rather than the pediatric population, probably owing to the small numbers of young people with SCI. The general recommendations for pressure injury prevention have been modified and are widely implemented in children, as follows.

Hygiene

Individualize bathing frequency to keep the skin clean and moisturized. Use a mild cleansing agent. Avoid hot water and excessive rubbing. Use a cream or ointment after bathing rather than a lotion that contains excessive water.

Bowel and bladder continence

Establish reliable and effective bowel and bladder programs. After bowel or bladder accidents, cleanse skin at the time of soiling and use a topical barrier to protect the skin. Select underpads or briefs that are absorbent and provide a quick drying surface to the skin (see also Chapter 11).

Moisturize skin

Use moisturizers for dry skin. Minimize environmental factors leading to dry skin such as low humidity and cold air.

Mechanical loading and support surfaces

During the acute and initial rehabilitation, a written repositioning schedule should be utilized. Patients should be repositioned in bed at least every 2 hours, and the head of the bed should be maintained at or below 30°. When using the side-lying position, positioning directly on the trochanter should be avoided. Pressure redistributing or air mattresses should be utilized as needed. Skin subjected to device-related pressure, such as from continuous positive airway pressure, electroencephalography leads, or pulse oximetry devices, should be padded and inspected regularly. Devices such as boots or pillows that eliminate pressure on the heels should be utilized. Pillows or foam wedges to keep bony prominences such as knees and ankles from direct contact with each other should also be utilized. Lifting devices to move patients during transfers and position changes should be used in order to decrease shearing injuries. Another important consideration is the use of pressure-redistributing devices in the operating room.

Weight shifts in the wheelchair should be performed every 15 to 30 minutes and consist of complete pressure relief on sitting surfaces. Wheelchair push-ups entail pushing up with both arms to lift the ischia completely off the wheelchair cushion. Side-to-side weight shifts are performed by leaning to one side, completely lifting one buttock off the wheelchair cushion for several minutes and then completing this process on the other side. Forward leaning or backward tilts accomplish the same outcome of relieving pressure off the sitting surfaces. Because wheelchair push-ups cause significant repetitive stress to the upper extremities with the potential for long-term musculoskeletal complications, lateral or forward-leaning techniques are preferable. A custom seating system that has options such as a tilt-in-space feature should be considered for patients who are unable to complete adequate pressure-relieving activities. Custom seating surfaces should be utilized, guided by pressure mapping, and equipment and cushions should be evaluated periodically, based on growth and physical changes, to keep equipment well fitted and in adequate working condition. Donut-type devices and sheepskin for pressure redistribution should be avoided. Sheepskin can trap heat and moisture and does not redistribute pressure as well as other products now available.

Pressure-relief surfaces

Choosing the appropriate support surface can be a daunting prospect, and should be implemented under the direction of a certified wound, ostomy, and continence nurse or qualified physical or occupational therapist. Support surfaces for beds and wheelchairs should keep pressures less than 30mmHg (see also Chapter 22). Although pressure-reduction surfaces have been shown to reduce pressure injuries compared with standard mattresses and surfaces, the importance of continued turning and repositioning cannot be overemphasized. Pressure-relief surfaces must be fitted and used properly.

Nutrition

It is vital to address nutrition in every child with an SCI and provide early identification and management of nutritional deficiencies (refer to Chapter 16 for additional information). A nutritional screen should be performed during hospitalizations, during follow-up visits, and if there is development of a pressure injury. If nutritional screening identifies the child as being at risk of developing pressure injuries, being malnourished, or nutritional deficiencies, then a more extensive nutritional assessment should be administered by a registered dietitian or a multidisciplinary nutritional team.

Patient, Family, and Caregiver Education

Education of patients and families is an essential element for successful pressure injury prevention and may be a challenge requiring the efforts of an interprofessional SCI team. Education should be initiated during the acute post-injury hospitalization and initial rehabilitation and be continued during out-patient follow-up visits. The importance of the prevention of pressure injuries cannot be overemphasized and it requires frequent reminders and integration into daily schedules. Barriers may exist related to the level of independence and reliance on family/caregivers for assistance for weight shifts and skin checks. Social barriers such as feeling embarrassed to complete weight shifts in public or in front of peers increase with age and throughout adolescence. Culture, primary language, educational level, and learning abilities must be assessed and integrated into individual teaching plans.

Educational programs for pressure injury prevention must be structured, organized, comprehensive, and directed at all levels of healthcare providers, patients, family, and caregivers. Education should be individualized and developmentally based. Educational programs should include information on etiology and risk factors for pressure ulcers, risk assessment tools and their application, skin assessment, support surfaces, nutritional support, and bowel and bladder programs (National Pressure Ulcer Advisory Panel 2007a).

Developmental Considerations for Prevention and Education

Pressure injury prevention is particularly challenging in children and adolescents with SCI. Dramatic developmental changes occur from infancy to adolescence with a shift from dependency to independence. These rapid changes create many physical, emotional, and psychosocial challenges for this population (Hickey et al 2000).

Infant

The infant is dependent upon caregivers and those around them for all of their needs. Routine skin checks and frequent positioning are required for infants. Bath time, diaper changes, and catheterizations are good times to conduct these activities. The back of the head and skin around medical devices are areas of risk, particularly during the acute phase of treatment. Between toes and under skin rolls should be assessed with special care to thoroughly dry these areas after bathing. Skin safety includes checking the temperature of water before bathing. Smoothing out diaper folds, clothing, and blankets are additional prevention measures. It is important to ensure that surfaces that the infant will have contact with are not hot, such as buckles on infant car seats. Measures should be implemented to protect the skin when the infant is able to roll or crawl because their knees, ankles, and feet are vulnerable to scraping, shearing, and pressure. Pool shoes should be worn to protect feet while in the pool. The best prevention from premature aging of the skin (and some cancers) is ultraviolet protection. The use of protective clothing and hats is recommended and the use of a sunscreen with a sun protection factor of at least 45 is recommended any time the infant is outside and should be reapplied every 2 hours and every 40 minutes if swimming.

Toddler

Toddlers desire more autonomy and need to explore their environment. Skin breakdown through shearing and friction can occur during scooting, crawling, and bumping, and skin should be protected during these activities. Shoes should be worn to protect the feet. Sunscreen should be applied during outdoor activities and supervised play is always recommended for this age group. Attention to sitting times and surface areas that may increase the risk of pressure injury is required. Playground equipment and car seats should be monitored for temperature and safe conditions. Skin checks should occur regularly throughout the day during diaper changes and bathing. Toddlers can begin to have increased responsibility for skin checks, pressure relief, and safe and proper transfers. Approaching the toddler at eye level is the best approach, utilizing age-appropriate teaching materials such as a favorite doll, picture books, or music.

School-aged children

School-aged children are increasing their independence and should assume more responsibility for self care including skin checks, weight shifts, and transfers. Depending on the level of injury and neurologic impairment, the goal may be independence or instructing others in necessary interventions. School-aged children will benefit from established routines incorporating skin-care activities. Utilization of alarms and watches may be helpful tools to assist the school-aged child with their routine. Mirrors may be utilized to assess areas not able to be directly visualized. Simple educational materials including pictures and diagrams can supplement learning for the school-aged child.

Hickey et al (2000) reported an increase in pressure injuries in 8- and 9-year-old children. The hypothesis was that parents/caregivers might develop a false sense of security that these children are completing self care related to the skin. Lapses in responsibility may lead to development of pressure injuries. There may be reluctance on the part of the young person to report the presence of a pressure injury to parents/caregivers. Parents/caregivers should maintain a supervisory role with the school-aged child with gradual transition of responsibility to the young person.

Adolescents

The adolescent years can be challenging for patients, parents, and healthcare providers. This is a time of struggle with body image, sexuality, peer pressure, and the desire to be independent from parents. Educating adolescents about pressure injuries and their prevention is extremely important and the healthcare team will need to be aggressive in this effort. Causes and consequences of pressure injuries should be highlighted, including the effect on their social life if they are restricted to bed rest to heal a pressure injury. Use of graphic pictures to display the extreme consequences of not preventing pressure injuries may be a useful teaching technique.

Privacy is essential to the adolescent, and one-to-one teaching with individualized prevention education should be implemented with every effort to connect and gain the adolescent's trust. As much as the adolescent can do independently should be incorporated into their plan, including instructing others to assist with weight shifts, skin checks, and transfers. Clear and concise educational materials that are age appropriate and not geared toward younger children are necessary. Tools to assist with schedules and routines, such as alarm watches, may be helpful.

Management of a pressure injury

A young person who develops pressure injuries must undergo comprehensive, individualized evaluation and management by an interprofessional team. The evaluation must address antecedent factors, both physical and psychosocial, that contributed to the development of the pressure injury as well as factors that will impact its management and prevention of future pressure injuries. A thorough evaluation should include functional assessment including mobility, activity status, the fit of the wheelchair and equipment, wheelchair cushion, and pressure relief and turning program.

Nutritional Interventions

All individuals with a pressure injury should be referred to a registered dietitian for early assessment and intervention of nutritional problems. Weight history and any significant loss from usual body weight should be assessed, such as a greater than 5% change in 30 days or greater than 10% change in 180 days (Dorner et al 2009). This assessment should include food, fluid, and oral supplements, as well as any enteral or parenteral feedings. If a child with an SCI is found to be undernourished, intervention is necessary to promote healing. While nutrition is multifactorial and should be individualized, interventions should include the provision of four key factors: sufficient calories, adequate protein, adequate daily fluid intake, and adequate vitamins and minerals. Please refer to Table 15.2 for nutrition recommendations.

Oxygenation

Oxygen is a prerequisite for successful wound healing owing to the increased demand for cell proliferation, bacterial defense, angiogenesis, and collagen synthesis. Wound healing has been

TABLE 15.2
Nutritional interventions in the child with a pressure injury

Sufficient calories	Ensure appropriate calories for wound-healing needs. Adjust formula based on weight loss, weight gain or level of obesity. Individuals who are underweight or who have had significant unintentional weight loss may need additional calories to cease weight loss and/or regain lost weight
	Revise and adjust dietary restrictions when restrictions result in decreased food and fluid intake. This should be done by a dietitian or medical professional
	Provide enhanced foods and/or oral supplements between meals if needed
	Consider nutritional support (enteral or parenteral nutrition) when oral intake is inadequate. This must be consistent with individual goals
Adequate protein	Offer 110–125% more protein for an individual with a pressure ulcer when compatible with goals of care, and reassess as condition changes
	Consider requirement of conditionally essential amino acids important for wound healing, such as arginine and glutamine
Adequate daily fluid intake	Monitor individuals for signs and symptoms of dehydration: changes in weight, skin turgor, urine output, elevated serum sodium, or calculated serum osmolality
	Provide additional fluid for individuals with dehydration, elevated temperature, vomiting, profuse sweating, diarrhea, or heavily draining wounds
Adequate vitamins and minerals	Encourage consumption of a balanced diet which includes good sources of vitamins and minerals
	Offer vitamin and mineral supplements when dietary intake is poor or deficiencies are confirmed or suspected. A dietitian or medical professional should assist in these recommendations

Adapted from National Pressure Ulcer Advisory Panel (2009) and Dorner et al (2009). Used with permission of the National Pressure Ulcer Advisory Panel, 22 May 2012.

shown to be impaired under hypoxic conditions. Smoking can contribute to impaired tissue oxygenation and smoking education/cessation should be provided to young people with SCI. Comorbidities that impact wound healing include pulmonary compromise (such as asthma), diabetes, cardiovascular disease, post-thrombotic syndrome, and venous/arterial stasis. These conditions and treatment plans should be evaluated frequently for impact on oxygenation.

Pressure Injury Evaluation

Thorough assessment and documentation of pressure injuries is another critical element of wound care. The examination of a pressure injury is critical to document occurrence and to monitor progress during treatment. The most commonly used system in the USA for standard assessment and description of pressure injuries is that developed by the National Pressure Ulcer Advisory Panel (2007b). These recommendations were updated in 2009 in collaboration with the European Ulcer Advisory Panel (Ayello et al 2009, National Pressure Ulcer Advisory Panel and European Ulcer Advisory Panel 2009). The National Pressure Ulcer Advisory Panel recommendations describe pressure injuries by progression or in stages. This staging was developed to describe the extent of tissue destruction and wound depth at the time the ulcer is assessed. The staging is labeled as stage 1 to stage 4, unstageable, and suspected deep tissue injury (Fig. 15.1). Staging a pressure injury takes a thorough understanding of the different stages and the practical experience of staging them. Institutional resources should be available to support the education, prevention, identification, and treatment of these injuries.

Differentiating pressure injuries from other wounds is important. Pressure injuries should not be confused with a skin tear, a burn, incontinence-associated diaper dermatitis, or other trauma to the skin. Nurses frequently examine the skin and are most likely to be the first professional to identify a skin lesion. However, all members of the SCI interprofessional team should be familiar with the initial identification, evaluation, and management of pressure ulcers.

Non-surgical Management

The key to treatment of pressure injuries is the relief of all pressure on affected tissues. Whenever redness is noted on a skin check, pressure on the site must be avoided until the redness is gone. Bed rest may be the most effective mode to offload pressure. While bed rest can interfere with participation in normal activities such as school and work, the earlier a pressure ulcer is treated, the less resting time will be required. There may be demands made to sit a patient on a red skin area during rehabilitation owing to the desire for active participation in rehabilitation by payors, family, the patient, or members of the treatment team, but there should be no exception to the 'no-sitting' policy. Additional requests may be presented to sit a patient on an ulcer that will be surgically repaired. The rationale may be that, since it is already a surgical ulcer, there is no harm in sitting. Unfortunately, additional damage to the tissue and underlying structures can occur, making surgical repair and healing more complex.

Wound Management

Wound management involves a comprehensive care plan with consideration of all factors contributing to and affecting the wound. Medical management of pressure ulcers is primarily determined by the stage of the wound, clinical presentation, and provider discretion.

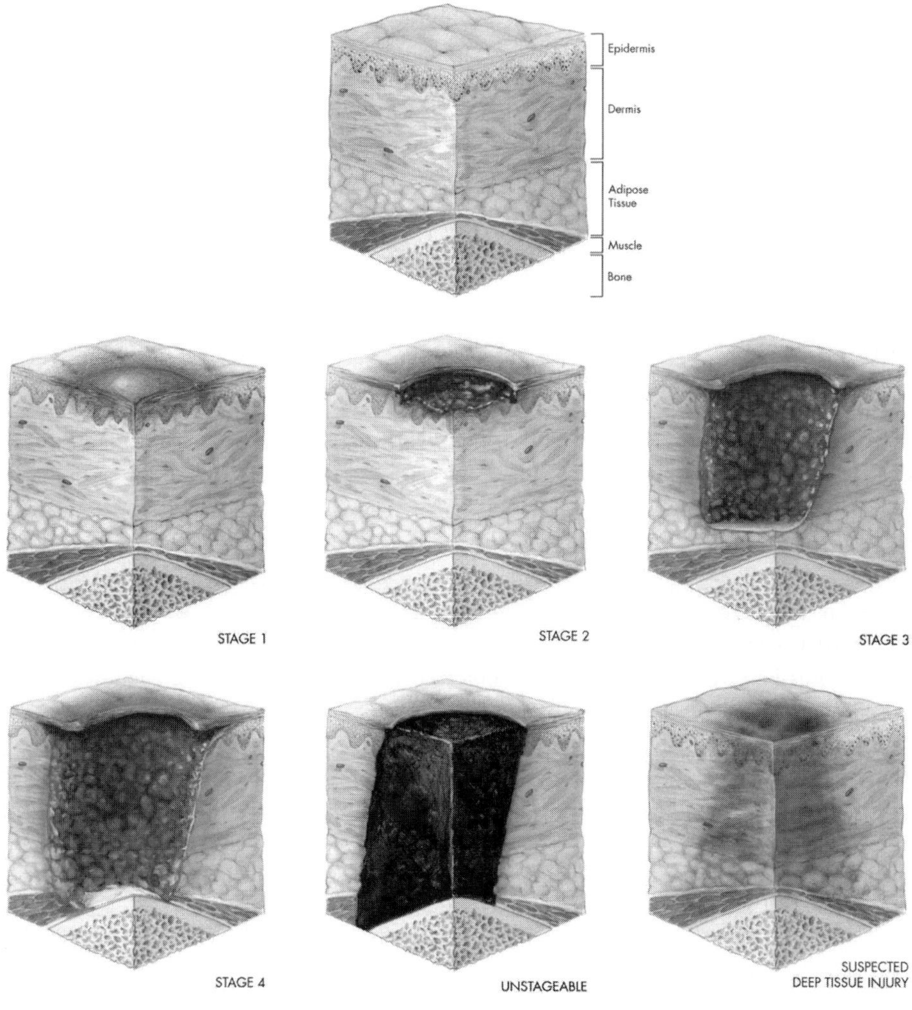

Fig. 15.1 Stage 1. Intact skin with non-blanchable redness of a localized area usually over a bony prominence. Darkly pigmented skin may not have visible blanching; its color may differ from the surrounding area. The area may be painful, firm, soft, warm, or cool compared with adjacent tissue. Stage 1 may be difficult to detect in individuals with dark skin tones. May indicate 'at risk' persons (a heralding sign of risk). **Stage 2.** Partial thickness loss of dermis presented as a shallow open ulcer with a red-pink wound bed, without slough. May also present as an intact or open/ruptured serum filled blister. Presents as a shiny or dry shallow ulcer without slough or bruising (bruising indicates suspected deep tissue injury). This stage should not be used to describe skin tears, tape burns, perineal dermatitis, maceration, or excoriation. **Stage 3.** Full thickness tissue loss. Subcutaneous fat may be visible but bone, tendon, or muscle is not exposed. Slough may be present but does not obscure the depth of tissue loss. May include undermining and tunneling. The depth of a stage 3 pressure injury varies by anatomical location. The bridge of the nose, ear, occiput, and malleolus do not have subcutaneous tissue and stage 3 ulcers can be shallow. In contrast, areas of significant adiposity can develop extremely deep stage 3 pressure ulcers. Bone/tendon is not visible or directly palpable. **Stage 4.** Full thickness tissue loss with exposed bone, tendon, or muscle. Slough or eschar may be present on some parts of the wound bed. Often include undermining and tunneling. The depth of a stage 4 pressure injury varies by anatomical location. The bridge of the nose, ear,

Cleansing

Wound cleansing is an important component of effective wound management. Maximal wound healing cannot occur until the wound is cleansed of all pro-inflammatory material and foreign bodies have been removed from the wound. Wound cleansing is a mechanical process that can be accomplished by gentle scrubbing with moistened gauze or low-pressure irrigation (4–15 pounds per square inch), and appropriate cleansing should be based on the type of wound. Typically, wounds are cleansed with normal saline, sterile water, or a pH-balanced wound cleanser.

Antiseptics such as bleach solutions (e.g. 0.25- to 0.5-strength Dakin's solution), povidone iodine, chlorhexidine, and hydrogen peroxide may be used but can be cytotoxic and should be used cautiously for short periods. Hydrogen peroxide has been used as a mechanical cleanser to flush dirty or necrotic wounds but should not be used for forceful irrigation owing to the potential for air emboli. Hydrogen peroxide is also cytotoxic and can damage new granulation tissue. Hydrogen peroxide and hypochlorites are not appropriate for clean granulating wounds. Although hypochlorites have their place in wound care, apart from wound cell toxicity and the depression of collagen synthesis, hypochlorites can cause burns, hypernatremia, hyperthermia, and localized edema.

Because wounds change as they progress through the healing cascade, a treatment modality used to start treatment is usually not the same as the one being used at the time the wound has healed. Understanding the basic principles of wound care will aid in the choice of a topical therapy (dressings) and address the needs of a wound. These basic principles entail providing an optimal environment for wound healing to take place. A good acronym to help remember these principles is TIME or DIME: T/D – tissue/debridement; I – infection/inflammation; M – moisture balance; E – edge affect/extracellular matrix.

Tissue debridement

It is important to optimize the wound-healing environment by maximizing tissue perfusion and nutritional status. Necrotic tissue must be debrided to eliminate the medium for bacterial growth and move the wound out of the inflammatory phase and into the proliferative phase of repair.

---

occiput, and malleolus do not have subcutaneous tissue and these ulcers can be shallow. Stage 4 ulcers can extend into muscle and/or supporting structures (e.g. fascia, tendon, or joint capsule) making osteomyelitis possible. Exposed bone/tendon is visible or directly palpable. **Unstageable.** Full thickness tissue loss in which the base of the ulcer is covered by slough (yellow, tan, gray, green, or brown) and/or eschar (tan, brown, or black) in the wound bed. Until enough slough and/or eschar is removed to expose the base of the wound, the true depth, and therefore the stage, cannot be determined. Stable (dry, adherent, intact without erythema or fluctuance) eschar on the heel serves as 'the body's natural (biological) cover' and should not be removed. **Suspected deep tissue injury.** Purple or maroon localized area of discolored intact skin or blood-filled blister owing to damage of underlying soft tissue from pressure and/or shear. The area may be preceded by tissue found to be painful, firm, mushy, boggy, warm or cool compared with adjacent tissue. Deep tissue injury may be difficult to detect in individuals with dark skin tones. Evolution may include a thin blister over a dark wound bed. The wound may further evolve and become covered by thin eschar. Evolution may be rapid, exposing additional layers of tissue even with optimal treatment. From National Pressure Ulcer Advisory Panel (2007b). Used with permission of the National Pressure Ulcer Advisory Panel, 22 May 2012. A color version of this figure is available in the color plate section.

Autolytic debridement utilizes white blood cells and enzymes in the patient's wound to digest necrotic tissue. Autolytic debridement requires a moisture-retentive dressing such as a transparent adhesive dressing to trap exudate in a dry wound, or an alginate, hydrocolloid, or foam dressing in an exudative wound.

Chemical or enzymatic debridement utilizes ointments or solutions to separate or break down necrotic tissue and can be useful in wounds that are infected, malodorous, or not appropriate for surgical debridement. Products such as Dakin's solution or collagenase are frequently utilized. It is important to protect the skin around the wound and use the products according to the manufacturer's instructions.

Other forms of debridement include hydrotherapy, which is most helpful in wounds with loose slough and/or large amounts of exudates. Biotherapeutic debridement utilizes maggots to selectively debride the wound.

Mechanical debridement can be accomplished in a number of ways including surgical debridement (see 'Surgical Intervention' section below) and a variety of dressings. Wet-to-dry dressings may provide mechanical separation of eschar, but the dressings can be painful, leave behind debris, lead to hypothermia of the wound, macerate healthy tissue, and, if allowed to dry, may damage newly formed viable tissue. Wet-to-dry debridement may be used with heavily necrotic or infected wounds without visible granulation tissue and should be utilized only if other options are not available.

Infection/inflammation

It is important to protect a healing wound from further trauma and secondary infection in addition to maintaining a normal temperature at the wound surface.

It is important to understand that all chronic wounds (such as pressure ulcers) are colonized with bacteria. Wound infection is defined as 'the presence of replicating microorganisms within the deep compartment of a wound' (Krasner et al 2007). Clinical signs, such as odor, increased pain, increased exudates, and absent or abnormal granulation tissue, indicate wound infection. Without intervention, wounds go through a stepwise process from contamination to colonization to critical colonization and ultimately to wound infection. The practitioner should identify and use topical or systemic agents to treat wound infections because they prolong the inflammatory phase and inhibit wound healing.

Moisture

A balanced (not too wet, not too dry) moist wound environment facilitates the wound-healing process by providing an optimal wound environment and enhancing angiogenesis. This moist wound surface promotes cell migration and prevents cell death from desiccation. Additionally, signaling proteins and cytokines present in wound exudate allow for pain reduction, especially in occluded moist wounds.

Excess exudates must, however, be absorbed. Exudates contain inflammatory mediators that can interfere with wound repair and can cause maceration of intact wound borders. Absorption of excess exudate can be accomplished by wicking moisture from dead space as opposed to 'packing' it. Overpacking can create additional pressure and generate an ischemic effect on the wound bed. The goal is to wick fluid from tunneled or undermined areas and to prevent premature closure of the wound at the surface. A dressing that will maintain a moisture-balanced wound surface without maceration or desiccation should be chosen. The challenge is to maximize healing with the control of exudate while maintaining the right level of wound fluid at the wound surface.

Edge affect/extracellular matrix

Much can be learned about the health of a wound by looking at its edges. A wound that is too wet has macerated edges and a wound that is too dry has hyperkeratotic and/or desiccated edges. Both can produce curled (epibole) edges. A macerated or desiccated epibole or hypergranulated wound will result in impairment of epithelialization of the wound.

Dressing selection presents one of the greatest challenges in wound care and the assistance of a certified wound-care specialist can be invaluable. Dressings do not heal wounds, but appropriately selected dressings can enhance the body's ability to heal the wound. It is beyond the scope of this chapter to review dressing selection for pressure ulcers (see Sussman and Bates-Jensen 2011).

Adjunctive Therapies

There are a myriad of adjunctive therapies for managing a pressure injury, but it is beyond the scope of this chapter to review them all. Some adjunctive therapies that may be beneficial include electromagnetic energy and ultraviolet-C light (Houghton et al 2013). Other adjunctive therapies that have insufficient evidence to allow them to be recommended include negative pressure wound therapy and ultrasound (Houghton et al 2013).

Surgical Intervention

When it is determined that the best solution to repair a pressure injury is surgical intervention, the patient and caregivers, the interprofessional SCI team, and the surgical team should arrive at a mutual understanding regarding the chosen treatment. Successful surgical outcomes are optimized by the interprofessional SCI team approach, including the expertise of a wound-care specialist. Management to address muscle spasticity and fixed contractures must occur preoperatively and continue at least until the wound is completely healed (Whitney et al 2006). The success of surgery is dependent on the preoperative condition of the patient, skill of the surgeon, diligence of the patient's postoperative care team, and commitment of the patient and caregivers to prevent recurrence of the wound. Surgical treatment of pressure wounds is a final invasive choice for wounds refractory to less aggressive care or for use when rapid closure is indicated (Whitney et al 2006). Once the child's medical conditions have been optimized and an acceptable postoperative plan has been made, corrective surgery can be scheduled.

Surgical debridement of devitalized tissue can be a vital first step to begin healing deep pressure wounds. Wounds, which contain necrotic tissue, support bacterial overgrowth, and require debridement to expose viable tissue. Sharp surgical debridement allows thorough wound exploration; allows evaluation for tunneling, fistulas, or abscess; and provides the surgeon with the opportunity to conceptualize surgical repair. A solution containing methylene blue dye can be instilled into the wound to define wound borders and to ensure that all areas of the wound have been excised. Tissue at the base of the wound should be sent for pathologic examination and microbiological analysis to determine the timing and extent of surgical repair. The presence of osteomyelitis may necessitate treatment with antibiotics before surgical repair.

Surgical repair of pressure wounds is aimed at filling a defect and providing durable coverage in an area that will probably need to continue to support pressure. Wound closure decreases protein and fluid loss, the possibility of wound infection, and the potential for later development of malignancy in the wound (Whitney et al 2006). The approach to closure depends on the size, location, wound depth, previous surgical repairs, and potential future surgical repairs. Surgical principles and guidelines indicate the use of the most durable, tension-free wound closure with the consideration that future repair in the same area may be needed. The most reliable repair fills the ulcer with bulk and provides padding over the underlying structures. Primary closure, skin grafts, and fasciocutaneous flaps may provide adequate coverage for small wounds and areas in which pressure can be effectively offloaded.

Surgical closure of pressure wounds must be based on both the patient and the location of the wound. Ischial pressure injuries are a result of seated positioning, and tend to recur most frequently. A posterior thigh flap such as a V-Y hamstring advancement flap is a good choice because it can be re-advanced in the case of recurrent ulceration. Medially based thigh flaps, gluteus maximus muscle flaps, island gluteus muscle flaps, gracilis rotation flap, and tensor fascia lata flaps can also be considered.

Sacral pressure injuries are most commonly caused by prolonged supine position, but also frequently occur as a result of seating and posture-related issues. The most commonly utilized musculocutaneous flaps are based on the gluteus maximus muscle, and can be rotated, advanced, or turned over. Lumbosacral muscle flaps based on lumbar perforating vessels can also be considered but, owing to the lack of bulk, are not as beneficial in deep defects.

Trochanteric pressure wounds frequently affect patients who have significant hip contractures or lie in a lateral decubitus position. The tensor fascia lata flap is usually a rotational flap based on its perforating vessels.

If local flaps are not available owing to previous use of adjacent tissue or extensive defects, distant free-vascular flaps may be an option. Free flaps are significantly more complex, as they require isolation of individual vessels and microsurgical anastomosis to keep the transplanted tissue viable. The patient must be able to undergo a prolonged surgical procedure and consideration must be given to the repair of the defect, which is created at the donor site.

Care after surgical repair of pressure injuries requires diligent and persistent monitoring to ensure adequate blood flow to the flap and to prevent contamination of the surgical repair with urine and stool. Patients initially require complete offloading of the surgical site, which can be accomplished with diligent positioning maneuvers and the use of an air-fluidized mattress. Pressure is incrementally increased after 14 days, and after 6 weeks patients may begin to return to weight bearing on the surgical site with close monitoring.

Young people with SCI with pressure injuries are at high risk of recurrence owing to the complexity involved in eliminating causative factors (Kierney et al 1998). Prevention of recurrent pressure ulcers after surgical repair is a lifelong process. Wheelchairs and other relevant equipment may need to be adjusted owing to anatomic variances created by the surgical intervention.

Summary

Prevention of pressure injuries is one of the most important aspects of managing a young person with an SCI and should be accomplished by a comprehensive interprofessional approach involving the patient and family as early as possible after sustaining an SCI. Prevention of pressure injuries is a lifelong process that must be tailored to each developmental stage of the young person as he or she progresses from infancy, through childhood and adolescence, to adulthood. It is critically important to provide comprehensive management of pressure injuries including nutritional and psychological support, assessment-based wound care, and ongoing evaluation of the response to therapy.

REFERENCES

Ayello EA, Capitulo KL, Fife CE et al (2009) Legal issues in the care of pressure ulcer patients: key concepts for health care providers: a consensus paper from the international expert wound care advisory panel. *J Palliat Med* 12: 995–1008. doi: 10.1089/jpm.2009.9939

Baharestani MM, Ratliff CR (2007) Pressure ulcers in neonates and children: an NPUAP white paper. *Adv Skin Wound Care* 20: 208–20. http://dx.doi.org/10.1097/01.ASW.0000266646.43159.99

Consortium for Spinal Cord Medicine (2000) *Pressure Ulcer Prevention and Treatment Following Spinal Cord Injury: A Clinical Practice Guideline for Healthcare Professionals*. Washington, DC: Paralyzed Veterans of America.

Consortium for Spinal Cord Medicine (2014) *Pressure Ulcer Prevention and Treatment Following Spinal Cord Injury: A Clinical Practice Guideline for Healthcare Professionals*. 2nd Ed. Washington, DC: Paralyzed Veterans of America (in preparation).

Dorner B, Posthauer ME, Thomas D (2009) The role of nutrition in pressure ulcer prevention and treatment: National Pressure Ulcer Advisory Panel white paper. Available at: http://www.npuap.org/Nutrition%20White%20Paper%20Website%20Version.pdf (accessed 26 May 2012).

Hickey KJ, Anderson CJ, Vogel LC (2000) Pressure ulcers in pediatric spinal cord injury. *Top Spinal Cord Inj Rehabil* 6(Suppl): 85–90. doi: 10.1310/1C86-7L96-1JAR-7Y3N

Houghton PE, Campbell KE, CPG Panel (2013) *Canadian Best Practice Guidelines for the Prevention and Management of Pressure Ulcers in People with Spinal Cord Injury. A Resource Handbook for Clinicians* [online]. Available at: http://www.onf.org.

Kierney PC, Engrav LH, Isik FF, Esselman P, Cardenas DD, Rand RP (1998) Results of 268 pressure sores in 158 patients managed jointly by plastic surgery and rehabilitation medicine. *Plast Reconstr Surg* 102: 765–72. http://dx.doi.org/10.1097/00006534-199809010-00022

Krasner DL, Rodeheaver GT, Sibbald RG (eds) (2007) *Chronic Wound Care: A Clinical Source Book for Healthcare Professionals*. 4th Ed. Malvern, PA: HMP Communications. doi: 10.1111/j.1742-481x.2007.00311.x

McLane KM, Bookout K, McCord S, McCain J, Jefferson LS (2004) The 2003 national pediatric pressure ulcer and skin breakdown prevalence. *J Wound Ostomy Continence Nurs* 31: 168–78. http://dx.doi.org/10.1097/00152192-200407000-00004

National Pressure Ulcer Advisory Panel (2007a) *Pressure Ulcer Prevention Points* [online]. Available at: www.npuap.org (accessed 26 May 2012).

National Pressure Ulcer Advisory Panel (2007b) *Updated Pressure Ulcer Stages* [online]. Available at: http://www.npuap.org (accessed 3 January 2011).

National Pressure Ulcer Advisory Panel, European Ulcer Advisory Panel (2009) *Prevention and Treatment of Pressure Ulcers: Clinical Practice Guideline* [online]. Available at: http://www.npuap.org (accessed 6 May 2012).

Schluer AB, Cignacco E, Muller M, Halfens RJ (2009) The prevalence of pressure ulcers in four paediatric institutions. *J Clin Nurs* 18: 3244–52. doi: 10.1111/j.1365-2702.2009.02951.x

Smith MEB, Totten A, Hickam DH et al (2013) Pressure ulcer treatment strategies. A systematic comparative effectiveness review. *Ann Intern Med* 159: 39–50. doi:10.7326/0003-4819-159-1-201307020-00007

Sussman C, Bates-Jensen B (eds) (2011) *Wound Care: A Collaborative Practice Manual for Health Professionals*. 4th Ed. Philadelphia, PA: Lippincott Williams & Wilkins. doi: 1608317153.9781608317158

Whitney J, Phillips L, Astani R et al (2006) Guidelines for the treatment of pressure ulcers. *Wound Repair Regen* 14: 663–79. doi: 10.1111/j.1524-475X.2006.00175.x

Wu SS, Ahn C, Emmons KR, Salcido RS (2009) Pressure ulcers in pediatric patients with spinal cord injury: a review of assessment, prevention, and topical management. *Adv Skin Wound Care* 22: 273–82. doi: 10.1097/01.ASW.0000305474.37745.55

16
METABOLIC COMPLICATIONS IN PEDIATRIC SPINAL CORD INJURY: COMBINING OPTIMAL EXERCISE AND NUTRITION TO PROMOTE HEALTH AND FITNESS

Craig M McDonald and Therese E Johnston

Case vignette

Erin is a 9-year-old female who sustained a T9 American Spinal Injury Association Impairment Scale A spinal cord injury when she was 8 years old. Before her injury she was a lean child and was active in soccer and beginning to play softball. Her parents are concerned that she may gain too much weight, since she is no longer active. They requested a nutritional consultation for an appropriate diet and an evaluation by a recreation therapist for an exercise program.

Introduction

In children and adults with spinal cord injury (SCI) and spina bifida, there is a high prevalence of obesity, deficits in lean tissue, impaired insulin resistance, hypertension, and hyperlipidemia; this group also exhibits impaired levels of fitness and they are at risk of a variety of adverse health conditions associated with a sedentary lifestyle. According to the Healthy Children 2010 report, children with disabilities are less likely to participate in sustained exercise than children with typical development (United States Department of Health and Human Services 2012). Obesity in those with spinal cord dysfunction is caused by lean tissue deficits with hypometabolic state along with reduced physical activity-associated energy expenditure and suboptimal energy balance. The increased fat tissue contributes to the development of metabolic syndrome, which ultimately places children at a long-term risk of cardiovascular disease, diabetes, and stroke. Since children with SCI have longer lifespans remaining after their injury than adults with SCI, they will be at risk of the negative health consequences of obesity and inactivity for a longer duration than adults.

The purpose of this chapter is to identify some of the potential issues related to metabolic complications, changes in body composition, and impaired fitness in pediatric SCI, and to report what is known about the effects of fitness-related interventions for children with SCI. In addition, literature on children with spina bifida will be included to provide insight into the effects of conditions impacting the spinal cord in children (collectively referred to as 'spinal cord dysfunction').

Obesity in children with spinal cord dysfunction

Children with SCI have limited mobility and physical activity, reduced total lean body mass, and reduced resting energy expenditure (REE), leading to an increased risk of obesity (Liusuwan et al 2004). These children with spinal cord dysfunction typically have reduced lean body mass in the lower extremities and increased abdominal and lower extremity fat tissue accumulation (Roberts et al 1991, Liusuwan et al 2004). Increased adiposity has been documented for many mobility-impaired children, and there is a high prevalence of obesity in children with spina bifida (Roberts et al 1991, McPherson et al 2013) and SCI (Liusuwan et al 2007). Deficits in lean muscle tissue have been documented in children with spina bifida (Shepherd et al 1991) and SCI (Liusuwan et al 2004, 2007). In spina bifida, the relative deficit in lean tissue increases with age beyond 4 years, owing to segmental retardation of growth of lower limbs and muscle hypoplasia (Shepherd et al 1991). This lean tissue deficit in children with spinal cord dysfunction contributes to reduced REE, placing these children at an increased risk of impaired energy balance with excessive caloric intake relative to caloric expenditure (Roberts et al 1991, Shepherd et al 1991).

Investigators have shown that body mass index (BMI) underestimates the percentage fat mass in children in a similar manner to adults with SCI (McDonald et al 2007). Thus, BMI is not an accurate surrogate for increasing adiposity in children with SCI. Yamaki et al (2011) found a tendency toward a higher prevalence of chronic health conditions in overweight adolescents with disability than in their healthy weight counterparts with disability.

Physical inactivity and reduced aerobic capacity in disabled children: potential impact on health and fitness

Widman et al (2007) have shown that a group of children with SCI and spina bifida had significantly reduced aerobic capacity ($\dot{V}O_2$/kg) compared with a comparison group of non-obese healthy children, but were not different from the non-disabled overweight participants. During the maximal exercise test, the children with spina bifida and SCI reached exhaustion at significantly lower workloads than both the comparison group of non-obese healthy children and the non-disabled overweight participants. Although comparison values for specific activities are not available for children with SCI, peak oxygen consumption data are available in the literature. Using a peak arm cranking test, in which power output was increased every minute, Johnston et al (2008) reported average peak oxygen uptake values of 14.0ml/kg/minute (SD 7.9) for children with motor complete SCI aged 5 to 13 years, and Widman et al (2007) reported average peak oxygen uptake values of 15.1ml/kg/minute (SD 6.5) for females and 19.0ml/kg/minute (SD 5.8) for males with complete and incomplete SCI aged 11 to 20 years. Johnston et al (2008) further defined these values based on the level of injury and found that children with tetraplegia had a peak oxygen uptake of 9.5ml/kg/minute (SD

3.9), those with high paraplegia had a peak of 13.4ml/kg/minute (SD 7.5), and those with low paraplegia had a peak of 18.2ml/kg/minute (SD 8.8). Widman et al (2007) further found that, during the maximal exercise test, the children with spina bifida and SCI reached exhaustion at significantly lower workloads than both the comparison group of non-obese healthy children and the non-disabled overweight participants. Overall, these studies indicate that children with SCI have decreased peak oxygen consumption, suggesting that children with SCI may have less respiratory capacity and may fatigue more quickly with submaximal tasks than children with typical development. Specifically, children with spina bifida and SCI had reduced aerobic capacity, which is associated with being overweight and having reduced upper extremity strength (Widman et al 2007).

A primary goal of many medical treatments and rehabilitation programs for disabled children is to restore patients' ability to be physically active and, hence, aerobic exercise and strengthening are important goals. Improvement in cardiopulmonary endurance, body composition, muscle strength and endurance, and flexibility are associated with reductions of risk factors associated with various disease stages. In adults, physical activity is well documented as being associated with the prevention and control of coronary artery disease, hypertension, non-insulin-dependent diabetes mellitus, osteoporosis, obesity, and mental health problems. Patterns of physical activity in childhood continue into adulthood and appear, in part, to determine adult levels of physical activity. The Allied Dunbar National Survey of Fitness and Physical Activity (2000), in which 600 people were surveyed, demonstrated that childhood activity is associated with the general level of physical activity in adulthood. Thus, improved physical activity in children with spinal cord dysfunction may have lasting health benefits.

Metabolic syndrome: importance of childhood prevention

Increased morbidity and mortality have been well documented in adults with four clustered risk factors: obesity, increased insulin resistance, dyslipidemia, and hypertension. Medical researchers refer to the clustering of these four risk factors as metabolic syndrome, insulin resistance syndrome, or syndrome X. More specifically, the central features of metabolic syndrome are abdominal adiposity, hypertension, increased fasting glucose concentrations/abnormal glucose tolerance, and dyslipidemia characterized by increased serum triglycerides, low serum high-density lipoprotein (HDL), and/or small dense low-density lipoprotein particles. These are known risk factors in children for the development of obesity, type 2 diabetes, and cardiovascular disease (Paulsen 1968, Srinivasan et al 2002, Steinberger and Daniels 2003). Most importantly, the metabolic syndrome has been shown to predict future cardiovascular and coronary heart disease mortality (Juonala et al 2005). Obesity has been implicated as the primary inciting factor of metabolic syndrome. It is likely that the serum triglyceride levels are found to be elevated owing to the accelerated lipogenesis, decreased lipoprotein lipase activity, and impaired clearance of triglycerides (Robertson and Grossman 1987).

Early identification and treatment of obesity and associated health risk factors during childhood is of critical importance. Evidence suggests that obesity established in childhood may be more harmful than obesity that has appeared in adulthood. In addition, weight reduction during adolescence may protect against the occurrence of metabolic syndrome in adulthood (Vanhala et al 1998). The metabolic syndrome variables are frequently manifested during childhood among obese able-bodied children. The Bogalusa Heart Study (Srinivasan et al 2002) found that childhood adiposity was associated with an increased incidence of the following variables of metabolic syndrome in adulthood: increased BMI, increased fasting insulin, increased systolic or mean arterial blood pressure, increased total cholesterol to HDL cholesterol ratio, and increased triglyceride to HDL cholesterol ratio. Csabi et al (2000) found 76.6% of obese children have two or more of these factors elevated, whereas 79.1% of the children in the comparison group had none elevated. Vanhala et al (1998) tracked 439 individuals from childhood to adulthood, and, of the 30 adults who were identified with metabolic syndrome, 28 were obese as adults and 21 had been obese as children.

Metabolic syndrome in adults and children with spinal cord dysfunction and spinal cord injury

Bauman and Spungen (1994) first reported an increased prevalence of metabolic syndrome in adults with SCI and showed that metabolic syndrome was directly associated with increased adiposity and the loss of lean tissue (muscle mass) secondary to paralysis, which is associated with increased insulin resistance. It is now well established that a state of insulin resistance, hyperinsulinemia, hyperlipidemia, and hypertension occurs in patients with chronic SCI. However, the relationship between obesity and increased risk factors for adverse health outcomes among children with spinal cord dysfunction has only been recently examined.

It has recently been shown by Nelson et al (2007) that children with SCI and spina bifida are at a particularly high risk of the development of early metabolic syndrome. In this study with 20 children (11–20y) with SCI, 11 were found to have metabolic syndrome, and all that were classified as obese had metabolic syndrome. The definition of metabolic syndrome in this study was the presence of at least three of the following: obesity (BMI z score>2), decreased HDL levels (<45mg/dl for males, <50mg/dl for females), elevated triglycerides (≥100mg/dl), high blood pressure (≥95th centile), and insulin resistance (based on the homeostatic model assessment [HOMA] measuring fasting insulin and glucose). Compared with obese able-bodied children, who are already at risk, children with SCI had increased trunk fat, increased total body fat, and decreased HDL levels. In another recent series by Mazur et al (2011), 51 out of 123 children with spina bifida (41.5%) were hypertensive. The presence of these conditions, in addition to the increased risk of metabolic syndrome, places these children with spinal cord dysfunction at an increased risk of cardiovascular disease, diabetes, and even stroke, which represents a serious concern for their long-term health as adults.

Casteels et al (2010) recently confirmed the prevalence of insulin resistance in individuals with both spina bifida and myogenic atrophy owing to muscular dystrophy. Study participants (n=42) had a mean age of 15 years 6 months, a short stature (height −2.4 SD), a relatively high BMI (+1.7 SD), and a high body fat fraction (41.9% or +2.8 SD). Abdominal computed tomography confirmed the high fat mass and disclosed a high fraction of visceral fat. As expected, insulin resistance was increased in these participants and benefits were observed with metformin treatment.

Resting energy expenditure in pediatric spinal cord injury: implications for development of obesity

For children with SCI, data from a study by Johnston et al (2009) showed an average REE of 3.0ml/kg/minute (SD 1.5) for children aged 5 to 13 years with motor complete SCI, a value below the normal range for children with typical development reported by Harrell et al (2005). For children aged 11 to 20 years with complete or incomplete SCI, REE has been reported to be 3.8ml/kg/minute (SD 0.8) for females and 4.1ml/kg/minute (SD 1.2) for males (Widman et al 2007), which is at the lower end (males) or below the range (females) of the values reported for children with typical development (Harrell et al 2005). Therefore, the data suggest that, similar to adults with SCI, children with SCI show a decreased REE. This finding is consistent with Liusuwan et al (2007a), who reported that a relationship exists between total lean body mass and REE in children with SCI (r=0.67), and that lean body tissue is also decreased in children with SCI.

Mechanisms of metabolic syndrome and impaired insulin resistance in spinal cord injury

The relationship between subcutaneous and visceral abdominal fat, thigh intramuscular adipose tissue, and insulin sensitivity was first described in healthy individuals in 1997 (Goodpaster et al 2000). In 1999, Bauman and colleagues reported that 27 out of 201 adults with SCI (13.4%) had diabetes mellitus and 56 (28.8%) had impaired glucose tolerance (Bauman et al 2009). The disorder of carbohydrate metabolism was directly associated with motor level and degree of paralysis (complete tetraplegia [73%], incomplete tetraplegia [44%], complete paraplegia [24%], incomplete paraplegia [31%]), and the impaired insulin resistance postulated to be due to both substantial muscle atrophy and increased intramuscular fat in SCI. Subsequently, Elder et al (2004) found that intramuscular fat measured by magnetic resonance imaging in adults with SCI is a good predictor of plasma glucose during an oral glucose tolerance test.

The increased prevalence of metabolic syndrome in SCI is thought to be due to inactivity, body composition changes of decreased skeletal muscle mass and increased adiposity seen in acquired paralysis. In addition to intramuscular fat, lipid around skeletal muscle accounted for about 70% of the variance in plasma glucose 120 minutes after ingesting 75g of glucose in individuals with SCI versus a control group (Elder et al 2004). It has been postulated that lipid accumulation and fatty acids arising from lipid metabolism may interfere with carbohydrate metabolism in skeletal muscle and subsequently create suboptimal gradients for carbohydrate entry into skeletal muscle, although a clear mechanism has not been established (Elder et al 2004).

Additional mechanisms involving glucose transport in the muscle after SCI are being increasingly understood. It is clear that skeletal muscle is the primary site of glucose disposal in the body. Glucose transport from the blood across the muscle cell membrane is the rate limiting step in glucose utilization and is dependent on facilitated diffusion involving two glucose transporter proteins in skeletal muscle: GLUT-4, involved in insulin- and exercise-stimulated glucose uptake; and GLUT-1, involved in glucose uptake in the basal, non-insulin-stimulated state. Alterations in these transport proteins therefore impact glucose tolerance and the risk of metabolic syndrome (Klip and Paquet 1990).

Bone health in pediatric spinal cord dysfunction

A lack of exercise and skeletal muscle paralysis produce reductions in bone mineral density (BMD) in SCI. For children, the effects of an SCI on the development of BMD and bone microarchitecture are just beginning to be understood. Lauer et al (2007) reported that children aged 5 to 13 years with SCI have decreased BMD at the hip compared with children with typical development. In comparing the BMD values of children with the adult fracture threshold of less than 0.78g/cm^2, children in Lauer's reported group had values below this threshold and thus may have an increased fracture risk.

Exercise and nutrition management to improve fitness in pediatric spinal cord dysfunction

Anthropometric Assessment

In able-bodied individuals, being overweight is defined as a having a BMI of 25 to 29.9kg/m^2 and obesity is defined as having a BMI greater than or equal to 30.0kg/m^2. As previously noted, several investigators have shown that BMI underestimates percentage fat mass in children with SCI (McDonald et al 2007). The ideal body weight (IBW) is determined by height. In non-ambulant individuals or those with contractures, ulnar length measurement can be used to estimate standing height using the formula described by Gauld et al (2004). Ulnar length is measured in millimeters from the distal tip of the styloid process to the tip of the olecranon using the Rosscraft segmometer (Rosscraft Innovations, Inc., Vancouver, BC, Canada). The IBW should be adjusted for body type (frame sizes: small, IBW 10% reduction; middle size, no changes required; large, IBW increased by 10%) and SCI (paraplegia, decrease IBW by 10–15%; tetraplegia, decrease IBW by 15–20%). The weight on acute admission is usually the most reliable measure of actual body weight (ABW).

To determine the weight which should be used on the nutritional calculations, first percentage IBW should be calculated using the following equation: percentage IBW=ABW/IBW × 100. If the ABW is less than the IBW, ABW is used to define the nutritional requirements. If ABW is greater than IBW, but less than 120%, it is necessary to determine nutritional needs using the adjusted relationship of body weight in the calculation needs: IBW + (ABW – IBW × 0.25). The nutritional status of patients can be categorized according to their ABW as a percentage of IBW as follows: over 200% of IBW (pathologic obesity), over 150% of IBW (obese), more than 120% IBW (overweight), 100% of IBW±10% (normal), 80% to 90% of IBW (mildly malnourished), 70% to 80% of IBW (moderately malnourished), less than 70% of IBW (severe nutritional deficiency – malnutrition) (Dawodu et al 2011). In general, anthropometric measures in persons with SCI tend to underestimate fat percentage when compared with able-bodied individuals.

Assessment of Energy Balance

Energy balance is equal to the difference between daily caloric intake and daily caloric expenditure. Mathematically, a positive energy balance as low as 50kcal/day may lead to an increase in body weight by 5lbs in one year (1lb=3500kcal). Therefore, monitoring daily caloric intake is an important factor in decreasing the risk of dyslipidemia, insulin resistance, postprandial hyperlipidemia, and inflammation. To accurately monitor caloric intake, many measure REE or basal metabolic rate after 10 to 12 hours of fasting. Lee et al (1985) determined that individuals with SCI with paraplegia who were hypometabolic (35% of total) were heavier in weight and their caloric intake was 25% greater than their basal metabolic rate.

Specific Nutrition Needs for Children with Spinal Cord Injury

Carbohydrates

Carbohydrates are organic compounds which provide the human body with high levels of energy for physical activity and organ function. The term carbohydrates refers to any food that is particularly rich in the complex carbohydrate starch (such as cereals, bread, and pasta) or simple carbohydrates, such as sugar (found in candy, jams, and desserts). A pediatric dietitian should be consulted to estimate the minimum intake of carbohydrate per day in children with SCI for essential functions and prevention of the consumption of endogenous protein. Reduction in physical activity will result in storage of glucose as fat and expansion of the storage of adipose tissue in non-adipose tissue sites. Adopting a standard diet protocol in which the carbohydrate constituent represents 45% may be beneficial to individuals with SCI and does not disrupt their body composition or metabolic profiles (Gorgey and Gater 2011).

Fiber is an important component in complex carbohydrates (such as whole grains, vegetables, and fruits) that aid in a healthy diet, reduce the chances of constipation, may help lower blood cholesterol and reduce the risk of coronary vascular diseases by binding to the cholesterol and removing it from the body as waste, and may reduce the risk of developing type II diabetes, all of which are common in patients with SCI. It is highly recommended that a child with SCI consumes sufficient grams of fiber daily. Dietary fiber intake should be adjusted as necessary to achieve the desired bowel function. Inadequate or excessive fiber may result in constipation, impaction, excessive flatulence, and abdominal distension (see Chapter 11).

Nitrogen balance and protein intake

Nitrogen balance is the relationship between the amount of nitrogen taken into the body, usually as food, and that excreted from the body in urine and feces. A negative nitrogen balance, which occurs when more nitrogen is excreted than is taken in, indicates wasting or destruction of tissue. The process of nitrogen balance is crucial for the mechanism of protein synthesis because most of the body's nitrogen is incorporated into protein. A positive nitrogen balance, which occurs when the intake of nitrogen is greater than its excretion, implies tissue formation and growth. There is an increase in urinary nitrogen output and protein catabolism after acute SCI (Khalil et al 2013). The process of negative nitrogen balance leads to significant skeletal muscle atrophy as described above in individuals with both complete and incomplete SCI. The accelerated catabolism of muscle mass results in a supply of amino acids for the acute phase of protein synthesis, gluconeogenesis, and the healing of wounds. In acute injury, despite the provision of sufficient quantities of calories and protein, a negative nitrogen balance usually occurs, which peaks during the third week after injury. Acute immobilization of paralyzed patients contributes to increased excretion of nitrogen, which starts about a week after paralysis and immobilization.

For individuals with SCI, a protein intake of 0.8 to 1.0g/kg of body weight is sufficient to maintain protein stores; however, this intake cannot offset the rapid decline in lean mass after injury (Khalil et al 2013). There is evidence to suggest that this protein intake should exceed 1.2g/kg in people with pressure ulcers and may reach up to 2g/kg with grade III and IV pressure ulcers. Considering these facts, dietitians in clinical settings commonly encourage the ingestion of high-protein supplements. These fluids are rich in leucine, which is one of the essential amino acids.

Specific proteins (albumin, transferrin, and pre-albumin) are biochemical indicators used for assessing nutritional status. The level of serum albumin is not a definitive measure of visceral protein status. Given the long half-life of 21 days, serum albumin cannot be effectively used for monitoring the acute response to nutritional therapy. Serum albumin levels can be included in the initial nutrition assessment and for monitoring trends of visceral protein or as an indicator of chronic nutritional status in the out-patient clinic. A more optimal protein biochemical indicator is pre-albumin, which has a very short half-life (2d), making it an excellent nutritional index and, for this reason, it is used as an indicator of response to nutritional therapy. The failure to increase pre-albumin above 11mg/dl with dietary therapy in patients is an indication that nutritional needs are not met (Dionyssiotis 2012). Concentrations should increase by about 1mg/dl per day or twice a week when dietary treatment is appropriate. A pre-albumin level above 30mg/dl is commonly recommended as a cut-off line for healthy nutritional and protein status.

Fats

Fats are organic compounds which belong to a group of substances called lipids and exist in liquid or solid form. All fats are combinations of saturated and unsaturated fatty acids. Fats are responsible for transporting certain vitamins, maintaining skin and hair, insulating the organs from shock, promoting healthy cell function, and maintaining body temperature. High-fat diets are not recommended in spinal cord dysfunction because excess fat is stored in adipose tissue which results in obesity and increases the likelihood of cardiovascular diseases and diabetes (Khalil et al 2013).

Reliance on a diet of saturated and polysaturated fat has atherogenic effects by increasing dyslipidemia, whereas intake of monounsaturated fatty acids have the opposite effect in individuals with disabilities. It has been recommended that persons with SCI should not consume more than 30% total fat and 10% saturated fat in their daily caloric intake (Tomey et al 2005).

Vitamins and minerals

Deficiencies of zinc, vitamin C, and vitamin D have been associated with patients with SCI (Dionyssiotis 2012). Deficiencies in zinc and vitamin C have been associated with poor wound healing. Zinc is often prescribed to improve pressure ulcers, and is known to be involved in the structural integrity of collagen. The role of vitamin C in collagen synthesis is also crucial. In addition, for neurogenic bladder, vitamin C and other supplements are helpful for the acidification of urine and the prevention of infections of the urinary tract.

Children with SCI may be deficient in vitamin D (25 hydroxyvitamin D [25(OH)D]). In patients with SCI, there is a negative correlation between serum levels of 25(OH)D and parathyroid hormone. Bone loss increases when there is secondary hyperparathyroidism, which worsens osteoporosis in these patients. In a series of 82 young people with SCI reported by Zebracki et al (2013), 79% had vitamin D deficiency or insufficiency. There were no differences in vitamin D status as a function of sex or level of injury. Adolescents, however, were more likely to exhibit deficiency than younger children. In view of the high prevalence of vitamin D insufficiency in young people with SCI and the risk of complications such as pathologic fractures, serum 25(OH)D levels should be routinely monitored.

Exercise interventions to promote improved body composition, reduce metabolic syndrome, and improve fitness

Of the programs designed for children or adolescents, only a few have addressed the special health, nutrition, and fitness needs of children and adolescents with mobility impairment (Ekblom and Lundberg 1968, Andrade et al 1991, Block et al 2005). In response to this need, McDonald and colleagues developed a pilot intervention referred to as the BENEfit program (Behavioral approach to Exercise and Nutrition Education to improve fitness) designed specifically to improve the health and fitness of children with mobility impairment by using nutrition and exercise education, aerobic and strengthening exercises, and behavior modification (Liusuwan et al 2007b). The program consisted of nine biweekly sessions covering 16 weeks with alternating topics of exercise education and nutrition concepts. Participants were given a schedule of aerobic and strengthening exercises and attended nutrition education and behavior modification sessions every other week along with their parent(s). McDonald and colleagues sought to determine if the health promotion activities conducted through the BENEfit program would reduce weight, improve body composition characteristics (increase lean muscle tissue and/or reduce fat tissue), increase strength, increase fitness, and improve nutritional understanding and food choice habits.

Shriners BENEfit Program for Children with Mobility Impairment

As described by Liusuwan et al (2007b) the structure of the BENEfit session was modeled after the Shapedown program (Mellin et al 1987) and included an interactive lecture on a specific nutrition or exercise concept followed by an activity designed to reinforce the concept in a visual or tactile mode. Games, rewards, and motivational tools were used to promote active participation in the nutrition and exercise curriculum. All participants were required to keep daily food records and complete nutrition and exercise assignments each week. In addition to the group sessions, participants completed a home-based exercise program of aerobic and resistance-training components designed to improve their strength and cardiovascular health. The home-based aerobic training program involved use of an arm ergometer (Widman et al

2006) connected to a video game (GameCycle™, Three Rivers, Mesa, AZ). The resistance level that elicited the heart rate and $\dot{V}O_2$ just below the participant's anaerobic threshold was designated as the starting resistance level.

The home-based resistance-training program consisted of upper extremity strengthening exercises using hand weights (dumbbells). The exercises were selected according to primary muscles involved in wheelchair propulsion and functional activities in patients using wheelchairs (Davis and Shephard 1990, Mulroy et al 1996). Participants were instructed to perform aerobic and resistance programs 3 days a week with alternating days. Resistance training was done at three sets of 10 repetitions with 1-minute rests between sets. Aerobic sessions started with 10 minutes per session for the first 2 weeks, increasing by 5 minutes every 2 weeks. For the aerobic program, the number of minutes and the level of exertion were recorded. For the resistance program, the weight used for each exercise was recorded along with the exertion scale score. An exertion score of 5 to 7 was the desired range and was used as a guideline for changing resistance. Weights between 1 and 10 pounds were changed in 2-pound increments, whereas weights over 10 pounds were modified in 5-pound increments. The progress logs for both programs were reviewed at each of the 16 biweekly BENEfit sessions. During each biweekly session, the physical therapist met individually with participants and parents to review the program and address any questions.

Results of the BENEfit program were encouraging. Liusuwan et al (2007b) reported that lean body tissue increased by 2.1% by dual-energy X-ray absorptiometry in this obese cohort with a concomitant, non-significant reduction in total body fat tissue (–2.1%). There was a 27% increase in oxygen uptake at rest ($\dot{V}O_{2rest}$), reflecting the increase in lean tissue. There was no significant change in $\dot{V}O_{2max}$ before and after the BENEfit program. However, the maximum power output (PO_{max}), which represents work capacity, increased by 22%. There was also a 35% increase in the aerobic efficiency as measured by the power output at the

TABLE 16.1
BENEfit class topics and the order in which they were presented

Session No	Topic	Related activity
1	Free, light, and junk food – descriptions	Food charades
2	Basic anatomy and physiology of exercise	Exercise pictionary
3	'FIT TV' video, hunger, and thirst cues	Food groups category
4	Strength training 101 – basics	Obstacle/relay race
5	Fast food dining – tips for eating at fast food restaurants	Choose a meal from the 'BENEfit menu' – figure out the fat and calories
6	Exercise myths and mysteries	Distance scavenger hunt
7	Portion distortion	Portion sizes exercise
8	Portion control for exercise/injury prevention and future exercise plans	How much, how far? (Calculating distance traveled and weight lifted during program)
9	Food choices	Make your own pizza

anaerobic threshold (Po_{AT}). Most of the participants improved their shoulder strength, with a 23% increase in peak shoulder extension. For the group, shoulder flexion strength increased by over 15%. There were no significant changes in mean values for total cholesterol, HDL, low-density lipoprotein, or triglycerides.

Functional Electrical Stimulation Cycling

Chilibeck et al (1999) first evaluated the effect of functional electrical stimulation (FES) exercise on insulin sensitivity and GLUT-1 and GLUT-4 transporter protein levels in paralyzed skeletal muscle for adults with chronic SCI after 8 weeks of training with an FES cycle. On muscle biopsy, GLUT-1 increased by 52% and GLUT-4 increased by 72% after training. In addition, there was an increase in muscle oxidative capacity as indicated by a 56% increase in citrate synthase activity and an improvement in the insulin sensitivity as determined by oral glucose tolerance tests. Johnston et al (2011) compared the effects of a 6-month home-based program of cycling with FES, passive cycling, and electrically stimulated exercise for children with SCI (aged 5–13y; C4–T11; 1–13y after injury). Children exercised at home for 1 hour, 3 days/week. Johnston et al (2011) reported increases in quadriceps muscle mass by dual-energy X-ray absorptiometry after training in children using electrical stimulation. Children cycling with FES showed increases of 24.4% (SD 15.0), whereas children exercising with electrical stimulation without cycling showed increases of 27.2% (SD 19.6). Increases in muscle volume such as those seen for the groups exercising with electrical stimulation are not seen in children with typical development, who typically increase strength by more synchronized neural recruitment rather than by muscle hypertrophy (Ramsay et al 1990). These gains in muscle mass reported by Johnston et al (2011) are clinically significant and may provide these children with a decreased risk of cardiovascular disease, insulin resistance, glucose intolerance, and type 2 diabetes.

After a 6-month program, unpublished data from Johnston and colleagues showed mean increases in REE of 26.3% (SD 36.8) for children cycling with FES and 23% (SD 58.9) for the children receiving electrically stimulated exercise without cycling. Children in the FES cycling and electrically stimulated exercise group also showed a significant increase in quadriceps muscle volume, suggesting that the changes in muscle mass helped to increase REE for the two groups who used electrical stimulation. Johnston et al (2009) also showed gains with FES cycling in children with SCI of 16.2% (SD 25.0) in peak oxygen consumption via arm crank testing. Increases in REE may decrease the risk of weight gain and obesity, and increases in oxygen consumption in deconditioned patients may allow more vigorous activities to be performed.

Johnston et al (2009) also reported no changes in lipid levels for those cycling with and without FES, but a decrease in total cholesterol level was seen for the group exercising with electrical stimulation (without cycling). Since some children studied did not have altered lipid levels at the start of the study, a meaningful change would not be anticipated. In Johnston et al (2009) and Liusuwan et al (2007a), HDL levels tended to run low or at the low end of the typical range in pediatric SCI; however, other lipid values were more variable in the two studies.

Impact of Functional Electrical Stimulation Exercise on Bone Health in Children

There are few data available on the impact of FES exercise on BMD for children with SCI. Lauer et al (2011) reported the effects of a 6-month program of cycling with FES, passive cycling, and electrically stimulated exercise for children with SCI. Although no significant differences were seen between groups over time, children cycling with FES had increases of 32.4%, 6.6%, and 10.3% at the hip, distal femur, and proximal tibia, respectively, and children cycling passively increased BMD at the hip by 29.2% with no changes seen at the knee. Children performing the electrically stimulated exercise (without cycling) had no changes at the hip or distal femur and a decline for the distal femur of 7.1%. Both children cycling with FES and children with passive cycling experienced a significant increase in hip BMD. Children with the lowest BMD experienced the greatest increases in BMD (Lauer et al 2011). Further research is needed to determine optimal dosing for providing the greatest impact on bone health.

Summary

Research since 2000 has brought a better understanding of how SCI or spinal cord dysfunction impacts the long-term health and fitness of children. Diabetes and metabolic disease are potentially serious concerns for children as they develop into adulthood, and spinal cord dysfunction-related complications of decreased bone health, decreased muscle mass, decreased glucose transport, insulin resistance, dyslipidemia, and obesity can all increase a child's or adolescent's risk of long-term morbidities.

It is highly recommended that nutrition assessment and management should be performed during acute, subacute, and chronic phases of rehabilitation after SCI. It is critical to establish a set of nutritional goals that address the adaptations in body composition, metabolism, and lifestyle after SCI. Caloric needs are estimated based on the measured basal metabolic rate. Caloric intake should be optimized to reduce the risk and burden of obesity. A properly planned diet program is also necessary for overweight and obese children with SCI to help them lose weight without deteriorating their overall health and lean mass.

Exercise interventions have had some success in addressing muscle mass and insulin sensitivity in patients with SCI, as well as some of the risks factors of obesity (i.e. reduced REE). Another significant health complication of SCI is the increased risk of fractures, often resulting from decreased weight bearing and low force activity from paralyzed muscle. Exercise interventions, specifically cycling with FES, have shown some positive effects on lean mass, REE, and BMD. Future research will need to evaluate dose–response relationships, and to develop strategies for lifelong recreational interventions that will keep children with spinal cord dysfunction physically active, fit, and participating optimally throughout childhood and adulthood.

REFERENCES

Activity and Health Research (1992) *Allied Dunbar National Fitness Survey*. London, UK: Health Education Authority/Sports Council.

Andrade CK, Kramer J, Garber M, Longmuir P (1991) Changes in self-concept, cardiovascular endurance and muscular strength of children with spina bifida aged 8 to 13 years in response to a 10-week physical-activity programme: a pilot study. *Child Care Health Dev* 17: 183–96. http://dx.doi.org/10.1111/j.1365-2214.1991.tb00689.x

Bauman WA, Spungen AM (1994) Disorders of carbohydrate and lipid metabolism in veterans with paraplegia or quadriplegia: a model of premature aging. *Metabolism* 43: 749–56. http://dx.doi.org/10.1016/0026-0495(94)90126-0

Bauman WA, Adkins RH, Spungen AM, Waters RL (1999) The effect of residual neurological deficit on oral glucose tolerance in persons with chronic spinal cord injury. *Spinal Cord* 37: 765–71. http://dx.doi.org/10.1038/sj.sc.3100893

Block P, Skeels SE, Keys CB, Rimmer JH (2005) Shake-It-Up: health promotion and capacity building for people with spinal cord injuries and related neurological disabilities. *Disabil Rehabil* 27: 185–90. doi:10.1080/09638280400019583

Casteels K, Fieuws S, van Helvoirt M et al (2010) Metformin therapy to reduce weight gain and visceral adiposity in children and adolescents with neurogenic or myogenic motor deficit. *Pediatr Diabetes* 11: 61–9. doi: 10.1155/2012/541363

Chilibeck PD, Bell G, Jeon J et al (1999) Functional electrical stimulation exercise increases GLUT-1 and GLUT-4 in paralyzed skeletal muscle. *Metabolism* 48: 1409–13. http://dx.doi.org/10.1016/S0026-0495(99)90151-8

Csabi G, Torok K, Jeges S, Molnar D (2000) Presence of metabolic cardiovascular syndrome in obese children. *Eur J Pediatr* 159: 91–4. http://dx.doi.org/10.1007/PL00013812

Davis GM, Shephard RJ (1990) Strength training for wheelchair users. *Br J Sports Med* 24: 25–30. http://dx.doi.org/10.1136/bjsm.24.1.25

Dawodu TS, Scott DD, Chase M (2011) *Nutritional Management in the Rehabilitation Setting* [online]. Available at: http://emedicine.medscape.com/article/318180-overview (accessed 5 August 2012).

Dionyssiotis Y (2012) Malnutrition in spinal cord injury: more than nutritional deficiency. *J Clin Med Res* 4: 227–36. doi: 10.4021/jocmr924w.

Ekblom B, Lundberg A (1968) Effect of physical training on adolescents with severe motor handicaps. *Acta Paediatr Scand* 57: 17–23. http://dx.doi.org/10.1111/j.1651-2227.1968.tb07280.x

Elder CP, Apple DF, Bickel CS, Meyer RA, Dudley GA (2004) Intramuscular fat and glucose tolerance after spinal cord injury – a cross-sectional study. *Spinal Cord* 42: 711–6. http://dx.doi.org/10.1038/sj.sc.3101652

Gauld LM, Kappers J, Carlin JB, Robertson CF (2004) Height prediction from ulna length. *Dev Med Child Neurol* 46: 475–80. http://dx.doi.org/10.1111/j.1469-8749.2004.tb00508.x

Goodpaster BH, Thaete FL, Kelley DE (2000). Thigh adipose tissue distribution is associated with insulin resistance in obesity and in type 2 diabetes mellitus. *Am J Clin Nutr* 71: 4885–92.

Gorgey AS, Gater DR (2011) Regional and relative adiposity patterns in relation to carbohydrate and lipid metabolism in men with spinal cord injury. *Appl Physiol Nutr Metab* 36: 107–14. doi: 10.1139/H10-091

Harrell JS, McMurray RG, Baggett CD, Pennell ML, Pearce PF, Bangdiwala SI (2005) Energy costs of physical activities in children and adolescents. *Med Sci Sports Exerc* 37: 329–36. http://dx.doi.org/10.1249/01.MSS.0000153115.33762.3F

Johnston TE, Smith BT, Betz RR, Lauer RT (2008) Exercise testing using upper extremity ergometer in pediatric spinal cord injury. *Pediatr Phys Ther* 20: 146–51. doi: 10.1097/PEP.0b013e318171faa1

Johnston TE, Smith BT, Mulcahey MJ, Betz RR, Lauer RT (2009) A randomized controlled trial on the effects of cycling with and without electrical stimulation on cardiorespiratory and vascular health in children with spinal cord injury. *Arch Phys Med Rehabil* 90: 1379–88. doi: 10.1016/j.apmr.2009.02.018

Johnston TE, Modlesky CM, Betz RR, Lauer RT (2011) Muscle changes following cycling and/or electrical stimulation in pediatric spinal cord injury. *Arch Phys Med Rehabil* 92: 1937–43. doi: 10.1016/j.apmr.2011.06.031

Juonala M, Jarvisalo MJ, Maki-Torkko N, Kahonen M, Viikari JS, Raitakari OT (2005) Risk factors identified in childhood and decreased carotid artery elasticity in adulthood: the Cardiovascular Risk in Young Finns Study. *Circulation* 112: 1486–93. http://dx.doi.org/10.1161/CIRCULATIONAHA.104.502161

Khalil RE, Gorgey AS, Janisko M, Dolbow DR, Moore JR, Gater DR (2013) The role of nutrition in health status after spinal cord injury. *Aging Dis* 4: 14–22.

Klip A, Paquet MR (1990) Glucose transport and glucose transporters in muscle and their metabolic regulation. *Diabetes Care* 13: 228–43. http://dx.doi.org/10.2337/diacare.13.3.228

Lauer R, Johnston TE, Smith BT, Mulcahey MJ, Betz RR, Maurer AH (2007) Bone mineral density of the hip and knee in children with spinal cord injury. *J Spinal Cord Med* 30(Suppl 1): S10–14.

Lauer RT, Smith BT, Mulcahey MJ, Betz RR, Johnston TE (2011) Effects of cycling and/or electrical stimulation on bone mineral density in children with spinal cord injury. *Spinal Cord* 49: 917–23. http://dx.doi.org/10.1038/sc.2011.19

Lee BY, Agarwal N, Corcoran L, Thoden WR, Del Guercio LR (1985) Assessment of nutritional and metabolic status of paraplegics. *J Rehabil Res Dev* 22: 11–17. http://dx.doi.org/10.1682/JRRD.1985.07.0011

Liusuwan A, Widman L, Abresch RT, McDonald CM (2004) Altered body composition affects resting energy expenditure and interpretation of body mass index in children with spinal cord injury. *J Spinal Cord Med* 27(Suppl 1): S24–8.

Liusuwan RA, Widman LM, Abresch RT, Styne DM, McDonald CM (2007a) Body composition and resting energy expenditure in patients aged 11 to 21 years with spinal cord dysfunction compared to controls: comparisons and relationships among the groups. *J Spinal Cord Med* 30(Suppl 1): S105–11.

Liusuwan RA, Widman LM, Abresch RT, Johnson AJ, McDonald CM (2007b) Behavioral intervention, exercise, and nutrition education to improve health and fitness (BENEfit) in adolescents with mobility impairment due to spinal cord dysfunction. *J Spinal Cord Med* 30(Suppl 1): S119–26.

McDonald CM, Abresch-Meyer AL, Nelson MD, Widman LM (2007) Body mass index and body composition measures by dual x-ray absorptiometry in patients aged 10 to 21 years with spinal cord injury. *J Spinal Cord* 30(Suppl 1): S97–104.

McPherson AC, Swift JA, Yung E, Lyons J, Church P (2013) The assessment of weight status in children and young people attending a spina bifida outpatient clinic: a retrospective medical record review. *Disabil Rehabil* 35: 2123–31. doi: 10.3109/09638288.2013.771705

Mazur L, Lacy B, Wilsford L (2011) The prevalence of hypertension in children with spina bifida. *Acta Paediatr* 100: e80–3. doi: 10.1111/j.1651-2227.2011.02225.x

Mellin LM, Silnkard LA, Irwin CE (1987) Adolescent obesity intervention: validation of the SHAPEDOWN program. *Am Diet Assoc* 87: 333–8.

Mulroy SJ, Gronley JK, Newsam DJ, Perry J (1996) Electromyographic activity of shoulder muscles during wheelchair propulsion by paraplegic persons. *Arch Phys Med Rehabil* 77: 187–93. http://dx.doi.org/10.1016/S0003-9993(96)90166-5

Nelson MD, Widman LM, Abresch RT et al (2007) Metabolic syndrome in adolescents with spinal cord dysfunction. *J Spinal Cord Med* 30(Suppl 1): S127–39.

Paulsen EP, Richenderfer L, Ginsberg-Fellner F (1968) Plasma glucose, free fatty acids, and immunoreactive insulin in sixty-six obese children. Studies in reference to a family history of diabetes mellitus. *Diabetes* 17: 261–9.

Ramsay JA, Blimkie CJ, Smith K, Garner S, MacDougall JD, Sale DG (1990) Strength training effects in prepubescent boys. *Med Sci Sports Exerc* 22: 605–14. http://dx.doi.org/10.1249/00005768-199010000-00011

Roberts D, Shepherd RW, Shepherd K (1991) Anthropometry and obesity in myelomeningocele. *J Paediatr Child Health* 27: 83–90. http://dx.doi.org/10.1111/j.1440-1754.1991.tb00358.x

Robertson CS, Grossman RG (1987) Protection against spinal cord ischemia with insulin-induced hypoglycemia. *J Neurosurg* 67: 739–44. http://dx.doi.org/10.3171/jns.1987.67.5.0739

Shepherd K, Roberts D, Golding S, Thomas BJ, Shepherd RW (1991) Body composition in myelomeningocele. *Am J Clin Nutr* 53: 1–6.

Srinivasan SR, Myers L, Berenson GS (2002) Predictability of childhood adiposity and insulin for developing insulin resistance syndrome (syndrome X) in young adulthood: the Bogalusa Heart Study. *Diabetes* 51: 204–9. http://dx.doi.org/10.2337/diabetes.51.1.204

Steinberger J, Daniels SR (2003) Obesity, insulin resistance, diabetes, and cardiovascular risk in children: an American Heart Association scientific statement from the Atherosclerosis, Hypertension, and Obesity in the Young Committee (Council on Cardiovascular Disease in the Young) and the Diabetes Committee (Council on Nutrition, Physical Activity, and Metabolism). *Circulation* 107: 1448–53. http://dx.doi.org/10.1161/01.CIR.0000060923.07573.F2

Tomey KM, Chen DM, Wang X, Braunschweig CL (2005) Dietary intake and nutritional status of urban community-dwelling men with paraplegia. *Arch Phys Med Rehabil* 86: 664–71. http://dx.doi.org/10.1016/j.apmr.2004.10.023

United States Department of Health and Human Services (2012) *Healthy People 2020* [online]. Available at: http://www.healthypeople.gov/2020/default.aspx (accessed 16 April 2012).

Vanhala M, Vanhala P, Kumpusalo E, Halonen P, Takala J (1998) Relation between obesity from childhood to adulthood and the metabolic syndrome: Population based study. *BMJ* 317: 319. http://dx.doi.org/10.1136/bmj.317.7154.319

Widman LM, McDonald CM, Abresch RT (2006) Effectiveness of an upper extremity exercise device integrated with computer gaming for aerobic training in adolescents with spinal cord dysfunction. *J Spinal Cord Med* 29: 363–70.
Widman LM, Abresch RT, Styne DM, McDonald CM (2007) Aerobic fitness and upper extremity strength in patients aged 11 to 21 years with spinal cord dysfunction as compared to ideal weight and overweight controls. *J Spinal Cord Med* 30(Suppl 1): S88–96.
Yamaki K, Rimmer JH, Lowry BD, Vogel LC (2011) Prevalence of obesity-related chronic health conditions in overweight adolescents with disabilities. *Res Dev Disabil* 32: 280–8. doi: 10.1016/j.ridd.2010.10.007
Zebracki K, Hwang M, Patt PL, Vogel LC (2013) Autonomic cardiovascular dysfunction and vitamin D deficiency in pediatric spinal cord injury. *J Pediatr Rehabil Med* 6: 45–52. doi: 10.3233/PRM-130236

17
PAIN

Thomas N Bryce and Tonya M Palermo

Case vignette

Andrew is a 17-year-old male who sustained a traumatic spinal cord injury after a motor vehicle crash 2 years ago. After being discharged from in-patient rehabilitation, Andrew developed pain that continued to worsen and is now present most days. He reports pain from just above the chest down to his feet. He describes the pain intensity as severe and the quality of the pain as burning, stabbing, and tingling. Andrew also complains of painful sensitivity in response to light touch or pressure on his lower extremities. His family has been concerned about his debilitating pain as well as his general adjustment to the spinal cord injury and his behavior. He seems depressed and withdrawn. He has very limited contact with peers. Because of the significant interference from the pain, Andrew stopped attending school and enrolled in an online school program to complete his high-school degree. He is refusing to participate in most physical and self-care activities. Family conflict has also increased considerably; his parents try to 'push' him to do more and they have become increasingly frustrated by what they perceive as a lack of motivation.

Intervention involved

1 Encouraging Andrew to set goals around valued activities in his life. Andrew is interested in computer programming but has not engaged in any computer-related projects in many months because he says it is too painful to work at the computer. He was taught several coping strategies including activity pacing to gradually increase his tolerance for sitting at a desk, which also encouraged task persistence.
2 Instructing Andrew in strategies to reduce his feelings of helplessness and his belief that the pain was uncontrollable. Andrew was also taught several relaxation strategies that were modified for his disability and was trained in self hypnosis.
3 Working with Andrew's parents on ways to support his independence and autonomy around pain management. They were instructed to not focus on pain and to eliminate their frequent 'check-ins', and instead allow Andrew to come and ask for help if needed. His parents were instructed to focus on supporting positive coping behaviors and encouraging the attainment of goals.

Introduction

Pain after spinal cord injury (SCI) is common. Approximately 65% of children with SCI report pain (Jan and Wilson 2004), whereas 70% of adults who sustained their injuries as children (Vogel et al 2002) and 80% of adults who sustained their injuries as adults report pain (Cardenas et al 2004). In persons injured when they are younger than 3 years, the prevalence of pain is 72%, which is similar to the prevalence in those children injured at older ages (Jan and Wilson 2004).

Pain is commonly defined as an unpleasant sensory and emotional experience associated with actual or potential tissue damage or is described in terms of such injury. Pain is usually categorized into one of two subtypes: either nociceptive pain or neuropathic pain. Nociceptive pain is defined as pain arising from the activation of peripheral nerve sensory receptors (nociceptors) capable of transducing and encoding noxious stimuli, whereas neuropathic pain is defined as pain caused by a lesion or disease of the somatosensory nervous system. The International SCI Pain (ISCIP) classification has been developed to help organize the different pain types experienced after SCI in an easily understandable format (see Table 17.1) (Bryce et al 2012). In the ISCIP classification, in addition to the nociceptive and neuropathic pain types, there is also a third type of pain, labeled as 'other' pain, which must be distinguished from these two types. This is pain that occurs in situations in which there is no identifiable noxious stimulus or any detectable inflammation or damage to the nervous system responsible for the pain. It is usually unclear what causes this latter category of pain to begin or persist. Established pain syndromes of unknown etiology which fall into this category include fibromyalgia and complex regional pain syndrome type I.

Persistent or chronic pain is defined as pain that occurs beyond the time of expected healing, most typically thought to be 3 months. Tremendous variation exists in the reported frequency, severity, and duration of pain complaints, both within children and between children.

TABLE 17.1
International spinal cord injury pain (ISCIP) classification

Tier 1: pain type	Tier 2: pain subtype	Tier 3: primary pain source and/or pathology (some examples)
Nociceptive pain	Musculoskeletal pain	lateral epicondylitis, comminuted femur fracture, quadratus lumborum muscle spasm
	Visceral pain	abdominal pain owing to bowel impaction, cholecystitis
	Other nociceptive pain	migraine headache, surgical skin incision
Neuropathic pain	At-level SCI pain	spinal cord compression, nerve root compression, cauda equina compression
	Below-level SCI pain	spinal cord ischemia, spinal cord compression
	Other neuropathic pain	carpal tunnel syndrome
Other pain		fibromyalgia, Complex Regional Pain Syndrome type I, interstitial cystitis, irritable bowel syndrome
Unknown pain		

Of concern for many children with recurrent and chronic pain is the potential for associated decrements in their ability to function in important life roles. Children may experience limitations in their ability to attend school and complete academic work as well as in their participation in physical, social, recreational, and peer activities. Chronic pain can also have a negative impact on family life, including increased stress and financial implications for parents.

The development of pain after SCI in children (similar to in other populations) is thought to involve biological, psychological, and social/environmental factors. Biological factors relate to the child's injury, impact of body positioning, and pain processing in the central nervous system (e.g. central sensitization) that may influence pain type and severity. Central sensitization refers to changes that occur in the brain in response to repeated nerve stimulation (repeated pain) that make the brain more excitable; this has now been identified as an important predictor of the development of chronic pain. Psychological factors, in particular children's anxiety and depressive symptoms, may influence both the child's pain experience and functional disability related to chronic pain. In particular, given that children may experience trauma related to the etiology of the SCI, anxiety and depressive symptoms are a critical area of potential influence. Parent factors have also been recognized in the broader pain literature as important in explaining the interindividual variability in children's response to pain. Much of the research on specific parent factors has focused on the role of parent behaviors, such as providing excessive attention to pain complaints.

Assessment

Children and adolescents have unique needs that should be considered in the assessment and management of pain, given the neurophysiology associated with development, the influence and involvement of their parents and families, and the differences in their methods of and abilities in communication. A thorough assessment of the child with pain takes into consideration pain characteristics as well as the broad impact of pain on the child's and family's daily lives, including emotional, physical, and social impact. Using a biopsychosocial assessment model, it is important to evaluate aspects of the child's physiology, psychological functioning, and social/environmental factors.

In evaluating pain itself, there are seven characteristics of pain that an assessor should elucidate. In evaluating a child with pain, the cognitive development of the child will guide the assessment, the specificity of the questions, and the answers obtained; however, optimally, all seven components should be addressed if possible. These components include the history of onset of the pain, the location on the body where the pain is felt, the temporal pattern of the pain presence, the quality of the pain, ameliorating and exacerbating factors for the pain, associated sensory disturbances (i.e. evoked pain), and the intensity of the pain.

The history of onset of the pain can link the SCI to the pain. A description of an inciting event can be useful in identifying the pain generator, especially if the pain developed after injury. The location of the pain can indicate a neuropathic type, occurring at or below the level of injury in a specific pattern, or a nociceptive type, where the specific pain location can allow one to hone in on the potential pain generators in that specific location of the body. The temporal pattern is useful for differentiating between nociceptive and neuropathic pains, as nociceptive pain is generally present only when there is stimulation of offending nociceptors, whereas neuropathic pain tends to be more persistent owing to the presence of nervous system damage or irritation. The quality of the pain can be useful in identifying the subtype, especially if a few specific descriptors such as 'burning' and 'electric shock-like' are specified, as these descriptors are more commonly seen in neuropathic types. However, one must be careful, as quite significant overlap and poor specificity of descriptors has been documented, even in adults. Ameliorating and exacerbating factors can be especially useful in differentiating nociceptive and neuropathic subtypes, especially if movement is involved, as a pain generator can often be localized by replicating exacerbating factors in these situations. Associated sensory disturbances, such as the presence of allodynia or hyperpathia, either noted on history or picked up on physical examination, are highly suggestive of neuropathic subtypes, although there is overlap and these findings can be seen in nociceptive subtypes as well. Finally, intensity is probably the best proxy of the severity of the pain and is the most commonly used measure of the effectiveness of treatment.

The developmental stage of the child, for which age is a good proxy, should guide the choice of the pain scale used, which is useful for indicating intensity. Children generally enter the Piaget stage of concrete operations by 7 to 11 years of age, whereupon they can perform serial ordering operations. At this age, a numeric rating scale (NRS) can be considered. This can be verbally administered without the use of physical materials. For the NRS-11 (named so because it uses 11 categories, from 0 to 10), the clinician asks the child how much pain or hurt he or she has using a number between 0 and 10, where 0 is no pain or hurt and 10 is the worst pain or hurt imaginable. The NRS-11 has been shown to be valid in children of these age groups (von Baeyer et al 2009) and is recommended as the preferred measure of intensity of pain for adults with SCI (Bryce et al 2007).

For children aged 4 to 6 years, who generally cannot perform serial ordering, facial expression scales, in which the child discriminates between different levels of pain depicted in a series of faces, are a common approach to pain assessment, and the best validated tool at present is the Faces Pain Scale Revised (Hicks et al 2001). This approach does not require the child to translate the pain experience into a numerical value; however, physical materials are required, for example a sign with the various faces illustrated. For children 3 to 4 years of age, the Poker Chip Tool, which consists of four red poker chips each representing a 'piece of hurt', from which the child chooses 'how many pieces of hurt' they have currently, has been shown to be valid (McGrath et al 2008).

For toddlers, infants, and those with developmental delays who are unable to speak, physiological and behavioral responses to pain must be relied upon. Recently, there has been considerable effort to develop multidimensional and evidence-based assessment instruments useful in home, clinical, and research settings to measure children's behavioral responses to pain. A number of inventories relying upon observation of the behavior of children and adults with significant neurologic disabilities or communication and cognitive impairments have demonstrated adequate reliability and validity (Valkenburg et al 2010).

Measurement of the impact of pain is equally important in a thorough clinical assessment of the child. Clinical interviews should cover important domains of daily life, including the impact of pain on the child's physical activities, sleep, peer activities, school functioning, emotional functioning, and daily family life (e.g. burden, stress).

Finally, in assessing a child with pain, it is important to understand parental, child, and caregiver beliefs about pain. This includes understanding beliefs about what is causing the pain, what the potential treatments for the pain are, and what the likelihood of pain control is. Parents and caregivers may evaluate a child's pain through their own understanding of pain, which probably has been nociceptive, related to an incident, and self-limited or cured. They may not understand that neuropathic pain may not serve a useful purpose (unlike acute nociceptive pain, which may serve as a signal to protect an injury) or have an effective treatment. Parents and children may search repeatedly for a cure and they often expect that the pain will disable them until they find that cure and that they have no ability to change the course of future pain and pain-related disability until that cure is found.

Nociceptive pain

In one study of 31 children with SCI, of whom 65% reported pain, 48% of the pains experienced were classified as nociceptive, whereas 19% were classified as neuropathic (Jan and Wilson 2004). Of the nociceptive pains reported by the children, approximately 80% were classified by the investigators as musculoskeletal, whereas the rest were thought to be visceral. The musculoskeletal pains were thought to include pains related to 'overuse syndromes, bone and joint problems, and painful muscle spasms'.

In a study of the long-term outcomes (average duration of injury 12y) of adults who had sustained their SCI when 18 years of age or younger (average age 14y), wrist, elbow, and shoulder pain were prevalent (Vogel et al 2011). Shoulder pain was present in nearly half (46%) of those with C1–C4 tetraplegia (American Spinal Injury Association Impairment Scale [AIS] A, B, or C [ABC]), and just over half (51%) of those with lower levels (C5–C8 and T1–T4 AIS ABC). Wrist pain was present in nearly a quarter (24%) of those with paraplegia (AIS ABC) and 9% in those with C5–C8 AIS ABC tetraplegia. It is likely that a proportion of the wrist pain was due to neuropathic causes, such as compressive neuropathy at the wrist, as well as musculoskeletal etiologies. Elbow pain prevalence ranged from 9% to 16% for the various groups, and was greatest in those with paraplegia. Similar prevalences for shoulder, wrist, and elbow pain were seen in those with functionally incomplete injuries (AIS D) at 40%, 8%, and 13%, respectively.

Musculoskeletal pain is pain which occurs in a region where there is at least *some* preserved sensation, including areas below the neurologic level of injury (NLI). It is believed to arise from stimulation of nociceptors within musculoskeletal structures (muscles, tendons, ligaments, joints, and bones). The degree of pain does not always correlate with the amount of damage within the structure stimulating the nociceptors; however, musculoskeletal pain typically changes in intensity with movement or palpation of the responsible structures. Appropriate imaging often shows musculoskeletal pathology consistent with the pain presentation. Musculoskeletal pain often responds better than other types of pain to anti-inflammatory or opioid medications, to physical measures such as stretching and massage, and to the modalities of heat and cold.

Shoulder Pain

Shoulder pain is prevalent in individuals with SCI who use all types of mobility devices ranging from power and manual wheelchairs to canes and crutches. There are a number of hypotheses for why persons with SCI develop shoulder pain. In the acute period after SCI, pain may develop owing to the high demand on unconditioned muscles. In the chronic period, pain is thought to be related to overuse. As persons use various mobility devices and load their shoulders repeatedly with their body weight, over time, degenerative changes ultimately take place. An imbalance of the shoulder and scapular stabilizing musculature is another key factor related to the development of pain in both the acute and chronic periods. This imbalance can be caused by the need to use different muscles, which are innervated, to perform tasks, because, in those with cervical injuries, all of the shoulder stabilizers may not be fully innervated. It can also be caused by the relative strengthening of certain muscles (e.g. increased abduction to adduction and internal rotation strength) during everyday activities such as transferring and wheelchair propulsion. Specific etiologies of chronic shoulder pain in adults, to which children with SCI may be expected to acquire, include rotator cuff impingement syndrome, subacromial bursitis, bicipital tendonitis, adhesive capsulitis, and osteoarthritis.

Prevention strategies for shoulder pain can be divided into two stages: (1) learning to minimize shoulder stress and (2) preparing the shoulders to accept the stresses that will be encountered. For children with tetraplegia with poor arm strength, strategies to minimize shoulder stress include avoiding lying directly on a shoulder in bed; always supporting the arms with pillows in bed, on arm rests or arm troughs, or using a tray table in the chair to avoid glenohumeral subluxation; and never allowing a caregiver to pull on an arm to change body position but to use the trunk instead.

For children with paraplegia, strategies to minimize shoulder stress include using long circular wheelchair propulsion patterns which maximize contact with and minimize force on the push rim; optimizing wheelchair seating posture to minimize the necessity for achieving positions of shoulder impingement with wheelchair propulsion and transfers; avoiding becoming overweight; provision of the lightest weight wheelchair that requires the least amount of force to propel and meets a person's needs; and changing the size of the wheelchair as the child grows to accommodate changing biomechanics (Paralyzed Veterans of America Consortium for Spinal Cord Medicine 2005) (see Chapter 22). Home modification should be done to limit the number of transfers needed daily, and proper transfer technique should be reviewed periodically in order to ensure that transfer is being done in the most efficient and least stressful manner. Activities which promote impingement, that is activities in which the arm is abducted or flexed more than 90 degrees, especially when combined with internal rotation, should be identified by a thorough functional evaluation, and alternatives should be sought and implemented.

For children with SCI, preparing shoulders to accept stress is done through exercise. For older adolescents, implementation of a formal regular exercise program is recommended. Strengthening of the dynamic shoulder stabilizers should occur in a balanced fashion. Effective programs used in adults with SCI have emphasized strengthening the posterior shoulder musculature, including the external rotators, the posterior scapular muscles (rhomboids and trapezius), and the adductors, as wheelchair use promotes strengthening of the antagonists to these muscles (i.e. the anterior shoulder musculature). Stretching of the dynamic shoulder stabilizers, especially the anterior shoulder musculature, which has often become hypertrophied and contracted through constant use during wheelchair propulsion and transfer activities, is also necessary to achieve a strength-balanced shoulder. In adults, several controlled studies of varied duration which concentrated on strengthening the shoulder stabilizers and stretching tight musculature in this fashion have been shown to be effective in decreasing long-standing shoulder pain (Curtis et al 1999, Serra-Ano et al 2012). In addition, as hand cycling has been shown both to load the shoulders less and to stress the rotator cuff muscles prone to overuse less than wheelchair propulsion under similar conditions of external power, hand cycling may be a better choice than wheelchair propulsion for regular aerobic exercise (Arnet et al 2012).

Adjuncts to the active treatment strategies for shoulder pain originating from the rotator cuff outlined above also include, as necessary, the application of ice, relative rest, the use of topical or oral non-steroidal anti-inflammatory drugs (NSAIDs), or, if other treatments are ineffective, bursal space injections of steroids.

Occasionally, shoulder pain is experienced by persons with tetraplegia where all the signs and symptoms point to musculoskeletal pathology as the cause. However, the actual primary pain generator is a tethered spinal cord or cord tissue compressed by a syrinx. Clues that the primary generator is actually the spinal cord may include the presence of allodynia or hyperpathia in the shoulder region and resistance to conventional musculoskeletal treatments.

Elbow and Wrist Pain

Common musculoskeletal causes of elbow pain in children and adolescents who utilize their arms as load-bearing structures include medial and lateral epicondylitis, and triceps tendonitis. Olecranon bursitis can occur in individuals who lean on their elbows for support for prolonged periods. The main methods of treatment of tendonitis/epicondylitis are stretching and gradual strengthening of involved muscles, relative rest, and a functional re-evaluation of activities that promote pain in these structures, which leads to the generation of new ways of performing activities with subsequent change in the performance of these activities. Ice and the use of NSAIDs are useful adjuncts. Avoiding weight bearing (leaning) on the elbows is the primary treatment for olecranon bursitis. Secondary treatments for olecranon bursitis include ice, cushioned elbow pads, and aspiration of an inflamed bursa with or without injection of corticosteroids.

Common musculoskeletal causes of wrist pain in adults include De Quervain tenosynovitis, inflammation/arthritis of the metacarpophalangeal joint of the thumb, and arthritis of the wrist. These typically are overuse injuries caused, for example, by repetitive grasping of a wheelchair pushrim during wheelchair propulsion or repetitive weight bearing on an extended wrist. Treatments include relative rest, splinting, ice, gentle stretching, a functional re-evaluation of causative actions and subsequent change in performance of activities, and anti-inflammatory administration (NSAIDs or local corticosteroid injections).

Back Pain

Musculoskeletal back pain in persons with SCI is common for a number of reasons, including a high prevalence of spinal surgeries, truncal muscle imbalances owing to spasticity and/or truncal weakness, and frequent dependence on wheelchairs. Nociceptive back pain generators include muscles, tendons, and ligaments; the facet joint; the intervertebral disk; the sacroiliac joint; and referred visceral sources. Pain caused by spinal instability or spinal hardware failure is primarily nociceptive. After a portion of the spine is fused, the spinal segments adjacent to the fusion often compensate for the lost motion of the fused segments and, over time, develop secondary degeneration and pain. Sitting in a wheelchair, especially sitting in a kyphotic posture, has been shown to induce back pain, in individuals both with and without SCI. The provision of lumbar lordotic support has been shown to diminish this pain. Conversely, if a child or adolescent in a wheelchair has a limited hip flexion range (less than 90 degrees, for instance) and they are sitting in a wheelchair with a seatback angle of 90 degrees, in order to accommodate to the chair, they will need to slide their buttocks forward, resulting in inadequate back support and a sitting posture which could lead to back pain. This problem is potentially corrected by adjusting the seatback angle of the chair. It is also likely that, in persons with SCI, whether they are ambulatory or wheelchair bound, the effects of spasticity on spinal biomechanics can cause musculoskeletal types of pain, especially if the spasticity is worse on one side of the body than the other. One such common type of pain is sacroiliac joint-related pain, with the distribution of pain usually localized to a vertical column extending from the posterior superior iliac spine caudally, associated with tenderness to palpation over this area. The pain is usually worse with extension of the lower spine and pelvis and is typically more severe on one side than the other. Treatments of sacroiliac joint pain need to address any underlying biomechanical imbalances precipitating the pain. Treatments aimed at addressing biomechanical abnormalities may include spasticity management with oral, intrathecal, or local injections of medication and strengthening of imbalanced core and extremity musculature.

Visceral Pain

In the study mentioned earlier by Jan and Wilson, of 31 children with SCI, approximately two-thirds of the nociceptive pains reported by the children were classified by the investigators as visceral (Jan and Wilson 2004). It is interesting to note that the prevalence of visceral pain (25%), at least in this small study, may be similar in children with SCI to that in adults, in whom the prevalence of visceral pain is up to 38% (Finnerup et al 2008). Visceral pain refers to pain located (usually) in the thorax, abdomen, or pelvis, which is believed to be primarily generated in visceral structures. Visceral pain often has a relationship to food intake or bowel function and may be associated with nausea or sweating. Tenderness to palpation of the abdomen and pain described as 'cramping', 'dull', or 'tender' are common. Appropriate imaging often shows visceral pathology consistent with the pain presentation (e.g. colonic distension by stool). Examples of visceral pain in children include pain resulting from urinary tract infection, ureteral calculus, or bowel impaction. Treatments depend on the cause. Ensuring a proper diet, avoidance of constipating medications, and daily bowel evacuations can help prevent visceral pain owing to bowel impaction or constipation.

Finally, if pain is localized to the thorax, abdomen, or pelvis but there is no link between this pain and any visceral function and there is no evidence of visceral pathology, at-level or below-level SCI pain should be considered the cause.

Other Nociceptive Pain

Other (nociceptive) pain refers to nociceptive pains that do not fall into the musculoskeletal or visceral categories. These pains may be indirectly related to the SCI (e.g. pain from pressure sores and autonomic dysreflexia headache) or may be unrelated to SCI (e.g. migraine headache).

Neuropathic pain

At-level and Below-level Spinal Cord Injury Pain

At-level SCI pain refers to neuropathic pain perceived within the dermatome of the NLI and/or within the three dermatomes below this level but not within any dermatomes four or more levels below the NLI and is thought by the assessor to be due to damage to the spinal cord or nerve roots. Neuropathic pain in this location, which cannot be attributed to spinal cord or nerve root damage, such as might occur with a focal peripheral nerve compression (e.g. symptomatic carpal tunnel syndrome in a person with a lower cervical injury), should be classified as 'other' neuropathic pain and not as at-level SCI pain. At-level SCI pain is suggested by altered sensation within the pain distribution, especially allodynia or hyperalgesia, and is often described as 'hot-burning', 'tingling', 'pricking', 'pins and needles', 'sharp', 'shooting', 'squeezing', 'painful cold', or 'electric shock-like' (Bryce et al 2012).

Below-level SCI pain refers to neuropathic pain perceived more than three dermatomes below the dermatome of the NLI with or without extension up to the NLI and thought by the assessor to be due to damage to the spinal cord. Similar to at-level SCI pain, neuropathic pain that occurs in this distribution that cannot be attributed to spinal cord damage should be classified as 'other' neuropathic pain and not as below-level SCI pain. Below-level SCI pain can occur in persons with complete or incomplete injuries and its descriptors are the same as those listed for at-level SCI pain. It is of note that neuropathic pain after SCI has not been shown to be more prevalent in any group stratified by neurologic level, sex, or degree of injury completeness (Dijkers et al 2009).

An evaluation to search for potentially treatable causes of neuropathic pain, such as nerve root or spinal cord compression, tethering, or syringomyelia, should be initiated when the cause is not clear, especially when neuropathic pain develops after SCI or there is worsening of pre-existing pain without a clear reason. It should be noted that other stressful or noxious stimuli such as may occur with urinary tract infections, constipation, or pressure ulcers may worsen the intensity of stable chronic pain. Pharmacologic and non-pharmacologic pain-relieving interventions can be initiated concurrently. The major pharmacologic classes of analgesics used to treat neuropathic pain after SCI in adults include antidepressants, specifically tricyclic antidepressants and selective serotonin and norepinephrine reuptake inhibitors; anticonvulsants; local anesthetics; and opioids. Use of pregabalin (Siddall et al 2006), gabapentin (Levendoglu et al 2004), amitriptyline (Rintala et al 2007), and tramadol (Norrbrink and Lundeberg 2009) have all shown greater efficacy than placebo for the treatment of neuropathic pain after SCI in adults. Use of these medications has been extrapolated to the pediatric population using dose equivalents. Additional considerations include the risk of suicide in children and adolescents that has been associated with the use of antidepressants, and the risks and benefits must be weighed carefully. As for most types of childhood chronic pain, there is a very limited evidence base for any class of medication, and pharmacologic treatment is largely based on anecdotal evidence or is derived from the adult literature rather than from controlled clinical studies in the pediatric population.

Cranial electrical stimulation is the application of a current delivered via ear clip electrodes or directly to the scalp. Small positive effects have been found in several studies treating adults with chronic pain after SCI, including spinal cord pain (Tan et al 2011). The long-term effects on the developing brain of this intervention are unclear and its use should be undertaken with caution in children. Spinal cord stimulation refers to the percutaneous implantation and electrical activation of single- or multiple-channel electrodes placed within the epidural space over the dorsum of the spinal cord. Case studies on the efficacy of this intervention in adults have not shown significant relief of neuropathic pain in persons with complete injuries, although some benefit has been reported in a minority of persons with incomplete injuries (Cruccu et al 2007).

Intrathecal drug delivery systems are implantable devices for medication administration via a catheter to the intrathecal space that can allow continuous and/or bolus dosing. In a study that evaluated the effect of intrathecal morphine, clonidine, and their combination on below-level and at-level neuropathic pain after SCI in adults, only the combination was found to be effective (Siddall et al 2000). Nevertheless, both these drugs are not uncommonly used in adults with chronic pain, including neuropathic pain, when the side effects of systemically administered medications outweigh the benefits. Intrathecal pumps can be implanted in children and adolescents of all ages and are not uncommonly utilized for the administration of baclofen for spasticity. However, since, in the literature, there is a lack of studies on the use of chronically administered intrathecal opioids, clonidine, or local anesthetics in children, except for a few case reports, the safety and efficacy of this indication is unknown.

Radiofrequency or laser coagulation destruction of the spinal cord dorsal root entry zone (DREZ) is an invasive procedure which may be somewhat effective for treating at-level SCI pain but not below-level SCI pain (Robert et al 2009). Sensation is lost through the destruction of the DREZ at those levels at which it is undertaken. When performed conventionally, the DREZ is coagulated two levels both above and below the level of injury. Alternatively, when performed with intramedullary electrical recording guidance, areas with abnormal spontaneous signals are selectively lesioned, causing potentially less sensory loss (Falci et al 2002). The literature on DREZ lesioning for the treatment of pain in children is lacking.

Psychological treatments have been used for many years to reduce pain sensations and modify situational, emotional, familial, and behavioral factors that contribute to pain-related disability in children. Cognitive behavioral therapy (CBT) interventions have been the most well studied to date. CBT includes a range of behavioral and cognitive strategies such as relaxation training, biofeedback, operant strategies to reinforce adaptive behaviors, hypnosis, and cognitive coping skills. The goals of CBT are typically to enhance children's coping skills, to instruct parents in strategies to increase adaptive child behaviors, and to minimize children's distress. In addition, specific areas of psychosocial functioning can also serve as therapeutic targets such as school avoidance or significant anxiety or depressive symptoms. Several meta-analytic reviews have documented the efficacy of psychological therapies for children with various chronic pain conditions with biofeedback, relaxation training, and CBT being most effective at reducing pain intensity in young people (Palermo et al 2010).

Psychological and behavioral interventions have also been studied in adults with SCI and chronic pain. Hypnosis and electromyogram biofeedback have both been shown to reduce pain intensity in a randomized trial with the treatment effect maintained at the 3-month point for those undergoing self hypnosis (Jensen et al 2009). CBT, which is focused on improving cognitive and behavioral reactions to pain, seems to be more effective for improving coping and for reducing interference with everyday function, mood, and sleep than for reducing pain severity in those with SCI (Gault et al 2009). On the basis of evidence in pediatric and adult pain studies, psychological interventions are considered appropriate for children and adolescents with any chronic pain condition, including young people with SCI.

Other Neuropathic Pain

Other neuropathic pain refers to neuropathic pain that is present above, at or below the NLI but is not directly related to the SCI. Examples include pain related to a brachial plexopathy or a compressive neuropathy. In adults, the incidence of pain at the wrist increases over time after the injury, and much of it is thought to be due to injury to the median nerve at the wrist. The pathophysiology is thought to be the result of a combination of repetitive trauma, as occurs with wheelchair propulsion, and ischemia from repetitive marked increases in carpal canal pressures, as occurs with upper limb loading during functional mobility.

Prevention and treatment of these repetitive contact neuropathies at the wrist include minimizing the force applied to the rim during wheelchair propulsion by using long, smooth wheelchair propulsive strokes; by avoiding being overweight or propeling a wheelchair that is heavier than necessary; and by using ergonomically designed hand rims. Push-up ischial pressure reliefs and weight bearing on an extended wrist should be avoided, and should be substituted with side-to-side or forward-lean ischial pressure reliefs and a neutral wrist position, respectively.

Complex Regional Pain Syndrome

Complex regional pain syndrome (CRPS) is a pain syndrome that often affects the extremities for which the pathophysiology is not well defined. Characteristics of CRPS include a severity of pain that is disproportionate to what is expected in relation to the purported inciting event, as well as signs and symptoms that fall within the following four categories: (1) sensory (e.g. allodynia and/or hyperesthesia), (2) vasomotor (e.g. skin temperature asymmetries and/or skin color changes), (3) sudomotor/edema (e.g. sweating abnormalities and/or edema of affected area), and (4) motor/trophic (e.g. motor dysfunction and/or trophic changes of the nails and/or skin) (Harden et al 2007). Pain is often characterized as burning. CRPS can be classified into one of two types: type 1 if there is no obvious nerve injury and type 2 if there is evidence of peripheral nerve injury.

By definition, SCI can result in changes within the sensory, vasomotor, sudomotor/edema, and motor realms in areas at or below the level of injury. As noted earlier, the ISCIP classification defines pain resulting from spinal cord or nerve root injury as either at-level or below-level SCI pain. At-level or below-level SCI pain can be further classified using autonomic features to clearly identify the subtypes of neuropathic pain that are consistent with CRPS. If the pain experienced by an individual occurs in an area innervated above the level of injury, the designation of CRPS is straightforward. However, signs and symptoms, which may otherwise be consistent with CRPS, that fall within the dermatomal innervations affected by the SCI renders a diagnosis of CRPS suspect. In this case, there is a neurologic etiology for the pain, and classifying the condition as at-level or below-level SCI pain with autonomic features is appropriate.

Nevertheless, with regard to treatment of at-level or below-level SCI pain, which includes a constellation of signs and symptoms similar to CRPS, it is reasonable to approach treatment as one might approach the treatment of CRPS. The main components of accepted physical treatments include intensive desensitization, edema control, and motor activities. Adjuvant pharmacologic treatments, for which there is some limited evidence of effectiveness in adults and for which use could potentially be extrapolated to children and adolescents, include a tapering course of corticosteroids for acute pain, and gabapentinoids and NSAIDs for symptomatic relief of pain. Mirror visual feedback can also be considered if symptoms are unilateral. The evidence for effectiveness for any of these treatments is limited.

Summary

Pain after SCI is as common in children as it is in adults and its treatment is often suboptimal. Although the ISCIP classification may provide a useful template for differentiating between types of pain, a thorough assessment of the child with pain must take into consideration the impact of the pain on the child and daily family life, in addition to elucidating the pain characteristics.

Certain types of pain can be prevented by minimizing the stress on the body caused by SCI through the provision of appropriate equipment and by learning proper techniques for performing physical activities. However, multimodal treatment strategies – including pharmacologic strategies, psychological treatments, physical therapy, complementary and alternative treatments, and their combination – may be needed to treat the most recalcitrant pains and to reduce the associated disability and dysfunction related to these pains. When available, children with complex and disabling chronic pain may benefit from pain evaluation and treatment through a specialized interdisciplinary pediatric pain clinic.

REFERENCES

Arnet U, van Drongelen S, Scheel-Sailer A, van der Woude LH, Veeger DH (2012) Shoulder load during synchronous handcycling and handrim wheelchair propulsion in persons with paraplegia. *J Rehab Med* 44: 222–8. doi: 10.2340/16501977-0929

Bryce TN, Budh CN, Cardenas DD et al (2007) Pain after spinal cord injury: an evidence-based review for clinical practice and research. Report of the National Institute on Disability and Rehabilitation Research Spinal Cord Injury Measures meeting. *J Spinal Cord Med* 30: 421–40.

Bryce TN, Biering-Sorensen F, Finnerup NB et al (2012) International spinal cord injury pain classification: part I. Background and description. *Spinal Cord* 50: 413–17. doi: 10.1038/sc.2011156

Cardenas DD, Bryce TN, Shem K, Richards JS, Elhefni H (2004) Gender and minority differences in the pain experience of people with spinal cord injury. *Arch Phys Med Rehabil* 85: 1774–81. doi: 10.1016/j.apmr.200404.027

Cruccu G, Aziz TZ, Garcia-Larrea L et al (2007) EFNS guidelines on neurostimulation therapy for neuropathic pain. *Eur J Neurol* 14: 952–70. http://dx.doi.org/10.1111/j.1468-1331.2007.01916.x

Curtis KA, Tyner TM, Zachary L et al (1999) Effect of a standard exercise protocol on shoulder pain in long-term wheelchair users. *Spinal Cord* 37: 421–9. doi: 10.1038/sj.sc.3100860

Dijkers M, Bryce T, Zanca J (2009) Prevalence of chronic pain after traumatic spinal cord injury: a systematic review *J Rehab Res Dev* 46: 13–29. doi: 10.1682/JRRD.2008.040053

Falci S, Best L, Bayles R, Lammertse D, Starnes C (2002) Dorsal root entry zone microcoagulation for spinal cord injury-related central pain: operative intramedullary electrophysiological guidance and clinical outcome *J Neurosurg Spine* 97: 193–200. doi: 10.3171/spi.200297.2.0193

Finnerup NB, Faaborg P, Krogh K, Jensen TS (2008) Abdominal pain in long-term spinal cord injury. *Spinal Cord* 46: 198–203. doi: 10.1038/sj.sc.3102097

Gault D, Morel-Fatio M, Albert T, Fattal C (2009) Chronic neuropathic pain of spinal cord injury: what is the effectiveness of psychocomportemental management? *Ann Phys Rehabil Med* 52: 167–72. doi: 10.1016/j.rehab.200812.007

Harden RN, Bruehl S, Stanton-Hicks M, Wilson PR (2007) Proposed new diagnostic criteria for complex regional pain syndrome. *Pain Med* 8: 326–31. http://dx.doi.org/10.1111/j.1526-4637.2006.00169.x

Hicks CL, von Baeyer CL, Spafford PA, van Korlaar I, Goodenough B (2001) The Faces Pain Scale-Revised: toward a common metric in pediatric pain measurement. *Pain* 93: 173–83. doi: 10.1016/S0304-3959(01)00314-1

Jan FK, Wilson PE (2004) A survey of chronic pain in the pediatric spinal cord injury population. *J Spinal Cord Med* 27(Suppl 1): S50–3. doi:10.1097/PEP.0b013e318181162a

Jensen MP, Barber J, Romano JM et al (2009) Effects of self-hypnosis training and EMG biofeedback relaxation training on chronic pain in persons with spinal-cord injury. *Int J Clin Exp Hypn* 57: 239–68. doi: 10.1080/00207140902881007

Levendoglu F, Ogun CO, Ozerbil O, Ogun TC, Ugurlu H (2004) Gabapentin is a first line drug for the treatment of neuropathic pain in spinal cord injury. *Spine* 29: 743–51. doi: 10.1097/01.BRS000011206816108.3A

McGrath PJ, Walco GA, Turk DC et al; PedIMMPACT (2008) Core outcome domains and measures for pediatric acute and chronic/recurrent pain clinical trials: PedIMMPACT recommendations. *J Pain* 9: 771–83. doi: 10.1016/j.jpain.200804.007

Norrbrink C, Lundeberg T (2009) Tramadol in neuropathic pain after spinal cord injury: a randomized double-blind placebo-controlled trial. *Clin J Pain* 25: 177–84. doi: 10.1097/AJP0b013e31818a744d

Palermo TM, Eccleston C, Lewandowski AS, Williams AC, Morley S (2010) Randomized controlled trials of psychological therapies for management of chronic pain in children and adolescents: an updated meta-analytic review. *Pain* 148: 387–97. doi: 10.1016/j.pain.200910.004

Paralyzed Veterans of America Consortium for Spinal Cord Medicine (2005) Preservation of upper limb function following spinal cord injury: a clinical practice guideline for health-care professionals. *J Spinal Cord Med* 28: 434–70. doi: 10.1043/1079-0268-31.4.408

Rintala DH, Holmes SA, Courtade D, Fiess RN, Tastard LV, Loubser PG (2007) Comparison of the effectiveness of amitriptyline and gabapentin on chronic neuropathic pain in persons with spinal cord injury. *Arch Phys Med Rehabil* 88: 1547–60. doi: 10.1016/j.apmr.200707.038

Robert R, Perrouin-Verbe B, Albert T, Bussel B, Hamel O (2009) Chronic neuropathic pain in spinal cord injured patients: what is the effectiveness of surgical treatments excluding central neurostimulations? *Ann Phys Rehabil Med* 52: 194–202. doi: 10.1016/j.rehab.200812.016

Serra-Ano P, Pellicer-Chenoll M, Garcia-Masso X, Morales J, Giner-Pascual M, Gonzalez LM (2012) Effects of resistance training on strength pain and shoulder functionality in paraplegics. *Spinal Cord* 50: 827. doi: 10.1038/sc.201232

Siddall PJ, Molloy AR, Walker S, Mather LE, Rutkowski SB, Cousins MJ (2000) The efficacy of intrathecal morphine and clonidine in the treatment of pain after spinal cord injury. *Anesth Analg* 91: 1493–8. doi: 10.1097/00000539-200012000-00037

Siddall PJ, Cousins MJ, Otte A, Griesing T, Chambers R, Murphy TK (2006) Pregabalin in central neuropathic pain associated with spinal cord injury: a placebo-controlled trial. *Neurology* 67: 1792–800. doi: 10.1212/01.wnl.0000244422.45278.ff

Tan G, Rintala DH, Jensen MP et al (2011) Efficacy of cranial electrotherapy stimulation for neuropathic pain following spinal cord injury: a multi-site randomized controlled trial with a secondary 6-month open-label phase *J Spinal Cord Med* 34: 285–96. doi: 10.1179/2045772311Y.0000000008

Valkenburg AJ, van Dijk M, de Klein A, van den Anker JN, Tibboel D (2010) Pain management in intellectually disabled children: assessment treatment and translational research. *Dev Disabil Res Rev* 16: 248–57. doi: 10.1002/ddrr.117

Vogel LC, Krajci KA, Anderson CJ (2002) Adults with pediatric-onset spinal cord injuries: part 3: impact of medical complications. *J Spinal Cord Med* 25: 297–305.

Vogel LC, Chlan KM, Zebracki K, Anderson CJ (2011) Long-term outcomes of adults with pediatric-onset spinal cord injuries as a function of neurological impairment. *J Spinal Cord Med* 34: 60–6. doi: 10.1179/107902610X12883422813787

von Baeyer CL, Spagrud LJ, McCormick JC, Choo E, Neville K, Connelly MA (2009) Three new datasets supporting use of the Numerical Rating Scale (NRS-11) for children's self-reports of pain intensity. *Pain* 143: 223–7. doi: 10.1016/j.pain.2009.03.002

Section 5 Neuromusculoskeletal Management

18
ORTHOPEDIC COMPLICATIONS

Randal R Betz and H Herndon Murray

Introduction

Musculoskeletal complications are the most frequent manifestations of secondary complications of pediatric spinal cord injury (SCI). They should be anticipated, and thus they require careful surveillance over the lifetime of the child. This chapter describes orthopedic complications of pediatric SCI, discusses treatment options, and, where available, provides outcomes of treatment. Neuromuscular scoliosis is discussed in relation to other orthopedic complications, but because of its high incidence and complexity with respect to prevention, management, and definitive treatment, Chapter 19 is devoted to this topic.

Hip instability

Hip dislocation, subluxation, and contractures are extremely common in pediatric SCI, especially among children injured at younger ages (Rink and Miller 1990, Betz and Mulcahey 1994, Miller and Betz 1996). In one series, hip instability was observed in 100% of children who were injured when they were younger than 5 years of age and in 93% of those injured when they were younger than 10 years (Fig. 18.1) (McCarthy and Betz 2006).

Development of hip instability occurs in patients with tetraplegia or paraplegia, in males and females, and in patients with flaccid and spastic SCI. In a patient who has gone through puberty, the most likely cause of a new hip dislocation is sepsis, and it is essential that any relatively acute, radiographically identified dislocated hip has an aspiration and adequate workup to rule out sepsis.

Because of the high incidence of hip instability and contractures in children injured when they are 10 years of age or younger, an aggressive prevention approach is recommended. This would include active soft tissue stretching, control of spasticity, prophylactic abduction bracing, and sleeping prone.

Indications for surgical management of hip instability are not entirely clear. With the development of functional electrical stimulation (FES) systems for standing and walking and the future possibility for spinal cord regeneration, aggressive prophylactic surgical treatment of hip instability should be considered (Weinstein 2001: p. 607, Betz et al 2001). If a patient has spasticity and there is opportunity for neurorecovery or future restoration with biological repairs or FES, then the hips should be aggressively prevented from being allowed to dislocate, including adequate control of severe spasticity with medication and/or a baclofen pump.

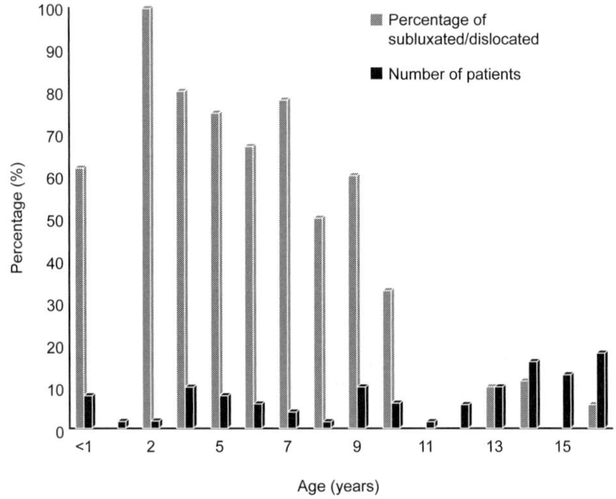

Fig. 18.1 Percentage of hips subluxated or dislocated plotted against age; 93% of those ≤10 years old at the time of SCI had subluxed or dislocated hips, versus only 9% of those >10 years old (McCarthy and Betz 2006).

Often it is the subluxing hip that causes the irritation which is exacerbating the spasticity. If the patient has flaccid paralysis, future biological repair of the SCI may not restore motor function; therefore, aggressive treatment of hip subluxations is not as urgent. Surgical treatment of patients with early subluxation is similar to that of patients who have low lumbar level myelodysplasia, especially if unilateral. Patients with lap belt injuries and low-level motor levels such as L3–L4 would be good candidates for keeping the hip reduced. A muscle balancing procedure is needed in addition to bony procedures in these patients with flaccid paralysis, such as the Lindseth external oblique muscle to the greater trochanter (Thomas et al 1950, Dias 1995).

Surgical treatment options for hip instability

A proximal femoral varus osteotomy is used to treat many subluxated hips, along with a Dega osteotomy for posterior augmentation of the acetabulum (Betz 1997, McCarthy and Betz 2006). Generally, most standard osteotomies used for congenitally dislocated hips are not adequate with regards to posterior coverage, as most of the subluxated and dislocated hips in these paralytic populations are unstable posteriorly. Additional acetabular procedures that do seem to be able to correct the posterior subluxation include a reverse triple innominate osteotomy or a Ganz osteotomy (Fig. 18.2a,b), or a posterior shelf osteotomy (Betz et al 2001).

In patients with flaccid paralysis who are having the hip reduced, a muscle transfer is needed to help maintain reduction of the hip. An external oblique transfer (Lindseth procedure) can be performed (see above). Although it may not always result in an active transfer, it may still be effective in maintaining hip stability, while functioning as a tenodesis. In patients with spastic SCI, a group that is treated almost the same as children with subluxated hips secondary

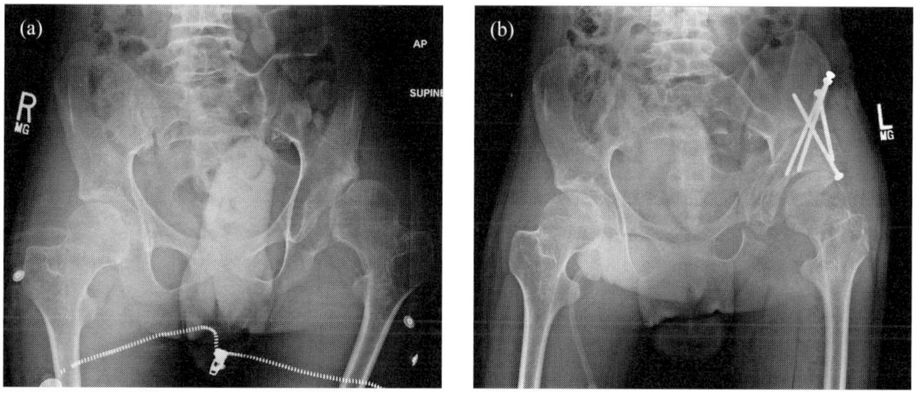

Fig. 18.2 (a) Preoperative anteroposterior view of hips showing subluxation of the left hip in a 15-year-old skeletally mature patient with thoracic level spinal cord injury. (b) Postoperative film showing excellent posterior coverage with a Ganz osteotomy (case courtesy of Dr Harold Van Bosse, photographs printed with permission).

to cerebral palsy, it is essential to control spasticity first before attempting to relocate the hip. Oral medication is tried first; however, it may be necessary to insert a baclofen pump. Complications unique to operating on the hip in children with SCI include development of heterotopic ossification around the operated hip. Prophylaxis with an anti-inflammatory drug (indomethacin 25mg three times per day or tolmetin sodium in children younger than 12 years) for 3 months after surgery has been useful. In addition, etidronate disodium is prescribed for 6 months.

Hip instability and scoliosis

Scoliosis that occurs concomitantly with a subluxated hip presents unique challenges in treatment. For example, complete correction of the scoliosis and pelvic obliquity helps to correct the early subluxation of the hip. After the spinal fusion is performed, hip contractures are often present and need to be released to help correct the hip subluxation and allow for proper sitting balance after scoliosis surgery.

Occasionally, scoliosis is caused by a pseudo hip flexion contracture (abduction contracture of the tensor fascia lata muscle and the gluteus medius). Pseudo hip flexion contracture can be identified by taking a hip that clearly shows a hip flexion contracture greater than 20 degrees and abducting the hip maximally, such that the hip flexion contracture almost disappears. This demonstrates tightness of the abductors and the tensor fascia femoris muscles and causes a pelvic obliquity (Fig. 18.3a–e). The modified Soutter release, which is a standard anterolateral approach to the hip that would be performed for osteotomies such as a Salter (Smith 1980), is a useful approach. The apophysis over the iliac wing is split anteriorly from approximately the mid-axillary line down to the anterior inferior iliac spine. The apophysis and gluteus muscles are stripped from the outer table of the ilium posteriorly enough that the muscle alignment is straight off the midline of the torso (no future flexion vector pull of the

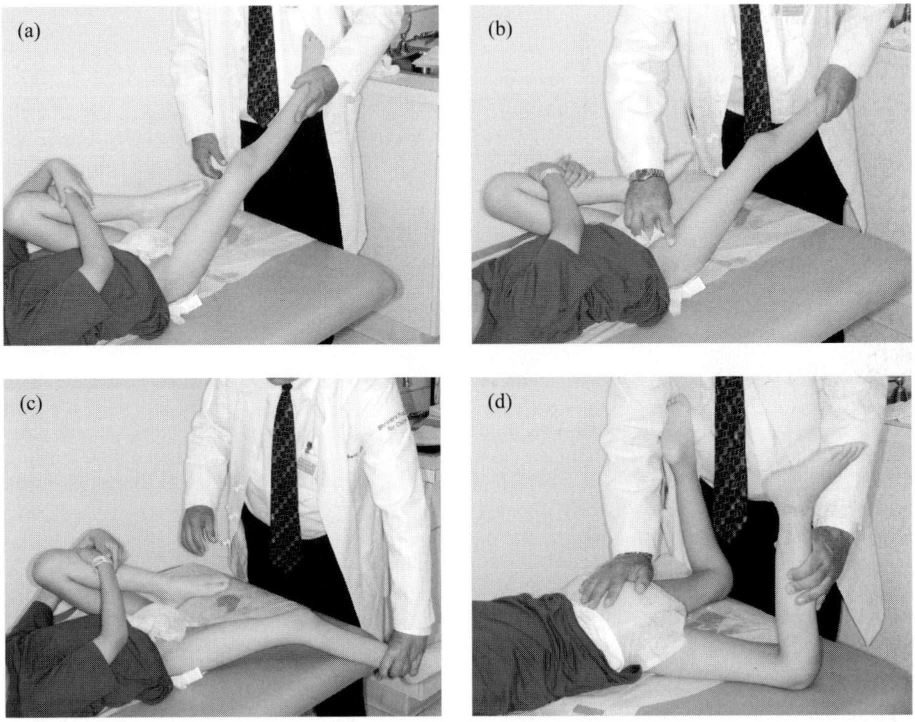

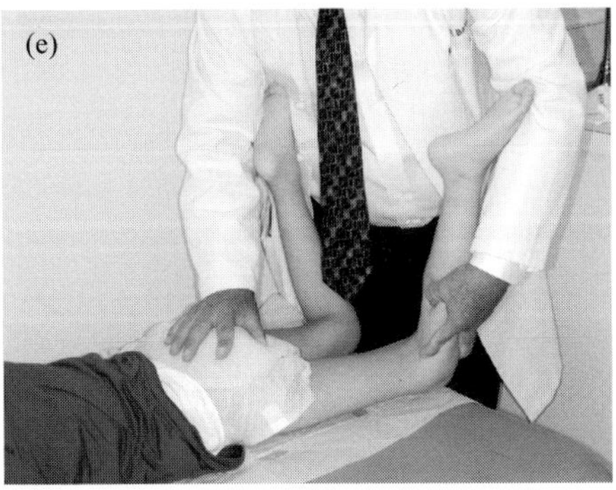

Fig. 18.3 Pseudo hip flexion contracture. (a) Flex opposite left hip to flatten the lumbar spine. (b) The right hip shows flexion contracture. Finger is on the tight tensor fascia femoris muscle. (c) The right hip is abducted and the flexion contracture is significantly reduced owing to the tight tensor fascia femoris and anterior gluteus medius muscle fibers becoming slack with abduction. (d,e) Non-operative treatment stretching. Prone position and stretch tensor fascia femoris and anterior gluteus medius.

muscles). The iliac crest is then trimmed, such that reattachment to bone cannot cause recurrence of the flexion contracture. This muscle release corrects the pelvic obliquity. The mild scoliosis can now be braced, and the risk of the opposite subluxated hip progressing to full subluxation or dislocation is reduced. A case example is shown in Figure 18.4a–d.

On some occasions the scoliosis needs surgical treatment, and the subluxated hip is so unstable that it must be surgically repaired as well. The overall principle here is to correct the spinal deformity (see Chapter 19) and pelvic obliquity completely before the surgery on the

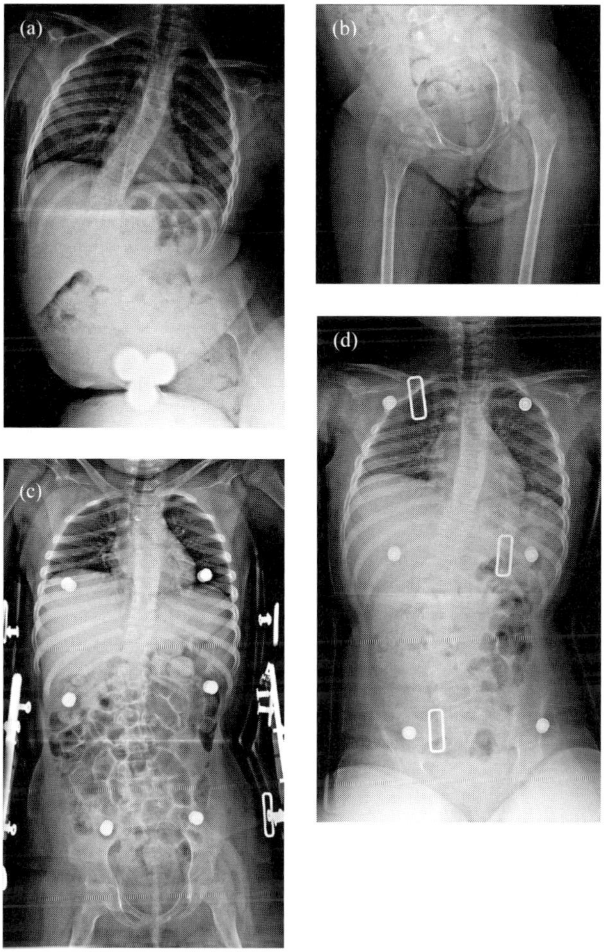

Fig. 18.4 (a) Anteroposterior view of the spine sitting: 9-year-old female after lap belt injury with T12 flaccid paralysis. She has severe scoliosis and pelvic obliquity. (b) Anteroposterior view of pelvis. The right hip has a very tight pseudo hip flexion contracture, which is felt to be causing the pelvic obliquity and aggravating the scoliosis. The left hip is then adducted, also now with fixed contracture and at risk of dislocating. (c) Anteroposterior view of spine and hips supine after bilateral hip releases: Soutter on the right hip and adductor/flexion release on the left hip. Scoliosis is corrected significantly and the hips are now not at risk. (d) Anteroposterior view of spine sitting in orthoses after hip releases. Patient could not have worn orthoses. There is considerable improvement compared with (a).

hip. The first reason is that, without correcting the pelvic obliquity first, the hip will not stay reduced for long because of the persistent adducted position secondary to the pelvic obliquity. The second reason for correcting the spine first is that there is very low prevalence of deep venous thrombosis (DVT) or pulmonary embolus after spine surgery in the SCI population. In contrast, surgery on the hip has a high prevalence of DVTs, even with prophylaxis. This makes it extremely difficult to operate on the spine after the hip because of the perioperative risk created by DVT prophylaxis and/or treatment, particularly if a DVT does occur.

Generally, the hip is treated a few weeks after the spine is corrected. After spine surgery, the patient is put on enoxaparin for DVT prophylaxis. Doppler studies to rule out DVTs are performed at least twice. If the spine wound is completely dry and without any evidence of draining hematoma or infection, approximately 2 to 3 weeks later it is generally appropriate to operate on the subluxated hip that needs treatment.

Soft tissue joint contractures

The prevalence of joint contractures has not been adequately studied in the pediatric population. In a study by Diong et al (2012) of 92 adult patients (over 18 years of age) who were followed prospectively, the proportion of all study patients who developed at least one contracture in any joint was 66% (95% CI 55–77%) (Diong et al 2012). The development of contracture was defined as a loss in range of motion of at least 10 degrees between the baseline and 1-year follow-up measurements. The proportion of participants with paraplegia who developed at least one contracture in any joint according to this definition of contracture was 47% (95% CI 31–64%). The proportion of participants with tetraplegia who developed at least one contracture in any joint according to this definition was 83% (95% CI 71–95%). In the study by Diong et al (2012), the incidence of contracture at each joint was the following: shoulder 43%, elbow and forearm 33%, wrist and hand 41%, hip 32%, knee 11%, and ankle 40%. Unfortunately, this study did not address clinically significant contractures (Diong et al 2012).

Hip contractures are common in children with SCI and can interfere with ambulation, particularly if they exceed 30 to 40 degrees. Unfortunately, just as in adults, stretching through physical therapy rarely results in improvement of joint range when dealing with a true joint contracture (Harvey et al 2011). Surgical releases are usually needed; however, recurrences are frequent (Lindseth 1996). The management of hip contractures must be individualized and based on the neurologic level, presence of hip dysplasia, and ambulation status. Hip contractures are generally managed by surgical releases and aggressive postoperative bracing and physical therapy. However, contracture releases should be limited to those with significant potential for continued ambulation with or without braces. Pseudo hip flexion contractures prevent erect standing and prevent the use of the reciprocating hip orthosis commonly used by patients with low lumbar level injuries. These pseudo hip flexion contractures can be released easily via a Soutter approach, as described in the earlier section 'Hip instability and scoliosis' in this chapter. Hip and knee contractures in older children are probably a consequence of disinterest in ambulation and increased use of wheeled mobility; therefore, contracture releases in these patients may not result in improved ambulation, and recurrence of the contractures are very common. For very severe knee flexion contractures preventing sitting and supine activities, the author has used bilateral femoral shortenings (over femoral nails) to accomplish improvement in joint range without the massive soft tissue destruction inherent in releases.

Heterotopic ossification

The incidence of heterotopic ossification in children with SCI is approximately 3% compared with approximately 20% in adults with SCI (Betz 1997, Garland 1991). Similar to adults, children and adolescents with SCI often experience hip problems. The average onset of heterotopic ossification is 14 months after injury for children and adolescents with SCI, compared with the typical onset of 1 to 4 months after injury in adults with SCI (Garland et al 1989).

Cipriano and colleagues studied various imaging techniques in the diagnosis of heterotopic ossification (Cipriano et al 2009), and it is recommended that the reader consult that reference for more details. The first author of this chapter (RRB) uses a three-phase bone scan using technetium Tc-99m-labeled methylene diphosphonate for early diagnosis where the blood phase can show a high probability of heterotopic ossification developing even before bone formation starts (Banovac et al 1997). The second author of this chapter (HHM) prefers magnetic resonance imaging (MRI) for early diagnosis when there is a clinical suggestion surrounding a particular joint. Argyropoulou et al (2006) found MRI to be more effective than radiography at demonstrating early heterotopic ossification in patients in the acute hospitalization setting. MRI was able to detect heterotopic ossification formation approximately 20 days after injury, confirming the diagnosis, on average, 1.4 days after the onset of clinical symptoms; radiography, however, did not detect evidence of heterotopic ossification until 23 days after the development of symptoms, on average. The earlier the diagnosis, the earlier treatment can start. More aggressive treatment such as radiation can be given when heterotopic ossification is occurring despite medical prophylaxis.

Prophylaxis for heterotopic ossification utilizing etidronate disodium (Banovac et al 1997) is not routinely used in the pediatric SCI population because of the relatively low risk of heterotopic ossification in pediatric patients (compared with 20% in adults [Garland 1991]).

In addition, etidronate disodium may be contraindicated in children before puberty because of the potential development of rachitic-like changes in the growth plates of long bones (Bellah et al 1992, Pazzaglia et al 1993, Silverman et al 1994). If there is evidence of early heterotopic ossification formation suspected clinically or diagnosed by a positive bone scan, ultrasound, MRI or computed tomography, an anti-inflammatory drug such as indomethacin or tolmetin sodium (which is approved for children younger than 12y) may be beneficial. In RRB's experience, almost every case of hip heterotopic ossification is concomitant with a sterile non-inflammatory knee effusion. It is conjectured that knee effusion may be a sympathetic response to the hip inflammation causing the heterotopic ossification.

The approach to management of heterotopic ossification in the pediatric SCI population is similar to that for adult SCI. Indications for surgical interventions would be significant functional deficits. Resection of heterotopic ossification probably should be undertaken approximately 1 year after its onset. The literature and our experience recommend no further delay in resection, so that progression of femoral neck osteoporosis and intra-articular fibrosis can be avoided (Garland 1991). A recommendation from 20 years ago suggested that surgery should be postponed until the bone scan and alkaline phosphatase are normal (Garland 1991, Freebourn et al 1999); however, this should not be followed. Instead, surgery should be considered once a functional problem exists, which may be only 1 year after onset. Severe osteoporosis can occur in the femoral neck region if one waits longer than 1 year. After surgery, prophylaxis is essential. Indomethacin (1–3mg/kg/day t.i.d. or q.i.d., maximum dose of 200mg/day) or tolmetin sodium is used in the postoperative period (Wick et al 1999). Postoperative use of radiation therapy is usually contraindicated as initial treatment in younger children because there are theoretical long-term consequences of radiation-induced sarcomas. However, for recurrences and severe cases of heterotopic ossification, radiation is the only prophylactic treatment that seems to work.

Long-bone fractures

Osteopenia begins immediately after sustaining an SCI and plateaus between 6 and 12 months after injury. Children and adolescents with SCI have bone densities of approximately 60% of age- and sex-matched individuals with typical development (Betz et al 1991, Moynahan et al 1996). In a study by Lauer and colleagues, a combination of standing, stepping, or cycling with FES has shown an increase in bone mineral density by approximately 25% (Lauer et al 2007).

Pathologic long-bone fractures occur as a consequence of loss of bone mineral density in approximately 14% of children and adolescents with SCI (Betz and Mulcahey 1994). In a study by Salkin and Betz et al (1988, unpublished material), the etiology in 40% of the patients included gait training, range of motion, and minor trauma. The etiology of the pathologic fractures in the remaining 60% of the patients was not identified. Patients with pathologic fractures typically present with fever and a swollen extremity. The most common sites of fracture are the supracondylar region of the femur and the proximal tibia. Initial radiologic findings may be subtle, and the diagnosis of a pathologic fracture in growing children may require a high index of suspicion. If there is a delayed diagnosis of a fracture through long-bone growth plates, an additional issue arises. This fracture through the growth plate, with its massive periosteal reaction, can radiographically appear similar to a malignant bone tumor (Wenger et al 1980). An experienced pediatric radiologist and pediatric orthopedist should be consulted so that children are not subjected to unwarranted biopsies or other tumor procedures.

Treatment of pathologic fractures should preferably consist of removable splints (Betz and Mulcahey 1994, Miller 1996). If casts are necessary, they must be well padded over all bony prominences and bivalved to enable skin inspection to prevent pressure ulcers. Because the bone is osteoporotic, it generally will not hold internal plates or external fixation devices very well; however, intramedullary nailing may be very helpful in preventing further deformity or shortening and allows for earlier mobilization. Fortunately, an exuberant callus develops within 3 to 4 weeks, at which time the splinting or casting can be minimized with resumption of range of motion. Ambulation with orthotics should be postponed for 6 to 8 weeks after sustaining a fracture.

Prevention of fractures is critical but may be particularly challenging in the pediatric SCI population because of risk-taking behavior observed in children and adolescents of different ages. Caregivers must focus on safety in risky activities. Bone mineral loss should be minimized by encouraging weight bearing with orthotics or FES. Good nutrition and adequate sunlight are important. Persons with SCI have been reported to have a higher prevalence of vitamin D deficiency than able-bodied persons, and an effective and safe vitamin D replacement protocol is necessary. One study found that 2000IU of vitamin D_3 generally raises levels from absolute or relative deficiency into an acceptable range in individuals who are supplemented with calcium (Bauman et al 2011). Although this study was not performed on children with SCI, it suggests that bisphosphonates such as alendronate do not reliably improve bone density in children and young adults with primarily neuromuscular disease (Dominguez-Bartmess et al 2012).

Spinal cord syrinx

Hydrosyringomyelia, or cystic formation in the spinal cord, may also be referred to as syringomyelia, hydromyelia, or syrinx (Isu et al 1990, Nohria and Oakes 1994, Menkes and Till 1995). Spinal cord syrinxes are prevalent in both children and adults after SCI, occurring in approximately 50% of adults (Hussey et al 1990) and children (Backe et al 1991). These syrinxes are generally asymptomatic but can clearly affect upper extremity function, and a pre-operative MRI is indicated in all patients considering upper extremity reconstructive surgery as a baseline to determine that there is not a large syrinx that currently or may in the future cause further motor neuron loss. The authors have seen an expanding syrinx in an individual cause a loss of function after tendon transfers.

Summary

Numerous orthopedic problems occur as children continue to grow after an SCI, including hip instability (43%), joint contractures (83%), heterotopic ossification (3.3%), pathologic long-bone fractures (14%), and spinal cord syrinx (51%). Conservative measures are the primary component of treatment. Surgery may be necessary on occasion for these orthopedic problems, but if done appropriately when indicated, it can have a significant positive outcome for these children.

REFERENCES

Argyropoulou MI, Kostandi E, Kosta P et al (2006) Heterotopic ossification of the knee joint in intensive care unit patients: early diagnosis with magnetic resonance imaging. *Crit Care* 10: R152. http://dx.doi.org/10.1097/BSD.0b013e31821fbf72

Backe HA, Betz RR, Mesgarzadeh M, Beck T, Clancy M (1991) Post-traumatic spinal cord cysts evaluated by magnetic resonance imaging. *Paraplegia* 29: 607–12. http://dx.doi.org/10.1038/sc.1991.89

Banovac K, Gonzalez F, Renfree KJ (1997) Treatment of heterotopic ossification after spinal cord injury. *J Spinal Cord Med* 20: 60–5.

Bauman WA, Emmons RR, Cirnigliaro CM, Kirshblum SC, Spungen AM (2011) An effective oral vitamin D replacement therapy in persons with spinal cord injury. *J Spinal Cord Med* 34: 455–60. http://dx.doi.org/10.1179/2045772311Y.0000000032

Bellah RD, Zawodniak L, Librizzi RJ, Harris MC (1992) Idiopathic arterial calcification of infancy: prenatal and postnatal effects of therapy in an infant. *J Pediatr* 121: 930–3. http://dx.doi.org/10.1016/S0022-3476(05)80345-2

Betz RR, Mulcahey MJ (2001) Spinal cord injury rehabilitation. In: Weinstein SL (ed.). *The Pediatric Spine: Principles and Practice*. 2nd Ed. Philadelphia, PA: Lippincott Williams & Wilkins, p. 607.

Betz RR, Triolo RJ, Hermida VM et al (1991) The effects of functional neuromuscular stimulation on the bone mineral content in the lower limbs of spinal cord injured children. *J Am Paraplegia Soc* 14: 65–6.

Betz RR, Mulcahey MJ, Smith BT, Triolo RJ, McCarthy JJ (2001) Implications of hip subluxation for FES-assisted mobility in patients with spinal cord injury. *Orthopedics* 24: 181–4.

Cipriano CA, Pill SG, Keenan MA (2009) Heterotopic ossification following traumatic brain injury and spinal cord injury. *J Am Acad Orthop Surg* 17: 689–97.

Dias LS (1995) Myelomeningocele. In: Canale ST, Beaty JH (eds). *Operative Pediatric Orthopaedics*. 2nd Ed. St. Louis, MO: C.V. Mosby. pp. 765–6.

Diong J, Harvey LA, Kwah LK et al (2012) Incidence and predictors of contracture after spinal cord injury – a prospective cohort study. *Spinal Cord* 50: 579–84. http://dx.doi.org/10.1038/sc.2012.25

Dominguez-Bartmess SN, Tandberg D, Cheema AM, Szalay EA (2012) Efficacy of alendronate in the treatment of low bone density in the pediatric and young adult population. *J Bone Joint Surg Am* 94: e621–6. http://dx.doi.org/10.2106/JBJS.K.00751

Freebourn TM, Barber DB, Able AC (1999) The treatment of immature heterotopic ossification in spinal cord injuries with combination surgery, radiation therapy and NSAID. *Spinal Cord* 37: 50–3. http://dx.doi.org/10.1038/sj.sc.3100719

Garland DE (1991) A clinical perspective on common forms of acquired heterotopic ossification. *Clin Orthop Rel Res* 263: 13–29. http://dx.doi.org/10.1097/00003086-199102000-00003

Garland DE, Shimoyama ST, Lugo C, Barras D, Gilgoff I (1989) Spinal cord insults and heterotopic ossification in the pediatric population. *Clin Orthop Rel Res* 245: 303–10. http://dx.doi.org/10.1097/00003086-198908000-00046

Harvey LA, Glinsky JA, Katalinic OM, Ben M (2011) Contracture management for people with spinal cord injuries. *NeuroRehabilitation* 28: 17–20. doi: 10.3233/NRE-2011-0627

Hussey RW, Ha C, Vijay M, Lipper M, Kubota R (1990) Prospective duty of the occurrence of posttraumatic cystic degeneration of the spinal cord utilizing magnetic resonance imaging. *J Am Paraplegia Soc* 13: 1–20 (abstract 41).

Isu T, Iwasaki Y, Akino M, Abe H (1990) Hydrosyringomyelia associated with a Chiari I malformation in children and adolescents. *Neurosurgery* 26: 591–6. http://dx.doi.org/10.1097/00006123-199004000-00006

Lauer R, Johnston TE, Smith BT, Mulcahey MJ, Betz RR, Maurer AH (2007) Bone mineral density of the hip and knee in children with spinal cord injury. *J Spinal Cord Med* 30(Suppl 1): S10–14.

Lindseth RE (1996) Myelomeningocele. In: Morrissy RT, Weinstein SL (eds). *Lovell & Winter's Pediatric Orthopaedics*. 4th Ed. Philadelphia, PA: Lippincott-Raven. pp. 503–35.

McCarthy JJ, Betz RR (2006) Hip disorders in children who have spinal cord injury. *Orthop Clin N Am* 37: 197–202. http://dx.doi.org/10.1016/j.ocl.2005.09.004

Menkes JH, Till K (1995) Malformations of the central nervous system. In: Menkes JH (ed.). *Textbook of Child Neurology*. 5th Ed. Baltimore, MD: Williams & Wilkins. pp. 240–324.

Miller F (1996) Pathologic long-bone fractures: diagnosis, etiology, management, and prevention. In: Betz RR, Mulcahey MJ (eds). *The Child With a Spinal Cord Injury.* Rosemont, IL: American Academy of Orthopaedic Surgeons. pp. 331–8.

Miller F, Betz RR (1996) Hip joint instability. In: Betz RR, Mulcahey MJ (eds). *The Child with a Spinal Cord Injury.* Rosemont, IL: American Academy of Orthopaedic Surgeons. pp. 353–61.

Moynahan M, Betz RR, Triolo RJ, Maurer AH (1996) Characterization of the bone mineral density of children with spinal cord injury. *J Spinal Cord Med* 19: 249–54.

Nohria V, Oakes WJ (1994) Chiari malformations, hydrosyringomyelia, and the tethered cord syndrome. In: Weinstein SL (ed.). *The Pediatric Spine: Principles and Practice.* New York, NY: Raven Press. pp. 685–705.

Pazzaglia UE, Beluffi G, Ravelli A, Zatti G, Martini A (1993) Chronic intoxication by ethane-1-hydroxy-1,1-diphosphonate (EHDP) in a child with myositis ossificans progressiva. *Pediatr Radiol* 23: 459–62. http://dx.doi.org/10.1007/BF02012453

Rink P, Miller F (1990) Hip instability in spinal cord injury patients. *J Pediatr Orthop* 10: 583–7. http://dx.doi.org/10.1097/01241398-199009000-00002

Silverman SL, Hurvitz EA, Nelson VS, Chiodo A (1994) Rachitic syndrome after disodium etidronate therapy in an adolescent. *Arch Phys Med Rehabil* 75: 118–20.

Smith H (1980) Ankylosis and deformity. In: Edmonson AS, Crenshaw AH (eds). *Campbell's Operative Orthopaedics*. 6th Ed. St. Louis, MO: The C.V. Mosby Co. p. 1153.

Thomas LI, Thompson TC, Straub LR (1950) Transplantation of the external oblique muscle for abductor paralysis. *J Bone Joint Surg Am* 32: 207–17.

Wenger DR, Jeffcoat BT, Herring JA (1980) The guarded prognosis of physeal injury in paraplegic children. *J Bone Joint Surg Am* 62: 241–6.

Wick M, Muller EJ, Hahn MP, Muhr G (1999) Surgical excision of heterotopic bone after hip surgery followed by oral indomethacin application: is there a clinical benefit for the patient? *Arch Orthop Trauma Surg* 119: 151–5. http://dx.doi.org/10.1007/s004020050379

19
NEUROMUSCULAR SCOLIOSIS

Joshua M Pahys, Randal R Betz and Amer F Samdani

Case vignette

Stephanie has C7 tetraplegia from a birth injury; he has spastic paralysis and is non-ambulatory. At 5 years of age, he presented with a 25-degree neuromuscular scoliosis and dislocation of his right hip; the left hip was tight but located. A thoracolumbosacral orthosis was prescribed for 23 hours a day to slow the progression of scoliosis. The right hip was managed surgically, and aggressive preventive measures were established to protect the left hip from dislocating, including prone sleeping, stretching, and pharmacologic management of the spasticity (see Chapter 18). Once he was cleared from postoperative hip precautions, a standing program was initiated and an upright mobility program was pursued (see Chapters 12 and 18). Stephanie was monitored every 6 months for the progression of scoliosis and for modifications to the thoracolumbosacral orthosis to accommodate growth and curve progression; the Cobb angle remained under 40 degrees until 11 years of age. Between 12 years and 13 years 7 months of age, the Cobb angle increased from 40 to 55 degrees over two visits. A spinal fusion was recommended to prevent further progression and functional decline; the family declined and requested continued surveillance of the curve. At 16 years of age, the Cobb angle measured 95 degrees; there was significant pelvic obliquity despite both hips being located, and Stephanie reported an inability to sit upright for more than 4 hours owing to breathing difficulties, necessitating a reclining chair at school. At 16 years 6 months of age, Stephanie underwent a definitive spinal fusion with instrumentation from T2 to the pelvis; the Cobb angle was reduced from 95 to 20 degrees, the pelvic obliquity was corrected, and, after 3 months of postoperative recovery, Stephanie was able to sit upright for 10 hours a day. After the fusion, Stephanie reported no decline in function and reported improved sitting balance and breathing.

Etiology

Spinal deformity as a result of spinal cord injury (SCI) most commonly affects children and adolescents, but may also affect adults. The coronal and/or sagittal plane deformity typically develops secondary to muscle weakness and imbalance. The development of progressive kyphosis alone can also present as a residual deformity after a fracture or can be iatrogenic secondary to a laminectomy possibly performed at the time of initial surgical stabilization (Mayfield et al 1981).

Prevalence

The prevalence of neuromuscular scoliosis in SCI is quite high, especially when an injury occurs in a younger patient. Lancourt et al (1981) reported that the prevalence of scoliosis was 100% in patients with SCI under the age of 10 years, 19% in patients aged from 11 to 16 years, and 12% in patients over 16 years of age. Dearolf et al (1990) found that the need for surgery for spinal deformity resulting from SCI was 67% if the injury occurred before maturity. In perhaps the largest cohort studied to date, Mulcahey et al (2013) reported that age at injury was the single predictive factor of scoliosis in children with SCI.

Problems associated with spinal deformity in spinal cord injury

A multitude of problems can be incurred as a result of spinal deformity in a patient with SCI. Most notably, the spinal deformity can lead to significant pelvic obliquity that results in poor sitting balance; this puts the patient at risk of pressure ulcerations from asymmetrical sitting. Furthermore, poor sitting ability can inhibit upper extremity function and lead to difficulties fitting and using lower extremity orthotics. It has been shown that gastrointestinal dysfunction can result from severe pelvic obliquity, and a patient's cardiopulmonary status can be negatively impacted when the spinal deformity progresses above 80 to 90 degrees (Driscoll and Skinner, 2008) (Fig. 19.1a–d).

Non-operative management

BRACING

Historically, the timing and efficacy of bracing for neuromuscular scoliosis have been debated. The standard bracing protocols for idiopathic scoliosis were often followed for patients with SCI, and bracing was initiated only after the curves progressed to more than 25 degrees in growing children. However, more recently, Mehta et al (2004) evaluated a more aggressive bracing regimen (Table 19.1). The study demonstrated a significant reduction in the need for surgery when brace treatment was initiated on curves of less than 20 degrees. There was a trend toward a reduction in the need for surgery if bracing was started when the curves measured 21 to 40 degrees, although this was not statistically significant (p=0.08). There was minimal to no effect on the need for surgery when bracing was initiated on curves of more than 40 degrees. The timing of surgery was also evaluated in the study, and similar trends were found with regards to earlier bracing (Table 19.2). There was a significantly prolonged delay in the need for surgery of over 4 years when patients were braced with a curve measuring less than 10 degrees. A 3-year delay was noted when bracing was initiated for curves between 11 and 20 degrees. Finally, only a 1-year delay in surgery was identified when bracing was started for curves between 21 and 40 degrees.

Compliance with brace wear can be a challenge for any pediatric patient (Miller et al 2012). However, this hurdle is increased for children with pre-existing functional limitations secondary to SCI. A study of pediatric patients with SCI demonstrated a 28% reduction in the

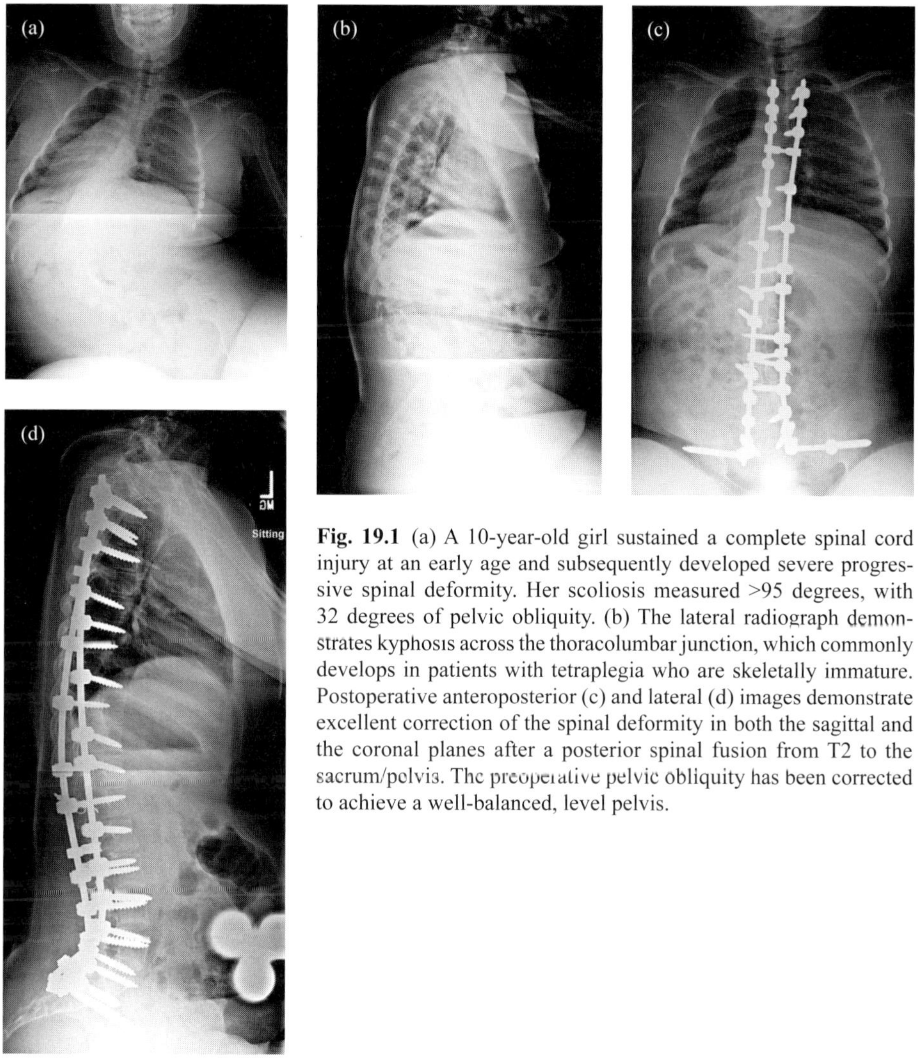

Fig. 19.1 (a) A 10-year-old girl sustained a complete spinal cord injury at an early age and subsequently developed severe progressive spinal deformity. Her scoliosis measured >95 degrees, with 32 degrees of pelvic obliquity. (b) The lateral radiograph demonstrates kyphosis across the thoracolumbar junction, which commonly develops in patients with tetraplegia who are skeletally immature. Postoperative anteroposterior (c) and lateral (d) images demonstrate excellent correction of the spinal deformity in both the sagittal and the coronal planes after a posterior spinal fusion from T2 to the sacrum/pelvis. The preoperative pelvic obliquity has been corrected to achieve a well-balanced, level pelvis.

TABLE 19.1
Number of patients requiring surgery (from Mehta et al [2004])

Group	*n*	Braced	Not braced	*p* value
I (<10°)	42	13/29	10/13	0.03
II (11–20°)	25	9/18	6/7	0.04
III (21–40°)	27	12/20	6/7	0.08

TABLE 19.2
Time to surgery from presentation (y:mo) (from Mehta et al [2004])

Group	*n*	Braced	Not braced	*p* value
I (<10°)	42	8:6	4:3	0.002
II (11–20°)	25	6:10	3:9	0.008
III (21–40°)	27	4:3	3:3	0.38

reachable workspace when the children were wearing the thoracolumbosacral orthosis (TLSO) (Sison-Williamson et al 2007). These potential limitations in upper extremity range of motion can compromise a patient's independence and may hinder his or her compliance. Preliminary studies have been underpowered, so that sufficient evidence on brace wear compliance in this patient population has not been provided. However, given that approximately two-thirds of all patients who sustain an SCI before maturity will require a spinal fusion, the practitioner must aggressively pursue and encourage non-operative management to potentially diminish and/or delay this unacceptably high risk of surgery.

Wheelchair Modifications

Additional and/or alternative options to the brace can be attempted by modifying the seating system of the wheelchair. Lateral supports on a wheelchair may or may not affect curve progression but can be useful for improving sitting balance and allowing the use of the arms. The patient's wheelchair should be intermittently pressure mapped to identify areas of increased dependence owing to pelvic obliquity. Variations can be made in seating materials, and custom molding can be used to attempt to reduce the development of pressure ulcerations.

Upright Mobility

Ambulation for children and adolescents with SCI is encouraged, noting that varying degrees of functional ambulation (i.e. using ambulation as the primary means of mobility) is highly dependent upon the neurologic and motor level of the SCI (see Chapter 22). Although not specifically evaluated in the pediatric SCI population, a relationship between cessation of walking and curve development and progression has been shown in patients with Duchenne muscular dystrophy (Smith et al 1989, Kinali et al 2007). The spinal orthosis can be utilized as the pelvic portion of a hip–knee–ankle–foot orthosis. Alternatively, the pelvic portion of the hip–knee–ankle–foot orthosis can be modified to fit over the spinal orthosis to allow concomitant wear of both braces.

Surgical management

Indications for Surgery

Surgical intervention is recommended for progressive spinal deformity secondary to SCI when the curvatures progress to more than 40 degrees and/or significant functional limitations are encountered related to the deformity. The nature of the procedure is dependent upon the patient's age and skeletal maturity. Typically, standard spinal fusions can be performed on children older than 10 years of age, whereas specialized instrumentation allowing for continued spine and chest wall growth is considered for patients younger than 10 years with significant deformities.

The threshold curve magnitude of greater than 40 degrees for surgical intervention in skeletally immature patients is derived, in part, from the study of patients with spina bifida. Muller and colleagues reported an average progression of 13 degrees per year once the curve exceeded 40 degrees in patients with spina bifida (Muller et al 1992). Complication rates have also been reported to be significantly higher for surgical intervention with larger spinal deformities (>70 degrees) (Samdani et al 2011).

Spinal fusion may also be considered for scoliosis in a skeletally mature patient with SCI if the deformity leads to significant functional limitations. Poor sitting balance can result in pressure ulcerations on the dependent buttocks and hip. Furthermore, sitting imbalance can restrict the maximal capacity of the patient's upper extremities. Finally, cardiopulmonary function has also been shown to be negatively affected by severe spinal deformity.

Growing Instrumentation

Standard spinal fusion is typically avoided in patients under the age of 10 years with curves of more than 40 degrees, as significant spinal height and chest wall growth remain in this age group. Two current options are growing rods and the vertical expandable prosthetic titanium rib, which can be lengthened at regular intervals during the child's growth. The growing rods are connected to the spine at the proximal and distal aspects of the construct with hooks and/or pedicle screws. The vertical expandable titanium rib differs from growing rods in that its proximal fixation point is out laterally on the rib, and not the spine. These systems have overlapping rods, which are progressively lengthened at regular intervals, typically every 6 months, to keep pace with the patient's spinal growth.

There are no studies that systematically evaluate the use of growing systems in patients with SCI. However, in longitudinal clinical registries, the complication rate is between 25% and 72% in the able-bodied population (Campbell et al 2004, Samdani et al 2009, Sankar et al 2010). Experience suggests that this risk is even higher in the SCI population. Children with SCI are already prone to urinary tract and respiratory infections. This risk is increased with the need for surgical lengthening procedures of the growing instrumentation every 6 months. Typically, most patients with growing systems will eventually undergo a spinal fusion.

Wedge Osteotomies

A vertebral wedge osteotomy has been previously described as a 'fusionless technique' for adolescent idiopathic scoliosis, in which a wedge of bone from each of the vertebral bodies in the curve is resected, but the disk space is preserved (Maruyama et al 2006). A modification to this technique was adapted to the SCI population in response to subjective reports of patient dissatisfaction with the rigidity associated with their spinal fusion.

An instrumentation system was developed that helped support the deformity correction while the osteotomy site heals. Biomechanical and preclinical studies of the wedge osteotomy were performed (Betz et al 2003) as well as a clinical series of 14 patients with myelodysplasia or SCI (Guille et al 2003), and then a 2-year follow-up of the same series (McCarthy et al 2010). There were no intra-operative complications or changes in neurologic level in the patients with myelodysplasia, and there was no loss of spasticity in those with SCI. Patients maintained the rod for approximately 12 weeks, and, upon rod removal at an average follow-up of 43 months after injury, 62% showed improvement, with 45% having maintained their Cobb angle and three individuals showing an increase in their Cobb angle (two of the three curves actually reversed and progressed in the opposite direction). Most importantly, the patients maintained their range of motion across the spinal surgery site, with an average of 43 degrees. The wedge osteotomy surgery needs further study with a Food and Drug Administration-approved device before it can be recommended. Currently, such a device is not available.

Preoperative workup

The preoperative evaluation includes a rigorous medical and anesthesia workup. A daily 30-minute Hibiclens back scrub starting 3 days before the operation is recommended. Many of these patients are on an every-other-day bowel program, and a bowel movement the day before surgery should be performed. Patients with SCI may develop deep venous thrombosis (DVT), and preoperative ultrasound of all four extremities is recommended. These usually reveal clinically insignificant chronic superficial vein thrombosis, which then provides a baseline for postoperative comparison. However, there have been reports of patients having clots in deep veins, which have delayed surgery (Jones et al 2005).

A preoperative evaluation with physical and occupational therapy is highly recommended. The purpose of this evaluation is multifold. First, the therapist educates the patient and family about the potential positive and negative functional consequences of a straighter, yet stiffer, spine. They emphasize the effect on activities of daily living that the patient currently performs. Part of this evaluation may include placing a rigid TLSO on the patient to emulate spine fusion. This is useful to patients who use limited ambulation to simulate their ability to ambulate postoperatively. In addition, the TLSO trial on patients with high tetraplegia can simulate function after a spinal fusion as a way to determine the degree to which a spine fusion may negatively impact compensatory strategies (i.e. hand to mouth). The preoperative physical therapy evaluation also covers the postoperative restrictions. Although there is not a consensus on postoperative restrictions of function, for a period, patients will not self-propel their wheelchair, assist in transfers, or flex their hips past 90 degrees. Factors that influence the duration of these restrictions include patient body habitus and bone quality.

The preoperative evaluation includes standard posteroanterior/lateral sitting full-spine radiographs (Fig. 19.1a,b) and supine full-spine bend or traction films. In particular, a high-quality sitting lateral radiograph is imperative, as these patients rely on an exaggerated kyphosis to permit the performance of activities of daily living, including self-catheterization and feeding. In a series of 30 patients with SCI, the usually neutral T10–L2 region measured a kyphosis of 19.8 degrees. Similarly, the lumbar lordosis was, on average, 9.8 degrees (Fayssoux et al 2007). Thus, fusing these patients with a 'normal' sagittal thoracic kyphosis and lumbar lordosis may prevent them from performing at their preoperative level. This is particularly true of patients with limited upper extremity functioning. It is very instructive for the surgeon to observe these patients performing activities of daily living to truly appreciate the importance of maintaining their kyphosis. When a patient with tetraplegia cannot sit up, the authors will make a temporary TLSO and see how the patient can function. If the patient does well in the TLSO, then a lateral radiograph in the TLSO is obtained and the rods bent to match. Sometimes, a malleable rod can be bent preoperatively against the film, sterilized, and inserted.

Intra-operative management

Similar to other patients with neuromuscular scoliosis, patients with SCI may benefit from the use of antifibrinolytics, although this should be weighed against the increased risk of DVT. The surgeon should also consider the use of a central line, as patients with cervical-level injuries may demonstrate hemodynamic instability secondary to autonomic dysfunction (Kassioukov and Claydon 2006). Furthermore, the anesthesia team should refrain from the use of succinylcholine, as it may cause the release of potassium and sudden cardiac arrest (Nash et al 1981).

The infection rate for scoliosis surgery in patients with SCI has been reported to be 16% in a recent large-volume retrospective study (Cahill et al 2010). Intra-operative antibiotics, therefore, should include strong coverage of Gram-positive and Gram-negative bacteria, as previously reported by others. We prefer cefazolin and gentamicin, with vancomycin substituting when there is a penicillin allergy. In addition, we mix vancomycin with the bone graft and/or use vancomycin powder spread on the wound surfaces before closure, as demonstrated by others, to decrease the incidence of infection (Borkhuu et al 2008, Sweet et al 2011).

Neuromonitoring is recommended for all individuals to include somatosensory evoked potentials and motor evoked potentials. Neurologic injury is a potentially devastating complication for individuals already suffering impairment. Loss of bladder control and protective sensation can compound the risk of decubiti in non-ambulatory patients. Intra-operative neuromonitoring is typically feasible in patients who are paralyzed with neuromuscular scoliosis, with the exception of monitoring neurologic function below the level of a complete SCI (Ashkenaze et al 1993, Schwartz et al 2011).

Traditionally, the entire thoracolumbar spine is fused from T2 to the sacrum/pelvis. This allows for complete control of the thoracolumbar spine as well as stabilization and correction of pelvic obliquity, which plays a significant role in sitting balance. Recent trends in instrumentation have shifted from 'unit rods' and sublaminar wires and hooks to segmental pedicle screw and iliac wing fixation. Pedicle screw instrumentation provides purchase into all three columns of the vertebra, resulting in a powerful corrective force (Clements et al 2009) (Fig. 19.1c,d). Conducting dual-energy X-ray absorptiometry preoperatively to assess a patient's bone mineral density can be considered. This may have an impact on the number and type (pedicle screws, hooks, wires, hybrid combination, etc.) of fixation points necessary to achieve a stable spinal fusion (Paxinos et al 2010).

Postoperative Care

Postoperatively, there are significant forces placed on the fixation of the spinal implants into the bone, especially rotation torques and lateral bends, which can, over time, allow for the development of a non-union. For this reason, we try to minimize these forces by requesting that, for 6 months, patients do not transfer independently and that they use a power wheelchair. Patients may be asked to wear a TLSO postoperatively to minimize motion across the fusion segment and reduce stress across the implants in severe deformity and/or osteoporotic bone.

Since many of these patients are not continent of urine or stool, covering the inferior one-third of the wound with a bioclusive dressing at all times for the first month after surgery should be enforced. The authors recommend initiating pharmacologic DVT treatment after the drains have been removed for a total of 6 weeks. Furthermore, the authors obtain postoperative Doppler ultrasounds of all four extremities between 1 and 2 weeks after surgery to evaluate for the presence of DVT.

Surgical outcomes

It has been shown that functional outcomes postoperatively can be significantly affected by overall alignment. The goals for spinal alignment include addressing the complications associated with scoliosis (poor sitting balance, poor breathing, risk of pressure sores) and recreating a comfortable, functional, and cosmetically pleasing position for the patient with balanced shoulders and an anatomically correct spine. An important consideration is proper weight distribution and prevention of pressure sores. Assuming that their preoperative pressure mapping is acceptable, reproducing their sagittal alignment should then maintain their pressure distribution postoperatively. In a study by Drummond and colleagues, weight distributions in normal sitting should be 21% in each posterior thigh, 18% over each ischial tuberosity, and 5% over the sacrum (Drummond et al 1982). It is important to do pressure mapping after spinal fusion when the patients first sit up to ensure that there are no abnormal high-pressure areas. It is critical to prevent pressure sores postoperatively not only for the patient's overall well-being but also specifically to prevent wound infection.

Furthermore, as described above, patients with higher cervical spine injuries may be reliant on some degree of kyphosis preoperatively to enable hand-to-mouth activities if there is limited upper extremity function. The surgeon must diligently preserve this functional sagittal profile to maintain the patient's independent capabilities. This has required, albeit infrequently, a potential return to the operating room to augment a patient's sagittal profile if a patient loses the ability to raise his or her hand to mouth owing to a fusion with hypokyphosis.

The risks and benefits of spinal fusion are discussed with patients. After surgery, patients may report a feeling of being 'stuck' or 'stiff', and caregivers may report an increased difficulty with transferring patients secondary to a rigid spine. These considerations are important to the informed consent process and must be balanced with conversations about the benefits of spinal fusion, particularly those associated with prevention of medical demise related to pressure sores owing to pelvis obliquity and respiratory compromise. Equally important is the conversation about how risks of surgery dramatically increase with curves that progress beyond 70 degrees (Samdani et al 2012). These elements will support the shared decision making regarding surgical management.

Complications of surgical management

Postoperative Infection

The treatment for postoperative spinal fusion infection typically involves a formal operative debridement(s) with or without the removal of the existing instrumentation. In the case of late-onset infections, or those refractory to antibiotic treatment alone, a staged approach with initial implant removal is followed by a period of antibiotic treatment. The spine can be reinstrumented after eradication of the infection if a pseudarthrosis is found during debridement, if the fusion mass is immature, and/or if the deformity has progressed (Clark and Shufflebarger 1999). The need for complete removal of the implants has been shown to be reduced in neuromuscular scoliosis with the use of negative pressure wound dressings after debridement (Canavese et al 2008). Single-stage exchange of instrumentation and replacement with titanium implants has also been recently suggested as an effective treatment (Muschik et al 2004).

Pseudarthrosis

A pseudarthrosis, or non-union of the spinal fusion, has been reported in 2% to 29% of patients with SCI (Tsirikos et al 2007). This may be identified by pain, progression of the deformity, and/or implant breakage. Treatment of the pseudarthrosis often requires revision instrumentation and fusion. Bone morphogenetic protein (BMP) has been used in recent years to help obtain an early fusion or as an adjunct for pseudarthrosis treatment. The use of BMP may be acceptable for patients with SCI several years after their initial injury. However, research has suggested that the use of BMP for a recent SCI may trigger detrimental changes and adversely affect functional recovery (Dmitriev et al 2011). The importance of this is probably more related to the use of BMP in the acute trauma setting, but further studies with chronic injuries are needed.

Spinal Charcot Arthropathy

Charcot arthropathy of the spine is a phenomenon unique to patients with SCI, which arises from the loss of joint sensation and proprioception. There is abnormal mechanical degeneration and destruction of the spine, which may be difficult to diagnose given the altered or complete lack of normal sensory feedback. Patients with SCI may present with ill-defined back pain, a loss of previous sitting balance, and/or neurologic changes including loss of previous spasticity. This complication can be devastating to a patient with SCI, as any loss of their already compromised neurologic function can significantly alter their independence and/or protective sensation (Brown et al 1992).

Usually with Charcot arthropathy of the spine there is abnormal mechanical degeneration and eventually joint/spine destruction. The clinical presentation makes it difficult to diagnose. The patients sometimes complain of ill-defined pain in their back. They may present with a loss of their previous sitting balance. They may describe a 'grinding' or 'popping' sound, and, if left untreated, they may develop neurologic changes which can be as severe as loss of spasticity (Fig. 19.2a–f). The differential diagnosis of a Charcot spine can be difficult, and the two main conditions to rule out include chronic infection and tumor (Jones et al 2000, Wagner et al 2000, Vialle et al 2005, Brousse et al 2008). Biopsies are clearly justified, and, in a literature review by Barrey and colleagues, 36% of the 109 patients had biopsies done to rule out infection or tumor (Barrey et al 2010). A biopsy is further justified in a suspected Charcot spine because, in the literature, infection and Charcot spine were both present in 14% of the patients (Mikawa et al 1989, Pritchard and Coscia 1993, Suda et al 2005, Morita et al 2008). This concomitant infection and Charcot spine may present together and may occur when a spinal infection erodes enough bone and disk to create instability and a Charcot spine.

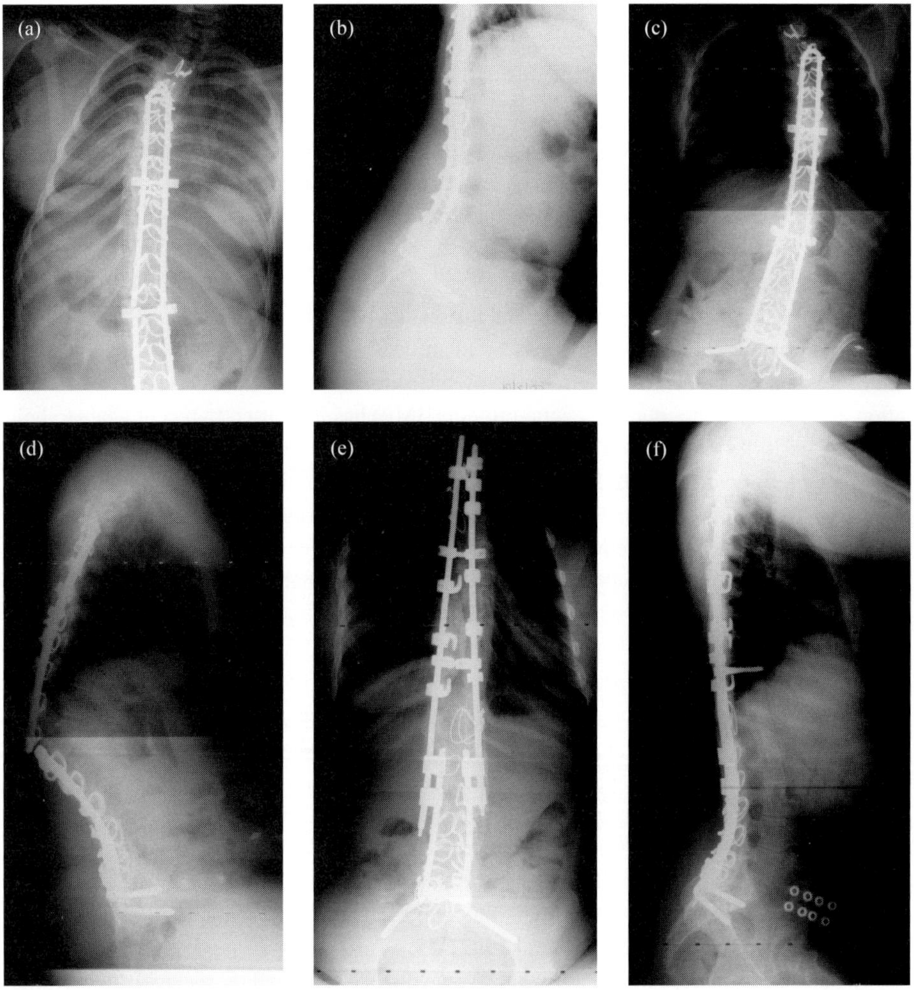

Fig. 19.2 Anteroposterior (a) and lateral (b) radiographs of a patient who had a fusion at 11 years of age. These radiographs reveal broken rods at T12–L1 that occurred 3 years 6 months later, after a traumatic event. Anteroposterior (c) and lateral (d) radiographs of the same patient. While waiting for surgery (within 3 months of the traumatic event), she presented with a loss of spasticity, as well as severe instability and a kyphotic deformity. Anteroposterior (e) and lateral (f) postoperative radiographs after extensive surgery and multiple implants to repair the non-union of the spine. In addition to the extensive posterior instrumentation, the patient had a vascularized rib graft placed anterolaterally across the spine to help healing.

Alternatively, the Charcot spine develops a pseudarthrosis with fluid development. The fluid swells, sometimes through the skin surface, creating a sinus tract, and the spine becomes secondarily infected. Treatment of both the Charcot spine and infection must be carried out concurrently. This condition typically requires both anterior and posterior fusions for adequate stabilization (Devlin et al 1991).

Summary

Patients with scoliosis secondary to SCI can benefit from different strategies such as prophylactic bracing, especially if started immediately after the injury. Aligning the spine during a fusion in a sitting posture and early fusion to minimize the complication risks should also be considered. Major problems do exist in managing the spinal care of patients with SCI, including failure to recognize the compensatory patterns that the patient may be utilizing before a spinal fusion. Spinal Charcot arthropathy can be a very elusive problem that is difficult to diagnose early. Spinal deformity will always be a problem, even when the biological treatment options for the SCI are used, since patients with incomplete injuries also develop paralytic scoliosis. For this reason, further efforts to develop fusionless treatments are warranted.

REFERENCES

Ashkenaze D, Mudiyam R, Boachie-Adjei O, Gilbert C (1993) Efficacy of spinal cord monitoring in neuromuscular scoliosis. *Spine (Phila Pa 1976)* 18: 1627–33. http://dx.doi.org/10.1097/00007632-199309000-00010

Barrey C, Massourides H, Cotton F, Perrin G, Rode G (2010) Charcot spine: two new case reports and a systematic review of 109 clinical cases from the literature. *Ann Phys Rehabil Med* 53: 200–20. doi: 10.1016/j.rehab.2009.11.008

Betz RR, Cunningham B, Selgrath C, Drewry T, Sherman MC (2003) Preclinical testing of a wedge-rod system for fusionless correction of scoliosis. *Spine (Phila Pa 1976)* 28: S275–8. http://dx.doi.org/10.1097/01.BRS.0000092486.61943.99

Borkhuu B, Borowski A, Shah SA, Littleton AG, Dabney KW, Miller F (2008) Antibiotic-loaded allograft decreases the rate of acute deep wound infection after spinal fusion in cerebral palsy. *Spine (Phila Pa 1976)* 33: 2300–4. http://dx.doi.org/10.1097/BRS.0b013e31818786ff

Brousse C, Montigny JP, Marroun I, Garreau de Loubresse C, Kahn JE (2008) [Charcot's disease of the lumbosacral joint in spinal cord injury: a case report]. [Article in French] *Ann Readapt Med Phys* 51: 734–7. doi: 10.1016/j.annrmp.2008.09.001

Brown CW, Jones B, Donaldson DH, Akmakjian J, Brugman JL (1992) Neuropathic (Charcot) arthropathy of the spine after traumatic spinal paraplegia. *Spine (Phila Pa 1976)* 17: S103–8. http://dx.doi.org/10.1097/00007632-199206001-00007

Cahill PJ, Warnick DE, Lee MJ et al (2010) Infection after spinal fusion for pediatric spinal deformity: thirty years of experience at a single institution. *Spine (Phila Pa 1976)* 35: 1211–17. http://dx.doi.org/10.1097/BRS.0b013e3181c212d1

Campbell RM Jr, Smith MD, Mayes TC et al (2004) The effect of opening wedge thoracostomy on thoracic insufficiency syndrome associated with fused ribs and congenital scoliosis. *J Bone Joint Surg Am* 86: 1659–74.

Canavese F, Gupta S, Krajbich JI, Emara KM (2008) Vacuum-assisted closure for deep infection after spinal instrumentation for scoliosis. *J Bone Joint Surg Br* 90: 377–81. http://dx.doi.org/10.1302/0301-620X.90B3.19890

Clark CE, Shufflebarger HL (1999) Late-developing infection in instrumented idiopathic scoliosis. *Spine (Phila Pa 1976)* 24: 1909–12. http://dx.doi.org/10.1097/00007632-199909150-00008

Clements DH, Betz RR, Newton PO, Rohmiller M, Marks MC, Bastrom T (2009) Correlation of scoliosis curve correction with the number and type of fixation anchors. *Spine (Phila Pa 1976)* 34: 2147–50. http://dx.doi.org/10.1097/BRS.0b013e3181adb35d

Dearolf WW 3rd, Betz RR, Vogel LC, Levin J, Clancy M, Steel HH (1990) Scoliosis in pediatric spinal cord-injured patients. *J Pediatr Orthop* 10: 214–18. http://dx.doi.org/10.1097/01241398-199010020-00016

Devlin VJ, Ogilvie JW, Transfeldt EE, Boachie-Adjei O, Bradford DS (1991) Surgical treatment of neuropathic spinal arthropathy. *J Spinal Disord* 4: 319–28. http://dx.doi.org/10.1097/00002517-199109000-00009

Dmitriev AE, Castner S, Lehman RA Jr, Ling GS, Symes AJ (2011) Alterations in recovery from spinal cord injury in rats treated with recombinant human bone morphogenetic protein-2 for posterolateral arthrodesis. *J Bone Joint Surg Am* 93: 1488–99. http://dx.doi.org/10.2106/JBJS.J.00904

Driscoll SW, Skinner J (2008) Musculoskeletal complications of neuromuscular disease in children. *Phys Med Rehabil Clin N Am* 19: 163–94. http://dx.doi.org/10.1016/j.pmr.2007.10.003

Drummond DS, Narechania RG, Rosenthal AN, Breed AL, Lange TA, Drummond DK (1982) A study of pressure distributions measured during balanced and unbalanced sitting. *J Bone Joint Surg Am* 64: 1034–9.

Fayssoux RS, Samdani AF, Asghar J, Mulcahey MJ, McCarthy JJ, Betz RR (2007) Sagittal profile of pediatric patients with spinal cord injury (SCI): a radiographic analysis. 14th International Meeting on Advanced Spine Techniques, Nassau, Bahamas. 11–14 July 2007.

Guille JT, Betz RR, Balsara RK, Mulcahey MJ, D'Andrea LP, Clements DH (2003) The feasibility, safety, and utility of vertebral wedge osteotomies for the fusionless treatment of paralytic scoliosis. *Spine (Phila Pa 1976)* 28: S266–74. http://dx.doi.org/10.1097/01.BRS.0000092485.40061.ED

Jones EA, Manaster BJ, May DA, Disler DG (2000) Neuropathic osteoarthropathy: diagnostic dilemmas and differential diagnosis. *Radiographics* 20: 279–93. http://dx.doi.org/10.1148/radiographics.20.suppl_1.g00oc22s279

Jones T, Ugalde V, Franks P, Zhou H, White RH (2005) Venous thromboembolism after spinal cord injury: incidence, time course, and associated risk factors in 16,240 adults and children. *Arch Phys Med Rehabil* 86: 2240–7. http://dx.doi.org/10.1016/j.apmr.2005.07.286

Kassioukov A, Claydon VE (2006) The clinical problems in cardiovascular control following spinal cord injury: an overview. *Prog Brain Res* 152: 223–9. http://dx.doi.org/10.1016/S0079-6123(05)52014-4

Kinali M, Main M, Eliahoo J et al (2007) Predictive factors for the development of scoliosis in Duchenne muscular dystrophy. *Eur J Paediatr Neurol* 11: 160–6. http://dx.doi.org/10.1016/j.ejpn.2006.12.002

Lancourt JE, Dickson JH, Carter RE (1981) Paralytic spinal deformity following traumatic spinal-cord injury in children and adolescents. *J Bone Joint Surg Am* 63: 47–53. http://dx.doi.org/10.1097/01241398-198111000-00058

McCarthy KP, Chafetz RS, Mulcahey MJ, Frisch RF, D'Andrea LP, Betz RR (2010) Clinical efficacy of the vertebral wedge osteotomy for the fusionless treatment of paralytic scoliosis. *Spine (Phila Pa 1976)* 35: 403–10. http://dx.doi.org/10.1097/BRS.0b013e3181c3e89a

Maruyama T, Kitagawa T, Takeshita K et al (2006) Fusionless surgery for scoliosis: 2–17 year radiographic and clinical follow-up. *Spine (Phila Pa 1976)* 31: 2310–15. http://dx.doi.org/10.1097/01.brs.0000238971.05671.d5

Mayfield JK, Erkkila JC, Winter RB (1981) Spine deformity subsequent to acquired childhood spinal cord injury. *J Bone Joint Surg Am* 63: 1401–11.

Mehta S, Betz RR, Mulcahey MJ, McDonald C, Vogel LC, Anderson C (2004) Effect of bracing on paralytic scoliosis secondary to spinal cord injury. *J Spinal Cord Med* 27: S88–92.

Mikawa Y, Watanabe R, Yamano Y, Morii S (1989) Infected Charcot spine following spinal cord injury. *Spine (Phila Pa 1976)* 14: 892–5. http://dx.doi.org/10.1097/00007632-198908000-00024

Miller DJ, Franzone JM, Matsumoto H et al (2012) Electronic monitoring improves brace-wearing compliance in patients with adolescent idiopathic scoliosis: a randomized clinical trial. *Spine (Phila Pa 1976)* 37: 717–21. http://dx.doi.org/10.1097/BRS.0b013e31822f4306

Morita M, Miyauchi A, Okuda S, Oda T, Yamamoto T, Iwasaki M (2008) Charcot spinal disease after spinal cord injury. *J Neurosurg Spine* 9: 419–26. doi: 10.3171/SPI.2008.9.11.419

Morrison WB, Przybylski GJ, Parker L (2000) Can imaging findings help differentiate spinal neuropathic arthropathy from disk space infection? Initial experience. *Radiology* 214: 693–9. http://dx.doi.org/10.1148/radiology.214.3.r00mr16693

Mulcahey MJ, Barakat N, Hunter L, Gaughan J, Betz R, Vogel L (2013) Neuromuscular scoliosis in children with spinal cord injury. *Top Spinal Cord Inj Rehab* 19: 96–103. http://dx.doi.org/10.1310/sci1902-96

Muller EB, Nordwall A, von Wendt L (1992) Influence of surgical treatment of scoliosis in children with spina bifida on ambulation and motoric skills. *Acta Paediatr Scand* 81: 173–6. http://dx.doi.org/10.1111/j.1651-2227.1992.tb12197.x

Muschik M, Luck W, Schlenzka D (2004) Implant removal for late developing infection after instrumented posterior spinal fusion: reinstrumentation reduces loss of correction. A retrospective analysis of 45 cases. *Eur Spine J* 13: 645–51. http://dx.doi.org/10.1007/s00586-004-0694-4

Nash CL Jr, Haller R, Brown RH (1981) Succinylcholine, paraplegia, and intraoperative cardiac arrest. A case report. *J Bone Joint Surg Am* 63: 1010–12.

Paxinos O, Tsitsopoulos PP, Zindrick MR et al (2010) Evaluation of pullout strength and failure mechanism of posterior instrumentation in normal and osteopenic thoracic vertebrae. *J Neurosurg Spine* 13: 469–76. http://dx.doi.org/10.3171/2010.4.SPINE09764

Pritchard JC, Coscia MF (1993) Infection of a Charcot spine. A case report. *Spine (Phila Pa 1976)* 18: 764–7. http://dx.doi.org/10.1097/00007632-199305000-00016

Samdani AF, Ranade A, Dolch HJ et al (2009) Bilateral use of the vertical expandable prosthetic titanium rib attached to the pelvis: a novel treatment for scoliosis in the growing spine. *J Neurosurg Spine* 10: 287–92. http://dx.doi.org/10.3171/2008.12.SPINE08427

Samdani AF, Cahill PJ, Hwang SW et al (2011) Larger curve magnitude is associated with markedly increased perioperative complications after scoliosis surgery in patients with spinal cord injury. 18th International Meeting on Advanced Spine Techniques, Copenhagen, Denmark. 13–16 July 2011.

Samdani AF, Belin EJ, Miyanji F et al (2012) Major perioperative complications after surgery for cerebral palsy: assessment of risk factors. 47th Scoliosis Research Society annual meeting, Chicago, IL. 5–8 September 2012.

Sankar WM, Acevedo DC, Skaggs DL (2010) Comparison of complications among growing spinal implants. *Spine (Phila Pa 1976)* 35: 2091–6. http://dx.doi.org/10.1097/BRS.0b013e3181c6edd7

Schwartz DM, Sestokas AK, Dormans JP et al (2011) Transcranial electric motor evoked potential monitoring during spine surgery: is it safe? *Spine (Phila Pa 1976)* 36: 1046–9. http://dx.doi.org/10.1097/BRS.0b013e3181ecbe77

Sison-Williamson M, Bagley A, Hongo A et al (2007) Effect of thoracolumbosacral orthoses on reachable workspace volumes in children with spinal cord injury. *J Spinal Cord Med* 30(Suppl 1): S184–91.

Smith AD, Koreska J, Moseley CF (1989) Progression of scoliosis in Duchenne muscular dystrophy. *J Bone Joint Surg Am* 71: 1066–74. Suda Y, Saito M, Shioda M, Kato H, Shibasaki K (2005) Infected Charcot spine. *Spinal Cord* 43: 256–9.

Suda Y, Saito M, Shioda M, Kato H, Shibasaki K (2005) Infected Charcot spine. *Spinal Cord* 43: 256–9. http://dx.doi.org/10.1038/sj.sc.3101687

Sweet FA, Roh M, Sliva C (2011) Intrawound application of vancomycin for prophylaxis in instrumented thoracolumbar fusions: efficacy, drug levels, and patient outcomes. *Spine (Phila Pa 1976)* 36: 2084–8. http://dx.doi.org/10.1097/BRS.0b013e3181ff2cb1

Tsirikos AI, Markham P, McMaster MJ (2007) Surgical correction of spinal deformities following spinal cord injury occurring in childhood. *J Surg Orthop Adv* 16: 174–86.

Vialle R, Mary P, Tassin JL, Parker F, Guillaumat M (2005) Charcot's disease of the spine: diagnosis and treatment. *Spine (Phila Pa 1976)* 30: E315–22.

20
UPPER EXTREMITY FUNCTION

MJ Mulcahey, Dan A Zlotolow and Scott H Kozin[a]

> **Case vignette**
> Adam sustained a birth injury resulting in C6 tetraplegia. Immediate management of his upper extremities included night-time padded hand splints that positoned the hands in an intrinsic-plus position, the wrist in a neutral position, and the arms in proper positioning to prevent elbow flexion and forearm supination contractures. Throughout the first 4 years of his life, Adam was trained to engage in play and self care (eating, teeth brushing) using custom-made universal cuffs (to hold a bottle or cup, a baby biscuit or child utensil, and a toothbrush); these cuffs were modified frequently to accommodate growth and development. Two-handed techniques were also used for play. Preventive night-time splinting continued. At 5 years of age, Adam underwent bilateral reconstruction to restore elbow extension (biceps to tricpes transfer), palmar grasp (radial wrist extensor to flexor digitorum profundus), and lateral pinch (brachioradialis to flexor pllicus longus); the surgical procedures were staged so that reconstruction of the right upper extremity occurred first and, 1 week later, reconstruction of the left upper extremity occurred. The goals of surgery included the ability to hold a crayon, marker, or pencil with one hand; the ability to hold utensils in both hands to cut food; a decreased effort needed for object manipulaiton; the ability to self-catheterize; and the ability to reach to write on a dry-erase board. Adam's arms were immobilized for 3 weeks; post-surgery therapy was initiated after cast removal, progressing from movement of the transfers in a gravity-eliminated position and partial range to full range against gravity. Therapy also included integration of new movements into activites and training in activities that were identified as goals of surgery. Around 6 months after surgery, Adam was able to use his new movement to accomplish the surgical goals. He reported less effort needed for most activities.

Introduction

Although the numbers vary based on the source, more spinal cord injuries (SCIs) occur at the cervical level than any other level of the vertebral column (DeVivo 2012), resulting in varying

a Jillian Strober-Horowitz also contributed to this chapter.

degrees of upper extremity impairment. In young children, injuries to the upper cervical levels (C1–C4) are most common (Brown et al 2001, Vogel et al 2012). Children and adolescents with tetraplegia require more care and have more difficulty being independent than those affected with lower extremity dysfunction alone (Allen et al 2009). Weakness in the hands and arms decreases the capacity for transfers, self-feeding, perineal care, self-catheterization, school, and play activities. For children, spontaneity and ease of activities are also associated with participation in activities and are compromised in children with tetraplegia (Mulcahey et al 2007). The limitations imposed on the upper extremities by cervical injuries are so pervasive that the majority of adults with tetraplegia prioritize improvements in upper limb function over bowel or bladder function, sexual function, or walking ability (Snoek et al 2004). This chapter discusses the management of upper extremities after SCI, with particularly emphasis on unique considerations in children.

Current practice guidelines for upper extremity function in spinal cord injury

Although they were not written specifically for children, the Paralyzed Veterans of America clinical practice guidelines for upper limb function after SCI (Consortium for Spinal Cord Medicine 2005) and outcomes after traumatic SCI (Consortium for Spinal Cord Medicine 1999) provide important treatment guidelines for rehabilitation of persons with tetraplegia. Clinicians working with persons with SCI should know and understand these practice guidelines and, as appropriate, integrate them into existing clinical pathways in their clinical setting. Modifications to the upper extremity guidelines may be necessary when working with younger children and exceptions to anticipated functional outcomes, as defined by the consortium, may be explained by management of secondary complications unique to pediatric SCI, such as neuromuscular scoliosis (Mulcahey et al 2013).

Unique considerations in children

The upper extremities of children with tetraplegia have similar features to those of patients with adult-onset SCI, with a few notable exceptions (Mulcahey 1997). Because of their small trunk size, younger children with tetraplegia are able to reach their mouths, their ears, and the top of their head using elbow flexion and little shoulder forward flexion; in essence, everything they need to access is within their immediate workspace. Since the need for active range of shoulder forward flexion and abduction is minimal in young children, they are at a greater risk of significant shoulder contractures. In addition, as children with tetraplegia grow, many take advantage of their neuromuscular scoliosis as a compensatory mechanism for weak and or contracted shoulder forward flexion and abduction. For those unfamiliar with pediatric SCI, the implications of these functional compensatory strategies may be underappreciated; shoulder contractures lead to significant pain and overuse of muscles and the majority of children with neuromuscular scoliosis will require a spinal fusion (Mulcahey et al 2013), resulting in a loss of the compensatory strategy. Thus, active or active-assisted range of motion of the shoulder should be performed during every diaper change or daily in preschool- and school-aged children. Anticipatory guidance about neuromuscular scoliosis should be provided to the parents and child on an ongoing basis.

Another common complication of the upper extremities that is associated with children injured less than 5 years of age with mid-cervical SCI is metacarpophalangeal (MCP) extension contractures. MCP extension contractures develop in children with low-level cervical injuries as a compensatory strategy for weak hand function; commonly, children will hold objects between their palms, with fingers extended. Although the compensatory strategy should be encouraged, prevention of MCP contractures is a priority and is achieved with prophylactic nap- and night-time splinting that holds the hand in an intrinsic-plus position (Fig. 20.1) (Mulcahey 1997).

Splinting and orthotic intervention

Detailed discussions about splinting and orthotic intervention for persons with SCI is beyond the scope of this chapter, but can be found in several notable references (Atkins et al 2003, Mulcahey 2008, 2009). For children, light, soft material and frequent modifications of splints and orthoses are needed to accommodate constant growth. However, with adequate design, children as young as 3 months of age are able to engage in developmentally important activities using upper extremity orthoses. Custom-made splints for function can be fabricated to assist with the grasp of bottles, biscuits, and other age-appropriate toys and tools (Figs 20.2 and 20.3). To avoid damage to the gums and teeth, when splints and orthoses are used with infants, close monitoring is recommended owing to infants' frequent 'mouthing' and 'teething' on the splints.

Serial casting interventions are used to enhance passive range of motion in patients with SCI with secondary joint tightness or recent contracture (Mulcahey et al 2007) and can be successfully used with children (Mulcahey 2009). An understanding of the functional implications of potentially elongating a tight joint in a child is important to assess because some may rely on that passive limitation for enhancing functional performance; the most common example of this in adults and children is tenodesis hand function (passive finger flexion with active wrist extension) where there is intentional tendon tightening to aid in passive grasp

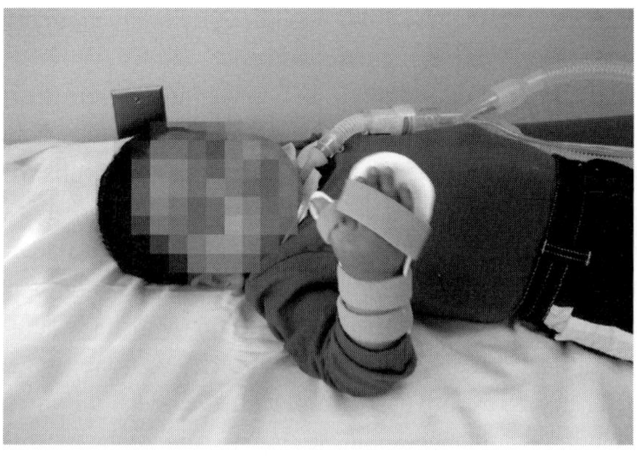

Fig. 20.1 Preventive splinting for a child with mid-level tetraplegia. Note the intrinsic-plus hand position to prevent metacarpophalangeal extension tightness. Splints should be worn at nap- and night-time.

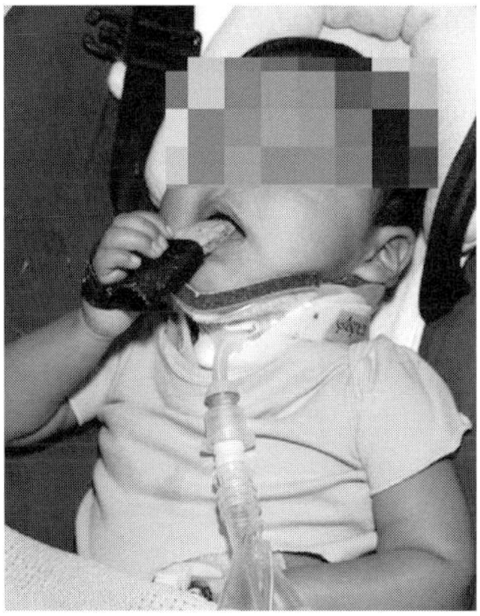

Fig. 20.2 Custom-fabricated universal cuff using soft material for child to hold a biscuit.

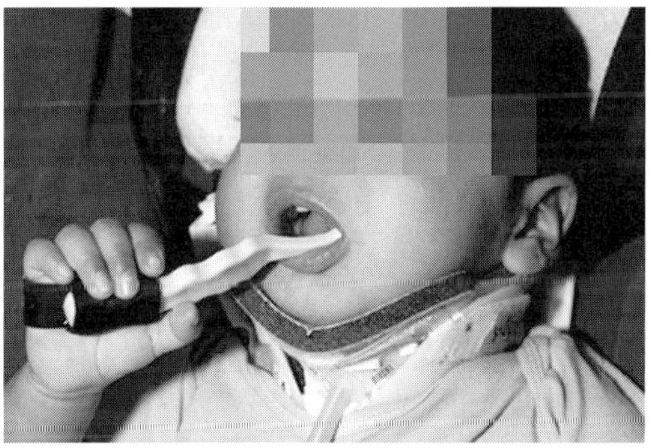

Fig. 20.3 Custom-fabricated universal cuff using soft material for child to hold a toothbrush.

function. In children, intentional tightening of forearm pronation has also been observed as a way to create a 'holding platform' for carrying objects. Contraindications for serial casting that are of particular relevance to children include a history of multiple pathologic or spontaneous fractures, pain, inability to comprehend the potential benefits of serial casting, and poor tolerance to immobilization.

Therapeutic and functional electrical stimulation

The principles of therapeutic and functional electrical stimulation for adults and children with SCI are similar (Bryden et al 2013). Modifications to stimulation parameters for children may be necessary to prevent hyperextension of joints, ensure tolerance to stimulation, and accommodate smaller muscle mass. There are conflicting reports on the effectiveness of therapeutic electrical stimulation on the upper limbs in adult populations (Beekhuizen and

Field-Fote 2008, Glinsky et al 2009, Harvey et al 2011), and there is one systematic report of positive findings with children with tetraplegia (Martin et al 2012). Additional studies are needed to inform the application of therapeutic electrical stimulation to the hand in children with tetraplegia. Outcomes of functional electrical stimulation systems in children have been described in detail and indicate long-term effectiveness (Mulcahey and Betz 1997, Mulcahey et al 2004). Pediatric clinicians should keep abreast of advancements currently under way in neurotechnology (Peckham and Kilgore 2013) and should advocate for full access to this technology for children with tetraplegia.

Surgical options for children with tetraplegia

Surgical guidelines for restoration of arm and hand function after SCI have been well described and are briefly addressed here, with particular relevance to children and young people. The underutilization of evidence-based surgical techniques is thought to be caused by misperceptions by both patients and their caregivers of available techniques and the results of upper limb reconstruction. Additionally, some patients do not want to potentially compromise their ultimate function in case a 'cure' is devised in their lifetime. This last concern is one that is shared by those who care for children, and great prudence is taken to only perform procedures that either are reversible or do not compromise function in case a patient fully recovers or a cure becomes available.

The potential risks of reconstructive surgery, even those that are long term, are low compared with the potential benefits (Anderson et al 2009). A recent review of over 500 adult patients who had restoration of elbow extension and pinch showed clinically significant improvements in overall upper limb function, including the ability to perform overhead activities (Hamou et al 2009). Published reports on children show similar results of high benefits with low complications (Mulcahey et al 1999, 2003).

When upper extremity surgery is being considered, in addition to the International Standards for Neurological Classification of Spinal Cord Injury (Kirshblum et al 2011, Mulcahey et al 2011), the International Classification for Surgery of the Hand in Tetraplegia (ICSHT) should be used to classify the neurologic consequence of the injury (Table 20.1). The ICSHT is a more precise guide for surgical planning and it describes the residual upper limb function. The higher the grade, the more function that the patient demonstrates, and the greater the surgical options that become available. For a child with an ICSHT grade 0 injury, no reconstructive procedures are possible to augment function. For patients with ICSHT 1, only passive pinch is possible, which is achievable by active wrist extension and passive finger flexion (tenodesis pinch). For patients with more motor function, active pinch, grasp, and thumb opposition are feasible, based on the ICSHT level of function. In addition to the more precise motor examination, the ICSHT also involves sensory evaluation (two-point discrimination) of the index finger and thumb.

The shoulder

In high cervical level SCI, the shoulder girdle muscles can be spastic, flaccid, or a combination of both. Weakness of the periscapular muscles can lead to painful scapular instability with winging (Fig. 20.4). Without a stable scapular platform, the already weakened glenohumeral

TABLE 20.1
International Classification for Surgery of the Hand in Tetraplegia (adapted from McDowell et al 1986)

		Sensibility motor description
Shoulder function[a]		**Ocular or cutaneous sensation group characteristics function**
	0	No muscles below elbow suitable for transfer Flexion/supination of elbow
Weak posterior deltoid Upper trapezius Latissimus dorsi External shoulder rotation	1	Brachioradialis
Reliable posterior deltoid Internal shoulder rotation Anterior deltoid Pectoralis major	2	Extensor carpi radialis longus Extension of wrist (weak or strong)
	3	Extensor carpi radialis brevis Extension of wrist
	4	Pronator teres Extension and pronation of wrist
	5	Flexor carpi radialis Flexion of wrist
	6	Finger extensors Extrinsic extension of fingers, partial or complete
	7	Thumb extension Extrinsic extension of the thumb
	8	Partial digital flexors Extrinsic flexion of the fingers, weak
	9	Lacks only intrinsic function Extrinsic flexion of the fingers
	X	Exceptions

[a]Shoulder function description from Kuz et al (1999).

muscles are less effective, further reducing abduction and flexion strength. Scapular winging also creates a bony prominence at the inferior pole, increasing the risk of pressure ulcers. In children, scapular winging may be worsened by neuromuscular scoliosis or spinal fusion for the correction of neuromuscular scoliosis. Stabilization of the scapula to the thorax has demonstrated reduced shoulder pain and modestly improved shoulder function (Pahys et al 2009).

Patients with periscapular control but rotator cuff denervation often develop painful pseudosubluxation of the glenohumeral joint. In addition, without a sufficient force couple,

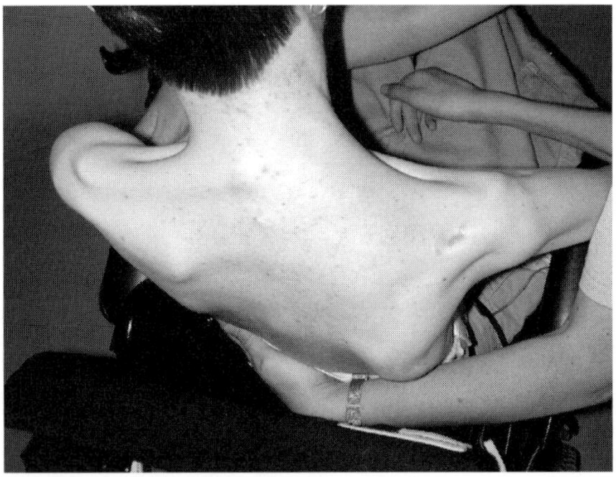

Fig. 20.4 Scapular winging can be seen with higher level cervical spinal cord injury if the periscapular muscles are denervated.

the bony and ligamentous anatomy is insufficient to maintain joint congruity. Increased shear forces across the joint combined with incomplete proprioception may lead to early joint degeneration (Lal 1998).

If the patient has good periscapular and glenohumeral joint function, the shoulders become their primary means of propulsion and weight bearing. This can lead to overuse syndromes including pain, tendonitis, and arthritis (Akbar et al 2010, Jain et al 2010). The problem of shoulder pain and overuse may be even more problematic in pediatric-onset SCI. Long-term follow-up of adults with pediatric-onset SCI reported a high degree of pain, including shoulder pain (Vogel et al 2002). Establishing exercise programs and diligence in appropriate wheelchair designs and configurations can reduce the risk of developing painful shoulders (Howarth et al 2010, Lin et al 2011, Giner-Pascual et al 2011, Norrbink et al 2012, Slowik and Neptune 2013). Early surgical correction of rotator cuff tears may also prevent the worsening of pain.

The elbow

Elbow extension is necessary for transfers, weight shifting, and overhead activities, as well as for more effective wheelchair propulsion. It has been said that the ability to extend the hand in space an additional 12 inches increases workspace of the hand by 800% (Hentz and LeClercq 2002). Posterior deltoid to triceps tendon transfer with use of a tendon graft has historically been the operation of choice for restoration of active elbow extension, expect in the presence of severe elbow flexion and supination spasticity in which the biceps-to-triceps transfer was the transfer of choice. More recently, the biceps-to-triceps transfer has been described as a primary surgery, even without spasticity (Kozin 2003).

In a randomized controlled study with children with SCI, better outcomes were seen after the biceps-to-triceps transfer than after the posterior deltoid-to-triceps transfer (Mulcahey et al 2003). Sufficient antigravity strength to enable overhead activities is not commonly achieved after transfer of the posterior deltoid, but grade 4/5 muscle strength is typical with the biceps-to-triceps transfer. Hutchinson and colleagues have shown that the biceps achieve phasic reversal when rerouted as an extensor (Hutchinson et al 2008). Occasionally, the biceps are only partially innervated and/or the patient may rely on the biceps as the primary flexors of the elbows. If the brachioradialis has poor tone or elbow flexion strength is not 5/5, the brachialis alone may be insufficient to power elbow flexion once the biceps are transferred. In these cases, the biceps-to-triceps transfer is contraindicated.

Experience with the biceps-to-triceps transfer in children has raised some concerns regarding long-term outcomes. In a recently published series of 68 patients, 75% of patients were able to achieve antigravity elbow extension (Kozin et al 2010). The remaining 25% of children have undergone a revision procedure or declined revision. In those children who have undergone revision, some of the transferred tendons have elongated, and have therefore lost the tension set at surgery, whereas other transfers have avulsed from their insertion site into the olecranon. In most cases, a discrete event occurred that resulted in loss of function, which was usually more than 3 months after surgery. Although there are no studies on the use of botulinum neurotoxin to weaken the biceps muscle while the transfer incorporates, this may prevent complications after tendon transfer, particularly during early mobilization and if the patient is prone to spasticity. The goal of early active motion is to minimize motion-limiting scars, encourage tendon collagen organization, and prevent late rupture.

Pinch and grasp

There is a well-established hierarchy of importance of upper limb function: (1) wrist extension, (2) pinch, (3) grasp, (4) finger and thumb extension, and (5) intrinsic function. For patients with an ICSHT grade 0 injury, there are no muscles/tendons available for transfer, thus there are no surgical options to improve upper limb function. Patients with an ICSHT grade 1 injury have a functioning brachioradialis, allowing restoration of wrist extension by brachioradialis to extensor carpi radialis brevis (ECRB) transfer (Freehafer and Mast 1967). Concurrent flexor pollicis longus (FPL) tenodesis to the radius or the ulna creates a weak pinch function. A split FPL transfer is necessary in almost all cases of passive and active pinch restoration to maximize FPL function in the absence of active intrinsic or extrinsic interphalangeal joint extension.

There is a difference between active and passive pinch function in terms of function for patients. Patients with active pinch are more likely to be able to self-catheterize and achieve a higher level of independence. For children, active pinch allows for unilateral grasp of a pencil or crayon and the ability to participate in bilateral play and school tasks. Patients with an ICSHT grade 2 injury can achieve active pinch via a brachioradialis to FLP transfer. The functioning extensor carpi radialis longus (ECRL) is maintained for wrist extension. If the ECRB is also innervated (ICSHT grade 3), crude grasp is possible by transferring the ECRL to the flexor digitorum profundus (FDP). Patients with full 5/5 wrist extension strength reliably have both ECRL and ECRB function, but patients with high 4/5 wrist strength may be candidates for a wake-up test to make sure that the ECRB is sufficiently strong to extend the wrist after the ECRL is tenotomized.

If the thumb does not line up with the proximal interphalangeal joint of the index finger during pinch, a thumb carpometacarpal arthrodesis may be needed. Typically, the position of fusion sets the thumb in pronation and slight abduction. A figure of eight tendon shortening suture in the index FDP tendon will flex the index finger slightly and create a broader platform for pinch. After tendon transfers for hand function, pinch and grasp force increases, performance on standardized tests improves, and children and their parents report better performance in and higher levels of satisfaction with their own goals (Mulcahey et al 1999).

Finger and thumb extension

Children with ICSHT grade 4 or greater injuries have more available tendon donors, raising the potential for higher functional goals. Surgical decision making therefore becomes more complicated and should be reserved for surgeons familiar with this patient population, in collaboration with the primary rehabilitation physician, child, parent(s), and occupational therapist. The addition of the pronator teres muscle as an available transfer donor adds active finger and thumb extension, allowing for greater ease in acquisition and release of objects in some patients. The brachioradialis can be transferred to the extensor digitorum communis and extensor pollicis longus tendons, the pronator teres to the FPL, and the ECRL to the FDP. If multiple tendon transfers are planned for opposing functions, a two-stage reconstruction is recommended, with the extensor procedures performed first. Extensor transfers can be unpredictable, however, particularly if there is insufficient wrist flexion to counteract the wrist extension created by restoration of finger extension.

If the flexor carpi radialis is functioning, active wrist flexion enhances active or passive acquisition and release and stabilizes the wrist if active finger and thumb extension is restored. Harvesting this tendon as a donor for any other function is not recommended given the importance of active wrist flexion in children for object acquisition. Tendon transfers for patients with ICSHT grade 5 injuries are therefore identical to those with grade 4 injuries.

Patients with ICSHT grade 6 and 7 injuries possess finger and thumb extensors, respectively. Patients in these groups typically have active elbow flexion and extension, forearm pronation and supination, wrist flexion and extension, and finger and/or thumb extension (Table 20.2). Missing functions are finger and thumb flexion, as well as intrinsic function. Finger and thumb flexion can be restored with brachioradialis to FPL and ECRL to FDP transfers. For those with grade 6 injuries, the extensor pollicis longus can be tethered to the extensor digitorum communis for thumb extension.

Intrinsic function

All patients with ICSHT grade 3 and higher injuries, for whom grasp is possible, should be considered for restoration of intrinsic function by either active transfers or tenodesis. Only those with grade 8 and 9 injuries have available donors for active intrinsic restoration. Other lower functioning groups may nonetheless benefit from passive intrinsic function, particularly in individuals who have extrinsic finger extension. There is a myriad of passive intrinsic reconstructions that have been described (Tse et al 2007). The technique described by Zancolli is preferred, whereby the flexor digitorum superficialis tendon is looped over the A1 pulley and sewn back to itself (Zancolli 1975).

TABLE 20.2
Segmental innervation of the upper extremity (adapted from Kuz et al [1999])

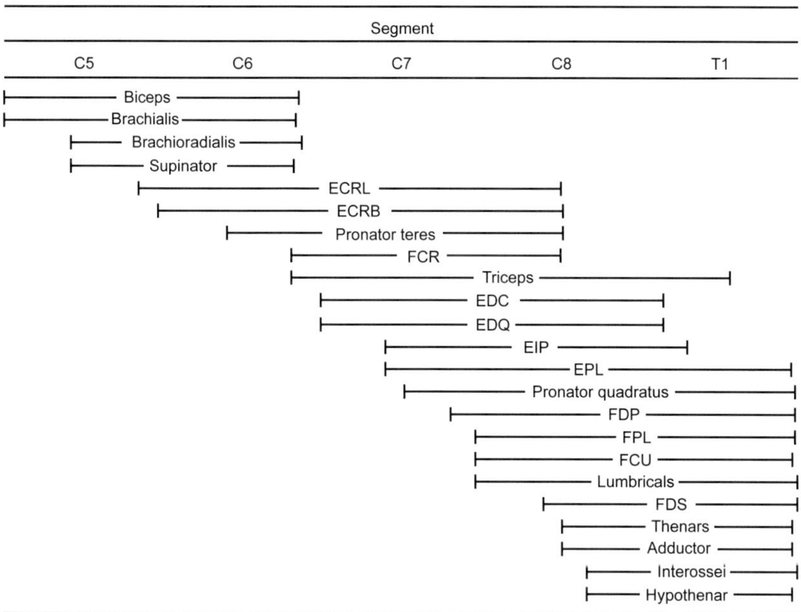

ECRL, extensor carpi radialis longus; ECRB, extensor carpi radialis brevis; FCR, flexor carpi radialis; EDC, extensor digitorum communis; EDQ, extensor digiti quinti; EIP, extensor indicis proprius; EPL, extensor pollicis longus; FDP, flexor digitorum profundus; FPL, flexor pollicis longus; FCU, flexor carpi ulnaris; FDS, flexor digitorum superficialis.

Rehabilitation associated with upper extremity reconstruction

Tendon transfer rehabilitation begins before surgery and involves the identification of desired outcomes (activity and participation) for reconstructive procedures, mobilization of tendons, muscle strengthening, and evaluation of equipment that may be needed during the immobilization period (Mulcahey 1997). Importantly, the preoperative therapy consultation is also used to ensure that the child is developmentally able to understand the surgical procedures and participate in the postoperative therapy requirements. Assuming there are no other mitigating cognitive, developmental, or behavioral factors, children as young as 4 to 5 years of age are typically able to participate. Child life and medical play are often provided by therapeutic recreation and are instrumental in the educational process and help to prepare the child and parents for the surgery and the follow-up program.

There are standard guidelines for tendon transfer rehabilitation and retraining (Mulcahey 1997, Hentz and Leclercq 2002, Mulcahey 2009). Play is an important modality to use with children to facilitate muscle re-education and transfer training. Children and parents must understand the precautions to be made in movement and activity and the role of protective splinting before discharge to out-patient therapy.

Summary

Like adults with SCI, children with tetraplegia are aware of their loss of independence, spontaneity, and ease of activity caused by upper extremity impairment. Although the management of the upper extremities in children is similar to that used with adults, there are considerations that are unique to children. Children are more prone to shoulder contractures and MCP extension contractures. Unlike adults with SCI, children develop neuromuscular scoliosis that may add to compensatory head-to-mouth function, but may also contribute to the risk of shoulder contractures, exaggerate scapular instability, and be progressive. Splinting and orthotic management is similar for children as that used for adults but, for the very young, custom fabrication using light, soft material with frequent modifications to accommodate growth is needed. The principles of surgical reconstruction for active arm and hand function are also similar to those used for adults. Reported outcomes of tendon transfers are positive and include increased pinch and grasp strength, restored unilateral function, and increased autonomy. The management of the upper limb after pediatric cervical SCI is paramount to a child's spontaneous and effortless function. Collectively, preventive, conservative, and surgical methods are effective techniques to achieve this goal.

REFERENCES

Akbar M, Balean G, Brunner M et al (2010) Prevalence of rotator cuff tear in paraplegic patients compared with controls. *J Bone Joint Surg Am* 92: 23–30. doi: 10.2106/JBJS.H.01373

Allen DD, Mulcahey MJ, Haley SM et al (2009) Motor scores on the functional independence measure after pediatric spinal cord injury. *Spinal Cord* 47: 213–17. doi: 10.1038/sc.2008.94

Anderson KD, Friden J, Lieber RL (2009) Acceptable benefits and risks associated with surgically improving arm function in individuals living with cervical spine injuries. *Spinal Cord* 47: 334–8. doi: 10.1038/sc.2008.148

Atkins M, Clark D, Waters R (2003) Upper limb orthoses. In: Lin VW (ed.). *Spinal Cord Medicine: Principles and Practice*. New York, NY: Demos Medical Publishing.

Beekhuizen KS, Field-Fote EC (2008) Sensory stimulation augments the effects of massed practice training in persons with tetraplegia. *Arch Phys Med Rehabil* 89: 602–8. doi: 10.1016/j.apmr.2007.11.021

Brown RL, Brunn MA, Garcia VF (2001) Cervical spine injuries in children: a review of 103 patients treated consecutively at a level 1 pediatric trauma center. *J Pediatric Surg* 36: 1107–14. http://dx.doi.org/10.1053/jpsu.2001.25665

Bryden AM, Ancans J, Mazurkiewicz J, McKnight A, Scholtens M (2012) Technology for spinal cord injury rehabilitation and its application to youth. *J Pediatr Rehabil Med* 5: 287–99. doi: 10.3233/PRM-2012-00227

Consortium for Spinal Cord Medicine (1999) *Outcomes Following Traumatic Spinal Cord Injury*. Washington, DC: Paralyzed Veterans of America.

Consortium for Spinal Cord Medicine (2005) Preservation of upper limb function following spinal cord injury: a clinical practice guideline for health care professionals. *J Spinal Cord Med* 5: 433–70.

DeVivo MJ (2012) Epidemiology of traumatic spinal cord injury: trends and future implications. *Spinal Cord* 50: 365–72. doi: 10.1038/sc.2011.178

Freehafer AA, Mast WA (1967) Transfer of the brachioradialis to improve wrist extension in high spinal-cord injury. *J Bone Joint Surg Am* 57: 648–52.

Giner-Pascual M, Alcanyis-Alberola M, Millan Gonzalez L, Aguilar-Rodriquez M, Querol F (2011) Shoulder pain in cases of spinal cord injury: influences on the position of the wheelchair seat. *Int J Rehabil Res* 34: 282–9. doi: 10.1097/MRR.0b013e32834a8fd9

Glinsky J, Harvey L, van Es P, Chee S, Gandevia SC (2009) The addition of electrical stimulation to progressive resistance training does not enhance wrist strength of people with tetraplegia: a randomized controlled trial. *Clin Rehabil* 23: 696–704. doi: 10.1177/0269215509104171

Hamou C, Shah NR, DiPonio L, Curtin CM (2009) Pinch and elbow extension restoration in people with tetraplegia: a systematic review of the literature. *J Hand Surg Am* 34: 692–9. doi: 10.1016/j.jhsa.2008.12.002

Harvey LA, Dunlop SA, Chutilov L, Hsueh YS, Galea MP (2011) Early intensive hand rehabilitation after spinal cord injury ('Hands ON'): a protocol for a randomized controlled trial. *Trials* 12: 14. doi: 10.1186/1745-6215-12-14

Hattrup SJ, Cofield RH (2010) Shoulder arthroplasty in the paraplegic patient. *J Shoulder Elbow Surg* 19: 434–8. doi:10.1016/j.jse.2009.07.003

Hentz VR, LeClercq C (2002) *Surgical Rehabilitation of the Upper Limb in Tetraplegia*. New York, NY: W.B. Saunders. doi: 10.1016/0363-5023(92)90478-8

Howarth SJ, Pronovost LM, Polgar JM, Dickerson CR, Callaghan JP (2010) Use of geared wheelchair wheel to reduce propulsive muscular demand during ramp ascent: analysis of muscle activation and kinematics. *Clin Biomech* 25: 21–8. doi: 10.1016/j.clinbiomech.2009.10.004

Hutchinson D, Kozin SH, Mayer N, Mulcahey MJ, Duffy T, Gaughan JP (2008) Dynamic electromyographic evaluation of adolescents with traumatic cervical injury after biceps to triceps transfer: the role of phasic contraction. *J Hand Surg Am* 33: 1331–6. doi: 10.1016/j.jhsa.2008.04.022

Jain NB, Higgins LD, Katz JN, Garshick E (2010) Association of shoulder pain with the use of mobility devices in persons with chronic spinal cord injury. *PM R* 2: 896–900. doi: 10.1016/j.pmrj.2010.05.004

Kirshblum SC, Waring W, Biering-Sorensen F et al (2011) Reference for the 2011 revision of the International Standards for Neurological Classification of Spinal Cord Injury. *J Spinal Cord Med* 34: 547–54. doi: 10.1179/107902611X13186000420242

Kozin SH (2003) Biceps-to-triceps transfer for restoration of elbow extension in tetraplegia. *Tech Hand Up Extrem Surg* 7: 43–51. doi: 10.1097/00130911-200306000-00001

Kozin SH, D'Addesi L, Chafetz RS, Ashworth S, Mulcahey MJ (2010) Biceps-to-triceps transfer for elbow extension in persons with tetraplegia. *J Hand Surg Am* 35: 968–75. doi: 10.1016/j.jhsa.2010.03.011

Kuz JE, Van Heest A, House JH (1999) Biceps-to-triceps transfer in tetraplegic patients: report of the medial routing technique and follow-up of three cases. *J Hand Surg Am* 24: 161–72. http://dx.doi.org/10.1053/jhsu.1999.jhsu24a0161

Lal S (1998) Premature degenerative shoulder changes in spinal cord injury patients. *Spinal Cord* 36: 186–9. doi: 10.1038/sj.sc.3100608

Lin CJ, Lin PC, Guo LY, Su FC (2011) Prediction of applied forces in handrim wheelchair propulsion. *J Biomech* 26: 352–7. doi: 10.1016/j.jbiomech.2010.09.029

McDowell CL, Moberg EA, House JH (1986) Proceedings: the second international conference on surgical rehabilitation of the upper limb in tetraplegia (quadriplegia). *J Hand Surg* 11: 604–8. http://dx.doi.org/10.1016/S0363-5023(86)80213-1

Martin R, Johnston K, Sadowsky C (2012) Neuromuscular electrical stimulation-assisted grasp training and restoration of function in the tetraplegic hand: a case series. *Am J Occup Ther* 66: 471–7. doi: 10.5014/ajot.2012.003004

Mulcahey MJ (1997) An overview of the upper extremity in pediatric spinal cord injury. *Top Spinal Cord Inj Rehabil* 3: 48–55.

Mulcahey MJ (2008) Upper limb orthoses for the person with spinal cord injury. In: Hsu J, Michael JW, Fisk JR (eds). *AAOS Atals of Orthoses and Assistive Devices*. 4th Ed. Philadelphia, PA: Mosby Elsevier.

Mulcahey MJ (2009) Management of the upper limb in individuals with tetraplegia. In: Sisto SA, Druin E, Silwinski MM (eds). *Spinal Cord Injuries. Management and Rehabilitation*. St Louis, MO: Mosby Elsevier. doi: 10.1016/B978-032300699-6.10010-3

Mulcahey MJ, Betz RR (1997) Upper and lower extremity applications of functional electrical stimulation: a decade of research with children and adolescents with spinal injuries. *Pediatr Phys Ther* 9: 113–22. doi: 10.1097/00001577-199700930-00005

Mulcahey MJ, Betz RR, Smith BT, Weiss AA (1999) A prospective study of the outcomes of tendon transfers with children with tetraplegia. *J Pediatr Orthop* 19: 319–28. http://dx.doi.org/10.1097/01241398-199905000-00008

Mulcahey MJ, Lutz C, Kozin SH, Betz RR (2003) Prospective evaluation of biceps to triceps and deltoid to triceps for elbow extension in tetraplegia. *J Hand Surg Am* 28: 964–71. doi: 10.1016/S0363-5023(03)00485-4

Mulcahey MJ, Betz RR, Kozin S, Smith BT, Hutchinson D, Lutz C (2004) Implantation of the Freehand system during initial rehabilitation using minimally invasive techniques. *Spinal Cord* 42: 146–55. doi: 10.1038/sj.sc.3101573

Mulcahey MJ, Hutchinson D, Kozin S (2007) Assessment of the upper limb in tetraplegia: consideration in evaluation and outcomes research. *J Rehabil Res Dev* 44: 91–102. doi: 10.1682/JRRD.2005.10.0167

Mulcahey MJ, Vogel L, Gaughan J (2011) The international standards for neurological classification of spinal cord injury: psychometric evaluation and guidelines for use with children and youth. *Phys Med Rehabil* 92: 1264–9. doi: 10.1016/j.apmr.2011.03.003

Mulcahey MJ, Gaughan JP, Betz RR, Samdani AF, Barakat N, Hunter LN (2013) Neuromuscular scoliosis in children with spinal cord injury. *Top Spinal Cord Inj Rehabil* 19: 96–103. doi: 10.1310/sci1902-96

Norrbrink C, Lindberg T, Wahman K, Bjerkefors A (2012) Effects of an exercise programme on musculoskeletal and neuropathic pain after spinal cord injury – results from a seated double-poling ergometer study. *Spinal Cord* 50: 457–61. doi: 10.1038/sc.2011.160

Pahys JM, Mulcahey MJ, Hutchinson D, Betz RR (2009) Scapular stabilization in patients with spinal cord injury. *J Spinal Cord Med* 32: 389–97.

Peckham PH, Kilgore KL (2013) Challenges and opportunities in restoring function after paralysis. *IEEE Trans Biomed Eng* 60: 602–9. doi: 10.1109/TBME.2013.2245128

Slowik JS, Neptune RR (2013) A theoretical analysis of the influence of wheelchair seat position on upper extremity demand. *Clin Biomech* 28: 378–85. doi: 10.1016/j.clinbiomech.2013.03.004

Snoek GJ, Ijzerman MJ, Hermens HJ, Maxwell D, Biering-Sørensen F (2004) Survey of the needs of patients with spinal cord injury: impact and priority for improvement in hand function in tetraplegics. *Spinal Cord* 42: 526–32. doi: 10.1038/sj.sc.3101638

Tse R, Hentz VR, Yao J (2007) Late reconstruction for ulnar nerve palsy. *Hand Clin* 23: 373–92. doi: 10.1016/j.hcl.2007.05.003

Vogel LC, Krajci KA, Anderson CJ (2002) Adults with pediatric onset spinal cord injury: part 2: musculoskeletal and neurological complications. *J Spinal Cord Med* 25: 117–23.

Vogel LC, Betz RR, Mulcahey MJ (2012) Spinal cord injuries in children and adolescents. *Hand Clinic Neurol* 109: 131–48. doi: 10.1016/B978-0-444-52137-8.00008-5

Zancolli E (1975) Surgery for the quadriplegic hand with strong wrist extension preserved—a study of 97 cases. *Clin Orthop* 112: 101–13. http://dx.doi.org/10.1097/00003086-197510000-00013

Section 6 Physical Rehabilitation

21
REHABILITATION

Pamela Wilson, Michael Dichiaro and Dennis J Matthews

Case vignette

Abby was 6 years old when she sustained a mid-cervical spinal cord injury (SCI) in a car crash. She spent 4 weeks in acute care where rehabilitation medicine specialists were consulted for the maintenance of range of motion, positioning, and equipment. She was admitted to the subacute rehabilitation unit where a multidisciplinary evaluation took place to define baseline neurologic function; to assess functional capacity, understanding of SCI, pre-injury roles (of child and parents), and developmental readiness for therapy; and to initiate discharge planning. Abby participated in 8 weeks of in-patient rehabilitation that included education about SCI (entire team); nutritional counseling and support (nursing and nutritionist); establishing a bladder and bowel program (nursing) and a skin maintenance program (nursing); breathing exercises and diaphragm-strengthening activities (respiratory and physical therapy); activities designed to increase tolerance to upright positions (entire team); functional mobility activities (including wheelchair and upright) (physical and occupational therapy); retraining in self care, play, and school activities (occupational therapy); experimenting with adaptive equipment for sports and leisure (occupational therapy and therapeutic recreation); and consultations regarding medicine, orthopedics, and psychology. Child Life specialists work closely with the nursing team to teach Abby about her medications and about intermittent catheterization and her bowel program. The social work and case management teams worked collaboratively to support the emotional and social recovery process and to prepare for Abby's discharge needs. The social work, case management, and physical and occupational therapy teams conducted a home visit and a school visit to identify social issues and any equipment needs and to determine community resources. The case management team worked with the school and confirmed a medical home for centralization and coordination of care. Abby was discharged from in-patient therapy and returned home and to her pre-injury first grade class. She has been participating in out-patient follow-up appointments every 6 months to monitor her rehabilitation and habilitation needs.

Introduction

Rehabilitation medicine is based on the premise of optimizing function, participation, and quality of life in those individuals who have impairments resulting from illness or trauma. It tends to be holistically oriented and patient centered. When treating children or adolescents with spinal cord injuries (SCIs) and illnesses, it is crucial to have a patient- and family-centered program in place. This care delivery system is based on the idea that the family is the primary source of support and strength and that the family's and child's perspectives must be incorporated into medical planning (Committee on Hospital Care and American Academy of Pediatrics 2003). Care delivery should be a collaborative effort between the family and health-care providers, as this type of care delivery tends to result in improved safety and outcomes, reduced cost of healthcare, and improved family satisfaction (Committee on Hospital Care and Institute For Patient- and Family-Centered Care 2012). Care delivery in a center that has expertise in spinal cord medicine is the optimal placement for a child or adolescent with this type of SCI. Analysis of the adult model systems suggests that early transfer to a specialty care center results in overall reduction in length of hospital stay and that complication and mortality rates are reduced (Parent et al 2011).

The multidisciplinary rehabilitation team

Spinal cord injury in children is a catastrophic event that often has a life-changing impact on the family and the child. The morbidity associated with SCI is highly multifactorial and, as such, there are physical, psychosocial, and emotional components that need to be identified and treated. To address these unique concerns, a team specifically trained in SCI medicine is ideal for evaluating rehabilitation needs (see Chapter 4) and providing a comprehensive care approach. This team incorporates multiple disciplines working together for a unified goal of ameliorating the impact of the SCI and maximizing functional potential. The interdisciplinary team members should include physicians from relevant disciplines such as physical medicine and rehabilitation, urology, orthopedics, neurosurgery, neurology, pulmonary medicine, and other consultation services. Just as critical to successful care are medical professionals from disciplines including rehabilitation nursing, therapy (physical, occupational, speech and therapeutic recreation), respiratory therapy, clinical psychology, nutrition, medical social worker/case management, child life, recreational and equipment specialists, and educational/vocational specialists.

The rehabilitation process of spinal cord injury

The acute rehabilitation of a child with an SCI can be divided into different phases. These phases include rehabilitation consultation during the acute medical admission, the initial evaluation upon rehabilitation admission, optimizing SCI-specific medical care and function, and discharge planning. The rehabilitation team often works in concert with the acute medical/surgical service to guide care related to the SCI before admission to the rehabilitation center. Acute care recommendations include defining the extent of the injury (International Standards for Neurological Classification of Spinal Cord Injury (ISNCSCI)) (American Spinal Injury Association 2011), the need for anticoagulation, the management of neurogenic bowel and bladder, identifying autonomic dysreflexia, skin care, maintaining range of motion, nutrition, respiratory care, and family/child education. Once medically stabilized, the child can be transferred to the rehabilitation specialty service where the initial evaluation by the complete rehabilitation team can occur. During the first few days of initial rehabilitation, it is essential to obtain a new baseline of preserved motor and sensory function. A repeat ISNCSCI examination will define what residual nervous function is present and also gives the team a template for setting goals for the rehabilitation stay. The ISNCSCI examination has utility in children as young as 6 years, as children of this age are able to follow appropriate testing; for those younger than 6 years, clinicians will need to use physical examination and observation to understand the extent of the injury (Mulcahey et al 2011; see also Chapter 4). Any individual with a traumatic injury should be screened for an associated brain injury. Information from the Spinal Cord Model Systems report indicates that 28.2% of individuals with an SCI have an associated brain injury (Go et al 1995). The choice of screening tools will be based on the developmental age of the child and residual motor skills. In addition, it is critical to get an idea of the extent of the patient and family education that has preceded the transfer to the rehabilitation unit. A solid background in simple pathophysiology is essential in developing an understanding of the overall implications of SCI. The rehabilitation philosophy is introduced, which includes moving young people and their families from an acute care model to one of active participation. Patients and families will be taught how to care for themselves and integrate themselves back into the home, school, and community environments.

In-patient rehabilitation treatment for spinal cord injury

The rehabilitation physician coordinates the interdisciplinary team, which together provides holistic care for the child with an SCI. Typical goals include medical stability, optimization of function and age-appropriate independence, bowel and bladder programs, skin management, provision of durable medical equipment needs, identification of home-care needs, and family education. Details of specific care plans for each child and family come from the nature of the SCI and the evaluations on admission to rehabilitation. Table 21.1 describes the expected function outcomes according to the level of SCI. For younger children, expected goals should take into consideration appropriate developmental milestones. In some instances, treatments to prevent complications from the SCI may also inhibit a child's ability to achieve their maximum level of function, for example the thoracolumbosacral orthosis for scoliosis (see Chapter 19).

Medical issues for a child with an SCI may be the more prominent focus early in the rehabilitation stay and are often similar to those encountered during the acute care. These are discussed in greater detail in Chapters 11 to 14. Once admitted to the rehabilitation center, these unique medical issues will be incorporated into the treatment programs.

Nurses with specialty SCI training will care for the child and family 24 hours per day and provide expertise and education on these SCI care issues. They will implement medical and nursing care plans and will also reinforce the therapy programs. In collaboration with the interdisciplinary team, nurses perform a large percentage of education and self-care training. Respiratory therapists are critical to the care of children with SCIs, especially those with high-thoracic and -cervical levels of injury. Their care may include both invasive and non-invasive techniques, from simple breathing treatments and percussion to managing long-term mechanical ventilation (see Chapter 9). For children who are not on ventilator support,

TABLE 21.1
Functional expectations for spinal cord levels

Level	Breathing	ADLs/self care	Mobility/transfers
C1–C3	Ventilator	Mouth stick or environmental controls	Power wheelchair with adapted access
C4	± ventilator. Ventilator early on	Environmental controls	Power wheelchair with adapted access
C5	Not usually required. Non-invasive ventilator for very young children	Assistance for ADLs such as feeding with adapted equipment and set-up. Assistance with dressing and bathing	Can use manual wheelchair-level surfaces. Power wheelchair for longer distances. Driving possible with modifications
C6	+	Assistance with or independent for most ADLs	Manual wheelchair; power wheelchair for longer distances. Sliding board transfers
C7	+	Can do most ADLs and household chores	Manual wheelchair; transfers
C8	+	Independent	Manual wheelchair; transfers
T1–T12	+	Independent	Manual wheelchair. Can stand with braces. Limited walking
L1–L2	+	Independent	Manual wheelchair; walking long-leg braces (therapy and home)
L3–L5	+	Independent	Manual wheelchair. Community ambulation
S1–S5	+	Independent	Community ambulation

ADLs, activities of daily living.

respiratory therapists work collaboratively with the interdisciplinary team on mechanisms to improve respiratory function. In addition to early mobilization, frequent position changes help children to keep their lungs free of secretions. Postural drainage positions can be used to maximize drainage at each segment of the lung (Frownfelter and Dean 2006). Other techniques addressed by the respiratory therapist include assisted cough (Kirby et al 1966, Braun et al 1984, Massery 1987) and breathing exercise (Frownfelter and Dean 2006).

The nutritional status of the child or adolescent needs to be followed closely, as this is very important to the healing and rehabilitation processes. Post-traumatic metabolic needs can vary based on the recovery process, and nutritional support services can guide the team in optimizing both nutrition and fluid needs. Nutritional parameters such as weights and nutritional lab values can assist in the initial and ongoing assessment of the child. Children with high-cervical injuries, swallow dysfunction, or multisystem trauma may require placement of nasogastric or gastrostomy tubes to optimize nutritional support. Bowel and bladder programs will be defined by the SCI team, and the patient and family will be trained on how to perform and manage these programs. With the bladder, the goals are to protect the kidney from high pressures and reflux and achieve social continence. Bowel programs are variable, but the end goal is to have predictable bowel movements for older children and to prevent constipation and diarrhea in young children (see Chapter 11). Autonomic dysreflexia can be life threatening and is often hard to identify in young children. It is common; it is found in approximately half of all pediatric patients with an injury at a T6 neurologic level and above. It is more common in children aged 6 to 13 years with complete injuries, especially those with complete cervical injuries (see Chapter 13). Autonomic dysfunction needs to be monitored throughout the rehabilitation process, as episodes of orthostatic hypotension and bradycardia are common.

The therapy team (physical therapy, occupational therapy, speech therapy, and therapeutic recreation) should have a complete understanding of SCI and functional considerations. Physical therapy emphasizes movement skills and lower extremity range of motion. In this context, research has identified 19 different treatment activities that physical therapy uses in daily therapy sessions for those with an SCI (Natale et al 2009). Therapy often begins with bed mobility, sitting, and transfers, and then progresses to ambulation with or without assistive devices, or mobility with a manual or power wheelchair. The means of mobility will vary depending on the residual motor function, and the goal is to achieve age-appropriate milestones (see Chapter 22). Physical therapy considers the child's or adolescent's developmental age and then employs different strategies to optimize strength, endurance, balance, upright positioning, and equipment needs.

Occupational therapy has 26 different skills that may be introduced during the rehabilitation process that include strength and range of motion in the upper extremities and activities of daily living such as feeding, grooming, bathing, dressing, transfers, and cooking (Ozelie et al 2009). The utilization of adaptive equipment and assistive devices often is needed to accomplish these goals. Occupational therapists works closely with the child and family to treat these deficits in an age-appropriate manner, considering the skills learned before the child's injury. Adaptive driving is an important skill for those who have already learned to drive. Hand controls can be modified to accommodate different levels of hand function. Driving training is typically performed by a driving specialist, often in conjunction with occupational therapists to help fit the car modifications to the adolescent.

In speech and language pathology, seven key treatment areas that are used in SCI therapy have been defined. Speech and language pathology specialists will diagnose and treat feeding difficulties, often in conjunction with the occupational therapist. In addition, speech and language pathology specializes in communication and language production. In high-level injuries, these specialists will assist in developing programs for vocalization and breathing support, and will identify assistive technology needs (see Chapter 9). They may also test children for concomitant brain injury and provide cognitive treatment interventions (Gordan et al 2009).

Therapeutic recreation has an important role in the treatment of SCI. These specialists are responsible not only for defining hospital-based recreation activities, but also for identifying community resources. Therapeutic recreation specialists help to define pre-injury lifestyles and then develop ways to include these in the therapeutic plan (see Chapter 26). How these goals will be incorporated will vary significantly depending on the patient's age, residual function, community setting, family structure, and philosophy (Cahow et al 2009). Rehabilitation psychology can be critical for the emotional well-being of the child or adolescent and family during the rehabilitation stay. The SCI may have an impact on all facets of the child's and family's lives and there is the potential for lifelong consequences for both. The evaluation of mood and the provision of skills for coping and adjustment are very important not only during the entire hospitalization, but also in the transition back home. Rehabilitation psychology can also offer neuropsychological testing to objectively test the cognitive abilities of children with SCI. This can be critical in understanding the ability of the child to learn new skills that can maximize the child's function, especially when there are premorbid intellectual disabilities or concerns because of concomitant traumatic brain injury.

Educational and vocational specialists are trained to continue the child's education during their in-patient rehabilitation stay and to help the child and family prepare for their return to school or work. Child life specialists work with children and families to assist with self-expression and coping with a new disability and the stress of hospitalization and painful procedures. Social workers play an important role with families who are dealing with a crisis in their lives. They are responsible for helping families to identify the psychological and social implications of the SCI. The case management team, on the other hand, specializes in resource utilization. They serve a vital role in interacting with insurance payers to ensure that these resources are optimally utilized and this team is also very important when alternative resources need to be identified. They assist with the logistical process of transitioning in-patient treatments and therapies to the out-patient setting.

Orthoses and assistive devices/durable medical equipment can be used to facilitate positioning and function. Orthoses have several potential uses including positioning, protecting a body segment, assisting a joint for functional use, or allowing for weight bearing (see Chapters 6 and 7). After the SCI, cervical and spinal orthoses may be utilized to immobilize the spine, allow for healing, and provide stabilization (see Chapter 6). Different neurologic injuries may benefit from a different combination of orthotics. For example, cervical-level SCI may utilize bracing of the wrist for position or to facilitate a tenodesis grasp, whereas a balanced forearm orthosis can be used to facilitate independent arm function for activities of daily living such as feeding (see Chapter 20). Lower extremities are braced to maintain position, to control upright posture, or for ambulation. These can be very extensive, such as hip–knee–ankle braces or reciprocal gait orthoses, or can be simple shoe inserts. Ankle–foot orthoses are commonly used to maintain the position of feet, to protect the feet, or for ambulation (see Chapter 22). Recently, the uses of robotic-type braces as an exoskeleton for support have been trialed in adults. Functional electrical stimulation and body weight-supported ambulation are two of several options for stimulating weak or paralyzed muscles. They have several physiological benefits and are discussed in detail in Chapters 22 and 28.

Assistive devices such as crutches and walkers may help support ambulation. Other equipment will augment self care and activities of daily living, such as modified eating utensils or bathing equipment. Durable medical equipment includes not only mobility-related devices, but also communication and environmental systems. The type of durable medical equipment ordered will be dictated by the age of the child and his or her residual function (http://www.asia-spinalinjury.org/rehab/dme_guide_public.php). High-level cervical injuries will need state-of-the-art technology to access and control the environment (see Chapter 9). Lower level injuries may not require any durable medical equipment. It is imperative that all providers of SCI medicine keep up to date on technology, durable medical equipment, and orthoses, as the field is rapidly expanding.

Developmental needs of children with spinal cord injury

The rehabilitation team must always take into consideration the developmental stage and needs of the child with an SCI. Physical, intellectual, emotional, and social development is dependent on age. Rehabilitation for infants with an SCI, for instance, will focus more on training of the family for functional needs, provision of medical care, and use of equipment. At an age when an uninjured child is walking, the ability to explore the environment is critical to a child's development. Therapy should focus on mobility, considering the use of adaptive equipment or a manual/power wheelchair. Activities of daily living should be addressed, with a greater focus on preschool- and early elementary school-aged children, as this is the time when uninjured peers will be progressing toward independence with activities of daily living. With appropriate upper extremity function and truncal balance/support, children can learn self-catheterization and begin to learn to insert a suppository with a bowel program as early as 6 years old (Molnar 1988). During the school years, education is vital for a child's development, and planning for their return to school is of the utmost importance. Teenagers are in a stage of development in which striving for independence is common. They should be encouraged to make choices in their rehabilitation, and to learn to direct caregivers to assist with any needs they cannot perform.

Discharge planning

The discharge planning aspects of the acute rehabilitation process begin on the first day of admission. In general, the patient-centered medical home model may be the most comprehensive approach. This medical home model is led by a primary care physician or SCI team that can provide and coordinate specialized levels of care in direct partnership with the child or adolescent and their family. It is an offshoot of the Healthy People 2010 (US Department of Health and Human Services 2000) ideology and emerged in response to increasing numbers of children with chronic conditions and fragmented medical care. The American Academy of Pediatrics defined, in 2002, the basic characteristics of the medical home model and consolidated them into the 'seven Cs' (continuous, comprehensive, coordinated, compassionate, culturally effective, family-centered, and accessible) (Medical Home Initiatives for Children With Special Needs Project Advisory Committee, American Academy of Pediatrics 2002).

Children with complex medical conditions and technology needs can be discharged home and back into the local community. Long gone are the days of discharges into congregate care centers (Murphy and Carbone 2011). A systematized approach will make sure all the bases are covered and ensure that there will be a smooth transition. Elias recently identified the critical elements as really understanding the family, child, home, and community dynamics; finding a medical home; training and education; home-care training; arranging home nursing and finding agencies; and availability of insurance resources (Elias and Murphy 2012). These approaches are described in more detail in Table 21.2. The impact of education and training by members of the medical team should not be underestimated, as it is one of the best predictors of discharge readiness. It has a positive impact on the family because it not only builds confidence, but also promotes that feeling of 'I'm ready' for the upcoming transition home (Weiss et al 2008).

Habilitation

Similar to all children with typical development, as children with SCI grow and develop, there is an expectation that they will achieve as much autonomy and independence in developmentally appropriate skills. Habilitation is the process of training children in new activities that have not been previously mastered owing to development. Moreover, changes in function are anticipated as children transition from one developmental stage to another; these changes should be monitored and, when appropriate, therapy should be provided to minimize the adverse impact they may have on independent functioning, quality of life, and solidifying skills required for the next developmental stage.

TABLE 21.2
Discharge elements

Education/ communication	Does the family/child understand spinal cord injury and the impact on function?
	Does the family understand the medical issues, including pulmonary, skin, bowel, and bladder management?
	Has the family/child been trained in healthcare tasks (this includes ventilator management, bowel programs, catheterization programs, skin care, treatment of autonomic dysreflexia)?
	Family knowledge of insurance benefits
Home evaluation	The home environment has been evaluated and adapted to be safe, accessible, and functional
Durable medical equipment / supplies	Equipment has been ordered (ventilators, mobility-related equipment, bathing supplies, bowel and bladder supplies, braces, equipment for activities of daily living and environmental control)
	Family has been trained in functional use of durable medical equipment
	Family knows who to call and where to get ongoing supplies/durable medical equipment
Medication	Family/child instruction in rational for medication
	Right dose, right route, right timing
	Knowledge of side effects
	Community pharmacy has been identified
Follow-up appointments, home care, school and community resources identified	Family understands what service will be provided in the out-patient setting (physical, occupational, and speech therapy)
	Home care has been arranged
	Schools have been contacted
	They have phone numbers and know who to contact for services and appointments
	They have a list of emergency services
	Primary physician or medical home has pertinent medical information
	Appointments for post-hospital care have been arranged
	Community resources have been identified

Summary

The rehabilitation and habilitation of children with SCI occurs within a family-centered approach by a multidisciplinary team that is fully competent in the care of children with SCI. Therapeutic interventions are highly dependent upon the level of injury, developmental age of the child, and coexisting medical complications that may be present. The goal of rehabilitation is to facilitate the child's functional recovery and emotional and social well-being so that he or she actively engages in typical childhood roles with enjoyment and competence, ultimately transitioning into productive adulthood.

REFERENCES

American Spinal Injury Association (2011) *International Standards for the Neurologic Classification of Spinal Cord Injury Revised 2011* (booklet). Atlanta, GA: American Spinal Injury Association.

Braun SR, Giovannoni R, O'Connor M (1984) Improving the cough in patients with spinal cord injury. *Am J Phys Med* 63: 1–10.

Cahow C, Skolnick S, Joyce J, Jug J, Dragon C, Gassaway J (2009) SCIRehab Project series: the therapeutic recreation taxonomy. *J Spinal Cord Med* 32: 298–306.

Committee on Hospital Care, American Academy of Pediatrics (2003) Family-centered care and the pediatrician's role. *Pediatrics* 112: 691–7. doi: 10.1542/peds.2011-3084

Committee on Hospital Care, Institute For Patient- and Family-Centered Care (2012) Patient- and family-centered care and the pediatrician's role. *Pediatrics* 129: 394–404. http://dx.doi.org/10.1542/peds.2011-3084

Elias ER, Murphy NA; Council on Children with Disabilities (2012) Home care of children and youth with complex health care needs and technology dependencies. *Pediatrics* 129: 996–1005. doi: 10.1542/peds.2012-0606

Frownfelter D, Dean E (2006) *Cardiovascular and Pulmonary Physical Therapy: Evidence and Practice*. 4th Ed. St Louis, MO: Mosby Elsevier.

Go BK, DeVivo MJ, Richards JS (1995) Epidemiology of spinal cord injury. In: Stover SL, DeLisa JA, Whiteneck GG (eds). *Spinal Cord Injury: Clinical Outcomes from the Model Systems*. Gaithersburg, MD: Aspen Publications. p. 355.

Gordan W, Spivak-David D, Adornato V et al (2009) SCIRehab Project series: the speech language pathology taxonomy. *J Spinal Cord Med* 32: 307–18.

Kirby NA, Barnerias MJ, Siebens AA (1966) An evaluation of assisted cough in quadriparetic patients. *Arch Med Phys Rehab* 47: 705–10.

Massery M (1987) An innovative approach to assistive cough techniques. *Top Acute Care Trauma Rehabil* 1: 73–85.

Medical Home Initiatives for Children With Special Needs Project Advisory Committee, American Academy of Pediatrics (2002) The medical home. *Pediatrics* 110: 184–6. http://dx.doi.org/10.1542/peds.110.1.184

Molnar GE (1988) A developmental perspective for the rehabilitation of children with physical disability. *Pediatr Ann* 17: 766, 8–71, 73–6.

Mulcahey MJ, Gaughan J, Chafetz RS, Vogel LC, Samdani AF, Betz RR (2011) Interrater reliability of the international standards for neurological classification of spinal cord injury in youths with chronic spinal cord injury. *Arch Phys Med Rehabil* 92: 1264–9. doi: 10.1016/j.apmr.201103.003

Murphy NA, Carbone PS; Council on Children With Disabilities; American Academy of Pediatrics (2011) Parent–provider–community partnerships: optimizing outcomes for children with disabilities. *Pediatrics* 128: 795–802. doi: 10.1542/peds.2011-1467

Natale A, Taylor S, LaBarbera J et al (2009) SCIRehab Project series: the physical therapy taxonomy. *J Spinal Cord Med* 32: 270–82.

Ozelie R, Sipple C, Foy T et al (2009) SCIRehab Project series: the occupational therapy taxonomy. *J Spinal Cord Med* 32: 283–97.

Parent S, Barchi S, LeBreton M, Casha S, Fehlings MG (2011) The impact of specialized centers of care for spinal cord injury on length of stay complications and mortality: a systematic review of the literature. *J Neurotrauma* 28: 1363–70. doi: 10.1089/neu.2009.1151

US Department of Health and Human Services (2000) *Healthy People 2010. With Understanding and Improving Health and Objectives for Improving Health*. 2nd Ed. Washington, DC: US Government Printing Office.

Weiss M, Johnson NL, Malin S, Jerofke T, Lang C, Sherburne E (2008) Readiness for discharge in parents of hospitalized children. *J Pediatr Nurs* 23: 282–95. doi: 10.1016/j.pedn.2007.10.005

22
MOBILITY FOR CHILDREN WITH SPINAL CORD INJURY

Christina L Calhoun and Lisa A Harvey

Case vignette: John

John is a 4-year-old male who sustained a C1–C3 spinal cord injury (SCI) in May 2002 secondary to a motor vehicle crash. He also sustained a ruptured spleen, fractured right femur, and closed head injury. John has a tracheostomy and is fully ventilatory dependent for breathing. His parents are fully independent in his respiratory and ventilator care. Before his SCI, he was a very healthy child with no acute or chronic illnesses and he achieved all of his developmental milestones on time. He currently receives 16 hours of home nursing care per day to support the care his parents provide him. After his SCI, John did not receive rehabilitation. He had some orthotic care at an out-patient rehabilitation facility where he received hand splints and ankle–foot orthoses. He recently spent 1 week at a specialized children's hospital for ventilator adjustments, evaluation, and rehabilitation (see Appendix 22.1).

Case vignette: Emma

Emma is a 13-year-old female who, at 3 years of age, sustained a T6 incomplete spinal cord injury of American Spinal Injury Association Impairment Scale grade B secondary to a motor vehicle crash. Emma's surgical history includes bilateral lower extremity osteotomies with external fixation and a posterior spinal fusion from T1 to the pelvis. She has a history of a stage IV sacral wound that required extensive hospitalization involving intravenous antibiotics, nasogastric nutrition, and negative pressure wound therapy to heal the wound. As a result of her spinal cord injury, Emma presents with flaccid lower extremity paralysis and impaired muscle function and movement and has absent sensation below the injury level. Functionally, Emma is non-ambulatory and requires a custom manual wheelchair as her primary means of mobility for home, school, and community environments (see Appendix 22.2).

Introduction

Mobility is integral to everything a child does and refers to free movement in all settings including in the home, school, the community, and the world at large. It enables learning, interaction with others, attendance at school, and participation in recreation, family life, and society. Mobility is particularly important for an infant and toddler because it allows for exploring of the environment, which is essential for the development of cognitive, social, and communication skills. However, it is also important as the child grows older and is central to the successful progression through childhood and adolescence into adulthood. It is therefore appropriate that the mobility of a child with a spinal cord injury (SCI) be given high priority.

The child with an SCI often uses more than one means of mobility at any stage in his or her development. For example, a child may primarily use a wheelchair while at school but use gait orthoses and mobility aids at home, or vice versa. In addition, often the type of mobility aids a child requires changes over time as the child's physical size, cognition, function, and social needs change. The type of mobility aids a child requires also changes in response to changing priorities and perspectives of the child and his or her family. The provision and revision of mobility aids is therefore a dynamic process throughout a child's development.

Most of what is known about mobility for children (and adults) comes from expert consensus rather than high-quality evidence (Fuhrer 2007). For example, there are no randomized controlled trials comparing different types of wheelchairs and there are few studies that identify the key determinants of mobility in children (Vogel and Lubicky 1995a,b, Schottler 2012). In the absence of this evidence, evidence about mobility from adults is applied to children, taking into account their special needs (Krey and Calhoun 2004). Similarly, there are no clinical practice guidelines about appropriate prescription of mobility equipment for children with SCI, but there are a few notable books, systematic reviews, guidelines, and recommendations for adults with SCI (Bergen 2000, Di Marco et al 2003, Michael et al 2007, EnableNSW and Lifetime Care and Support Authority 2011).

The first step in determining the appropriate form of mobility for a child is a comprehensive assessment. This includes assessing a child's functional abilities and limitations, neuromusculoskeletal and developmental status, and home, community, and school environments (see Chapter 4).

Wheelchairs

Children are typically prescribed a wheelchair during the initial in-patient rehabilitation. If it is anticipated that a child's neurologic status will markedly change, then it is often best to postpone the prescription of the definitive wheelchair and instead provide the child with a temporary wheelchair. The wheelchair needs to be properly configured and set up for the child. In addition, both the child and the child's parents need to be educated about its maintenance, care, assembly, disassembly, set-up, and use.

There are many different types of wheelchairs that come with an array of different seating systems. All need to be considered. A child should be provided with the opportunity to try out several types of appropriate wheelchairs and seating systems before making a final decision. The choice between a power and a manual wheelchair depends on many factors, as outlined below. Often a child will require both.

Power mobility

Power mobility is often recommended for those with motor complete injuries between C1 and C6 (Consortium for Spinal Cord Medicine 1999). However, power mobility is also recommended for children with lower lesions if (1) they are unable to push a manual wheelchair, (2) pushing a manual wheelchair is considerably more laborious and inefficient than mobilizing in a power wheelchair, or (3) pushing a manual wheelchair causes pain.

A power wheelchair can be front-, center-, mid-, or rear-wheel drive. There are advantages and disadvantages of each (Table 22.1). There are many different ways to drive and control a power wheelchair including, but not limited to, head and hand switches, sip and puff controls, head arrays, mini proportional joysticks, and standard hand joysticks. Those with sufficient hand function typically use the standard hand joystick. Those with very limited upper limb function use the other types of control mechanisms (Table 22.2). Power wheelchairs can have power tilt or power tilt and recline. These are recommended for the child with more severe disabilities who is unable to independently lift his or her body and reposition in the wheelchair. Tilt or power tilt and recline enables the child to independently relieve and redistribute

TABLE 22.1
Power wheelchair bases

Drive type	Description	Strengths	Limitations
Front	Main drive wheel is located anteriorly More of a pulling motion User's center of gravity is just posterior to the drive axle	Stable on up and down inclines Will not tip forward on a decline or with sudden stops	Slower speed compared with mid-, center-, or rear-wheel drives May be least intuitive to drive
Mid	Main drive wheel is located centrally under the user	Provides smallest turning radius Increased maneuverability in tight spaces Decreased need for spatial awareness or judgment when maneuvering	Requires a front stabilizer Increased potential to rock forward on declines and with sudden stops
Center	Like a mid-wheel drive, the main drive wheel is located centrally under the user All six wheels are in contact with the ground	Increased stability compared with mid-wheel because the front stabilizing wheels are in constant contact with the ground Provides smallest turning radius Increased maneuverability in tight spaces Decreased need for spatial awareness or judgment when maneuvering	
Rear	Main drive wheel is located posteriorly More of a pushing motion User's center of gravity is just anterior to the drive axle	May be the most intuitive to drive and easiest to learn to maneuver Provides the highest speeds with the most control Moderate ability to negotiate terrain and obstacles	Largest turning radius Potential to rock forward when maneuvering down an elevation or obstacle

TABLE 22.2

Power wheelchair drive controls. All (except conventional hand-operative joysticks) are appropriate for people with very poor or no upper limb and hand function (i.e. typically those with motor complete C1–C4 tetraplegia). The conventional hand-operative joystick is appropriate for everyone else

Drive control type	Description	Strengths	Limitations
Proportional drive controls: the user pushes the joystick or head array in the direction they want to go. The harder the user pushes, the faster he or she goes			
Conventional hand-operated joystick	The user controls the wheelchair with the hand through a gimbal knob	Widely available and relatively inexpensive The control mechanism is relatively easy to use	The user requires at least some upper limb and hand function
Compact chin-operated joystick	The user controls the wheelchair by the chin through a small cap that is mounted on a swing-away mechanism	This mechanism is the least expensive of all the options for individuals with no hand or upper limb function	The user needs to be well positioned in the wheelchair so that the chin easily makes contact with the drive mechanism The mechanism is bulky and sits in front of the user The arm of the mechanism can easily bend or become loose The mechanism needs to be removed or swung away each time the individual gets in and out of the wheelchair
Head array	The user controls the wheelchair with a headpiece that wraps behind and slightly lateral to each side of the head. The user pushes the head into the left side of the headpiece to move left and into the right side of the headpiece to move right. To move forwards or backwards the user pushes the head backwards into the headpiece. A switch determines whether backward movement of the head moves the wheelchair forwards or backwards	The head array is cosmetically and functionally superior to a chin-control mechanism because there is nothing in front of the user's face The head array is less sensitive to the position of the user and the headset	The user needs to activate a switch each time he or she wants to move between forwards and backwards
Non-proportional drive controls: the user does not need to apply pressure to move the wheelchair. Instead, the user only needs to move some part of his or her body			
Head control	Similar to the proportional head array, but the user does not need to maintain pressure to move the wheelchair. Instead, the user makes single movements of the head to set the wheelchair in motion	The user does not need to maintain constant pressure on the head control mechanism to keep the wheelchair moving	The headrest cannot be used to rest the head unless the wheelchair is turned off The user can not adjust the speed of the wheelchair while moving it

TABLE 22.2
(Continued)

Drive control type	Description	Strengths	Limitations
Sip and puff	The user controls the wheelchair by either sucking air or sipping air in and out of a small plastic tube similar to a straw The control mechanism can be set up so that different combinations and different strengths of sip and puff can move the wheelchair in different ways	The small plastic tube is less obtrusive than a chin-control mechanism	The user requires extensive training and practice to use this mechanism effectively and safely The user cannot speak while controlling the wheelchair The user constantly has the small plastic tube in his or her mouth The plastic tube in the mouth can be unhygienic

pressure and offers good stability and comfort. If the child requires ventilator support, then a ventilator tray needs to be attached to the wheelchair. It is important to ensure the ventilator and its tray do not impede the tilt of the wheelchair. Some wheelchairs have the capacity to bring a child into standing. This is an expensive additional option but has the obvious benefits associated with being in an upright position. Alternatively, it is possible to purchase power wheelchairs that allow the seat to be raised and lowered while the child remains in a seated position. These types of wheelchairs provide greater access to different environments and can facilitate peer interaction. For example, a child can raise the wheelchair to write on a blackboard at school and lower the wheelchair when sitting around a dining room table with family. Wheelchairs may also allow the seat to lower all the way to the ground to enable a child to crawl into them or be at the same level as his or her peers.

Children, like adults, need to receive training in the use of power mobility. There are various skills they need to master, including safely descending cambered slopes, negotiating doors and obstacles, and traversing uneven ground (Axelson et al 2002). There is no set age to initiate power mobility training for a child and chronologic age alone should not determine when a child is ready to use power mobility (Rosen et al 2009). Instead, the decision should be based on cognition and developmental age. Children without cognitive disabilities as young as 18 to 24 months can learn quickly to use a powered mobility device safely with supervision (Fig. 22.1) (Butler et al 1983, 1984, Corfman et al 2003, Lynch et al 2009). Historically, therapists have considered the use of powered mobility as the ability to independently and safely drive a chair in all situations (Kangas 1997). However, this seems unreasonable because no one expects a young child to walk and run independently and safely in all situations. Nor should they expect a young child to mobilize in a power wheelchair in all situations. Just as a child learns to walk over time, a child should be able to learn to move in a power wheelchair over time. Power mobility for a young and otherwise dependent child should be seen as a high priority because it promotes psychosocial development, reduces learned helplessness, and facilitates social and educational integration and independence (Rosen et al 2009).

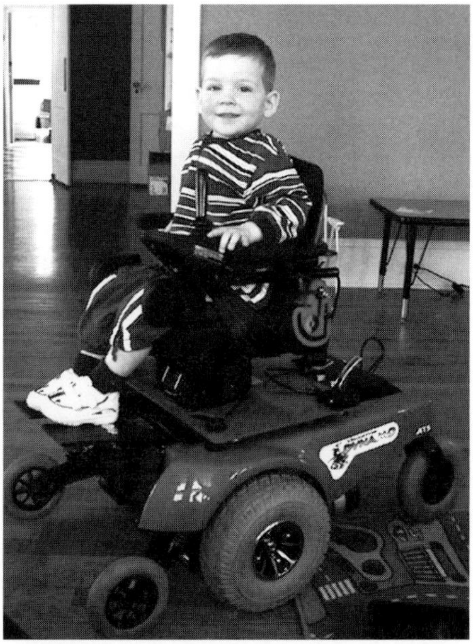

Fig. 22.1 Even very young children can learn to use a power wheelchair. This child sustained his SCI during birth and was evaluated for the use of power mobility at about 18 months of age. With training and age-appropriate supervision, he was able to use a joystick-controlled power wheelchair to move about with his ambulatory peers. Photograph printed with consent.

All children who use powered mobility require a backup manual wheelchair. For more impaired children, this should have the capacity to tilt in space for the same reasons that a power wheelchair should have this capacity. A backup manual wheelchair is essential because, invariably, power wheelchairs malfunction or require service (McClure et al 2009). Without a backup wheelchair, the child is restricted to bed. Backup manual wheelchairs are also often required when using cars, taxis, and trains because it is not possible to lift a power wheelchair because they are too heavy.

Sometimes it is appropriate to provide a child with a power sit-on scooter. However, scooters do not have good pressure-relieving qualities or back support. Nor can they be readily driven with poor upper limb function. Therefore, they are not typically appropriate for a child with motor complete tetraplegia. Instead, they are prescribed for the child who has reasonably good trunk control and who gets very tired pushing a manual wheelchair or walking long distances, although children with these characteristics are rare.

Manual mobility

Children with injuries from C7 to T12 typically use manual wheelchairs as their primary form of mobility (Consortium for Spinal Cord Medicine 1999). Similarly, those who primarily ambulate (i.e. those with incomplete lesions or lesions below T12) may require a manual wheelchair for traversing long distances (Axelson et al 1998, Best et al 2005). Similar to power mobility, children as young as 18 months of age should be encouraged to utilize a wheelchair to facilitate independence. However, it is also appropriate that infants and toddlers with SCI be provided with appropriate strollers for when they need to be pushed, just as children without SCI need a stroller.

Manual wheelchairs can have either a rigid or a folding frame. The main implication of the wheelchair frame is for stowing. For example, rigid-frame wheelchairs are stowed by removing the wheels, whereas folding-frame wheelchairs are stowed by folding the frame in half via a cross brace often without removing the wheels. Some like the ability to fold the wheelchair but these wheelchairs tend to be heavier than rigid-frame wheelchairs and less durable because of the moveable parts. In addition, the type of frame has implications for attaching swing away footplates and cambered wheels (wheels that are tilted with the top part of the wheel closer to the frame than the bottom part). The clinician, child, and child's family need to weigh up the pros and cons of each type of frame.

Regardless of whether a child is prescribed a fixed- or folding-frame wheelchair (Table 22.3), it is generally recommended that the wheelchair be strong, light, and fully customizable. In the absence of specific guidelines on wheelchair prescription for children, it is probably reasonable to adapt the key recommendations contained in the adult guidelines to the needs of children (Consortium for Spinal Cord Medicine 2005). One of the key recommendations in the adult guidelines, which is perhaps even more pertinent to children, is that a wheelchair be as light as possible to decrease the risk of shoulder and musculoskeletal injury and to decrease the effort associated with pushing (Boninger et al 2000).

It is not sufficient simply to provide a lightweight wheelchair. The child and his or her parents also need to be educated and trained in an effective and optimal propulsion technique (Boninger et al 2003). Heavy bags should not be placed on the back of a child's wheelchair because they increase the overall weight. These measures are all particularly important for children because they have many years ahead of them and need to ensure that their shoulders and upper limbs see them through adult life. Children also need to be taught wheelchair skills. These are important for independence. Initial evidence from clinical trials involving adults highlights the importance of structured training to facilitate the learning of wheelchair skills (Best et al 2005). It is no doubt equally important for children. There are excellent training manuals and web-based resources to guide training (Axelson et al 1998, Faculty of Medicine

TABLE 22.3
Fixed and folding manual wheelchair frames

Frame type	Description	Strengths	Limitations
Fixed	Frame does not fold in half Some have the ability for the back to fold down on the seat	Lighter than folding frames More durable than folding frames Better suited as a chair for wheelchair sports	Footplates must be fixed Wheels must be removed to stow
Folding	Frame has the ability to fold in half via a cross base under the seating system	Best for stowing and transport Allows for swing-away footplates	Contains more adjustable and removable parts, thus decreasing durability

Dalhousie University 2005, www.elearnsci.org). Spotter straps can be used for additional safety while children are learning wheelchair skills.

Clinicians face many challenges when prescribing a manual wheelchair for the growing child. The wheelchair needs to be highly adjustable to accommodate factors such as changing height, body weight, arm-to-trunk ratio, hip width, and strength. For example, the seat depth and width needs to be adjustable to ensure optimal fit is maintained as the child grows. In addition, the wheelchair needs to have an adjustable axle so that the position of the wheels on the frame can be changed. This can be used to change seat height and thereby change the distance between the tops of the wheels and the child's shoulders, which is an important consideration for optimal pushing technique. The tops of the wheels may also be brought closer to the child by increasing the camber of the wheels, although this also increases the overall width of the wheelchair. It is also important to consider the size of the wheels, wheel rims, and castors and the placement of wheel locks. Sometimes a child will need rims with projections or modifications to enable the child to push the chair. In the same way, a child may require brake extensions to ensure that he or she can engage and disengage the breaks. Anti-tippers are necessary to prevent the wheelchair from tipping backwards and hill holders are advantageous to prevent the wheelchair from rolling backwards on inclines.

Power-assisted mobility

It is possible to provide children with manual wheelchairs that have small motors in the wheels. The child pushes the wheelchair like a manual wheelchair but the motors provide varying amounts of assistance. The motors activate and increase power in response to the propulsion force from the child (Giacobbi et al 2010). These wheelchairs provide a good option for a child who has the potential to push a manual wheelchair but tires easily and requires some assistance. They do not have tilt features, so the child must be capable of some form of pressure relief. In addition, the child must be capable of propeling a manual wheelchair at least in a limited way. These wheelchairs are therefore typically recommended for children with injuries from C6 to T1.

Seating

All wheelchairs need to be fitted with an appropriate seating system. A seating system refers to the backrest, seat, trunk support, and cushion. The seating system on a child's wheelchair, whether power or manual, should promote appropriate posture, provide stability, minimize moisture, and provide pressure relief and pressure distribution. The need for stability should be weighed up against the need for freedom of movement. The balance between the two depends on the child's strength, ability to sit, and level of function (Consortium for Spinal Cord Medicine 1999). Some manufacturers provide wheelchairs with a soft canvas backrest and seat. These are generally not recommended. Instead, it is recommended that they be replaced with a solid seat pan (or rigidizer) and a solid backrest. The clinician needs to match the key features of a backrest to the needs of a child. Important considerations are height and back angle. Decisions on both should be based on the child's trunk strength and balance.

The cushion a child sits upon is central to effective skin management and requires careful consideration and monitoring. Cushions can be air-, foam-, or gel-based, and can be purchased from commercial suppliers or tailor-made by seating specialists. The most important feature of a cushion is its ability to reduce pressure under the ischial tuberosities; the area most vulnerable to pressure ulcers from prolonged sitting (Tam et al 2003, European Pressure Ulcer Advisory Panel and National Pressure Ulcer Advisory Panel 2009, Regan et al 2010). However, cushions influence seating stability and weight of a wheelchair. For some children, an important consideration is the effect of the cushion on a child's ability to transfer. Generally, firmer and flatter cushions are easier to transfer off than softer and shaped cushions, although the former would only be considered if they also provided adequate skin protection. Additional seating accessories, which are dependent on the child's needs, include a head rest or support, chest and/or lateral supports, lower and upper extremity supports, and a pelvic belt (Table 22.4).

Upright mobility with standers and orthoses

Walking may be used as an adjunct to a wheelchair for exercise and therapeutic purposes, or it may be used instead of a wheelchair as a child's primary form of mobility. Sometimes a

TABLE 22.4
Seating system accessories

Accessory	Justification and features
Pelvic belt	Necessary to maintain proper seated posture in the wheelchair
	May be padded to prevent bruising, which could occur with extensor spasms
	May be dual or single pull to further assist with proper positioning in the wheelchair
	Necessary for the individual who will be transported in a wheelchair
Head rest	Necessary to provide proper head placement and positioning
	Necessary for the individual who will be transported in a wheelchair
Arm supports	Necessary to provide support and maintain proper position of the upper extremities for individuals with high cervical-level spinal cord injury
Chest harness/ support	Necessary to provide support for individuals with decreased trunk balance
	Necessary to prevent falling forward
	Necessary to assist with maintenance of vertical alignment
	Necessary for the individual who will be transported in a wheelchair
Lateral trunk guides/support	Necessary to provide support for individuals with decreased lateral trunk balance
	Necessary to prevent falling to the right or left
	Necessary to assist with maintenance of vertical alignment
Hip guides	Necessary to maintain lower extremity positioning
	Necessary to prevent excessive hip abduction
Hip abductor pommel	Necessary to maintain lower extremity positioning
	Necessary to prevent excessive hip adduction
	May be recommended for the child with hip adductor spasticity to prevent hip subluxation and dislocation
	May be flip down/away to assist with transfers
Ankle positioners	Necessary to maintain proper foot positioning
	May reduce lower extremity extensor spasms while seated in the wheelchair

child may walk around the home and school but use a wheelchair for long distances. Before recommending any type of device or orthosis, a realistic goal for its use should be determined and agreed upon by all SCI team members, the parents, and the child (Chaftez et al 2008).

Whenever and wherever possible, children should be given the option to at least stand. Regular standing in children with lower limb paralysis is believed to have the same benefits as regular standing in adults with lower limb paralysis, namely to prevent osteoporosis and contractures, improve bladder and bowel function, reduce incidence of pressure ulcers, and aid psychological well-being (Eng et al 2001, Caulton et al 2004). Although these beliefs have not yet been substantiated in clinical trials, there is a sound rationale to believe that standing is beneficial (Glickman et al 2010). However, it is not clear how much standing a child needs to do to reap these possible therapeutic benefits. Regardless, it is generally assumed that standing in children should be encouraged. It is also often important for a child's parents to see their child stand and, if possible, to see their child attempt walking. In this way, parents can gain comfort knowing that walking was attempted, even if it was not a viable long-term solution. All children can be given the option to stand regardless of injury. The most widely used method of standing is with static standers that do not enable the child to move about. These include tilt tables and different types of wheelchairs that use hydraulic or electric lifts to bring the child into a standing position. Some include a seat that the child transfers onto, whereas others enable a child to stand directly from his or her own wheelchair with the use of a pelvic strap. Lower extremity, trunk, chest, and upper extremity supports are sometimes required. Other types of standers include mobile or active standers. A mobile stander has wheels that allow the child to propel from a standing position, whereas an active stander allows the child to exercise the upper limbs from a standing position (Fig. 22.2). All standers can provide an effective way of increasing upper limb strength and lower limb range of motion. In addition, there are devices called parapodiums (Fig. 22.3). These are orthotic devices that are used in very young children with paraplegia. They are designed for standing and moving short distances without the use of a mobility aid, thus freeing up the child's arms and hands for functional use. The hip and knee joints of the parapodium flex allow the child to sit in the device.

If a child is to walk, then he or she will usually require some type of orthosis and mobility aid, such as crutches or a walker. There are many different types of orthoses ranging from small shoe inserts to large hip–knee–ankle–foot orthoses (HKAFOs). It is important that orthoses be as least cumbersome as possible while still providing appropriate support. Children with the potential to walk often initially progress to less supportive orthotic devices and mobility aids as they improve, mature, and learn to use them. Children who are injured at a young age, especially those injured before 5 years of age, are more likely to attain functional levels of ambulation and are more likely to stay ambulating into adolescence and beyond than those injured later in childhood (Vogel et al 2007). However, it is not unusual for children to stop walking and opt for a wheelchair as they grow older, as this enables them to keep up with peers and to increase mobility and independence. In most cases, this should be viewed as a natural progression and not as a failure, because children should not be expected to continue walking into adulthood unless it provides an efficient way of moving about and facilitates independence.

Children with complete injuries above C5 cannot walk. Children with low levels of motor complete tetraplegia can be assisted in walking in a limited way around the home, provided they have extensive orthotic support and a mobility aid. However, this is not

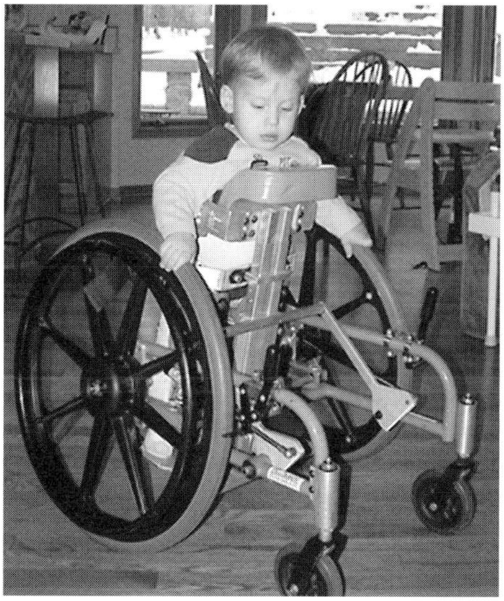

Fig. 22.2 This young child is able to move about his home in his mobile stander. Photograph printed with consent.

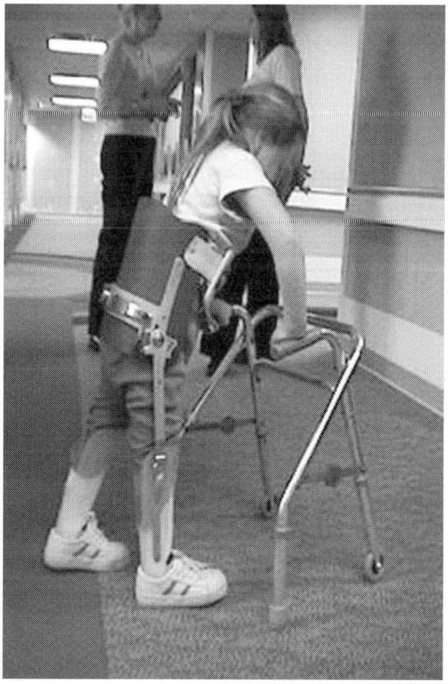

Fig. 22.3 In a reciprocal gait orthosis, this young female is able to ambulate using a reciprocal pattern. The reciprocal hip motion is achieved by shifting weight from one leg to the other while extending the trunk on the standing leg. Photograph printed with consent.

generally encouraged because it is costly, rarely continued, and exhausting for the child, and does not provide a functional form of mobility. Instead, walking is generally reserved for those with lesions below T1 (Consortium for Spinal Cord Medicine 1999, Vogel et al 2007) or for those with incomplete lesions. Children with motor complete injuries from T1 to T9 require orthoses, mobility aids, and assistance to ambulate. They typically use either bilateral knee–ankle–foot orthoses (KAFOs) or a HKAFO, depending on strength and balance. These children rarely ambulate in a functional way or with a reciprocal gait pattern. Instead, they predominantly ambulate for its therapeutic benefits or as a form of exercise using a swing to or swing through gait pattern. Both gait patterns involve pushing down into mobility aids positioned in front of the child and swinging the legs together as though jumping.

Unlike KAFOs, HKAFOs stabilize the hips in addition to the knee, ankle, and foot. There are many different types of HKAFOs including reciprocal gait orthoses (Fig. 22.4), parawalkers, walkabout orthoses, and hip guidance orthoses (Harvey et al 1997, Katz et al 1997, Robb et al 1999). They all incorporate some type of hip joint that is attached either laterally or medially to two KAFOs. Some have an additional trunk orthoses and/or pelvic band. All can be used to provide a swing to, swing through, or reciprocal gait pattern. In some of the HKAFOs, the hip joint can be locked providing support in the transverse and sagittal planes. This makes it easier for a child to use the swing to or swing through gait pattern. With the hip component unlocked, the child can use a reciprocal gait pattern; however, they still receive stability in the transverse plane. Reciprocal gait orthoses and isocentric reciprocal gait orthoses were once commonly used in children with paraplegia, but, like all HKAFOs, they are now less commonly prescribed. All HFAFOs are more difficult to put on and take off than KAFOs, especially if they include a bilateral leg pelvic attachment. There are numerous types of hip, knee, and ankle joints that can be incorporated into KAFOs and HKAFOs for those with incomplete lesions and varying patterns of lower limb paralysis. Any type of orthoses that helps maintain the knee in extension during stance but allows flexion during swing is called a stance control orthosis. One study found an increased walking speed, improved gait kinematics, and decreased oxygen consumption and energy cost when novice ambulators used a stance control orthosis compared with a KAFO (Irby et al 2005).

Children with motor complete injuries from T10 to L1 usually require the same level of orthotic support as children with lesions from T1 to T9. Some have sufficient strength around the trunk and hips to walk without assistance around the home provided they have a mobility aid. Most, however, walk or stand primarily for its therapeutic benefits and as a form of exercise. Children with injuries from L2 to S5 usually walk around the home and often around the community with assistance. However, they require orthotic support and a mobility aid. The level of orthotic support depends on the extent of paralysis but most require at least ankle–foot orthoses (AFOs) if not KAFOs. An AFO is primarily prescribed for children with isolated paralysis or weakness around the ankle. Numerous types of AFOs are available. All provide different levels and types of support. Some are adjustable whereas others are fixed depending on the child's strength and level of function. They may attach to a shoe or be used as an insert into a shoe. AFOs may be fabricated from carbon fiber, plastic, metal, or a combination of these materials. Some AFOs are aligned specifically to provide stability to the knee during stance. These are a type of stance control orthosis and are used in children with weakness around the knee but with sufficient strength to walk without a KAFO.

Upright mobility with functional electrical stimulation

Functional electrical stimulation (FES) can be used in addition to (or sometimes instead of) orthoses to enable children to stand and/or walk. FES requires an intact lower motor neuron to stimulate the muscles. When FES is used with orthoses, the combination is called a hybrid system. For example, FES can be used in combination with a HKAFO or bilateral KAFOs. FES is now being more commonly used to assist gait in children with less extensive paralysis. For example, FES is being used to stimulate the ankle dorsiflexor and evertor muscles during swing or to help maintain knee extension during stance. Sometimes it is used to assist the partially paralyzed hamstring muscles to flex the knee during swing and control the knee during stance. FES is typically activated through switches in the heels of shoes or in the handles of mobility aids. This triggers the FES and synchronizes it with the gait cycle. FES is typically applied through commercially available surface FES systems, although these are not always available in all pediatric sizes. Work with implantable FES for ambulation has remained in the research phase and is primarily focusing on adults with SCI (Bryden et al 2012).

In recent years, there has been a rapid increase in the use of technology to help children with SCI or spinal cord dysfunction to stand and walk. For example, there are robotic devices and training machines that enable children to practice either walking or elliptical stepping motions. These are sometimes used in combination with FES. They do not provide children with the ability to walk functionally, but they do provide children with the opportunity to experience upright posture and to practice using the legs. There are also a few different types of commercially available exoskeletons, but these are available only in small adult sizes. They have small batteries that help power the legs enabling individuals to walk short distances with mobility aids. They are currently very expensive but no doubt over coming years they will become less expensive and available in pediatric sizes. Ultimately, it is hoped that technology will become more refined and provide children with viable alternatives to wheelchairs.

Restraining children with spinal cord injury in vehicles

Individuals of all ages with SCI or spinal cord dysfunction should be properly restrained in motor vehicles. For example, infants and toddlers should be restrained in car seats and young children should be put on booster seats. Children with poor trunk or neck control require specialized three-point restraint systems. Children remaining in their wheelchairs while traveling in vehicles need to be appropriately restrained within their wheelchairs and the wheelchairs need to be fitted with headrests, pelvic belts, and chest supports. In addition, wheelchairs need to be locked onto the floor using approved restraint systems. It is important to an adolescent's independence to be able to access and use public and private transport without assistance if possible. Adolescents with paraplegia can transfer independently from their manual wheelchair to the driver's seat of a motor vehicle and then lift the wheelchair into the car. Most adolescents with tetraplegia, especially those who utilize power wheelchairs, will need an adapted van with a wheelchair lift and an automatic locking system for their wheelchairs. Vans can be adapted to enable an adolescent to drive while seated in his or her wheelchair. All children should sit on their pressure-reducing seating systems while traveling in vehicles, regardless of whether or not they remain within their wheelchairs. Although individuals with lesions as high as C5 are capable of driving an appropriately adapted motor vehicle, it is imperative that they receive a formal driving evaluation and obtain appropriate prescriptions for motor vehicle adaptations. The age at which adolescents can obtain a driver's permit varies from country to country, and even within different regions of the same country, but is generally 16 to 18 years.

Summary

This chapter addressed the considerations in the evaluation, provision, and training of mobility devices for children with SCI including wheeled mobility, upright mobility, and transport by vehicle. Emerging technologies were noted as being on the horizon with promise for future clinical applicability. Level of injury, age, mobility goals, and cognitive development are primary factors in the consideration of mobility.

REFERENCES

Axelson P, Chesny D, Minkel J, Perr A (1998) *The Manual Wheelchair Training Guide*. Santa Cruz, CA: PAX Press.

Axelson P, Minkel J, Perr A, Yamada D (2002) *The Powered Wheelchair Training Guide*. Minden, NV: PAX press.

Bergen AF (2000) The prescriptive wheelchair: an orthotic device. In: O'Sullivan SB, Schmitz TJ (eds). *Physical Rehabilitation: Assessment and Treatment*. Philadelphia, PA: F.A. Davis Company. pp. 1061–92.

Best KL, Kirby RL, Smith C, MacLeod DA (2005) Wheelchair skills training for community-based manual wheelchair users: a randomized controlled trial. *Arch Phys Med Rehabil* 86: 2316–23. doi: 10.1016/j.apmr.2005.07.300

Boninger ML, Baldwin M, Cooper RA, Koontz A, Chan L (2000) Manual wheelchair pushrim biomechanics and axle position. *Arch Phys Med Rehabil* 81: 608–13. doi: 10.1016/S0003-9993(00)90043-1

Boninger ML, Dicianno BE, Cooper RA, Towers JD, Koontz AM, Souza AL (2003) Shoulder magnetic resonance imaging abnormalities, wheelchair propulsion, and gender. *Arch Phys Med Rehabil* 84: 1615–20. doi: 10.1053/S0003-9993(03)00282-X

Bryden AM, Ancans J, Mazurkiewicz J, McKnight A, Scholtens M (2012) Technology for spinal cord injury rehabilitation and its application to youth. *J Pediatr Rehabil Med* 5: 287–99. doi: 10.3233/PRM-2012-00227

Butler C, Okamoto GA, McKay TM (1983) Powered mobility for very young disabled children. *Dev Med Child Neurol* 25: 472–4. doi: 10.1111/j.1469-8749.1983.tb13792.x

Butler C, Okamoto GA, McKay TM (1984) Motorized wheelchair driving by disabled children. *Arch Phys Med Rehabil* 65: 95–7.

Caulton JM, Ward KA, Alsop CW, Dunn G, Adams JE, Mughal MZ (2004) A randomised controlled trial of standing programme on bone mineral density in non-ambulant children with cerebral palsy. *Arch Dis Child* 89: 131–5. doi: 10.1136/adc.2002.009316

Chaftez RS, Johnston TE, Calhoun CL (2008) Lower limb orthoses for persons with spinal cord injury. In: Hsu JD, Michael J, Fisk, J (eds). *AAOS Atlas of Orthoses and Assistive Devices*. 4th Ed. Philadelphia, PA: Mosby Elsevier. pp. 357–71.

Consortium for Spinal Cord Medicine (1999) *Outcomes Following Traumatic Spinal Cord Injury*. Washington, DC: Paralyzed Veterans of America.

Consortium for Spinal Cord Medicine (2005) *Preservation of Upper Limb Function Following Spinal Cord Injury*. Washington, DC: Paralyzed Veterans of America.

Corfman TA, Cooper RA, Boninger ML, Koontz AM, Fitzgerald SG (2003) Range of motion and stroke frequency differences between manual wheelchair propulsion and pushrim-activated power-assisted wheelchair propulsion. *J Spinal Cord Med* 26: 135–40.

Di Marco A, Russell M, Masters M (2003) Standards for wheelchair prescription. *Aust Occup Ther J* 50: 30–9. http://dx.doi.org/10.1046/j.1440-1630.2003.00316.x

EnableNSW, Lifetime Care and Support Authority (2011) *Guidelines for the Prescription of a Seated Wheelchair or Mobility Scooter for People with Traumatic Brain Injury or Spinal Cord Injury*. Sydney, Australia: EnableNSW, LTCSA.

Eng JJ, Levins SM, Townson AF, Mah-Jones D, Bremner J, Huston G (2001) Use of prolonged standing for individuals with spinal cord injuries. *Phys Ther* 81: 1392–9.

European Pressure Ulcer Advisory Panel, National Pressure Ulcer Advisory Panel (2009) *Prevention and Treatment of Pressure Ulcers: Quick Reference Guide*. Washington, DC: National Pressure Ulcer Advisory Panel.

Faculty of Medicine Dalhousie University (2005) *Wheelchair Skills Program* [online]. Available at: http://www.wheelchairskillsprogram.ca (accessed 30 June 2012).

Fuhrer MJ (2007) Assessing the efficacy, effectiveness, and cost-effectiveness of assistive technology interventions for enhancing mobility. *Disabil Rehabil Assist Technol* 2: 149–58. http://dx.doi.org/10.1080/17483100701374355

Giacobbi PR, Levy CE, Dietrich FD, Winkler SH, Tillman MD, Chow JW (2010) Wheelchair users' perceptions of and experiences with power assist wheels. *Am J Phys Med Rehabil* 89: 225–34. doi: 10.1097/PHM.0b013e3181c9d7df

Glickman LB, Geigle PR, Paleg GS (2010) A systematic review of supported standing programs. *J Pediatr Rehabil Med* 3: 197–213. doi: 10.3233/PRM-2010-0129

Harvey LA, Smith MB, Davis GM, Engel S (1997) Functional outcomes attained by T9–12 paraplegic patients with the walkabout and the isocentric reciprocal gait orthoses. *Arch Phys Med Rehabil* 78: 706–11. doi: 10.1016/S0003-9993(97)90077-0

Irby SE, Bernhardt KA, Kaufman KR (2005) Gait of stance control orthosis users: the dynamic knee brace system. *Prosthet Orthot Int* 29: 269–82. doi: 10.1080/03093640500238915

Kangas K (1997) Clinical assessment and training strategies for the child's mastery of independent powered mobility. In: Furumasu J (ed.). *Pediatric Powered Mobility: Developmental Perspectives, Technical Issues, Clinical Approaches*. Arlington, VA: Rehabilitation Engineering and Assistive Technology Society of North America.

Katz DE, Haideri N, Song K, Wyrick P (1997) Comparative study of conventional hip-knee-ankle-foot orthoses versus reciprocating-gait orthoses for children with high-level paraparesis. *J Pediatr Orthop* 17: 377–86. http://dx.doi.org/10.1097/01241398-199705000-00020

Krey CH, Calhoun CL (2004) Utilizing research in wheelchair and seating selection and configuration for children with injury/dysfunction of the spinal cord. *J Spinal Cord Med* 27(Suppl 1): S29–37.

Lynch A, Ryu JC, Agrawal S, Galloway JC (2009) Power mobility training for a 7 month old infant with spina bifida. *Pediatr Phys Ther* 21: 362–8. doi: 10.1097/PEP.0b013e3181bfae4c

McClure LA, Boninger ML, Oyster ML et al (2009) Wheelchair repairs, breakdown, and adverse consequences for people with traumatic spinal cord injury. *Arch Phys Med Rehabil* 90: 2034–8. doi: 10.1016/j.apmr.2009.07.020

Michael S, Porter D, Pountney T (2007) Tilted seat position for non-ambulant individuals with neurological and neuromuscular impairment: a systematic review [with consumer summary]. *Clin Rehabil* 21: 1063–74. http://dx.doi.org/10.1177/0269215507082338

Regan M, Teasell RW, Keast D, Aubut JL, Foulon BL, Mehta S (2010) Pressure ulcers following spinal cord injury. In: Eng JJ, Teasell RW, Miller WC et al (eds). *Spinal Cord Injury Rehabilitation Evidence. Version 3.0*. Vancouver, BC, Canada: SCIRE.

Robb JE, Gordon L, Ferguson D, Dunhill Z, Elton RA, Minns RA (1999) A comparison of hip guidance with reciprocating gait orthoses in children with spinal paraplegia: results of a ten-year prospective study. *Eur J Pediatr Surg* 9(Suppl 1): S15–18. doi: 10.1055/s-2008-1072305

Rosen L, Arva J, Furumasu J et al (2009) RESNA position on the application of power wheelchairs for pediatric users. *Assist Technol* 21: 218–25. doi: 10.1080/10400430903246076

Schottler J, Vogel LC, Sturm P (2012) Spinal cord injuries in young children: a review of children injured at five years of age and younger. *Dev Med Child Neurol* 54: 1138–43. doi: 10.1111/j.1469-8749.201204411.x

Tam EW, Mak AF, Lam WN, Evans JH, Chow YY (2003) Pelvic movement and interface pressure distribution during manual wheelchair propulsion. *Arch Phys Med Rehabil* 84: 1466–72. doi: 10.1016/S0003-9993(03)00269-7

Vogel LC, Lubicky JP (1995a) Ambulation in children and adolescents with spinal cord injuries. *J Pediatr Orthop* 15: 510–16. http://dx.doi.org/10.1097/01241398-199507000-00020

Vogel LC, Lubicky JP (1995b) Ambulation with parapodia and reciprocating gait orthoses in pediatric spinal cord injury. *Dev Med Child Neurol* 37: 957–64. doi: 10.1111/j.1469-8749.1995tb11950x

Vogel LC, Mendoza MM, Schottler JC, Chlan KM, Anderson CJ (2007) Ambulation in children and youth with spinal cord injuries. *J Spinal Cord Med* 30(Suppl 1): S158–64.

Appendix 22.1 Power wheelchair letter of medical necessity

LETTER OF MEDICAL NECESSITY
Name: John _________
DOB:
Date of report:
Physician:
Therapists:
Others present:
Primary diagnosis: C1 spinal cord injury with resultant tetraplegia and tracheostomy, and is ventilator dependent

Background information/medical history, and client and parental concerns
Upon examination, John presents with absent motor strength and control in his upper and lower extremities and trunk. He has absent sensation from his neck down, putting him at increased risk of pressure ulcers and skin damage. He has spasms throughout his upper and lower extremities. John is completely dependent on his caregivers including all aspects of mobilization in his wheelchair. Currently, John's parents are using a [enter type] manual wheelchair for all of John's mobility. This wheelchair and seating system do not provide John with any independent mobility or a means to move throughout his environment or to interact with others.

Orthopedic and postural alignment problems

- Absent motor strength and motor control in his upper and lower extremities and trunk.
- Absent sensation in his upper and lower extremities and trunk.
- Increased tone in his upper and lower extremities.
- Absent trunk strength and motor control, resulting in poor balance.
- Decreased head control and decreased neck musculature strength.
- Limited muscle extensibility especially of the hamstring, hip adductor, hip flexor, and heel cord musculature.

Functional limitations

- Inability to sit independently.
- Inability to roll independently.
- Inability to stand independently.
- Inability to ambulate with or without assistive device.
- Inability to transfer or transition without complete dependence on a caregiver.
- Dependent on caregivers to complete activities of daily living such as feeding, hygiene activities, and dressing.
- Inability to move around home environment and keep up with siblings and peers.

Current status
Currently, John has no means of appropriate independent mobility. For all movement in the household, community, and school, as well as recreational and long-distance movement, John is pushed by his parents in a manual wheelchair. This does not provide him with independent mobility that would allow him to move throughout his environment for activities of daily living, functional mobility, play, school, and social interactions.

Caretaker's participation
John's mother and father were present for an examination and a trial power-mobility session. They agreed with the prescribed equipment and demonstrated their ability, willingness, and motivation to properly use and care for the prescribed equipment in conjunction with the plan of care.

During a complete evaluation in the seating and wheelchair clinic, John had the opportunity to trial a power wheelchair with a mini proportional joystick using his chin and mouth to maneuver it. During this time, he demonstrated the ability to start and stop the power wheelchair, drive in a forward direction, as well as turn to the left and right. After this examination and power-mobility session with the patient, his mother and father, and the physical therapist, the following power wheelchair and seating system was prescribed as medically necessary for John.

[In this section, clearly state all aspects of the wheelchair that are necessary, often directly from the order form. Anything that is not standard or includes an additional charge will need to be justified.]

[Enter type of power wheelchair] is necessary for John because it will provide him with a means of independent mobility required throughout his home, community, and school settings. This power wheelchair will allow increased independence with mobility and keeping up with his peers. Mobility is an important component of one's life; mobility provides a means to learn, interact with others, attend school and work, and participate in society. Research studies have shown that the ability to move independently facilitates all aspects of development and has an impact on cognitive, social, and communication skills. Over the past 25 years, multiple studies have linked the fields of psychology and rehabilitation regarding the relationship between physical and psychological development. An individual's early experiences influence all subsequent development. If there is a delay in mobility and motor development, all other development is delayed. If a child does not have a means of independent mobility, the result is different experiences than a child with typically developing motor skills. If a child is unable to independently move about his or her environment, an alternate means of mobility is necessary. Negative consequences of restricted or lost mobility include decreased ability to learn, decreased socialization, and learned helplessness due to decreased ability to have an impact on his or her environment. In contemporary psychology, there is widespread agreement that locomotion induces or accelerates important developmental changes. Self-produced locomotion has been theoretically linked to the growth of brain structures, the ability to cope with environmental stressors, a new level of self-awareness, shifts in patterns of attachment and interaction with caregivers, the emergence of a sense of competence and initiative, and the development of cognition.

Color: yellow.

Batteries, sealed gel, installed: necessary for powering the wheelchair.

Control module system with mini proportional joystick: necessary to allow John to access and maneuver the power wheelchair. The joystick enables John to control the wheelchair with his chin or mouth. This is necessary because John does not have any upper limb movement.

Attendant control: necessary to provide John's parents with a means to operate the power wheelchair if he is unable to. This will also provide a means for his parents to stop the chair during his initial power mobility training, serving as a safety mechanism.

Seating system: including the seating system, power tilt system, adjustable seat frame, adjustable backrest and leg rest angle, positioning belt, and one-piece footrest, which is necessary for the following reasons:

- The seating system will provide the pressure relief and postural support necessary for John. This is considered essential for people who rely on a power wheelchair as their primary means of mobility.
- The adjustable seat frame and backrest angle will allow for growth and proper placement to accommodate for John's size.
- The power tilt is necessary to provide John with a means of pressure relief, since he has absent sensation and is at high risk of pressure ulcers and skin damage.

__″ width × __″ height backrest: necessary to accommodate John's back width and back height, and to provide pressure relief and postural support.

__″ width × __″ depth fabric seating sizing: necessary to provide a surface for John to sit on that will provide pressure relief and postural support.

__″ fabric armrests for the right and left: necessary to provide support and proper positioning to John's upper extremities.

Legrests

Fabric lateral supports: necessary to provide trunk support, prevent falling to either side, and ensure that John maintains a vertical alignment while in his power wheelchair.

Thigh support fabric: necessary to maintain lower extremity position and prevent excessive abduction, especially when John has lower extremity spasms.

Abductor kit on flip down hardware: necessary to maintain lower extremity position and prevent excessive adduction, especially when John has lower extremity spasms.

Removable push handles: necessary to provide a means of pushing the power wheelchair at times when John is unable to drive it.

__″ width × __″ depth cushion: necessary to provide pressure relief and postural support in the seated position, as well as to help prevent pressure ulcers and skin damage.

Proportional mini joystick swivel-mounting hardware: necessary to provide and maintain placement of the mini proportional joystick, allowing John access for driving the power wheelchair.

Contoured headrest: necessary to ensure proper head placement and maintenance of head position, as John has no head control.

Body point chest harness: necessary to maintain proper trunk alignment and prevent John falling anteriorly.

Padded push button pelvic belt: necessary to maintain proper alignment and prevent bruising, which could occur owing to increased extensor tone and spasms.

Ankle positioners: necessary to maintain proper foot positioning and reduce lower extremity extensor patterns while sitting in the wheelchair.

Ventilator tray with attaching hardware: necessary to provide a secure place to mount John's ventilator, which he requires at all times to maintain respiratory and breathing function.

Oxygen tank holder: necessary to provide a secure place to mount John's oxygen tank, which he requires at all times to maintain respiratory and breathing function.

Tray: necessary to provide a place for John's caregivers to feed him, and any additional equipment he requires for school, and recreational and functional activities.

Other equipment that was considered and rejected because they did not meet John's seating and mobility needs:

- Stroller: does not provide John with independent mobility.
- Manual wheelchair: does not provide John with independent mobility.

How the prescribed equipment will curtail future medical costs: it will help prevent orthopedic deformities, particularly thoracic kyphosis, pelvic deformity, neck extensor muscle contractures, and lower extremity muscle contractures.

Assessment: the [enter type of power wheelchair] and seating system will provide increased independence with mobility, increased participation and independence with activities of daily living, improved postural support and alignment, and improved upper extremity and hand use.

Rehabilitation potential: excellent.

Plan of care

Treatment modality: power wheelchair, seating system, and equipment listed above to provide a means to drive and access the power wheelchair, while maintaining stable medical status.

Frequency/duration: minimum of one additional visit to provide the wheelchair, make adjustments, and ensure that John and his parents are educated in the use of the wheelchair. John will also require additional visits to learn how to manage the wheelchair in different environments.

Short-term goal: the therapist, vendor, and physician will work together and follow up as necessary to obtain authorization for the purchase of prescribed power wheelchair and seating system.

Long-term goals:

- Therapist and vendor to custom fit power wheelchair and seating system to meet John's needs on delivery.
- Therapist and vendor to train John and caregivers in proper use and care of power wheelchair and seating system.
- Additional power mobility training sessions as needed.
- Follow-up as needed with John and caregivers if problems arise after delivery.
- John will independently and successfully use the power wheelchair and seating system in all environments with follow-up modifications and adjustments as needed.

Please do not make any substitutions to this prescription without written consent of the evaluating team. All components have been specifically chosen to best meet the patient's medical and positioning needs.

Thank you for your prompt attention to this matter. Should any further information be required or questions arise, please contact [name and phone number].

[Enter the names and signatures of the patient's physician; all individuals involved in prescribing the wheelchair and seating system should sign and date this letter.]

Appendix 22.2 Example manual wheelchair letter of medical necessity

Date:

Patient Name: Emma _______

Patient Date of Birth:

To whom it may concern

Emma currently utilizes a [enter type] manual wheelchair [enter serial number] with a [enter type] cushion and [enter type] back. This wheelchair is over 5 years old; it is too small for her and very well worn. Emma has had good success with the [enter type] cushion she utilizes. After the healing of her stage IV sacral wound she was pressure mapped on many types of cushions, including foam, air, gel, and honeycomb, and she pressure mapped best on this cushion. In addition, she has not had any type of skin breakdown since using the [enter type] cushion. For an individual that requires a manual wheelchair as Emma does, it is critical that she utilizes an ultra-lightweight wheelchair. Over time, because wheelchair propulsion is a repetitive motion, Emma is at an increased risk of shoulder and upper extremity overuse injuries. This is well documented in the evidence-based literature and these studies show that degenerative changes to the shoulder and wrist can occur after only 3 years of utilizing a manual wheelchair. Therefore, she requires an ultra-lightweight chair as a preventive measure for possible shoulder, wrist, and upper extremity injuries. Emma has had her spinal cord injury for 10 years and will continue to require wheeled mobility for the rest of her life. It is medically necessary that she use an ultra-lightweight manual wheelchair.

During Emma's most recent visit at [enter wheelchair clinic or hospital name], a complete wheelchair and seating evaluation was performed. After a complete assessment with Emma, her parents, and [list all those involved such as physical and/or occupational therapist, vendor or manufacturer representative, physician, assistive technology provider], and based on the above stated reasons, it was determined that the following wheelchair frame and seating system will best meet Emma's seating and mobility needs

[In this section, clearly state all aspects of the wheelchair that are necessary, often directly from the order form. Anything that is not standard or includes an additional charge will need to be justified.]

[Enter type] manual wheelchair: this wheelchair is necessary because it will provide Emma with a means of independent mobility. This manual wheelchair is durable but also lightweight, which is critical for someone who uses a manual wheelchair as a primary means of mobility.

Wheelchair characteristics:

- __ degree fixed front frame
- __″ frame inset
- Classic frame, light shock
- __″ seat width
- __″ seat depth
- __″ front seat height
- __″ low profile polyurethane caster wheels

- Short caster fork
- Aluminum tubular with flat cover footrest
- __″ rear seat height
- __″ mag rear wheels
- Pneumatic airless inserts: necessary to prevent the potential for a flat tire
- Aluminum anodized handrim
- Quick release steel axle
- Standard short axle plates
- 101# to 190# rear suspension rating
- __ degrees camber
- __ center of gravity preset
- Folding lockdown angle adjustable back rest type
- __″ back height
- Omit back upholstery
- Padded swing-away adult armrests with standard hardware: necessary to provide upper extremity support as well as a means of completing pressure reliefs, which is critical for a patient with a spinal cord injury
- High mount push to lock wheels
- Grade aid: necessary to prevent the chair from rolling backwards in between pushes when Emma is ascending a ramp or hill
- Rear anti-tips: necessary to prevent Emma from falling backward should her center of gravity fall behind her; this serves as a safety mechanism
- Frame color

Seating system

__″ width × __″ depth (type) cushion: necessary to provide a seating surface with proper pressure relief, as well as provide the contouring necessary for positioning. After wound closure, Emma trialed and was pressure mapped on several types of cushions. This cushion provided the best pressure distribution and, since acquiring this cushion, Emma has not had any issues with skin integrity.

__″ width (type) back: necessary to provide postural support and pressure distribution of her back while in the seated position.
Auto style pelvic belt: required to maintain neutral pelvic alignment.

Please do not make any substitutions to this prescription without written consent of the prescribing physicians and physical therapist. All components have been specifically chosen to best meet the patient's medical and positioning needs.

Thank you for your prompt attention to this matter. Should any further information be required or questions arise, please contact [enter name and phone number].
[Enter the names and signatures of the patient's physician; all individuals involved in prescribing the wheelchair and seating system should sign and date this letter.]

Section 7 Psychosocial Issues

23 EDUCATIONAL AND VOCATIONAL ISSUES FOR CHILDREN WITH SPINAL CORD INJURY

Maria R Reyes, Teresa L Massagli and Kurt L Johnson

One of the most important roles that a child or adolescent fulfills is being a student. When a child sustains a spinal cord injury (SCI), there are significant implications for the provision of educational services and success at school. Success at school fosters educational and social development and is a key determinant of employment. This chapter will describe the preparation that takes place for returning to school during acute rehabilitation, barriers and support to educational re-entry, transitions from secondary to post-secondary education, barriers and support to employment, and rights and access to services in the USA and Canada. Other countries have similar processes for assisting a child with SCI in reintegrating into school and transitioning to work (see Bickenbach et al 2013).

Education and planning for school reintegration during acute rehabilitation

Education

Educational services are part of the acute rehabilitation program for school-aged children and adolescents who sustain an SCI (Fig. 23.1). Once the child is medically stable and has the endurance to participate in all rehabilitation therapies, it is essential to begin an educational assessment and provide some tutorial support. Some pediatric hospitals and rehabilitation centers have in-house teachers, whereas others may have contracts with local school districts to serve in-patient children and adolescents with SCI. With the consent of the child's legal guardian, the teacher will obtain school records from the home district to assess the child's learning history and act as a liaison to the home school district. The home schools may provide materials for the child to continue to work on during the rehabilitation hospitalization. Assessment of the child's current abilities by an educator may be augmented by assessments from a communication disorders specialist, pediatric psychologist, or pediatric neuropsychologist. These additional assessments are particularly helpful for a child with an SCI who has difficulty speaking owing to the presence of a tracheostomy or for formulating an educational plan for the cognitive communication needs of a child who sustained a concurrent traumatic brain injury (see Chapter 10). Educational assessments and tutorial support can begin at the bedside until the child has sufficient ability to sit upright in a wheelchair. When the child is able to sit, more traditional table-top or schoolroom environments can be used. The educational process will frequently be supported by email and web-based interactions with the home

During in-patient rehabilitation: early phase

- Educator requests consent of child's legal guardian to obtain home school district records
- If indicated, specialist evaluation by communications disorder specialist, pediatric psychologist, or pediatric neuropsychologist
- Bedside assessment and tutorial support begins, including assigned school work
- When wheelchair sitting tolerance is adequate, schoolroom or table-top school work commences
- Children with impaired hand function may require assistance for turning pages, transcribing written work, or computer/electronic access

During in-patient rehabilitation: preceding discharge

- School personnel (educators/nurses/therapists) may visit to become familiar with the child's needs
- If feasible, perform a home school visit with the child
    - Evaluate physical accessibility of school environment
    - Reacquaint teachers and peers with student
- Rehabilitation medical provider defines school health plan (including bladder care, respiratory, medication, and nutritional needs)
- Rehabilitation staff refer the student for Special Education services and accommodations

Special Education services planning

- Multidisciplinary school team reviews Special Education referral and determines if additional assessments are required
- If eligible under Individuals with Disabilities Education Act, school proceeds with individualized education plan (IEP) development
- For transition-aged children, Division/Department of Vocational Rehabilitation (DVR) involvement recommended with IEP development
- Special Education sites of service
    - 0–3 years: individual family service plan at birth to three center or home
    - 3–5 years: public preschool program
    - >5 years: public school system

During school

- Ongoing reassessments and modifications to IEP goals and services
- Regular rehabilitation medicine provider appointments to monitor and manage medical issues
- Assign home chores appropriate for age and ability

Age 16–21 years

- Active DVR involvement for educational/vocational transition planning
- Student prepares resume with assistance of transition team
- Encourage student to network with family and friends for potential job placement
- Determine eligibilty for graduation or continued school or community-based IEP services until age 21 or 22 years
- Review relevant disability laws with student
- If pursuing post-secondary education, encourage a school visit to evaluate accessibility, and determine necessary accommodations
- Prepare for transition to adult healthcare services, including establishing care with an adult spinal cord injury rehabilitation provider and transferring medical records

Fig. 23.1 Transition timeline for educational services after pediatric spinal cord injury.

school. The child's classroom teachers can email materials for the child, and the hospital can set up video conferencing using laptop computers to allow the child in the hospital to interact with classmates.

Planning for School Re-entry

The focus of acute in-patient rehabilitation for a child with SCI is developing competence in basic mobility and self-care skills that will be essential for community and school re-entry. A child with paraplegia should be able to rapidly progress to handling and using typical classroom materials such as books, paper, writing instruments, and keyboards/computers. A child with tetraplegia will need more physical assistance for turning pages and transcribing written work, and will need training in alternative ways to use a computer, such as the use of dictation software or a specialized mouse.

If the child lives within a reasonable distance of the hospital, a visit to the home school serves several goals. The rehabilitation team can evaluate physical accessibility of the building and classroom, and the teachers and classmates can become reacquainted with the student with SCI. Similarly, school personnel such as a teacher, school nurse, or physical or occupational therapist benefit from a visit to the rehabilitation center to observe the child's function and care needs and to meet with the rehabilitation team (Knight et al 2008). With all of the other rehabilitation goals, it will not be possible for a child to keep up with all assignments from their home school. Nevertheless, by the time of discharge, the child should have attempted some current school work, learned basic self-advocacy skills (directing set-up and care needs) and have had sufficient exposure to school services, adaptive technologies, and compensatory strategies to ensure that he or she has the confidence to transition back to the home school.

The types of educational services provided to students with SCI depend on the child's age, level of function, services available in the school district, and whether the child had a concurrent traumatic brain injury. Before discharge from the hospital, the rehabilitation program will make a referral to the child's school for special education services or accommodations. A multidisciplinary school team will review the referral to determine if assessments are needed in cognition, language, or sensory or motor areas that may require related therapy services. Schools are often able to use the assessments performed by the rehabilitation team. In the USA, students in private schools are also eligible to receive educational support or related therapy services from their local public school.

Many children continue to require out-patient physical or occupational therapy services, and therefore will require planning to coordinate both their return to school and their attendance at out-patient therapies. Out-patient therapies are used to address functional needs that are not education related when schools lack the resources to provide therapies at school. Related services such as physical or occupational therapy may also be provided at school to address disabilities that are specifically related to the child's educational needs. A school physical therapist may address wheelchair use or other mobility aids in the school setting or adaptive physical education, but other ongoing goals such as range of motion exercises, general strengthening, advanced wheelchair skills, or ambulation training would be managed via home or out-patient therapies. Similarly, the school occupational therapist may monitor the use of hand splints, assist with keyboard training, or help with fine motor skills as they are needed at school, but might not work on activities such as dressing, bathing, or functional transfers. Therapies provided at school are generally limited in frequency and duration, and may change to being consultative only, depending on the child's level of independence in the school environment. The school's therapists can help assess the access into and within the school building, to multiple levels within a building, to bathrooms, and to play areas; develop an evacuation plan; and assess classroom furniture (e.g. table height) to accommodate a wheelchair or other mobility devices.

The rehabilitation physician will need to work with the school nurse to define a health plan for the child with SCI at school. This includes activity restrictions or guidelines for participation in physical education and sports activities; assistance during recess; prescriptions for medications to be administered at school; emergency orders for medical complications, such as airway issues or autonomic dysreflexia; and plans for catheterization and pressure relief. Catheterization at school may require the use of an accessible toilet, or access to a lift, and the use of a transfer board and mat for the child to be positioned on. School nurses may require training if they have not had recent experience with intermittent catheterization, autonomic dysreflexia, pressure relief, or other medical issues. School nurses or instructional aides may provide or assist with personal care for students, including catheterization, pressure relief, or tube feedings. However, more complicated care, such as for the child with a tracheostomy or ventilator, necessitates one-on-one care, typically provided by families or nurses paid for through medical insurance.

Addressing barriers to school reintegration

A significant barrier to school participation includes inadequate preparation for the re-entry. Receiving schools will benefit from written information, such as that provided by the Stoke Mandeville Hospital Teaching Service in the form of a guide for schools, to support young people with SCI returning to school (Blueprint online). The following factors need to be considered in the planning and preparation for school reintegration of children and young people with SCI.

Accessibility

The physical and functional accessibility of the school for the child (see above regarding the school visit), as well as their transportation needs to and from school and for school trips should be addressed (Knight et al 2008).

Emotional

School-aged young people with SCI have reported educational re-entry concerns related to self-image, reactions of peers, and teachers' expectations (Mulcahey 1991). Encouraging continued communication between the child and school staff and peers, and an escorted school visit, prepares the child with SCI for formally returning to the school environment. Ongoing emotional monitoring and support should be provided at school for both the young person with SCI and any siblings they may have, and the child should be encouraged to request help or share concerns with school staff. A qualitative study from the UK found that the level or severity of SCI did not correlate with the perception of inclusion, suggesting that addressing attitudinal barriers would promote greater satisfaction in the process of returning to school (Knight et al 2008).

Training

School reintegration should be addressed as part of the transition process toward the conclusion of the in-patient rehabilitation program. Healthcare providers managing the SCI care of school-aged children and young people should assist the school with identification and anticipation of their special care needs while at school. Direct training of school therapists, nurses, and educational aides; videotaping of the child's function; and a school visit are strategies that can help schools prepare for the child's return. Rehabilitation treatment should include training in self-advocacy skills and tailoring care needs as appropriate for the child's age. Delays in school re-entry may be related to the unavailability of suitably trained staff to assist the child in school, requiring family support to facilitate timely reintegration.

Medical

Dropout from school has been attributed to medical reasons such as suboptimal control of pain and spasticity and inaccessibility of classrooms, with probable contribution from other premorbid factors (Graham et al 1991). Healthcare providers should address the management of continence, nutrition, respiratory needs, pain, and spasticity to maximize attendance and participation in school.

Modifications

Modifications for school re-entry often include provision of extended time for completion of class work, adjustment of assignments, and changing class location to improve access. Special or 'related' services such as physical and occupational therapies, use of an educational aide, and the need for a full-time private nurse may be required (Massagli et al 1996). Teaching both reading and writing skills to students who are unable to manipulate print material or use a pen or pencil may require technologies such as laptop computers or tablets. Assistive technologies such as voice recognition software or specialized computer-access tools may also be required.

Educational and vocational legislation in the USA

Children and young adults with SCI should learn about disability law so they can become effective self-advocates as they transition into adulthood. Article 24 of the United Nations *Conventions on the Rights of Persons with Disabilities* stresses the importance that governments provide equal access to the educational system for all individuals and at all levels, and provide reasonable accommodations to support learning (United Nations General Assembly 2006). The relevant US legislation is discussed below.

Americans with Disabilities Act (ADA)

All people with disabilities in the USA are guaranteed equal access to programs and services and are protected from discrimination by the Americans with Disabilities Act (ADA 1990). The major principles of this legislation are protection against discrimination based on disability, and assurance of equal opportunity to participate in education. The ADA requires that most private and public entities, ranging from movie theaters and physicians' offices to local and state government agencies, make reasonable accommodations to ensure that there is adequate access for people with disabilities.

To assure equal opportunities for all, schools are required to make reasonable accommodations or modifications to services, buildings, and instructions, unless the school can prove that it would be an undue hardship or require a fundamental alteration of the program. The ADA also prohibits discrimination against people with disabilities in the workplace if the individual can do the 'essential functions' of the job with or without 'reasonable accommodation'.

Section 504

The language used and obligations stated in Section 504 are included under the ADA. The definition found in this act of a qualified individual with a disability also applies to students. All children with disabilities in schools are covered by Section 504 of the Rehabilitation Act (1973), regardless of whether they receive special education services. Under Section 504, school districts in the USA are required to identify students with disabilities, evaluate them, and develop a written Section 504 plan that specifies any accommodations they may require. Schools are required to ensure that students with disabilities have the same access to educational opportunities as students in general in both academic and extracurricular arenas. This requirement, that is access to free and appropriate public education, must be provided in the least restrictive environment, that is students are to participate in mainstream classrooms and activities to the greatest extent possible.

Individuals with Disabilities Education Act

The Individuals with Disabilities Education Act (IDEA, 2004) covers students with disabilities who require a fundamental alteration to the educational program, such as specialized instruction, or a modification of the curriculum and/or related services, such as physical therapy, occupational therapy, and speech and language pathology. This is federal 'special education', includes all the obligations of Section 504, and requires that schools provide additional services and program modifications to the student. The federal eligibility categories for special education that apply to children with SCI include 'orthopedic impairment', 'other health impairment', or 'traumatic brain injury' for those with a dual diagnosis. When a child is found to be eligible for services under IDEA, an individualized education plan (IEP) is developed and revised periodically by the school district team, family, and any other related providers that may be helpful. The IEP sets the educational goals, which may include independent living and employment; the services that are needed to achieve those goals; who will provide those services; and how progress will be assessed. Under IDEA, children from birth to 3 years of age with SCI are eligible to receive special education or related services through an individual family service plan. These services may be provided in 'birth to three' centers, or in the home, with a focus on training parents/caregivers. From 3 to 5 years of age, children with SCI are eligible for special education or related services through public preschool programs, and, beyond 5 years of age, are eligible through the public school system.

When a student is on an IEP, the student may graduate based on completing the academic requirements (which may take additional time because of missed school and/or reduced class load), or the student may instead graduate based on completing the IEP goals. In either case, students may remain in school in order to continue receiving these services until the year of their 21st or 22nd birthday, depending on their state of residence. Often, students may receive the IEP services in community-based settings, including employment, rather than at the school.

Issues in transition to post-secondary education in the USA

Many students with SCI may transition from high school to vocational technical schools, community colleges, or 4-year universities. For some adolescents, this will represent a change in their previously anticipated career path. Consultation with a rehabilitation (vocational) counselor may help the adolescent to evaluate and understand the physical requirements of potential careers.

These transitions beyond high school are often difficult for other reasons as well. First, the legal obligations of post-secondary institutions are different from those in primary and secondary education. Although post-secondary institutions are covered by Section 504 and the ADA, they have no obligations under IDEA. Students also must initiate requests for accommodations and may be required to provide medical evidence to support their request. Post-secondary institutions in the USA are not required to provide assistive technologies for students with disabilities unless they provide similar technology to all students. Similarly, specialized assistance in studying and tutoring received by many students on an IEP in high school are not generally provided at the post-secondary level. Post-secondary institutions are not required to provide any kind of personal care assistance such as for toileting. Post-secondary education also generally requires that students function at a much higher level of independence than in high school, often in campuses that are larger and require more traveling between classes. It may be very helpful for students with SCI considering post-secondary education to visit the campus, travel between buildings, sit in on a class, meet with disability services personnel and an academic advisor, and even have a meal to get a sense for campus life.

Barriers to employment after pediatric-onset spinal cord injury

Educational participation is regarded as an essential preparatory phase for employment. SCI often significantly disrupts education, and may delay or disrupt the transition from primary and secondary education to post-secondary education or employment. In young people with SCI, the impact may be magnified because logistical factors or fatigue may limit opportunities to acquire early employment skills typically developed by working student jobs while in high school.

The most commonly cited reasons for non-employment in those with pediatric-onset SCI include health complications, transportation and accessibility issues, financial disincentives, decreased motivation, and reduced educational achievement (Anderson and Vogel 2002). Adults with pediatric-onset SCI face transportation challenges, including a lower likelihood of driving independently than the healthy population (Vogel et al 2011).

Systemic issues rather than individual factors can serve as formidable barriers to employment for people with disabilities, including people with SCI acquired when they were a child or adolescent. Work incentive programs available through the social security administration allow a person with a disability to maintain eligibility for financial subsidy and healthcare coverage while working, but these can be difficult to implement and are not widely used. The limited earnings potential of people living with SCI, coupled with the high cost of care, particularly for individuals without adequate educational preparation and with significant functional limitations, can lead to difficulty in generating an income sufficient for financial independence (Johnson 2010).

People with SCI who are employed report higher levels of psychological adjustment, satisfaction with life, independence, and general health (Hess et al 2004). Gainful employment is also linked to a greater likelihood of living and driving independently (Anderson and Vogel 2002). Therefore, successful school re-entry and maintaining school participation through to graduation are critical goals to enhance the vocational and psychological outcomes and future participation of people with pediatric-onset SCI.

Promoting favorable employment outcomes: vocational rehabilitation in the USA

Every state in the USA has a division or department of vocational rehabilitation, often known as DVR. DVR is funded as a federal and state partnership. Individuals with disabilities are eligible for DVR services if they have a disability that interferes with their ability to work. Most services are available without reference to family income and include counseling and guidance, career assessment, vocational evaluation, job placement, job retention services, and assistive technologies. DVR may subsidize the costs of training or post-secondary education. Under US federal law, DVR is required to provide services to young people with disabilities who are in transition, although many agencies are not involved until graduation nears. DVR should be involved in the development of an IEP for students who are beginning the transition into adult life, to provide guidance regarding the realities of adult services and employment, and to determine the nature and timing of future DVR services. When the need for DVR services exceeds available funding, DVR is permitted under federal law to enter an 'order of selection' in which clients with the most severe disabilities are served first. In general, young people with SCI will meet these criteria, but it is important for the rehabilitation team to ensure that they have thoroughly described the range of functional limitations, including neurocognitive (including premorbid conditions such as learning disabilities) and psychological barriers.

Transition services for young people and adolescents with SCI should include vocational education, development and training, community and paid work experiences, and training in daily living skills (Massagli et al 1996).

Although DVR and the school transition team (e.g. special educator, school psychologist, physical or occupational therapist, as appropriate) may assist young people with SCI in getting a job, the process will be improved greatly when a network of family and friends is activated to help the student first acquire real work experience. The student should create a resume with appropriate assistance from the team, and should meet with family and friends to network about employment options. Because finding and maintaining employment is more difficult for people with disabilities, it is important to incorporate natural supports into the process to enable the student to solve problems or issues arising from work with a trusted advisor. Although a 'first job' is important, planning for transition should include a strong focus on career development and planning for the future. Successive approximations to employment should be supported and failure to get a job or job loss should be reframed by the supporting community as part of the normal developmental process in obtaining employment.

To improve future employability after pediatric-onset SCI, healthcare providers, families, and educators should promptly establish and promote an outlook inclusive of the expectation of post-secondary education (if appropriate) and future employment (Anderson and Vogel 2002). Consistent with this strategy, children and adolescents with SCI should be assigned age-appropriate household chores in preparation for this. Exposure to 'real work in the work place' helps students anticipate employment. Previous research suggests that paid work experience for disabled high-school students was associated with improved future employment outcome (Hasazi et al 1989). Health promotion via complication prevention, as well as interventions to improve functional independence, is critical to surmount the barriers to employment. Interventions should address the most prevalent conditions that impact long-term functional outcomes in those with pediatric-onset SCI, such as pressure ulcers, urinary control and infection rates, bowel continence, and prevention of upper limb overuse injuries and pain (Vogel et al 2011).

The Canadian experience: education and vocation after pediatric spinal cord injury

More than half of participants in a workforce survey by the Canadian Paraplegic Association reported being injured between 15 and 24 years of age (Canadian Paraplegic Association 2000). Canadian children with SCI share many similar experiences with their American peers in preparation for educational re-entry while receiving acute rehabilitation (Vancouver School Board 2012a,b). However, the related legislative basis and processes surrounding school re-entry and employment differ. In Canada, where national programs are not legislatively mandated, differences are apparent between provinces and even at the local level. In British Columbia, for example, the provincial special education law requires many similar components to IDEA, including an IEP, inclusion in the least restrictive environment, and transition planning. It does not, however, require the provision of related services (e.g. physical, occupational, and speech therapy) as part of the educational process. These therapy services would typically be covered via other healthcare funding. Students seeking career counseling may return to out-patient services at the SCI center for assistance (Vancouver School Board 2012b, J Cobb personal communication 2012).

The responsibility for labor market training transitioned from the Canadian federal government to the provincial level between 1997 and 2000. In Canada, as was noted in the USA, the employment outcomes for people with SCI are poor. National workforce survey data revealed that only 38% of Canadians with SCI between the ages of 15 and 64 years were working (Canadian Paraplegic Association 2000, Jongbloed et al 2007). Similar individual and systemic barriers as in the USA have been reported in Canada. In the absence of a national vocational rehabilitation system, assistance with employment for people with SCI is determined by the mechanism of injury (e.g. work related, motor vehicle crash), and the type of individual insurance coverage (e.g. long-term disability insurance). Since most school-aged children with SCI are not eligible for worker's compensation rehabilitation or for vocational rehabilitation under long-term disability policies, other funding sources are often necessary for such programs. Injuries resulting from a motor vehicle crash may have vocational rehabilitation covered under insurance. Otherwise, individuals with disability may depend on the Canadian pension plan, which results in a similar predicament as in the USA, wherein program eligibility can only be maintained if the personal income limit is not exceeded.

The story of Rose: an example of educational and vocational issues after spinal cord injury

Rose was injured in a motor vehicle crash at 16 years of age and sustained a C6 American Spinal Injury Association Impairment Scale (AIS) B SCI. After her acute care stabilization, she was hospitalized for in-patient rehabilitation for 10 weeks before being discharged. During her first week of rehabilitation, the hospital schoolteacher contacted her school and obtained an academic performance history as well as assignments that Rose could work on during the hospitalization. In addition to her rehabilitation therapies, her weekday schedule included daily 45- to 60-minute sessions of tutorial support. She began work on writing words and brief phrases using a tenodesis splint and an adapted pen, and on turning single pages in her texts. She also engaged in schoolwork for 60 minutes each evening. During the hospitalization, she maintained coursework in three of her five main classes. She applied occupational therapy training to the use of a computer and, by the time of her discharge, was able to type slowly, and use dictation software to complete written work. When she was discharged, she was independent – using a power wheelchair indoors and in the community – and was working on use of a manual wheelchair for indoor mobility. School was on summer break at the time of her discharge, and after the summer break, she returned to school. She received outpatient physical and occupational therapy at a local clinic to continue work on activities of daily living, mobility, and transfers.

In order to prepare for school, she awoke 1.5 hours earlier than previously, to allow time for dressing, bathing, bowel program, and catheterization before traveling to school. The school provided door-to-door transportation via a wheelchair-accessible bus. The school also provided an instructional assistant, who assisted Rose with managing her wheelchair in difficult areas, with intermittent catheterization, with cutting food and set-up of adaptive devices to eat lunch, and with manipulating texts and taking notes or writing to dictation. At the start of the school year, Rose received physical therapy at school for 45 minutes once a week to progress her skills in wheelchair mobility on uneven terrain on the school campus. She continued out-patient physical therapy to supplement this, working on manual wheelchair mobility and transfers. She also received occupational therapy at school for 60 minutes a week to work on fine motor skills related to education, such as handwriting, typing, and use of a computer. School-based physical therapy was discontinued after 4 months and occupational therapy was discontinued after 6 months, as she had met her goals. Rose's accommodations in the school included the instructional assistant and physical therapy as described above. She also received access to space where she could dictate notes into her voice recognition system without disturbing others and a modification of the curriculum to allow her to substitute her therapies for the physical education requirement.

At approximately 1 year after her injury, Rose had surgery to perform a right brachioradialis to flexor pollicis longus transfer to improve her tenodesis grasp, with one goal being to allow her to complete self-catheterization. At 18 months after her injury, she underwent a Mitrofanoff procedure so that she could perform intermittent catheterization with set-up, without the need to transfer from her wheelchair. At 1 year after her injury, Rose's IEP team also began planning for her transition out of school. A referral to the DVR was made and the DVR counselor participated in the planning. She was found to be eligible for services, and DVR agreed to fund a portion of her post-secondary education, as long as there was an anticipated employment outcome. Rose and her family expected her to transition into post-secondary education. Rose visited both 2- and 4-year campuses in the area to find out about accessibility, disability student services, curriculum, and the social context. She selected a 4-year institution. The team worked with her to request accommodations for the university college entrance examination, including extended testing time and using a scribe to record her responses.

Around 2 years after her injury, she completed training to drive a lift-equipped van using hand controls and she graduated from high school and enrolled at university. At that time, she was independent with sliding board transfers, used a manual wheelchair for limited outdoor community mobility and a power wheelchair for longer distances and on uneven terrain at the university. She hired an attendant to assist with her bowel program, lower body dressing, transfers to the bathtub, and pushing her wheelchair on hills, as well as for housekeeping.

Although Rose was able to graduate from the university, she was not able to secure employment that paid a high enough wage that she could live independently. With DVR assistance, she found part-time employment as an hourly administrative assistant for a small law office. The job provided enough supplemental income to improve her quality of life, but she had to remain on a subsidy. She requested, and was provided, accommodations, including flexibility in hours to accommodate changes in health status, and bowel and bladder care needs; a raised desk to accommodate her wheelchair; a monitor on an adjustable arm; her preferred mouse; voice recognition for text entry and computer commands; a voice-activated telephone; and dialing through her computer. Currently she is considering returning to graduate school to see if she can qualify for higher paying jobs in the future.

Summary

Given that one of the major roles that a child fulfills is being a student, the rehabilitation process should address return-to-school issues as soon as possible in acute rehabilitation. The rehabilitation team can work with the child's caregivers to recognize barriers to educational and vocational participation, and identify equipment, technologies, physical assistance, and medical management that will inform the receiving school on how to facilitate school attendance and participation. In the USA and other countries, federal and regional laws influence the provision of education and vocational services. Children with SCIs and their families need to become acquainted with these laws in order to become advocates for accommodations and services, and to reduce barriers to success at school and in the workplace.

REFERENCES

Americans with Disabilities Act (1990) 42 USC § 12101 et seq.

Anderson CJ, Vogel LC (2002) Employment outcomes of adults who sustained spinal cord injuries as children or adolescents. *Arch Phys Med Rehabil* 83: 791–801. doi: 10.1053/apmr.2002.32742

Bickenbach J, Bodine C, Brown D et al (2013) *International Perspectives on Spinal Cord Injury.* Geneva, Switzerland: World Health Organization (WHO) Press. Available at: http://apps.who.int/iris/bitstream/10665/94190/1/9789241564663_eng.pdf (accessed 7 March 2014).

Blueprint (online) Blueprint Short Stay School Hospital Teaching Service and Stoke Mandeville Hospital. Going back to school. Supporting young people returning to school with spinal cord injury: a guide for schools. Available at: http://www.blueprint.org.uk (accessed on 17 September 2012).

Canadian Paraplegic Association (2000) Workforce participation survey of Canadians with spinal cord injuries. Available at: http://sci-bc-database.ca/employment/reports-and-surveys/workforce-participation-survey-of-canadians-with-spinal-cord-injuries/ (accessed 25 September 2012).

Graham P, Weingarden S, Murphy P (1991) School reintegration: a rehabilitation goal for spinal cord injured adolescents. *Rehabil Nurs* 16: 122–7. doi: 10.1002/j.2048-7940.1991.tb01196.x

Hasazi S, Johnson R, Hasazi J, Gordon L, Hull M (1989) Employment of youth with and without handicaps following high school: outcomes and correlates. *J Spec Educ* 23: 243–55. doi: 10.1177/002246698902300302

Hess DW, Meade MA, Forchheimer M, Tate DG (2004) Psychological well-being and intensity of employment in individuals with spinal cord injury. *Top Spinal Cord Inj Rehabil* 9: 1–10. http://dx.doi.org/10.1310/UYQV-7KL9-QLPR-TWYH

Individuals with Disabilities Education Improvement Act (2004) 20 USC § 1400 et seq.

Johnson KL (2010) Vocational rehabilitation and spinal cord injury. In: Lin V (ed.). *Spinal Cord Medicine: Principles and Practice.* 2nd Ed. New York, NY: Demos. pp. 819–25.

Jongbloed L, Backman C, Forwell S, Carpenter C (2007) Employment after spinal cord injury: the impact of government policies in Canada. *Work* 29: 145–54.

Knight A, Petrie P, Potts P, Zuurmond M (2008) *The School Lives of Children and Young People with a Spinal Cord Injury: Report to the Back-Up Trust.* London, UK: Thomas Coram Research Unit, Institute of Education, University of London. pp. 1–88. Available at: http://www.ioe.ac.uk (accessed on 20 September 2012).

Massagli TL, Dudgeon BJ, Ross BW (1996) Educational performance and participation after spinal cord injury in childhood. *Arch Phys Med Rehabil* 77: 995–9. doi: 10.1016/S0003-9993(96)90058-1

Mulcahey MJ (1991) Returning to school after a spinal cord injury: perspectives from four adolescents. *Am J Occup Ther* 46: 305–32. doi:10.5014/ajot.46.4.305

Rehabilitation Act (1973) § 504 29 USC Section 794 et seq.

United Nations General Assembly (2006) *Convention on the Rights of Persons with Disabilities* A/RES/61/106. Available at: http://www.un.org/disabilities/documents/convention/convoptprot-e.pdf (accessed 7 March 2014).

Vancouver School Board (2012a) BC Children's Hospital – School Program. Available at: http://www.vsb.bc.ca/programs/bc-childrens-hospital-school-program (accessed on 26 September 2012).

Vancouver School Board (2012b) G F Strong – School Program. Available at: http://www.vsb.bc.ca/programs/gf-strong-school-program (accessed on 20 September 2012).

Vogel LC, Chlan KM, Zebracki D, Anderson CJ (2011) Long-term outcomes of adults with pediatric-onset spinal cord injuries as a function of neurologic impairment. *J Spinal Cord Med* 34: 60–6. doi: 10.1179/107902610X12883422813787

24
AN OVERVIEW OF PSYCHOSOCIAL ADJUSTMENT AFTER PEDIATRIC SPINAL CORD INJURY

Zoë Chevalier, Erin H Kelly and Kevin Jones

Psychosocial adjustment to pediatric spinal cord injury (SCI) is complicated by the reality that the experience of sustaining and living with this injury is highly individualized and influenced by a wide range of biopsychosocial factors including pre-injury characteristics, injury-related factors, stressors and coping approaches, family characteristics, access to resources, the quality of social supports, and the accessibility of the child's home, school, and community environments (Webster 2008). Furthermore, one factor distinguishing young people with SCI from their adult counterparts is the developmental context of childhood; as a result, developmental issues are paramount in the rehabilitation process (Vogel 1997).

This chapter provides an overview of the research literature pertaining to psychosocial considerations after pediatric-onset SCI, followed by a discussion of adaptive adjustment and positive emotional functioning among young people with SCI aged 0 to 5 years, 6 to 12 years, and 13 to 18 years. Each age-specific section includes a description of key developmental issues and a case vignette. For a more in-depth review of the literature, please refer to Webster (2008).

Pediatric spinal cord injury

The impact of SCI on the child is wide-reaching and includes the impact of the trauma itself; pain and abnormal sensations; alterations to bodily functions; separation from normal routines and home when initially hospitalized; disruption of the normal trajectory of growth, independence, and development; concerns about pursuing current hobbies and hopes for the future; parental and family distress; body image concerns and a desire to appear 'normal'; a need for safety; and the impact of being cared for by, and dependent on, others.

There is no set pattern to emotional and behavioral adjustment; responses are unique to the child and his or her circumstances. Most children and parents adjust well to injury and report positive psychosocial outcomes, such as increased self confidence (Augustis et al 2007). Nevertheless, young people with SCI face a significant challenge in that they must cope with their SCI while at the same time negotiate development through childhood and adolescence into adulthood. For these reasons, a developmental and lifespan perspective is imperative. Furthermore, a transitional approach will be necessary to best support the child and his or her family at each point of transition: from hospital to home, from home to school, and from home to community (Labhard 2010). The following section gives an overview of the key points of adjustment for the child and his or her family.

Psychosocial adjustment

A small but growing body of research has begun investigating psychosocial outcomes among young people with SCI. In general, this research highlights characteristics associated with mental health (including anxiety, depression, and post-traumatic stress disorder [PTSD]), quality of life (QOL), and participation in school and community activities of young people.

Although outcomes vary, in general, when compared with existing population norms, young people with SCI have been found to experience relatively typical levels of anxiety and depression (Anderson et al 2009), but increased levels of PTSD (Boyer et al 2000), decreased QOL (Garma et al 2011), and reduced community participation (Anderson et al 2004). Although having any type of chronic illness or disability may pose an additional risk of developing psychosocial problems, it is important to emphasize that only a minority experience clinical levels of distress (Barlow and Ellard 2006), and the majority of children with SCI do well in terms of emotional and psychological adjustment (e.g. Anderson et al 2004). In addition, although different methodologies were employed, levels of depression reported in adults with pediatric-onset SCI seem considerably lower than levels reported for those with adult-onset SCI (Duff and Kennedy 2003, Anderson et al 2007). This may indicate that individuals who acquire injuries at a younger age experience better adjustment, but further research is needed to draw solid conclusions.

Specific to PTSD, Boyer et al (2000) reported 25% of the children with SCI met the *Diagnostic and Statistical Manual of Mental Disorders*, fourth edition, criteria for current PTSD. An additional 31% of their sample experienced symptoms of post-traumatic stress but did not meet the full diagnostic criteria for the disorder. Aside from the potential trauma of the event causing the injury, the subsequent medical care and rehabilitation may also be traumatizing in its own right, as ongoing invasive medical treatments have been linked to post-traumatic stress (Boyer et al 2000). This emphasizes the importance of reviewing how hospitalization and rehabilitation are approached and managed for children and families.

Young people with SCI have also been found to have lower QOL than uninjured children; this finding persists across both child self-reports and caregiver proxy-reports (Garma et al 2011). Greater levels of anxiety and depression have been associated with lower QOL, highlighting the links between psychological functioning, adjustment, and longer term outcomes (Garma et al 2011). In terms of participation, young people with disabilities have been found to participate in more informal, sedentary activities, such as playing board or card games, talking on the phone, and reading, and fewer 'formal' activities, such as playing team sports, taking singing or music lessons, and going on outings (Brown and Gordon 1987, Johnson and Klaas 2007, Klaas et al 2010). This is problematic, particularly as formal participation seems to serve as a gateway to other networks of support, for example through exposure to interacting with a more diverse social group and being involved in activities further from home (Klaas et al 2010); these experiences may help foster increased independence and confidence. Research has (retrospectively) addressed the participation of young people with SCI in educational activities, uncovering relatively high rates of educational attainment of individuals with pediatric-onset SCI (Anderson et al 2004). However, of particular concern is the strikingly high unemployment rate for these individuals (43%), particularly given their educational success (Anderson et al 2004). However, of particular concern is the strikingly high rate of under- or unemployment for adults with pediatric-onset SCI (Andersen et al 2004); this is particularly true for those without a college degree (Hwang et al 2014).

Positive Psychological Outcomes

To date, the research literature regarding psychosocial outcomes after pediatric-onset SCI has mainly focused on the negative impact on and outcomes of children with SCI. As the majority of children and parents adjust well to SCI and report positive psychosocial outcomes, research studies to support and explore the anecdotal and clinical evidence regarding post-traumatic growth and resilience after pediatric-onset SCI are needed. Such research could help identify factors related to positive outcomes: factors that could then be facilitated through intervention.

Coping and Appraisals

Investigations of coping among young people with SCI have found relationships between the use of specific coping strategies and participation in community activities (Lindwall et al 2012). In particular, higher levels of social support and cognitive restructuring (which involves identifying false or maladaptive cognitions and replacing them with more accurate or adaptive beliefs) and lower levels of self-criticism, social withdrawal, and blaming others were linked to more positive participation outcomes, including participating in more activities with a more diverse group of people (Lindwall et al 2012). However, little is known about patterns of coping or whether coping can be changed through intervention; this is an area for future research.

In the adult SCI literature, the importance of appraisals in emotional adjustment after SCI has been highlighted (Chevalier et al 2009). Within this context, 'appraisals' refer to the subjective evaluations an individual makes regarding a situation or event, and the extent to which they perceive themselves as possessing the necessary resources to cope with or manage the situation (Lazarus and Folkman 1984). The relationship between appraisals and coping is dynamic in nature, as how an individual appraises a situation will influence how they cope, and how they cope will influence their reappraisal of the situation. Current thinking is that clinical intervention should focus on techniques to identify an individual's appraisals of their SCI, and engender adaptive perceptions of their current situation as being manageable and controllable (Chevalier et al 2009). This is an under-researched area in pediatric SCI.

Appraisals and coping have implications for both short- and long-term adjustment. This is shown in the diagrammatic model of children's psychosocial adjustment after pediatric-onset SCI, proposed by Webster (2008), found in Figure 24.1. In the model, Webster (2008) distinguishes between problem- and emotion-focused coping. Problem-focused support is recommended to target modifiable stresses, and includes looking for practical ways to increase control; enhancing participation and maximizing independence; encouraging adherence to treatment and routines and engagement in rehabilitation; increasing functional independence by developing self-management skills and providing functional aids; providing psychological

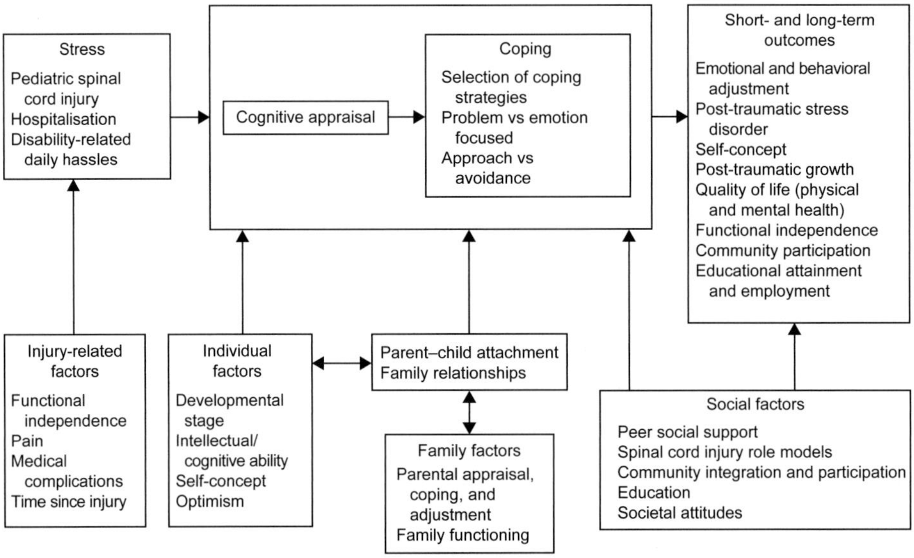

Fig. 24.1 Proposed model of children's psychosocial adjustment following pediatric SCI (Webster 2008; reproduced with author's permission).

support via psycho-education to increase problem-solving skills; family support for parents and siblings; and peer contact to meet and learn from other children with similar experiences. Emotion-focused support is necessary to address uncontrollable or unchangeable stresses, and includes facilitating the development and maintenance of social support; relaxation; reframing; distraction; normalizing; and supporting the expression of emotion (including via verbal and non-verbal practices such as play, music, drama, and art).

Family Functioning and Adjustment

The impact of pediatric SCI radiates throughout the child's network of support, including parents, other caregivers, and siblings. A significant minority of caregivers of young people with SCI have been found to experience anxiety, depression, and PTSD (Boyer et al 2000, Kelly et al 2011), and have reported that their child's injury negatively affected their personal relationships (Anderson et al 1994). Research that has been conducted examining family adjustment after pediatric trauma establishes connections between the adjustment of each individual in the family unit (Killen 1990, Boyer et al 2000, Kelly et al 2011). Because of the mutual interaction between the members of the family, consideration of parental issues is important for the well-being of both caregivers and the injured child. A social–ecological approach offers a framework by which to organize the family and other contextual influences impacting upon a child with SCI (Kazak et al 2009).

Webster (2008) reported that protective factors for positive parental adjustment after a child's traumatic injury included having strong social support, talking openly about the child's condition, and remaining optimistic. Risk factors included an increased number of hospitalizations, and the child having less functioning and needing more assistance (Webster 2008). Specific to the level of functioning, other research has found no relationships between injury level and parent mental health (Kelly et al 2011). A better understanding of the factors related to parental adjustment can help to identify groups at risk of poor outcomes, and develop effective interventions to address their needs.

Although research has begun examining the parental outcomes of young people sustaining an SCI, there is a paucity of research on understanding the psychological consequences for siblings. To date, only one published study has examined healthy siblings of children with SCI (Akhtar et al 2012). This qualitative research highlighted that these children do have particular psychological and emotional needs that should be attended to. The authors emphasized the need to maintain normal routines and sibling relationships, and also to ensure that undue responsibility and burden are not placed upon the healthy sibling.

Summary

It is important to identify risk and protective factors for psychosocial adjustment, and develop approaches to eliminate barriers to adjustment and bolster facilitators of psychosocial health. An individual's adjustment to pediatric SCI can be influenced by individual, injury-related, social, family, and environmental variables. As such, intervention and treatment approaches should be multilevel and address factors falling within each of these categories.

Developmental considerations

Several critical themes have emerged in the pediatric SCI literature: the importance of peer support, cognitive appraisal, and coping; the need to engage young people in their treatment; the attitudes of others toward disability; and how the SCI impacts the entire family system (Webster 2008). These factors necessitate consideration when striving to understand the context of pediatric SCI. Moreover, the interaction between the injury and the child's continuing growth and development is paramount and a developmental approach is therefore essential. The following section presents the unique developmental issues that should be considered for young people with SCI aged 0 to 5 years, 6 to 12 years, and 13 to 18 years.

Early Childhood: 0 to 5 Years

Case vignette: a 4-year-old child

Ben, aged 4 years, sustained a T4 complete injury in a car crash. His father was driving and his younger brother Owen was also in the car; both were relatively unhurt.

Case conceptualization

Ben has just entered into the rehabilitation phase of his hospital stay and is finding physical interventions distressing: he is shouting at and hitting ward staff. His parents are distressed and anxious and Ben's father, in particular, feels guilty about having survived the crash without long-term injury. Both parents are under pressure, feeling the need to support Ben in hospital but also care for their other child at home.

Intervention strategies

1 The hospital play specialist worked with Ben on a one-to-one basis, and the nursing team helped to develop the family's understanding of spinal cord injury, the rehabilitation process, and functional abilities using age-appropriate resources such as models of the body, picture books, toys, and so forth.
2 A team approach was employed to consider how to incorporate fun and play approaches necessary for physical interventions. For example, the physiotherapist used games such as building a tower and playing catch to help Ben to develop skills with balance and coordination.
3 Ben's parents were encouraged to bring in items from home (such as bedding, toys, posters, and photographs) to help foster a friendlier environment in hospital.
4 The multidisciplinary team was aware of the importance of allowing Ben control and choice within his environment; for example, Ben could choose which activity to work on from a choice of two options at the start of each occupational therapy session.
5 The nature of the specialist spinal injuries children's ward enabled Ben to have space for play and social interaction with similarly injured children in hospital and for Ben's parents to interact with other parents in a similar position.
6 Day trips away from the ward and hospital were encouraged so that Ben and his family could spend quality time together outside of a healthcare setting and maintain their individual relationship needs.
7 Ben's parents worked with the clinical psychologist on a regular basis and sessions focused on providing space to process their own trauma reactions and reflect on loss and fears for the future. Additional work with his parents addressed how to maintain parenting when emotional resources are low, and how to respond to Ben's questions and behavior using developmentally appropriate terms and being guided by Ben in terms of the time and place for such discussions.

Developmental theory

Young people aged 0 to 5 years cycle through three distinct developmental stages, with each stage having different implications for rehabilitation. Erikson (as seen in Carr 2006) proposes that the stage of infancy (typically birth to 1y) is characterized by the development of trust versus mistrust. Trust primarily revolves around parental caregivers and, during this time, infants face particular difficulties when separated from these caregivers. In order to support infants throughout this developmental stage, rehabilitation should focus on including parents in the continued care of their child and familiar routines should be encouraged as much as possible.

Toddlers (2–3y) begin to explore their environment through play. The goal in this stage is for the child to develop a sense of self-control without loss of self-esteem (Carr 2006). Building on the natural tools of this stage of development, rehabilitation should foster play, and provide appropriate adaptations for children to explore their environment in fun ways. Therapy-based games to assess function and work therapeutically with children could involve favorite games or toys from home, for example blowing bubbles to help assess respiratory function.

Finally, children in early childhood (4–5y) strive to achieve direction and purpose in their activities (Carr 2006). This stage also sees a time in which cognitive development is characterized by egocentric and imaginative thinking. Crucial to the adjustment of children is their capacity to make sense of what they see; egocentric and magical thinking, combined with a lack of information, can contribute to erroneous beliefs that their thoughts, wishes, and behaviors may have an influence on their injury or rehabilitation (e.g. 'I'm hurt because I was naughty', 'If I am good I will get better'). In order to avoid misperceptions about the cause of their injury or the reason for various (at times painful) hospital procedures, children should be given clear, age-appropriate information about their injury and related treatments (Webster 2008). It may also be comforting to a young hospitalized child for parents to bring in favorite toys or familiar bed linens from home.

Intervention

In terms of fostering positive outcomes, in addition to the age-specific suggestions above, children should be supported to follow normal developmental trajectories. For example, children should be encouraged to be independent in their mobility as early as 12 to 18 months of age, as this is consistent with when children with typical development master walking; however, research has found practice to fall short of this recommendation (Schottler et al 2012). Children should also be supported in participating in school and community activities, similar to the experience of a child with typical development. Likewise, although rehabilitation for children of this young age will primarily involve the education of parents, children should be encouraged to learn self-care techniques independently whenever it is developmentally appropriate. For example, children can be taught bowel and bladder management techniques around 5 years of age (Webster 2008). Although these young children will still require supervision and assistance, including them in the rehabilitation process from a young age can help children feel like active participants in the management of their injury and, more generally, their health.

Research suggests that children injured at younger ages fare better in terms of psychosocial outcomes than those injured later in childhood (Warschwausky et al 1996, Nelson et al 2000). However, most of what is known about outcomes of the youngest children is based upon parent reports. Parental reports of child outcomes provide valuable information, particularly for these youngest children who are often unable to verbalize their needs and concerns. In addition, parent perspectives probably drive treatment decisions for their children and, for this reason, should be closely attended to. However, research has found discrepancies between parent and child reports of child outcomes (Barlow and Ellard 2006, Johnston et al 2006, Garma et al 2011). In general, as early as possible, child reports should be gathered to complement parent reports. For example, pain assessments have been conducted in children as young as 4 years of age (Webster 2008). To be effective, assessments with young children may need to involve use of non-traditional methods including detailed interviewing and behavioral observation instead of predetermined standardized tools (Kortesluoma and Nikkonen 2006).

Research affirms that children who acquire an SCI at a young age experience relatively long life expectancies (Shavelle et al 2007); as such, rehabilitation must be adaptive, responsive, and anticipatory to their needs. Planning for future transitions, for example to high school, adulthood, and employment, should begin immediately (Anderson and Vogel 2000). At this young age, parents should be given information on what they should expect for their child, including information on education, fertility and sexuality, future employment, and transition to independent living (Mulcahey et al 2004). Normalizing the exchange of such information can help foster realistic expectations and set in place a reasonable plan for transition.

Middle to Late Childhood: 6 to 12 Years

Case vignette: a 10-year-old child

Just before her ninth birthday, Chloe developed sudden-onset incomplete paralysis at neurologic level T12, attributed to transverse myelitis.

Case conceptualization

Chloe's mother is concerned about Chloe's adjustment since she returned home from hospital 1 year ago. Her mother reports that Chloe regularly 'acts out' and she is unsure how to handle this. When her parents try to help Chloe around the house, this often ends in arguments. Chloe's younger brother told his parents he feels Chloe is able to 'get away with anything now'. Chloe says she feels frustrated and upset as she cannot access certain parts of the house and feels her parents 'take over' and do things their way. Chloe is currently refusing to undertake certain standing routines and wear ankle and foot splints as advised when she was in hospital.

Intervention strategies

1 The clinical psychologist formulated and normalized the family's responses: Chloe's parents were helped to see that her 'acting out' at home was her way of reacting to the understandable frustrations of not being able to access her previous way of coping and calming down, which was to go to her bedroom (upstairs) for some time alone.

2 Chloe's parents were encouraged to consider strategies to increase Chloe's independence with her rehabilitation skills at home, such as her mother and father remaining mindful to give Chloe choices and actively support and encourage her verbal or physical independence with regards to her routines. Additionally, the family was helped to consider which age-appropriate household chores could belong to Chloe. It was also suggested to the family that they make a room downstairs accessible for Chloe so she could have readily available access to some personal space.

3 After discussions with Chloe, the clinical psychologist contacted Chloe's school and facilitated the allocation of a named teacher for Chloe to talk to at school. It was agreed upon that this arrangement would be at Chloe's request, as and when she felt she needed this additional level of support.

4 The clinical psychologist adopted a family approach to consider the needs of Chloe's parents and brother, including advice for Chloe's parents about long-term coping and adjustment, reinforcing the need to keep boundaries, and resources to help address the needs of siblings, including a leaflet on supporting child relatives and an invitation to a workshop for siblings of children with SCI.

Developmental theory

A focus on productivity and skill mastery is often seen in middle childhood (Erikson, as seen in Carr 2006). A sense of accomplishment, competence, and self-efficacy is derived through the development and use of new skills to achieve meaningful and rewarding goals. Cognitive development facilitates a greater, more sophisticated understanding of SCI and rehabilitation. Furthermore, school-aged children begin to develop their problem-solving abilities, applying logic and intuition to solve concrete problems (Piaget, as seen in Carr 2006).

Peer relationships assume greater importance in middle childhood, and children often describe themselves in terms of class membership and personal traits, giving them a sense of self-identity (e.g. 'I am a member of a dance school and I am a good tap dancer'). Children with SCI may need support to rethink some goals and activities, and re-evaluate their dreams in order to achieve a redeveloped sense of identity. This may be particularly important during acute treatment, as children find themselves suddenly removed from the social context of school, community activities, and other experiences that provide their sense of identity (Vogel et al 2004).

Throughout middle childhood and onwards the development of complex emotions such as envy, embarrassment, pride, shame, and guilt emerge alongside the child's ability to see the world from another's perspective. By middle childhood, children start to be able to regulate emotions by changing their thoughts in addition to their actions (Carr 2006). Insight regarding the experience of mixed feelings or emotional ambivalence also develops around this time, and emotional development can be facilitated by encouraging the child to relate his or her experiences about having a disability, and helping the child make links between the sophisticated interaction of thoughts, feelings, and behaviors.

Intervention

There is a developmental need for age-appropriate independence and, as part of their rehabilitation, children should be educated about their injury, and encouraged to actively participate in self-care, with rehabilitation staff providing plenty of opportunities for skill development and mastery (Vogel et al 2004). School-aged children should be encouraged to participate in decision making by being offered choices or being helped with interacting directly with healthcare professionals in order to develop their ability to negotiate their own care, advocate for themselves, and access information and resources (Vogel et al 2004). Children in middle childhood may be able to perform self-care activities, such as their bowel regime, with assistance, and should be encouraged and supported to assume self care with privacy and dignity. Independence in verbally directing, or physically undertaking, the stages of self-intermittent catheterization can also be achieved by those children who are able to tell the time and follow step-by-step instructions.

A goal of rehabilitation is to help the child to return to active participation in his or her life at home, at school, and in the community. Hobbies and play time should be encouraged, and children should be included in a range of social activities such as birthday parties, family or peer social gatherings, sleepovers, visits to playgrounds, summer camps, and playing or attending sports events (e.g. Vogel et al 2004, House et al 2009). Children growing up with SCI also need to keep up with their peers by doing activities that develop work skills. As children grow into school age, their chores become more complex in preparation for adolescence and adulthood (Anderson and Vogel 2000). It can be helpful for families to have input from healthcare professionals to generate ideas for appropriate chores, problem-solving resources, and any adaptations that may be necessary.

Good communication between rehabilitation and school professionals can support reintegration to school and minimize the impact of the disability on the child's access to education (see Chapter 23). Outside of the family, school may be the most influential social system in the life of a child; however, unfortunately, school is a place where prejudiced views of disability are often reproduced (Antle 2004). It would be useful for rehabilitation staff to share with the school the child's progress in rehabilitation, and help school officials consider how the child's needs could be met in the school environment. Rehabilitation professionals should promote a healthy and positive image of the child's future in terms of participation and future employment (Anderson and Vogel 2000, Klaas et al 2010). The child may also want the support of a member of the school staff to help explain to his or her class about SCI. However, it is important that this decision is made by the child and his or her family, and that everyone is aware of what has or has not been said. Having an allocated teacher or personal tutor in the school to speak to in confidence, and peer or 'buddy' support, may help support the child's emotional needs. Emotional development is also supported by inclusion on school trips and access to clubs, sports, and extracurricular activities. Access to more specialist input such as school counseling services, educational psychologists, or child-clinical psychologists in the community should be facilitated as needed.

Depending on the level of injury, the child may require additional support in the classroom (e.g. from a learning support assistant) to meet his or her learning needs, and carer support to meet his or her SCI needs. Privacy and time alone with peers are both important issues, and adult carers need to be mindful of, and sensitive to, these needs. For example, the carer might assist with personal care or a standing regime but then retreat to allow the child to mix, for example at lunch or social break times. The carer–child relationship requires regular reviews involving the child, parents, schools, and carers.

Children are inquisitive, and it is natural for children of this age to ask questions about sexuality. From this age onwards, as children progress through adolescence, to help with body image, self-esteem, and sex-specific sexuality issues, it is critical to educate children and their parents in a timely, responsive, and positive manner regarding the effects of SCI, which may include changes to sexual function. A developmental approach is needed to deliver appropriate and accurate sex education (see Beck and DiGiovanni 2010). Some parents and children may wonder about the future after SCI, in terms of whether it is possible to go on to form romantic relationships, be able to have sex, build a family, and have children. It is important to share clinical and research evidence showing that this is possible and to outline what help or options exist to support relationship building when the time is right. Furthermore, rehabilitation professionals should support the development of positive body image and self-esteem through modeling positive attitudes toward disability, encouraging a healthy interest in appearance, facilitating participation in adaptive activities and sports, and supporting young people to help them embrace the attributes of their disability that affect their appearance, for example by customizing adaptive equipment.

Adolescence: 13 to 18 Years

Case vignette: a 15-year-old adolescent
Around 4 years ago, Alex, aged 15 years, developed a C4 incomplete spinal cord injury secondary to a spinal tumor. He lives with his mother and his sister, aged 12 years.

Case conceptualization
At review clinic, Alex describes being low in mood. He feels frustrated and angry about certain daily procedures and routines, and the amount of forward planning and lack of spontaneity these bring. He particularly dislikes the fact that he has to rely on the support of carers. His friends are starting to go on dates, and talk about learning to drive and going to college. Alex feels 'left out' and 'left behind'. He lacks confidence about the way he looks and his disability. He has started to withdraw socially and has a limited number of hobbies. He is also unsure what job he could do in the future. At times he wonders to himself, 'What's the point?'

Intervention strategies

1. The clinical psychologist assessed Alex's current mood, risk of self-harm, and suicidal ideation using formal measures and interviewing techniques and referred him on to local services for ongoing counseling and monitoring.
2. Emotion-focused work was undertaken to acknowledge Alex's emotional reactions to losses and those aspects of his life that have changed, and to help Alex to express and manage his responses.
3. Problem-solving approaches were used to generate mutual ideas to solve specific issues such as ideas to increase social support; gain personal space and privacy; increase engagement in pleasurable activities; develop self- and body confidence via social participation activities; and consider options for the future in terms of driving, vocational opportunities, and so forth.
4. The clinical psychologist helped Alex to identify specific appraisals he held regarding his injury. Various sessions focused on explicitly identifying and addressing aspects which he viewed in terms of representing a loss or threat and as being unmanageable, and building on aspects which he perceived as a challenge.

Developmental theory

Adolescence is a time of significant biological, cognitive, and psychosocial change. Research indicates that the brain is still maturing in the adolescent years and that reasoning and judgment are developing well into the early- to mid-20s. Cognitively, adolescents gradually increase their ability to understand complex problems, abstract issues, and hypothetical situations, and develop an increasing meta-cognitive awareness of their own thought processes (Carr 2006). Psychosocially, adolescents face the task of developing a clear sense of identity (Newman and Newman 2011). Concerns regarding body image, sexuality, and group membership are typical, and adolescents with SCI may already be experiencing psychological challenges similar to those experienced by their peers, including low self-esteem, negative feelings toward their body, and isolation (Anderson 1997). The successful resolution of these challenges can lead to the development of a positive sense of self, realistic goals, greater independence, and increased resilience (Carr 2006).

Intervention

For adolescents, the demands of managing the physiological consequences of an SCI and the potential restrictions this poses upon an adolescent's lifestyle has the potential to increase dependence on the family at a time when dependence should be decreasing. Although adolescents report finding parental support important during rehabilitation (e.g. parents may take on the role of advocate and morale booster, and facilitate discussions about feelings and coping; see Augutis et al 2007), there is a need to strike a balance between appropriate parental support and over-involvement, particularly with regard to personal care activities.

A key challenge for rehabilitation professionals is thus to support the young person and his or her family in maintaining a developmentally appropriate level of independence and autonomy at a time when this may be emotionally challenging for all concerned. In practice, throughout adolescence, young people should be given increasing responsibility for managing their SCI. This may include increasing independence in making decisions regarding treatment, rehabilitation, care management, and future planning. Adolescents should have the opportunity to meet with healthcare professionals independently of their parents for at least part of any appointment. Furthermore, similar to other stages of childhood, adolescence is a time of unique transition in a young person's life, and in adolescence this relates to education, employment, healthcare, leaving home, and becoming an independent adult. Health professionals have a responsibility to contribute to the process of planning and managing successful transitions in these areas and the reader is referred to Labhard (2010) for a detailed discussion of the key issues that should be considered and recommendations for practice.

Facilitating the maintenance of friendships during rehabilitation should also be a key concern, as evidence suggests that children are at risk of losing friendships because of the challenges of maintaining contact while in hospital, and because of peers' lack of understanding of SCI (Webster 2008). In addition, from the perspective of the adolescent with SCI, the medical management of their injury may be perceived as a barrier that separates them from their peers. Friends have been reported as being important to adolescents with SCI in maintaining links with home while hospitalized, and in motivating adolescents to access the community at a time when they may have significant concerns regarding their body image and identity (Augutis et al 2007). Adolescents and families should be supported to help develop their confidence in managing peers' questions about SCI, and opportunities for young people to spend leisure time with their friends should be facilitated, whether in the hospital or community.

Similarly, maintaining links with the school, ensuring successful inclusion, and minimizing disruptions to educational progress are of significant importance. Adolescence is a time of important decisions and experiences with regard to qualifications, education, and career choices: these are decisions and choices that will have a lasting impact upon an individual's life.

Commonly reported negative emotional responses to injury during post-acute rehabilitation include anger and frustration, particularly toward parents and professionals; shame or disgust, particularly in relation to personal care; and attempts to gain control over the situation and assert independence (Augutis et al 2007). Although such emotions and behaviors (and related issues such as non-adherence to aspects of rehabilitation) present a significant concern for rehabilitation professionals, these are often developmentally appropriate expressions. Care must be taken to strike a balance between ensuring adolescents receive appropriate psychological support regarding emotional and adjustment issues, while avoiding pathologizing potential developmentally appropriate behaviors. In this way, intervention may also focus on reappraising and indeed normalizing such negative emotions. For example, anger and stubbornness may be reappraised as evidence of having a 'fighting spirit' and being helpful in attempts to persevere and manage the situation (Augutis et al 2007).

Finally, sexuality is a key issue for adolescents. Research indicates that adolescents with SCI do perceive themselves as sexually attractive, although have concerns regarding others' negative attitudes toward disability, and have ambivalent feelings regarding their body image (Potgieter and Khan 2005). During post acute rehabilitation, adolescents reported feeling physically unattractive owing to restrictions on clothing, difficulties maintaining personal appearance in hospital, and the need to use functional aids (Augutis et al 2007). Adolescents have further been shown to make efforts to hide bladder and bowel problems and changes in appearance owing to muscle loss, and have reported disliking rehabilitation aids that highlighted their disability (Dewis 1989). Collectively, this research highlights the importance of addressing issues relating to sexuality, intimacy, self-esteem, and body image early in the rehabilitation process. Recommendations pertaining to sexuality in the middle childhood section above continue to apply through adolescence.

Future directions

There is a lack of information on how best to intervene to foster psychosocial health in pediatric SCI. The current literature focuses on identifying psychosocial outcomes and outlining how things change after injury; however, this research base is still developing. Although Figure 24.1 includes a hypothesized model of the relationships between the multitude of factors impacting the adjustment of young people, few of these pathways have been established empirically. In addition, although the majority of young people with SCI and their caregivers adjust well after injury, there is a lack of information about resilience in this population. Of particular interest are the factors which facilitate positive adjustment, and whether these factors can be developed or enhanced through training, counseling, or resource sharing as part

TABLE 24.1
Psychosocial adjustment: key issues

Developmental consideration	Early childhood (0–5y)	Middle childhood (6–12y)	Adolescence (13–18y)
Cognitive	Provide age-appropriate information about SCI to avoid misconceptions	Provide opportunities for skill development and mastery through increasing participation in self care and other daily activities	Allow for greater autonomy and independence in all aspects of rehabilitation and future planning
Emotional	Foster play and employ appropriate adaptations to allow the child to explore his or her environment	Encourage the child to relate to his or her experiences regarding SCI and make links between specific thoughts, feelings, and behaviors	Avoid pathologizing emotional and behavioral issues (e.g. non-adherence) and aim to support young people with typical developmental issues regarding identity, body image, and self-esteem, which may be complicated by their SCI
Social and peer relationships	Facilitate maintenance of friendships and engagement in typical activities with peers (e.g. birthday parties)	Encourage hobbies and participation in social activities; facilitate contact with peers, including providing opportunities for the child to spend time alone with peers; and educate the wider system about opportunities for participation and inclusion	In addition to aforementioned strategies, support adolescents with issues related to intimate relationships
School and vocation	Support participation in school and community activities	Foster good communication between rehabilitation and school professionals, including providing education about SCI and support at school. Help children and families generate ideas for appropriate chores	In addition to aforementioned strategies, consider support from patient organizations and career planning services, and facilitating contact with role models with SCI
Responsibility and independence	Include parents in the care of their child and encourage familiar routines	Offer choices and support the child to help him or her interact directly with healthcare professionals to negotiate his or her own care where appropriate	Allow greater autonomy and independence with regard to decisions about treatment, rehabilitation, and future management (with regard to this, there may be a developmental requirement for increased flexibility and negotiation with respect to rules)
Transitions	Provide information to parents regarding expectations about education, future employment, and transition from home	Ensure good communication and planning for school transitions	Provide opportunities for career planning and ensure system-wide collaboration with regard to transitions between care teams and from home to independent living
Sexuality	Provide parents with information about sexuality and fertility	Provide parents and child with age-appropriate information about sexuality topics	Address issues regarding body image and sexuality early in rehabilitation; foster a positive attitude toward disability, encourage a healthy interest in appearance, and support young people to help them embrace attributes of their disability that affect their appearance (e.g. customize equipment)

SCI, spinal cord injury.

of the initial rehabilitation process. In the future, researchers, clinicians, young people with SCI, and their families should work in partnership to evaluate existing forms of treatment and develop new interventions to best support the adjustment of young people and their families after injury.

Summary

Although young people with SCI and their caregivers may be at an increased risk of poor psychosocial outcomes, many young people and caregivers adjust well after injury. Approaches to assessment and intervention will vary according to the child's age and stage of development. The key developmental considerations for enhancing psychosocial adjustment at different ages and stages are summarized in Table 24.1. A family-systems approach should be adopted and both young people and their families/caregivers should be encouraged to be actively involved in rehabilitation. Assessment and intervention should be considered a lifelong process for young people with SCI and their families/caregivers.

REFERENCES

Akhtar M, Kennedy P, Webster G, Graham A (2012) What about us? Children's experiences of living with a sibling with spinal cord injury. *J Pediatr Rehabil Med* 5: 301–13. doi: 10.3233/PRM-2012-00226

Anderson CJ (1997) Unique management needs of paediatric spinal cord injury patients: Psychosocial issues. *J Spinal Cord Med* 20: 21–3.

Anderson CJ, Vogel L (2000) Preparation for employment in children and adolescents with spinal cord injuries. *Top Spinal Cord Inj Rehabil* 6(supplement): 170–5. doi: 10.1310/3VMV-C31B-0AW2-YJF6

Anderson CJ, Lubicky JP, Vogel LC (1994) Impact of paediatric spinal cord injury on family adjustment: parents' perspective. *J Am Paraplegia Soc* 17: 102.

Anderson CJ, Vogel LC, Betz RR, Willis KM (2004) Overview of adult outcomes in paediatric-onset spinal cord injuries: implications for transition to adulthood. *J Spinal Cord Med* 27(Suppl): S98–106.

Anderson CJ, Vogel LC, Chlan KM, Betz RR, McDonald CM (2007) Depression in adults who sustained spinal cord injuries as children or adolescents. *J Spinal Cord Med* 30(Suppl 1): S76–82.

Anderson CJ, Kelly EH, Klaas SJ, Russell H, Daharsh E, Vogel L (2009) Anxiety and depression in children and adolescents with spinal cord injuries. *Dev Med Child Neurol* 51: 826–32. doi.org/10.1111/j.1469-8749.2009.03268.x

Antle BJ (2004) Factors associated with self-worth in young people with physical disabilities. *Health Soc Work* 29: 167–75. doi: 10.1093/hsw/29.3.167

Augutis M, Levi R, Asplund K, Berg-Kelly K (2007) Psychosocial aspects of traumatic spinal cord injury with onset during adolescence: a qualitative study. *J Spinal Cord Med* 30(S1): S55–64.

Barlow JH, Ellard DR (2006) The psychosocial well-being of children with chronic disease, their parents and siblings: an overview of the research evidence base. *Child Care Health Dev* 32: 19–31. doi: 10.1111/j.1365-2214.2006.00591.x

Beck T, DiGiovanni L (2010) Developmental approach to sexuality and intimacy. *Top Spinal Cord Inj Rehabil* 16: 48–54. doi: 10.1310/sci1601-48

Boyer BA, Knolls ML, Kafkalas CM, Tollen LG (2000) What *is* the trauma? Patients', mothers', and fathers' fear and helplessness related to posttraumatic aspects of paediatric spinal cord injury. *Top Spinal Cord Inj Rehabil* 6(Suppl): 134–47. http://dx.doi.org/10.1310/H5UP-12BM-7LE7-VBXR

Brown M, Gordon WA (1987) Impact of impairment on activity patterns of children. *Arch Phys Med Rehabil* 68: 828–32.

Carr A (2006) *The Handbook of Child and Adolescent Clinical Psychology*. 2nd Ed. London: Routledge.

Chevalier Z, Kennedy P, Sherlock O (2009) Spinal cord injury, coping and psychological adjustment: a literature review. *Spinal Cord* 47: 778–82. doi: 10.1038/sc.2009.60

Dewis ME (1989) Spinal cord injured adolescents and young adults: the meaning of body changes. *J Adv Nurs* 14: 389–96. doi: 10.1111/j.1365-2648.1989.tb01546.x

Duff J, Kennedy P (2003) Spinal cord injury. In: Llewelyn S, Kennedy P (eds). *Handbook of Clinical Health Psychology*. Chichester, UK: John Wiley & Sons Ltd. pp. 251–75. doi: 10.1002/0470013389.ch14

Garma SI, Kelly EH, Daharsh EZ, Vogel LC (2011) Health-related quality of life after paediatric spinal cord injury. *J Pediatr Psychol* 36: 226–36. doi: 10.1093/jpepsy/jsq037

House LA, Russell HF, Kelly EH, Gerson A, Vogel LC (2009) Rehabilitation and future participation of youth following spinal cord injury: caregiver perspectives. *Spinal Cord* 47: 882–6. doi: 10.1038/sc.2009.64

Hwang M, Zebracki K, Chlan K, Vogel L (2014) Longitudinal employment outcomes in adults with pediatric-onset spinal cord injury. *Spinal Cord* 52: 477–82. http://dx.doi.org/10.1038/sc.2014.32

Johnson KA, Klaas SJ (2007) The changing nature of play: implications for paediatric spinal cord injury. *J Spinal Cord Med* 30(Suppl 1): S71–5.

Johnston T, Lauer RT, Smith BT (2006) Differences in scores between children with spinal cord injury and their parents using the Paediatric Quality of Life Inventory. *Pediatr Phys Ther* 18: 94–5. doi: 10.1097/00001577-200601810-00046

Kazak AE, Rourke MT, Navsaria N (2009) Families and other systems in pediatric psychology. In Roberts MC, Steele RG (eds). *Handbook of Pediatric Psychology*. New York, NY: Guilford Press. pp. 656–71.

Kelly EH, Anderson CJ, Garma SI et al (2011) Relationships between the psychological characteristics of youth with spinal cord injury and their primary caregivers. *Spinal Cord* 49: 200–5. doi: 10.1038/sc.2010.78

Killen JM (1990) Role stabilization in families after spinal cord injury. *Rehabil Nurs* 15: 19–21. doi: 10.1002/j.2048-7940.1990.tb01148.x

Klaas SJ, Kelly EH, Gorzkowski J, Homko E, Vogel LC (2010) Assessing patterns of participation and enjoyment in children with spinal cord injury. *Dev Med Child Neurol* 52: 468–74. doi: 10.1111/j.1469-8749.2009.03552.x

Kortesluoma RL, Nikkonen M (2006) 'The most disgusting ever': children's pain descriptions and views of the purpose of pain. *J Child Health Care* 10: 213–27. http://dx.doi.org/10.1177/1367493506066482

Labhard S (2010) Transitioning to adulthood with disabilities: a holistic approach. *Top Spinal Cord Inj Rehabil* 16: 1–16. doi: 10.1310/sci1601-1

Lazarus RS, Folkman S (1984) *Stress Appraisal and Coping*. New York, NY: Springer.

Lindwall JJ, Russell HF, Kelly EH et al (2012) Coping and participation in youth with spinal cord injury. *Top Spinal Cord Inj Rehabil* 18: 220. doi: 10.1310/sci1803-220

Mulcahey MJ, Anderson CJ, Vogel LC, Devivo MJ, Betz RR, McDonald C (2004) Paediatric spinal cord injury: evidence-based practice and outcomes. *Top Spinal Cord Inj Rehabil* 10: 69–78. doi: 10.1310/MYWE-9RFA-BRYY-KAET

Nelson VS, Warschausky SA, Brennan PJ, Hurvitz EA, Hernandez M (2000) Long-term quality of life outcomes in ventilator-assisted, spinal-cord-injured children. *Top Spinal Cord Inj Rehabil* 6(Suppl): 246–7.

Newman B, Newman P (2011) *Development Through Life*. 11th Ed. Pacific Grove, CA: Brooks/Cole.

Potgieter CA, Khan G (2005) Sexual self-esteem and body image of South African spinal cord injured adolescents. *Sex Disabil* 23: 1–20. doi: 10.1007/s11195-004-2076-6

Schottler J, Vogel LC, Sturm P (2012) Spinal cord injuries in young children: a review of children injured at five years of age and younger. *Dev Med Child Neurol* 54: 1138–43. doi: 10.1111/j.1469-8749.2012.04411.x

Shavelle RM, DeVivo MJ, Paculdo DR, Vogel LC, Strauss DJ (2007) Long-term survival after childhood spinal cord injury. *J Spinal Cord Med* 30: S48–54. doi: 10.1097/00006416-200409000-00004

Vogel LC (1997) Unique management needs of paediatric spinal cord injury patients: introduction. *J Spinal Cord Med* 20: 9.

Vogel LC, Hickey KJ, Klaas SJ, Anderson CJ (2004) Unique issues in paediatric spinal cord injury. *Orthop Nurs* 23: 300–8. http://dx.doi.org/10.1097/00006416-200409000-00004

Warschwausky S, Engel L, Kewman D, Nelson VS (1996) Psychosocial factors in rehabilitation of the child with a spinal cord injury. In: Betz RR, Mulcahey MJ (eds). *The Child with a Spinal Cord Injury*. Rosemont, IL: American Academy of Orthopaedic Surgeons. pp. 471–82.

Webster G (2008) Paediatric spinal cord injury: impact on children and families. In: Craig A, Tran Y (eds). *Psychological Aspects Associated with Spinal Cord Injury: New Directions and Best Evidence*. London: Nova Science Publishers, Inc. pp. 89–131.

25
LONG-TERM OUTCOMES OF PEDIATRIC-ONSET SPINAL CORD INJURY

Kathy Zebracki, Kathleen Chlan and Lawrence C Vogel

Case vignette
Michael was a previously healthy male who sustained a C6 American Spinal Injury Association Impairment Scale A spinal cord injury at age 16 years in a motorcycle crash. He is now 30 years old and has been battling a pressure ulcer on his sacrum for the past 3 years. He worked part-time in insurance sales but was made redundant 2 years ago because of budget cuts, and since then he has been unable to find work. He lives independently with attendant care; however, he is socially isolated owing to sitting restrictions secondary to the pressure ulcer and transportation difficulties. He experiences moderate to severe depressive symptoms and attributes this to his inability to leave his home and do something meaningful in his day.

> If I had to change one thing in my life, yes, I wouldn't have dived into that pool, but in many ways [the incident] has made me who I am today. I used to be a bit of a troublemaker – as a teenager, I hung around with the wrong crowd – since my accident, I am a different, a better person. Sure, some things can be a challenge, but who doesn't have bad days? I have a good family and network of friends, who are patient and help me get through it. I can't change what has happened, so why dwell on it? Move on. I just want to live my life.
>
> Samantha, aged 34 years, injured at age 17 years

Introduction

Childhood and adolescence are developmental periods marked by significant changes in biological, psychological, cognitive, and social functioning. A spinal cord injury (SCI) produces immediate and wide-ranging effects on the individual's life. Specifically, a pediatric-onset SCI temporarily disrupts the normative trajectory of development. Consequently, one goal for caring for young people with an SCI is to facilitate positive adjustment and attainment of critical developmental milestones within the context of living life with an SCI. The ultimate aim of the rehabilitation process is for these young people to make a seamless transition to adulthood and function at an optimal level, fully participating in their community and experiencing a high quality of life.

Owing to the wide-ranging effects of SCI, understanding the outcomes of pediatric-onset SCI requires a multidimensional, biopsychosocial approach. Using the International Classification of Functioning, Disability and Health as a framework, a variety of outcomes need to be assessed throughout the lifespan of the individual with an SCI. These include secondary health conditions, emotional well-being, social and community participation, vocation, and overall life satisfaction. Moreover, other factors interact with SCI-specific outcomes, including normative developmental and environmental changes, such as intrapersonal factors, medical and technological advances, and the general aging process, all of which have an impact on outcomes.

Delineating the natural course of pediatric-onset SCI and major life outcomes can identify factors that promote resilience and are associated with optimal outcomes. Interventions can then target these factors, with the assumption that the earlier the intervention, the greater the impact. In addition, understanding the long-term outcomes of adults with pediatric-onset SCI will help define the minimum expectations for an individual with a given neurologic level and severity of injury. Therefore, the purpose of this chapter is to describe the outcomes of adults who have been living with SCI since childhood, including secondary health conditions, psychological functioning, and community integration, based on data from an ongoing longitudinal study on pediatric-onset SCI.

Study background

This ongoing study began in 1996 and involves current or former patients at one of the three pediatric SCI specialty programs at Shriners Hospitals for Children: Chicago, Philadelphia, and Northern California (www.clinicaltrials.gov). Participants are at least 19 years of age, sustained an SCI before 19 years of age, do not have a significant brain injury, and speak English. In-person or telephone interviews occur every year from initial enrollment. The sample currently consists of 457 participants, aged 19 to 48 years, and over 1950 interviews. Overall, 30 participants completed at least one interview but were deceased at the time of the follow-up interview. Additional information regarding this longitudinal study are available elsewhere (Zebracki et al 2010, Vogel et al 2011). Data reported in this chapter are cross-sectional and are from the participants' most recent interviews. Demographic and injury characteristics of the sample are shown in Table 25.1.

A structured questionnaire designed for this study assesses demographic, injury-related, medical, and social factors. Several standardized measures are included to assess outcomes; however, only measures for which data are reported in this chapter are described.

Health Condition

Impairment is measured using neurologic level and the American Spinal Injury Association (ASIA) Impairment Scale (AIS) as defined by the International Standards for the Neurological Classification of Spinal Cord Injury (American Spinal Injury Association 2011). Functional status and disability are assessed using the FIM® instrument[a] (Uniform Data System for Medical Rehabilitation, Amherst, NY, USA). The measure consists of two subscales – motor and socio-cognitive – and items are scored on a Likert scale ranging from 1 (total assistance) to 7 (complete independence). The Pittsburgh Sleep Quality Index measures sleep quality and sleep disturbances retrospectively for the previous 1-month period (Buysse et al 1989).

Psychological Functioning

The Patient Health Questionnaire 9 (PHQ-9) assesses depressive symptoms using the diagnostic criteria for major depressive disorder in accordance with the *Diagnostic and Statistical Manual of Mental Disorders*, fourth edition (Kroenke et al 2001). Anxiety symptoms are measured using the short self-report Beck Anxiety Inventory (Beck et al 1988). The Brief COPE measures both adaptive and maladaptive coping skills and was modified to measure selective coping strategies relevant to coping with an SCI (Carver 1997). The SF-12® Health Survey (QualityMetric Incorporated, Lincoln, RI, USA) assesses the individual's perception of his or her health-related quality of life (Ware et al 1996). The General Happiness Scale is a global measure of subjective happiness (Lyubomirsky and Lepper 1999). The Satisfaction with Life Scale measures global life satisfaction (Diener et al 1985).

Participation

The Craig Handicap Assessment and Recording Technique assesses community participation and consists of six separate subscales of physical independence, cognitive independence, mobility, occupation, social integration, and economic self-sufficiency (Whiteneck et al 1992).

Secondary health conditions

Secondary health conditions are physical or psychological health conditions that are influenced directly or indirectly by the presence of a disability or underlying physical impairment (Jensen et al 2012). Owing to their longer duration of living with an SCI, accelerated aging, and relatively sedentary lives with limited opportunities for aerobic activity, adults with pediatric onset SCI are at risk of experiencing a variety of secondary health conditions. These are attributed to SCI-specific factors, such as pressure ulcers and overuse syndrome, as well as age-related chronic health conditions and comorbidities, such as obesity, cardiovascular disease, and hypertension. The likelihood of developing a secondary health condition varies over time and among severity groups (Hwang et al 2014). Secondary health conditions may occur in able-bodied individuals; however, they are more likely to occur at a younger age and with greater severity in individuals with SCI (Jensen et al 2012). In adults with pediatric-onset SCI, secondary health conditions have been found to negatively impact several facets of life, including participation, life satisfaction, employment, income, and independent living (Vogel

a FIM is a trademark of Uniform Data System for Medical Rehabilitation (UDSMR), a division of UB Foundation Activities, Inc. The use of the FIM instrument to collect data for this research study was authorized and conducted in accordance with the terms of a special purpose license granted to the licensee by UDSMR. The patient data collected in the course of this research study have not been processed by UDSMR and there is no implication that such data have been or will be subjected to UDSMR's standard data processing procedures or that they are otherwise comparable to data processed by UDSMR.

TABLE 25.1
Characteristics of participants

Characteristic	All groups (*N*=457)	Neurologic impairment: C1–C4 ABC (*n*=66)	C5–C8 ABC (*n*=159)	T1–S5 ABC (*n*=191)	AIS D (*n*=41)
Demographic					
Male, *n* (%)	289 (63)	55 (83)	102 (64)	108 (56)	24 (59)
Caucasian, *n* (%)	387 (85)	55 (83)	135 (85)	162 (85)	35 (85)
Mean age at interview, y:mo (SD)	31:3 (5:11)	32:8 (6:0)	31:8 (6:2)	30:2 (5:6)	31:9 (5:3)
Age at interview, *n* (%)					
19–24y	43 (9)	2 (3)	14 (9)	23 (12)	4 (10)
25–29y	166 (36)	21 (32)	56 (35)	77 (40)	12 (29)
30–34y	119 (26)	18 (27)	40 (25)	48 (25)	13 (32)
35–40y	96 (21)	18 (27)	35 (22)	33 (17)	10 (24)
41–44y	22 (5)	5 (8)	9 (6)	6 (3)	2 (5)
45–48y	11 (2)	2 (3)	5 (3)	4 (2)	0
Spinal cord injury characteristics					
Age at injury, y:mo (SD) (range)	13:9 (4:5) (0–18)	15:1 (2:6) (7–18)	14:9 (3:2) (0–18)	12:6 (5:5) (0–18)	13:9 (3:8) (0–18)
Duration of injury, y:mo (SD) (range)	17:0 (6:9) (2–42)	17:1 (6:1) (3–31)	16:6 (6:3) (2–30)	17:3 (7:7) (2–42)	17:6 (5:8) (6–28)
Etiology of spinal cord injury, n *(%)*					
Motor vehicle	226 (50)	23 (35)	70 (44)	120 (63)	13 (32)
Sports	111 (24)	29 (44)	61 (38)	9 (5)	12 (29)
Medical/surgical	41 (9)	3 (5)	4 (3)	28 (15)	6 (15)
Violence	40 (9)	3 (5)	11 (7)	23 (12)	3 (7)
Falls	30 (7)	6 (9)	11 (7)	8 (4)	5 (12)
Other/unknown	9 (2)	2 (3)	2 (1)	3 (2)	2 (5)
FIM® motor score (SD)	59.2 (23.9)	25.5 (13.8)	46.5 (18.7)	76.9 (6.9)	77.9 (17.0)

AIS, American Spinal Injury Association Impairment Scale.

et al 2002a, Vogel and Anderson 2005). Consequently, preventing these conditions is a major focus of caring for individuals with SCI.

The prevalence of the most common secondary health conditions in our study population are listed in Table 25.2.

TABLE 25.2
Secondary health conditions

Condition	All groups (N=457)	Neurologic impairment C1–C4 ABC (n=66)	C5–C8 ABC (n=159)	T1–S5 ABC (n=191)	AIS D (n=41)
Physical[a], n *(%)*					
Autonomic dysreflexia[b]	215 (66), N=328	45 (68), n=66	118 (74), n=159	44 (60), n=74	8 (28), n=29
Bladder incontinence[c]	172 (38)	16 (24)	64 (40)	80 (42)	12 (29)
Bladder/kidney stones	45 (10)	11 (17)	18 (11)	15 (8)	1 (2)
Bowel incontinence[c]	63 (14)	10 (15)	22 (14)	29 (15)	2 (5)
Bone fractures	25 (6)	2 (3)	13 (8)	9 (5)	1 (2)
Cardiovascular disease	27 (6)	6 (9)	5 (3)	13 (7)	3 (7)
Hyperhidrosis	79 (17)	8 (12)	35 (22)	34 (18)	2 (5)
Pain					
Shoulder pain[a], *n* (%)	236 (52)	45 (68)	77 (48)	98 (51)	16 (39)
Elbow pain[a], *n* (%)	77 (17)	9 (14)	27 (17)	35 (18)	6 (15)
Wrist pain[a], *n* (%)	103 (23)	5 (8)	29 (18)	57 (30)	12 (29)
Current level of pain (SD) (range=0–10)[d]	2.3 (2.5)	2.5 (2.7)	2.8 (2.8)	1.8 (2.1)	3.2 (2.9)
Pressure ulcer, *n* (%)	150 (33)	34 (52)	56 (35)	52 (27)	9 (22)
Respiratory complications, *n* (%)	15 (3)	3 (5)	7 (5)	4 (2)	1 (2)
Sleep difficulties[c], *n* (%)	67 (43), N=157	14 (58), n=24	24 (45), n=53	24 (39), n=61	5 (56), n=9
Mean PSQI global score (SD) (range=0–16)[d]	5.9 (3.3)	7.1 (3.5)	6.0 (3.4)	5.0 (2.7)	7.4 (4.0)
Spasticity, *n* (%)	213 (47)	46 (70)	97 (61)	59 (31)	11 (27)
UTIs, *n* (%)	322 (71)	50 (76)	122 (77)	130 (68)	20 (49)
Mean number of UTIs per year (SD) (range=1–24)[e]	3.6 (3.4)	3.0 (2.7)	4.0 (3.4)	3.7 (3.7)	2.3 (1.7)
Mean SF-12® physical component score (SD) (range=14–63)[e]	45.0 (10.4)	41.2 (10.6)	42.7 (11.0)	48.0 (8.9)	45.9 (10.2)
Mean number of medications (SD)	4.1 (2.4)	5.6 (2.7)	4.7 (2.3)	3.2 (1.9)	3.0 (1.4)
Psychological					
Mean Beck Anxiety Inventory score (SD) (range=0–37)[d]	3.7 (6.4), N=157	6.5 (8.9), n=25	4.1 (7.3), n=56	2.2 (3.2), n=67	4.8 (8.1), n=9
Mild (8–15), *n* (%)	18 (11)	5 (20)	7 (13)	5 (7)	1 (11)
Moderate/severe (≥16), *n* (%)	7 (4)	2 (8)	4 (7)	0	1 (11)

TABLE 25.2
(Continued)

Condition	All groups (*N*=457)	Neurologic impairment C1–C4 ABC (*n*=66)	C5–C8 ABC (*n*=159)	T1–S5 ABC (*n*=191)	AIS D (*n*=41)
Depression: mean PHQ-9 score (SD) (range 0–23)[d]	3.2 (4.3), *N*=351	3.4 (4.5), *n*=51	3.3 (4.3), *n*=127	3.0 (4.3), *n*=147	4.0 (4.4), *n*=26
Mild (5–9), *n* (%)	59 (17)	9 (18)	19 (15)	24 (16)	7 (30)
Moderate/severe (≥10), *n* (%)	28 (8)	4 (8)	11 (9)	11 (7)	2 (8)
Mean General Happiness Scale score (SD) (range=1–7)[f]	5.6 (1.2), *N*=157	5.6 (1.1), *n*=25	5.8 (1.1), *n*=56	5.6 (1.1), *n*=67	5.1 (1.9), *n*=9
Mean satisfaction score with Life Scale (SD) (range=5–35)[f]	24.2 (7.7)	22.0 (8.0)	23.1 (8.0)	25.9 (6.9)	24.2 (7.5)
Mean SF-12® mental component score (SD) (range=13–74)[f]	53.3 (8.9)	53.1 (9.7)	52.8 (9.6)	53.6 (8.2)	54.1 (8.3)

[a]Occurring in the last year unless otherwise noted. [b]T6 and higher. [c]Occurring at least monthly. [d]Higher score = worse functioning. [e]SF-12 physical component scores range from 0 to 100, with 100 the highest level of physical health. [f]Higher score = better functioning. AIS, American Spinal Injury Association Impairment Scale; UTIs, urinary tract infections.

Physical Health Conditions

Autonomic dysfunction

Within our sample, the prevalence of autonomic dysfunction in adults with pediatric-onset SCI at or above T6 is 66%, with 7% of participants regularly taking an antihypertensive. This rate is slightly higher than the 54% prevalence of autonomic dysfunction among 157 participants (at or above T6) previously reported from this study population (Vogel et al 2002b). The prevelance of autonomic dysfunction in the adult SCI population ranges widely from 11% to 80% (McKinley et al 1999). In comparison, the prevalence of autonomic dysfunction in young people ranges from 40% to 51% (Hickey et al 2004, Schottler et al 2009). Data from our sample found that, when examining autonomic dysfunction by impairment level, individuals with cervical-level injuries (ABC groups) had an increased risk of autonomic dysfunction occurrence over time (Hwang et al 2014).

Bone fractures

In our sample, 6% of participants had developed a pathologic fracture over the past year. Our previous research has shown that those who develop fractures are more likely to be older, have a longer injury duration, and have C5–C8 ABC injuries (Vogel et al 2002c).

Cardiovascular disease

The prevalence of cardiovascular disease in the current patient population is 7%. Previous research has reported an increased risk of cardiovascular diseases (e.g. coronary heart disease, cerebrovascular disease, dysrhythmias) with increasing age, increasing rostral level of injury, and greater severity of SCI (Groah et al 2001). Our work has found that adults with pediatric-onset C1–C4 ABC SCI are at a significantly increased risk of hypertension/cardiac disease than other groups with neurologic impairment (Hwang et al 2014).

Neurogenic bladder and bowel

Bladder and bowel management are major challenges for individuals with SCI. Continence is essential for independence in adult life as well as participation in employment and the community; however, the prevalence of bladder and bowel incontinence (i.e. at least one incontinent episode per month) is common at 38% and 14% for the bladder and bowel, respectively. With the exception of bowel incontinence in those with AIS D, bladder and bowel incontinence is common for all groups with neurologic impairment (Vogel et al 2011). The most common bladder program is intermittent catheterization (51%), followed by indwelling urethral catheter and catheter free with external collector (each 10%), and continent diversions (e.g. Mitrofanoff, stoma; 8%). In regards to bowel programs, 1% have a Malone antegrade continence enema, 5% have a colostomy, and 31% use digital rectal stimulation/manual evacuation. The duration of bowel programs was 60 minutes or more for 29%, 31 to 60 minutes for 32%, and 30 minutes or less for 38%. Many of our participants regularly take bladder (e.g. oxybutynin; 48%) and bowel (e.g. docusate; 46%) medications.

Urinary tract infections (UTIs) are common, with most (71%) participants experiencing at least one UTI in the previous year (Vogel et al 2002b, 2011). Individuals with AIS D are the least likely to have UTIs; however, they are still common at 41% (Vogel et al 2011). Among those with a history of UTI, the average number of yearly infections is 3.6; 13% are prescribed a prophylactic antibiotic, 13% required hospitalization, and another 19% required intravenous antibiotics without hospitalization for treatment of the UTI. In previous work, we found that severe UTI (requiring intravenous antibiotics and/or hospitalization) was associated with decreased participation (total Craig Handicap Assessment and Recording Technique score) (Vogel et al 2002b) and an increased risk of occurrence over time in those with C1–C4 ABC (Hwang et al 2014).

Bladder or kidney stones affect 10% of our participants. Although this is a 15% decrease from previous findings (Vogel et al 2002b), longitudinal analyses suggest a decrease in prevalence over time (Hwang et al 2014). In previous work, we have found that individuals with stones had more severe neurologic deficits, lower mean AIS motor grade, and lower total and motor FIM scores, as well as an indwelling catheter (Vogel et al 2002b).

Pressure ulcers

One-third of our sample experienced pressure ulcers over the past year, with 2% requiring hospitalization and/or surgery for treatment of the pressure ulcer. Rates are generally higher than those reported for adult SCI populations (McKinley et al 1999). Occurrence varies among groups with various levels of impairment, with those with C1–C4 ABC at the greatest risk (Vogel et al 2011). The risk of developing pressure ulcers is stable over time, except for those with AIS D injuries, for whom the odds decrease over time (Hwang et al 2014). The high incidence of spine deformities (Dearolf et al 1990) and hip subluxation in individuals who sustained their SCI before puberty (Rink and Miller 1990) may result in sitting irregularities that in turn contribute to this heightened risk of pressure ulcers in adults with pediatric-onset SCI. Our previous work also found that males, those who are not white, and individuals with a sports-related etiology were more likely to have pressure ulcers than their counterparts (Vogel et al 2002b).

Pain

Pain has a significant impact on many spheres of life. A longitudinal study of adults with SCI found that 81% experience pain and 58% describe their pain as severe or excruciating (Siddall et al 2003). As young people with SCI age, they are prone to prematurely develop degenerative upper extremity joint arthropathy secondary to their excessive use of upper extremities for wheelchair propulsion and transfers. Within our sample, 76% report pain, with shoulder pain being the most common (55%), followed by neck (43%) and lower back pain (40%). These prevalence rates are comparable to those with adult-onset SCI (Dalyan et al 1999). Overall, pain is mild but frequent, with 42% reporting daily pain. Pain tends to last a few hours (26%) to most of the day (22%) and interferes at least a little with day-to-day activities (55%) and sleep (59%). In total, 24% are regularly taking either over-the-counter or prescription medications to treat pain; however, only 44% report that over-the-counter medications are helpful and even fewer (30%) report that prescription medication successfully manages pain. Moreover, the likelihood of upper extremity joint pain increases over time regardless of injury severity (Hwang et al 2014).

Respiratory complications

Among our sample, only 3% experienced pneumonia over the last year and 0.2% required the use of a ventilator. The risk of pneumonia or respiratory failure increases over time for individuals with C1–C8 ABC injuries (Hwang et al 2014). Our previous work found that those who experience pneumonia or respiratory failure are more likely to be older, have a longer injury duration, have more severe neurologic impairments, be unemployed, and have decreased life satisfaction (Vogel et al 2002b).

Sleep

Dysfunctional sleep may contribute to poor health outcomes over and above the effects of the SCI (Jensen et al 2009). There is a high prevalence of sleep apnea (40–50%) in the adult SCI population and of dysfunctional sleep (when unrelated to apnea) in veterans with SCI (49%) (Lavela et al 2012). In our sample, 43% endorse sleep difficulties ('poor sleepers'), with 37% having difficulty falling asleep within 30 minutes, and half experience nightwakings several nights a week. On average, individuals obtain 6.6 hours of sleep per night and 6% use sleeping medicines to facilitate sleep onset.

Spasticity

Compared with the adult-onset SCI population, spasticity in pediatric-onset SCI is less common (Vogel and Anderson 2003). In our sample, 47% report spasticity requiring treatment.

The risk of occurrence increases over time in those with C1–C4 ABC injuries; however, the risk decreases in those with T1–S5 ABC and AIS D injuries (Hwang et al 2014). Our previous work has also shown significant associations between spasticity and older age at injury, sports-related SCI, cervical injuries, lower AIS motor grades, and lower total and motor FIM scores (Vogel et al 2002c).

Perceived physical well-being

Individuals with paraplegia and AIS D demonstrate normative levels of perceived physical well-being; however, those with tetraplegia report lower levels (Vogel et al 2011). Cervical injury, severe UTI, and shoulder pain have been associated with decreased physical well-being (Vogel et al 2002a).

Psychological Health Conditions

Living with SCI places considerable psychological demands on the individual. Consequently, continuous assessment of well-being is critical in individuals with SCI. SCI has been associated with an increased risk of psychological morbidity, diminished life satisfaction and quality of life, and substance use (Post and Van Leeuwn 2012). Despite facing a variety of challenges, the majority of individuals with SCI are able to successfully surmount these obstacles and demonstrate resilience and positive psychological functioning and outcomes (Kortte et al 2010, White et al 2010, Sakakibara et al 2012). Research on adults with SCI experiencing positive outcomes found that, while the realities of daily life were altered after injury, these individuals maintained their same goals and values as before their injury. Moreover, factors such as social support, positive and challenge-focused appraisals, and meaningful participation were critical in attaining favorable outcomes and decreasing psychological distress (Griffiths and Kennedy 2012).

Anxiety

The lifetime prevalence of anxiety disorders (i.e. generalized anxiety disorder, post-traumatic stress disorder, phobias, and separation anxiety disorders) in the general US population is 15%, whereas the annual prevalence is 10% (Kessler et al 2009). Rates of clinically significant symptoms of anxiety in adult-onset SCI range from 13% to 40% (Post and Van Leeuwn 2012), with an inconsistent course over time (Kennedy and Rogers 2000). Little is known, however, about anxiety in pediatric-onset SCI. One study found a prevalence rate of 13% in young people with SCI (Klaas et al 2014). In our sample, 11% of adults with pediatric-onset SCI showed mild symptoms of anxiety and 4% showed moderate to severe symptoms. Regular use of anxiolytics was reported by 14% of our sample.

Depression

Major depressive disorder is one of the most common mental disorders in the USA. In the general population, the prevalence rate is 7%, and, for those classified as severe, the prevalence is 2% (Kessler et al 2005). Correspondingly, depression is the most common form of psychopathology in individuals with SCI and has been associated with numerous secondary health outcomes, such as pressure ulcers, UTIs, lower perceived health, fewer occasions of and less meaningful participation in social and leisure activities, and mortality (Bombardier et al 2004, Krause et al 2008, Saunders et al 2012). The prevalence of depression in adults with SCI typically ranges from 10% to 38% (Bombardier et al 2004, Fann et al 2011, Saunders et al 2012). Similarly, in our sample, 17% endorsed mild depressive symptoms (i.e. PHQ-9 total score between 5 and 9) and 8% endorsed moderate to severe symptoms (i.e. PHQ-9 total score ≥10). In regards to suicidal ideation, 7% had experienced thoughts of hurting themselves or death over the past 2 weeks, compared with 4% of the general US population. Moreover, 18% of our sample reported regular use of antidepressants. Factors linked with depressive symptoms include incomplete injury, secondary health conditions (i.e. pressure ulcers, shoulder pain), unemployment, low income, and poor perceived mental health (Anderson et al 2007). In addition, factors associated with suicidal ideation include lower AIS motor grades, being male, being unemployed, not living independently, lower satisfaction with life, and poor perceived mental health (Anderson et al 2007). The course of depression remains unclear. Data from the SCI Model Systems suggest a decrease in symptoms over many years (Richardson and Richards 2008). Our results suggest that there are small fluctuations in depression symptoms over time (i.e. a slow decrease after injury, then an increase, followed by another gradual decrease [January et al 2014]).

General happiness

Subjective happiness (i.e. experiencing frequent positive affect and infrequent negative emotion) as reported by our sample (mean=5.6) is comparable to that of the general US population (mean=4.8). Global subjective assessment has been associated with positive social rewards and work outcomes, participation in rewarding activities, greater physical health, and adaptive coping (Lyubormirsky et al 2005).

Life satisfaction

Although life satisfaction tends to improve from an initial low point after injury, it stabilizes in individuals with adult-onset SCI to a level below that of the general population (Post and Van Leeuwn 2012). In contrast, levels of life satisfaction in our sample of adults with pediatric-onset SCI is similar to that of the general population, irrespective of impairment level (Anderson et al 2002, Vogel et al 2011). We have found that life satisfaction is significantly higher for women and married persons, those who have an advanced degree, and those who are employed. Moreover, life satisfaction is positively related to younger injury age and fewer secondary health complications (e.g. severe UTIs, pressure ulcers, respiratory problems) (Anderson et al 2002, Vogel et al 2002a,b). Over time, individuals who feel unsatisfied are likely to stay unsatisfied if critical life factors remain unchanged in their life (Chen et al 2008).

Perceived mental well-being

Perceived mental well-being is comparable to normative data, regardless of impairment level (Vogel et al 2011). Shoulder and back pain have been associated with decreased mental well-being (Vogel et al 2002a).

Coping

Adaptive coping is associated with positive outcomes in young people with SCI. For example, higher levels of cognitive restructuring and lower levels of self-criticism and blaming others predict favorable outcomes (Lindwall et al 2012). In our sample of adults with pediatric-onset SCI, acceptance is the most used form of coping, followed by positive reframing and active coping. With regard to negative strategies, 15% use substances as a coping strategy. Alcohol (33%) was the most common substance used, followed by marijuana (14%) and tobacco (12%). Use of alcohol (55%) and tobacco (28%) is higher among young adults (ages 21–25y) (Hwang et al 2012). Our previous research has found that frequent use of adaptive coping (i.e. emotional support, acceptance, and religion) and infrequent use of maladaptive coping (i.e. substance use) are associated with greater life satisfaction (Anderson et al 2008, Chlan et al 2011).

Participation

Participation, defined by the World Health Organization as involvement in a life situation, is an essential component of living a meaningful and successful life. Participation characteristics of our study population are listed in Table 25.3.

Education

Educational attainment and employment are quintessential milestones of adult development and integral to self-identity, independent living, financial autonomy, socialization, emotional well-being, and life satisfaction (Anderson and Vogel 2002, Vogel and Anderson 2005, Anderson et al 2006). Moreover, educational attainment is associated with decreased mortality in individuals with SCI (Krause et al 2011). Between 2007 and 2011, in the general US population, 28% of adults over the age of 24 years attained a bachelor's degree or higher. In adults with pediatric-onset SCI, this rate is significantly greater, with 41% of our current sample having at least a bachelor's degree. When taking into consideration neurologic and impairment levels, educational attainment continues to be comparable to the general population or greater for all four groups of various levels of neurologic impairment (28–39%) (Vogel et al 2011).

Economic life

Despite being well educated, individuals with SCI are less likely to be employed than their able-bodied peers (Anderson and Vogel 2002) but are more likely to be employed than the overall population of individuals with a disability (defined as impairments in the areas of hearing, vision, cognition, and ambulation). According to US national data from 2011, 70% of the general population was employed compared with only 27% of individuals with a disability. Longitudinal studies of individuals with adult-onset SCI found employment rates of 35% (National Spinal Cord Injury Statistical Center 2012), whereas rates for adults with pediatric-onset SCI appear to be higher (Anderson and Vogel 2002, Vogel et al 2011). Among the participants of our study, 47% are employed and, of those employed, 40% are in full-time work (≥35h/wk). Factors associated with employment include white skin color, higher educational attainment, thoracic injury level, independent physical mobility and driving, greater perceived social support, and fewer secondary health complications, depressive symptoms,

TABLE 25.3
Participation

Area of participation	All groups (N=457)	Neurologic impairment C1–C4 ABC (n=66)	C5–C8 ABC (n=159)	T1–S5 ABC (n=191)	AIS D (n=41)
Education, n *(%)*					
High school diploma or equivalent	442 (97)	65 (99)	158 (99)	181 (95)	38 (93)
Bachelor's degree or higher	189 (41)	32 (49)	67 (42)	74 (39)	16 (39)
Economic life					
Employment status, *n* (%)					
Employed (full- or part-time)	214 (47)	24 (36)	64 (40)	102 (53)	24 (59)
Student	54 (12)	8 (12)	20 (13)	24 (13)	2 (5)
Homemaker	30 (7)	2 (3)	9 (6)	15 (8)	4 (10)
Unemployed	154 (34)	31 (47)	66 (42)	47 (25)	10 (24)
Personal annual income, median US$	19 000	12 000	14 900	24 000	25 000
Household annual income, median US$	33 600	25 400	29 000	40 000	40 000
Personal maintenance					
Lives independently, *n* (%)	299 (65%)	32 (49%)	94 (59%)	145 (76%)	28 (68%)
Paid attendant care, *n* (%)	165 (36%)	54 (82%)	92 (58%)	13 (6%)	6 (15%)
Mean h/d (SD) (range)	4.5 (4.2) (1–24)	5.9 (5.4) (1–24)	4.0 (3.4) (1–24)	2.8 (1.9) (1–7)	2.8 (1.7) (1–5)
Mobility, n *(%)*					
Wheelchair use[a]					
Manual wheelchair	267 (58)	6 (9)	65 (41)	178 (93)	18 (44)
Power wheelchair	167 (37)	59 (89)	92 (58)	9 (5)	7 (17)
Does not use wheelchair	15 (3)	0	0	0	15 (37)
Drives motor vehicle	287 (63)	13 (20)	83 (52)	161 (84)	30 (73)
Social					
Married/domestic partner, *n* (%)	116 (25)	9 (14)	35 (22)	59 (31)	13 (32)
CHART scores (SD)[b]					
Physical	91.3 (12.9)	78.2 (17.6)	86.9 (12.5)	98.2 (4.6)	96.6 (9.2)
Cognitive	97.7 (4.9)	96.7 (6.8)	97.6 (5.3)	98.1 (3.9)	97.1 (3.9)
Mobility	88.7 (17.9)	78.3 (20.7)	87.3 (19.7)	93.0 (13.7)	91.2 (15.1)

TABLE 25.3
(Continued)

		Neurologic impairment			
Area of participation	**All groups (*N*=457)**	**C1–C4 ABC (*n*=66)**	**C5–C8 ABC (*n*=159)**	**T1–S5 ABC (*n*=191)**	**AIS D (*n*=41)**
Occupation	74.7 (31.3)	64.4 (32.8)	69.9 (31.8)	80.4 (28.9)	83.3 (30.4)
Social integration	90.7 (15.3)	88.0 (18.0)	89.6 (16.8)	92.4 (13.3)	91.1 (12.0)
Economic	73.0 (34.2)	64.8 (35.9)	69.1 (35.4)	76.9 (32.6)	79.3 (32.8)

[a]Wheelchair used >50% of the time. [b]Higher score = better functioning. AIS, American Spinal Injury Association Impairment Scale.

and access-related barriers (Krause et al 1998, Vogel et al 1998, Anderson and Vogel 2002, Anderson et al 2006). Barriers to employment include secondary health conditions, challenges with transportation and accessibility, financial disincentives, and a lack of motivation (Anderson and Vogel 2002). In view of the discrepancy between high educational achievement and lower employment rate, young people with SCI must be encouraged to concentrate on educational activities that are directly linked to future employment.

Economic factors, such as income, may serve as a proxy for access to healthcare, assistance with activities of daily living, and overall living conditions. Life expectancy of adults with SCI varies as a function of household income, with mortality rates lowest in the highest income categories (>$75 000) (Krause et al 2011). In our sample, median personal and household incomes are $19 000 and $33 600, respectively, and 20% have household incomes greater than $75 000. In 2011, the poverty threshold for a one-person household was $10 890 and the median household income was $50 054.

Personal maintenance

Living independently is a goal for all adults, including the vast majority of adults with a chronic health condition and/or physical disability. Our work has found that living independently is associated with physical independence, employment, active participation in the community, and life satisfaction (Anderson et al 2004, 2006). Compared with the general population of 25- to 34-year-old individuals, 84% to 90% of whom live independently, adults with pediatric-onset SCI, regardless of their impairment level, were less likely to live independently (42–70%) (Vogel et al 2011). In our current sample, 65% live independently (i.e. without parents or a guardian). Nearly all (98%) live in a private residence and 35% have paid attendant care (mean=4.5h/d, range=1–24).

Mobility

The majority of our sample (87%) always uses a wheelchair for mobility; 58% use a manual wheelchair and 37% use a power wheelchair more than 50% of the time. Obtaining a drivers' license is a rite of passage for most adolescents and driving a motor vehicle is a sign of continuing independence in senior adults; however, these tasks are a significant challenge to those with SCI. Although individuals with injuries as high as C5 are capable of driving an appropriately adapted motor vehicle, they are less likely to drive than their able-bodied peers (Vogel et al 2011). In the general US population, 46% of individuals under 19 years of age are licensed drivers. This increases to 81% for those aged 20 to 24 years and to over 90% in those aged between 35 and 69 years (Federal Highway Administration 2010). In a survey of individuals aged 16 to 21 years with SCI, 52% drove independently (Anderson et al 1996). In our sample, 63% drive independently, which is comparable to the 65% national rate of all drivers of age with a disability (Federal Highway Administration 2010). Notably, however, a long-term outcome study conducted in the UK found that, although 54% of adults with a chronic physical disability had a license, only 19% were actually driving, with medical or financial reasons the main deterrents (Oakeshott and Hunt 2003). Additional factors associated with the inability to drive independently include higher neurologic level, pressure ulcers, and lack of higher education (Vogel et al 2002a). The outlook for independent driving is therefore limited, compelling individuals with SCI to rely heavily on others for essential transportation.

Social relationships

Peer relationships and healthy romantic experiences are crucial factors for positive development and promoting self-identity (e.g. self-concept, self-esteem) and interpersonal skills (e.g. communication, trust), and are particularly important for young people with chronic health conditions, including SCI, as these relationships may facilitate adjustment to the chronic condition, promote medical adherence, serve as a source of emotional support, and improve life satisfaction (Anderson et al 2008). For individuals with SCI, marriage serves as a major source of support, provides economic resources, and offers increased regulation of health behavior (Holicky and Charlifue 1999). Moreover, being married is associated with increased life satisfaction and emotional well-being and decreased depressive symptoms over time (Kalpakjian et al 2011, Chlan et al 2013). Estimates of marriage rates for adults with adult-onset SCI vary from 31% to 66% (Post and Van Leeuwn 2012). Within our sample, 25% are married and, of those who are single, 40% are dating.

Summary

This chapter provides an overview of an ongoing study of adults with pediatric-onset SCI and their long-term outcomes of secondary health conditions (i.e. physical and psychological health) and participation in education, employment, independent living, transportation, and social relationships. The ultimate outcome of caring for young people with SCI is that, throughout their lifespan from injury to later adulthood, they function at optimal physical and psychological levels, participate fully in their community, and experience a high quality of life. Delineating long-term outcomes can identify facilitators of positive outcomes as well as risks of poorer outcomes. This knowledge can be utilized to implement appropriate interventions and rehabilitation strategies for children and adolescents, thereby better preparing them for their future. Additionally, understanding the long-term outcomes of adults with pediatric-onset SCI will help to define expectations for an individual with a given neurologic level and severity of injury.

REFERENCES

American Spinal Injury Association (2011) *International Standards for the Neurologic Classification of Spinal Cord Injury Revised 2011* (booklet). Atlanta, GA: American Spinal Injury Association.

Anderson C, Vogel L (2002) Employment outcomes of adults who sustained spinal cord injuries as children or adolescents. *Arch Phys Med Rehabil* 83: 791–801. http://dx.doi.org/10.1053/apmr.2002.32742

Anderson CJ, Wright G, Vogel LC (1996) Driving issues for young adults with pediatric spinal cord injuries. *J Spinal Cord Med* 19: 115.

Anderson C, Krajci K, Vogel L (2002) Life satisfaction in adults with pediatric-onset spinal cord injuries. *J Spinal Cord Med* 25: 184–90.

Anderson CJ, Vogel LC, Betz RR, Willis KM (2004) Overview of adult outcomes in pediatric-onset spinal cord injuries: implications for transition to adulthood. *J Spinal Cord Med* 27: S98–106.

Anderson CJ, Vogel LC, Willis KM, Betz RR (2006) Stability of transition to adulthood among individuals with pediatric-onset spinal cord injuries. *J Spinal Cord Med* 29: 46–56.

Anderson CJ, Vogel LC, Chlan KM, Betz RR, Mcdonald CM (2007) Depression in adults who sustained spinal cord injuries as children or adolescents. *J Spinal Cord Med* 30: S76–82.

Anderson C, Vogel L, Chlan K, Betz R (2008) Coping with spinal cord injury: strategies used by adults who sustained their injuries as children or adolescents. *Spinal Cord Medicine* 31: 290–6.

Beck AT, Epstein N, Brown G, Steer RA (1988) An inventory for measuring clinical anxiety: psychometric properties. *J Consult Clin Psychol* 56: 893–7. http://dx.doi.org/10.1037/0022-006X.56.6.893

Bombardier CH, Richards JS, Krause JS, Tulsky D, Tate DG (2004) Symptoms of major depression in people with spinal cord injury: implications for screening. *Arch Phys Med Rehabil* 85: 1749–56. http://dx.doi.org/10.1016/j.apmr.2004.07.348

Buysse DJ, Reynolds CF 3rd, Monk TH, Berman SR, Kupfer DJ (1989) The Pittsburgh sleep quality index: a new instrument for psychiatric practice and research. *Psychiatry Res* 28: 193–213. http://dx.doi.org/10.1016/0165-1781(89)90047-4

Carver CS (1997) You want to measure coping but your protocol's too long: consider the Brief COPE. *Int J Behav Med* 4: 92–100. http://dx.doi.org/10.1207/s15327558ijbm0401_6

Chen Y, Anderson CJ, Vogel LC, Chlan KM, Betz RR, McDonald CM (2008) Change in life satisfaction of adults with pediatric-onset spinal cord injury. *Arch Phys Med Rehabil* 89: 2285–92. doi: 10.1016/j.apmr.200806.008

Chlan KM, Zebracki K, Vogel LC (2011) Spirituality and life satisfaction in adults with pediatric-onset spinal cord injury. *Spinal Cord* 49: 371–5. doi: 10.1038/sc.201080

Chlan K, Zebracki K, Vogel L (2013) Sexual intimacy in adults with pediatric-onset spinal cord injury. *Top Spinal Cord Inj Rehab* 19: 10.

Dalyan M, Cardenas D, Gerard B (1999) Upper extremity pain after spinal cord injury. *Spinal Cord* 37: 191–5. http://dx.doi.org/10.1038/sj.sc.3100802

Dearolf WW, Betz RR, Vogel LC, Levin J, Clancy MC, Steel HH (1990) Scoliosis in pediatric spinal-cord injured patients. *J Pediatr Orthop* 10: 214–18. http://dx.doi.org/10.1097/01241398-199003000-00016

Diener E, Emmons R, Larsen J, Griffin S (1985) The Satisfaction With Life Scale. *J Pers Assess* 49: 71–5. http://dx.doi.org/10.1207/s15327752jpa4901_13

Fann JR, Bombardier CH, Richards JS et al (2011) Depression after spinal cord injury: comorbidities mental health service use and adequacy of treatment. *Arch Phys Med Rehabil* 92: 352–60. doi: 10.1016/j.apmr.201005.016

Federal Highway Administration (2010) *Distribution of Licensed Drivers 2008 Highway Statistics*. Washington DC: US Department of Transportation.

Griffiths HC, Kennedy P (2012) Continuing with life as normal: positive psychological outcomes following spinal cord injury. *Top Spinal Cord Inj Rehab* 18: 241–52. doi: 10.1310/sci1803-241

Groah S, Weitzankamp D, Sett P, Soni B, Savic G (2001) The relationship between neurological level of injury and symptomatic cardiovascular disease risk in the aging spinal injured. *Spinal Cord* 39: 310–17. http://dx.doi.org/10.1038/sj.sc.3101162

Hickey K, Vogel L, Willis K, Anderson C (2004) Prevalence and etiology of autonomic dysreflexia in children with spinal cord injuries. *J Spinal Cord Med* 27: S54–60.

Holicky R, Charlifue S (1999) Ageing with spinal cord injury: the impact of spousal support. *Disabil Rehabil* 21: 250–7. http://dx.doi.org/10.1080/096382899297675

Hwang M, Chlan KM, Vogel LC, Zebracki K (2012) Substance use in young adults with pediatric-onset spinal cord injury. *Spinal Cord* 50: 497–501. doi: 10.1038/sc.20128

Hwang M, Zebracki K, Chlan K, Vogel L (2014) Longitudinal changes in medical complications in adults with pediatric-onset spinal cord injury. *J Spinal Cord Med* 37: 171–8. doi: 10.1179/2045772313Y.0000000150

January A, Zebracki K, Chlan K, Vogel L (2014) Symptoms of depression over time for individuals with pediatric-onset spinal cord injury. *Arch Phys Med Rehabil* 95: 447–54. doi: 10.1016/j.ampr.2013.11.011

Jensen MP, Hirsh AT, Molton IR, Bamer AM (2009) Sleep problems in individuals with spinal cord injury: frequency and age effects. *Rehabil Psychol* 54: 323–31. doi: 10.1037/a0016345

Jensen M, Molton I, Groah S et al (2012) Secondary health conditions in individuals aging with SCI: terminology concepts and analytic approaches. *Spinal Cord* 50: 373–8. doi: 10.1038/sc.2011150

Kalpakjian CZ, Houlihan B, Meade MA et al (2011) Marital status marital transition well-being and spinal cord injury: an examination of the effects of sex and time. *Arch Phys Med Rehabil* 92: 433–40. doi: 10.1016/j.apmr.201007.239

Kennedy P, Rogers BA (2000) Anxiety and depression after spinal cord injury: a longitudinal analysis. *Arch Phys Med Rehabil* 81: 932–7. http://dx.doi.org/10.1053/apmr.2000.5580

Kessler R, Chiu W, Demler O, Walters E (2005) Prevalence, severity, and comorbidity of 12-month DSM-IV disorders in the National Comorbidity Survey Replication (NCS-R). *Arch Gen Psychiatry* 62: 617–27. http://dx.doi.org/10.1001/archpsyc.62.6.617

Kessler R, Aguilar-Gaxiola S, Alonso J et al (2009) The global burden of mental disorders: an update from the WHO, World Mental Health (WMH) surveys. *Epidemiol Psichiatr Soc* 18: 23–33. http://dx.doi.org/10.1017/S1121189X00001421

Klaas S, Kelly E, Anderson C, Vogel L (2014) Depression and anxiety in adolescents with pediatric-onset spinal cord injury. *Top Spinal Cord Inj Rehab* 20: 13–22. doi: 10.1310/sci2001-13

Kortte KB, Gilbert M, Gorman P, Wegener ST (2010) Positive psychological variables in the prediction of life satisfaction after spinal cord injury. *Rehabil Psychol* 55: 40–7. doi: 10.1037/a0018624

Krause JS, Sternberg M, Maides J, Lottes S (1998) Employment after spinal cord injury: differences related to geographic region gender and race. *Arch Phys Med Rehabil* 79: 615–24. http://dx.doi.org/10.1016/S0003-9993(98)90033-8

Krause J, Carter R, Pickelsimer E, Wilson D (2008) A prospective study of health and risk of mortality after spinal cord injury. *Arch Phys Med Rehabil* 89: 1482–91. doi: 10.1016/j.apmr.200711.062

Krause JS, Saunders LL, Devivo MJ (2011) Income and risk of mortality after spinal cord injury. *Arch Phys Med Rehabil* 92: 339–45. doi: 10.1016/j.apmr.201009.032

Kroenke K, Spitzer RL, Williams JBW (2001) The PHQ-9: validity of a brief depression severity measure. *J Gen Intern Med* 16: 606–13. doi: 10.1046/j.1525-14972001016009606.x

Lavela SL, Burns SP, Goldstein B, Miskevics S, Smith B, Weaver FM (2012) Dysfunctional sleep in persons with spinal cord injuries and disorders. *Spinal Cord* 50: 682–5. doi: 10.1038/sc.201231

Lindwall J, Russell H, Kelly E et al (2012) Coping and participation in youth with spinal cord injury. *Top Spinal Cord Inj Rehab* 18: 220–31. doi: 10.1310/sci1803-220

Lyubomirsky S, Lepper H (1999) A measure of subjective happiness: preliminary reliability and construct validation. *Soc Indic Res* 46: 137–55. http://dx.doi.org/10.1023/A:1006824100041

Lyubormirsky S, King L, Diener E (2005) The benefits of frequent positive affect: does happiness lead to success? *Psychol Bull* 131: 803–55. http://dx.doi.org/10.1037/0033-2909.131.6.803

McKinley WO, Jackson AB, Cardenas DD, Devivo MJ (1999) Long-term medical complications after traumatic spinal cord injury: a regional model systems analysis. *Arch Phys Med Rehabil* 80: 1402–10. http://dx.doi.org/10.1016/S0003-9993(99)90251-4

National Spinal Cord Injury Statistical Center (2012) Spinal cord injury facts and figures at a glance. *J Spinal Cord Med* 35: 197–8. http://dx.doi.org/10.1179/1079026812Z.00000000063

Oakeshott P, Hunt GM (2003) Long-term outcome in open spina bifida. *Br J Gen Pract* 53: 632–6.

Post M, Van Leeuwn C (2012) Psychosocial issues in spinal cord injury: a review. *Spinal Cord* 50: 382–9. doi: 10.1038/sc.201118

Richardson E, Richards J (2008) Factor structure of the PHQ-9 screen for depression across time since injury among persons with spinal cord injury. *Rehabil Psychol* 53: 243–9. doi: 10.1037/0090-5550.53.2.243

Rink P, Miller F (1990) Hip instability in spinal cord injury patients. *J Pediatr Orthop* 10: 583–7. http://dx.doi.org/10.1097/01241398-199009000-00002

Sakakibara BM, Hitzig SL, Miller WC, Eng JJ (2012) An evidence-based review on the influence of aging with a spinal cord injury on subjective quality of life. *Spinal Cord* 50: 570–8. doi: 10.1038/sc.201219

Saunders LL, Krause JS, Focht KL (2012) A longitudinal study of depression in survivors of spinal cord injury. *Spinal Cord* 50: 72–7. doi: 10.1038/sc.201183
Schottler J, Vogel L, Chafetz R, Mulcahey MJ (2009) Patient and caregiver knowledge of autonomic dysreflexia among youth with spinal cord injury. *Spinal Cord* 47: 681–6. doi: 10.1038/sc.200912
Siddall PJ, Mcclelland JM, Rutkowski SB, Cousins MJ (2003) A longitudinal study of the prevalence and characteristics of pain in the first 5 years following spinal cord injury. *Pain* 103: 249–57. http://dx.doi.org/10.1016/S0304-3959(02)00452-9
Uniform Data System for Medical Rehabilitation (1997) *The Guide for Uniform Data Set for Medical Rehabilitation (including the FIM™ Instrument)*. Buffalo, NY: UDSMR.
Vogel LC, Anderson CJ (2003) Spinal cord injuries in children and adolescents: a review. *J Spinal Cord Med* 26: 193–203.
Vogel L, Anderson C (2005) Outcomes of adults with pediatric onset spinal cord injury. *Top Spinal Cord Inj Rehab* 10: 109–15. doi: 10.1310/V3E8-3M03-FHCM-YWRG
Vogel LC, Klaas SJ, Lubicky JP, Anderson CJ (1998) Long-term outcomes and life satisfaction of adults who had pediatric spinal cord injuries. *Arch Phys Med Rehabil* 79: 1496–503. http://dx.doi.org/10.1016/S0003-9993(98)90409-9
Vogel LC, Krajci KA, Anderson CJ (2002a) Adults with pediatric-onset spinal cord injuries. Part 3: impact of medical complications. *J Spinal Cord Med* 25: 297–305.
Vogel LC, Krajci KA, Anderson CJ (2002b) Adults with pediatric-onset spinal cord injury. Part 1: prevalence of medical complications. *J Spinal Cord Med* 25: 106–16.
Vogel LC, Krajci KA, Anderson CJ (2002c) Adults with pediatric-onset spinal cord injury. Part 2: musculoskeletal and neurological complications. *J Spinal Cord Med* 25: 117–23.
Vogel LC, Chlan KM, Zebracki K, Anderson CJ (2011) Long-term outcomes of adults with pediatric-onset spinal cord injuries as a function of neurological impairment. *J Spinal Cord Med* 34: 60–6. doi: 10.1179/107902610X12883422813787
Ware JE, Kosinski M, Keller SD (1996) A 12-item short-form health survey: construction of scales and preliminary tests of reliability and validity. *Med Care* 34: 220–33. http://dx.doi.org/10.1097/00005650-199603000-00003
White B, Driver S, Warren AM (2010) Resilience and indicators of adjustment during rehabilitation from a spinal cord injury. *Rehabil Psychol* 55: 23–32. doi: 10.1037/a0018451
Whiteneck GG, Charlifue SW, Gerhart KA, Overhosler JD, Richardson GN (1992) Quantifying handicap: a new measure of long-term rehabilitation outcomes. *Arch Phys Med Rehabil* 73: 519–26.
Zebracki K, Anderson CJ, Chlan C, Vogel L (2010) Outcomes of adults with pediatric-onset spinal cord injury: longitudinal findings and implications on transition to adulthood. *Top Spinal Cord Inj Rehab* 16: 17–25. doi: 10.1310/sci1601-17

26
LEISURE AND RECREATIONAL ACTIVITIES

Deepan C Kamaraj, Kathy Zebracki, Sara J Klaas and Rory A Cooper

Case vignette

Growing up in Innsbruck, Austria, Lukas was a competitive Alpine skier from an early age. By age 17 years, he had two top-15 finishes in Giant Slalom at the World Junior Alpine Skiing Championships. Shortly after his 18th birthday, he was involved in a motor vehicle crash and sustained a C8 spinal cord injury. He primarily uses a manual wheelchair for mobility, but also has a power-assist system for long distances or when navigating challenging terrains. About 18 months after his injury, Lukas returned to skiing and racing using a bi-ski and outriggers. Lukas reported that his desire to return to skiing was a motivating factor during his rehabilitation. When asked what he tells newly injured individuals, he says 'Always keep trying. Don't let the disability stop you from doing what you want to do'.

Overview

Spinal cord injury (SCI) brings physical, psychological, and social changes to all areas of everyday life. The approach of rehabilitation interventions for individuals with SCI is a holistic one and includes improving and optimizing daily functioning, engagement in life, and well-being (Gorter 2009). This is especially crucial among children with SCI, as the challenges they face are unique because of the injury and the dynamic growth and development that occurs during childhood (Zebracki et al 2010). Studies on child development reinforce the important role that play, leisure, and recreation have on health and well-being, and it is known that engagement in recreational activities is a key element to the development of children (Shikako-Thomas et al 2013). In addition, recent studies have also shown that parents, young people, and professionals consider enhanced participation in leisure time activities as one of the most important outcomes of rehabilitation interventions (Vargus-Adams and Martin 2011). This chapter embraces an evidence-based approach in examining the various opportunities and barriers that may be faced by children and young adults with SCI and the role of their family, friends, and professionals working with them as they venture into leisure and recreational activities.

With the growing advancements in assistive technology, the spectrum of leisure time activities in which a child can participate has been expanding. Van Naarden Braun and colleagues proposed that leisure time activities can be represented by three general categories: (1) organized group activities (e.g. going to a religious service, playing an organized sport, participating in wheelchair ballet); (2) informal social activities (e.g. getting together with friends, going out to eat or on a date); and (3) informal individual activities (e.g. reading a book, doing a hobby) (Van Naarden Braun et al 2006). Although specific research examining the influence of informal social or individual activities on the lives of individuals with SCI has been limited, the impact and positive influence of organized group activities – specifically organized sports – on individuals with SCI and other neurologic disabilities has been well documented (Ittenbach et al 1993). Overall, young adults participating in sporting activities may garner more benefits from having a richer diversity of experiences than those with a limited number of leisure time activities (Nash 2005).

Benefits of leisure and recreational activities after spinal cord injury

Medical/Physiological Implications

As discussed throughout this book, individuals with SCI are highly susceptible to medical complications and secondary chronic conditions. Promoting leisure time and physical activity can help prevent such conditions, enhance functional abilities, and increase quality of life and social integration (Kehn and Kroll 2009). Although scientific research has been limited, a few specific studies have demonstrated the significant positive impact on health due to participation in organized recreational physical activity (Slater and Meade 2004). Specifically, studies have shown that there are considerable positive improvements in the cardiovascular, respiratory, and metabolic systems of people with SCI (e.g. Muraki et al 2000, Fernhall et al 2008, Jacobs 2009).

Jacobs (2009) demonstrated that individuals with paraplegia increased their $\dot{V}O_{2peak}$ by 15% after a short-term resistance-training program. Muraki et al (2000) established that the number of days per week a person with SCI is physically active is strongly related to physical work capacity. Moreover, vigorously active wheelchair athletes with SCI have been found to have higher levels of high-density lipoprotein than their sedentary peers (Brenes et al 1986). Improving physical work capacity or increasing physical activity in persons with SCI has also been shown to improve lipid profiles, particularly high-density lipoprotein cholesterol over time (Dallmeijer et al 1999). Considering low high-density lipoprotein cholesterol is common among individuals with SCI, the side effects related to this, such as cardiovascular morbidity, could be potentially avoided. In addition, participants of wheelchair sport were found to have fewer kidney infections and pressure sores requiring long-term hospitalizations than their inactive counterparts (Fernhall et al 2008).

Psychosocial Implications

Similar to the general population, individuals with long-term neurologic conditions perceive recreational exercise as beneficial to physical, psychological, and social functioning, with some individuals reporting that it provides hope, purpose, a sense of identity, and vitality

(Mulligan et al 2012). Recreational and leisure activities have also been associated with a higher perceived quality of life, increased self-esteem, and reduction in anger, confusion, fatigue, and stress among individuals with SCI (Clayton and Chubon 1994, Mulligan et al 2012).

Participation in leisure and recreational activities

With advancements in assistive technology and better awareness of disability, the variety of sports and leisure activities available for children with physical disabilities such as SCI have increased tremendously, for both individual and team activities (King et al 2002, Cooper 2012). These advancements have also led to the development of many national and international sporting events such as the Paralympics. Despite these advancements, however, participation rates have failed to increase, indicating that we have a long road ahead. Rimmer and colleagues reported that 56% of adults with disabilities do not engage in any leisure time physical activity compared with 36% of adults without disabilities (Rimmer et al 2004). Moreover, the physical activity level of children with disabilities is 17% lower than that of children without disabilities (Rimmer 2008).

Multiple reasons may contribute to the low rates of participation. Martin Ginis et al (2012) classified barriers and facilitators to participation as interpersonal, systemic, and informational (Tables 26.1 and 26.2). Bult et al (2011) identified key factors affecting participation rates among young individuals with SCI, which included current health status, medical

TABLE 26.1
Barriers to physical activity for persons with spinal cord injury

Type	Barrier	Description
Intrapersonal	Physical health factors	Autonomic dysreflexia, thermal dysregulation, circulatory dysregulation, musculoskeletal injury, recurring infections
	Psychological factors	Depression, lack of motivation, lack of energy, lack of time, lack of activity skills, lack of interest, lack of self-confidence, fear of pain and injury, fear of failure, fear of embarrassment, fear of conspicuous or unfriendly exercise environments, worry concerning physical limitations, perception of exercise as boring or too difficult, dislike of exercise
Systemic	Accessibility	Equipment (e.g. inadequate transfer space, difficulty operating equipment independently), facilities (e.g. small space, heavy doors), outdoor environment (e.g. steep or uneven terrain, lack of sidewalks, poorly maintained sidewalks, lack of curb cuts, inclement weather, neighborhood crime rate), limited accessible transportation
	Financial cost	High cost of transportation, programs, equipment, and membership
Informational	Lack of knowledge	Development of an exercise program to meet guidelines about types of activities that are appropriate, execution of exercises, play of adapted sport
	Lack of awareness	Exercise program availability, adapted sport availability
	Experts	Failure of physicians to discuss physical activity, fitness professionals lack of spinal cord injury-specific physical activity knowledge

TABLE 26.2
Facilitators of physical activity for persons with spinal cord injury

Type	Facilitator	Description and/or examples
Intrapersonal	Action planning	Specifying where, when, and how to engage in physical activity
	Coping planning	Planning ways to manage anticipated barriers to physical activity to achieve goals
	Goal setting	Using SMART goals: specific, measurable, accomplishment oriented, realistic, time bound
	Seeking social support	Sources: physicians, health and fitness professionals, rehabilitation staff, team mates, family, friends, caregivers
Systemic	Advocacy and support organizations	Canadian Paraplegic Association, Spinal Cord Injury Action Canada, Swedish Sports Organization for the Disabled, Canadian Paralympic Committee, Swedish Paralympic Committee, NCHPAD, Canadian Wheelchair Sports Association, Christopher and Dana Reeve Foundation
	Physical activity counseling services	NCHPAD, Get in Motion
	Building codes	Establish and enforce policies to reduce accessibility issues
	Subsidized fitness memberships	Adjust costs for individuals with disabilities based upon limited access to certain facilities
Informational	Evidence-based resources	Manuals, videos, guides, websites (http://nchpad.org/; http://sciactioncanada.ca)
	Awareness of local resources	Alternatives to gyms or health clubs: shopping malls or outdoor tracks
	Experts	Clinicians talk to patients about physical activity; health and fitness professionals trained to provide exercise assistance and resources to people with spinal cord injury

NCHPAD, National Center on Health, Physical Activity and Disability.

complications and comorbidities, personal factors (e.g. age and sex), and environmental factors (e.g. attending school and continued rehabilitation services). Furthermore, Klaas et al (2010) identified that higher caregiver education was associated with increased participation in more organized leisure activities.

A team approach

The multitude of barriers and facilitators to participation highlights the necessity for an interprofessional approach to improving participation among individuals with SCI. The transition from the rehabilitation setting to the community is an elaborate process involving the child or young adult, healthcare provider, therapists, family, and friends, as well as the community (King et al 2002). This section describes the roles of several members of the rehabilitation team in identifying and adapting the needs of the child to promote better participation in leisure and recreational activities. The process begins with identifying the activity in which the child with SCI would like to participate, followed by an evaluation with a recreational therapist.

Recreational Therapist

The recreational therapist conducts a thorough clinical evaluation to identify the needs of the child or young adult. The clinical assessment should include appraisals and examinations of cognitive, motor, sensory, and other perceptual functional factors to determine the exact needs of the individual (King et al 2002). Based on the assessment, a rational approach should be established early in the rehabilitation process; afterwards, continued follow-up visits should occur periodically, ranging from 6 months to 1 year depending upon the growth needs of the child. It is essential that the therapist assumes the role of facilitator, while the child with SCI participates independently. Furthermore, it is of utmost importance that family and friends are involved early in the process to facilitate maximum participation by the child.

Family and Friends

Social support from important people in the child's life may be a significant factor in determining adjustment to SCI. McGowan and Roth (1987) found that individuals with SCI who perceive the family environment as affectionately responsive, open in communication, and clear in delineation of responsibility demonstrated greater self-initiation in activities, increased social involvement, and higher overall levels of independence. Pachalski and Pachalska (1984) also indicated that children whose families have been involved in rehabilitation described their adaptation to society as 'good' or 'very good'. These children had increased feelings of positive self-worth, decreased feelings of guilt and fear, and increased participation in recreation and leisure activities. In combination, these studies show the positive effects that family participation in recreation has on the rehabilitation process.

Community and Legislation

Community support in terms of support groups and peer support plays a crucial role in assisting children with SCI to participate in recreational and leisure time activities. Although there are a number of organizations and associations that are geared toward providing community support for individuals with SCI (Table 26.3), community integration begins during initial rehabilitation. For example, trips outside of the hospital setting are an initial and crucial step in community integration. Such excursions prevent the child from developing facility-specific skills, which may or may not transfer to their community or home environment upon discharge, and promote confidence building and problem-solving skills concerning overcoming environmental barriers (Johnson and Klaas 2000).

As mentioned previously, multiple physical and environmental factors may serve as potential barriers to participation. Extensive study among researchers and policy makers is being done to address barriers and promote better participation among individuals with disabilities. The relative inactivity among children and young adults with disabilities makes clear the need for public policy that addresses adaptive sports for these individuals. Although the topic of adaptive sports for children with disabilities is not explicitly addressed in federal public policy in the USA, equality of access to sports for children with disabilities (e.g. SCI) is broadly addressed in federal civil rights, rehabilitation, and education legislation.

The Americans with Disabilities Act (ADA) of 1990, the Individuals with Disabilities Education Act of 2004, and Section 504 of the Rehabilitation Act of 1973 protect rights of

TABLE 26.3
Examples of organizations promoting sports for individuals with disabilities

Organization	Website
Blaze Sports America	www.blazesports.org
British Wheelchair Athletic Association	www.bwaa.co.uk
British Wheelchair Racing Association	www.bwra.co.uk
Disability Sports Australia	www.sports.org.au
Disabled Sports USA	www.dsusa.org
English Federation of Disability Sport	www.efds.co.uk
International Sports Federation for Para-athletes with an Intellectual Disability	www.inas.org
International Paralympic Committee	www.paralympic.org
International Wheelchair and Amputee Sports Federation	www.iwasf.com
International Wheelchair Basketball Federation	www.iwbf.org
International Wheelchair Rugby Federation	www.iwrf.com
National Ability Center	www.discovernac.org
National Center on Health, Physical Activity and Disability	www.nchpad.org
Special Olympics Great Britain	www.specialolympicsgb.org.uk
Special Olympics International	www.specialolympics.org
WheelPower	www.wheelpower.org.uk
Wheelchair and Ambulatory Sports USA	www.wsusa.org
Wheelchair Sports WA	www.wheelchairsportswa.org.au

equal access and educational participation of students with disabilities and provide safeguards that ensure their participation in school athletics (see Chapter 23). Both the ADA and Section 504 of the Rehabilitation Act prohibit discrimination based on disability and require that public schools ensure that students with disabilities have equal access to all school programs and activities. The Individuals with Disabilities Education Act requires states and schools to guarantee that, within a school setting, children with and without disabilities have the same access to physical education and other extracurricular activities (US Department of Education 2011). Therefore, some students with disabilities may have individual education plans that outline specific physical education instructional strategies to facilitate this equality of opportunity.

Starting in 1999, the National Center on Physical Activity and Disability (NCPAD), funded by the US Centers for Disease Control and Prevention, was created and charged with addressing access concerns related to recreation. Additionally, in 2002, the US Access Board – under the purview of the National Center on Accessibility – issued guidelines for recreation facilities under the ADA and addressed the activities of amusement park rides, golf and miniature golf, boating, fishing, and community sporting facilities. Just before the National Center's guidance, the US Access Board offered a set of similar guidelines for recreational and sporting facilities starting in 2000 under the banner of ADA accessibility guidelines for play areas.

Although the three aforementioned pieces of federal policy provide broad access protection, they are relatively silent on the topic of specific adaptation in sports for children with disabilities. Federal legislation on assistive technology (i.e. the Assistive Technology Act of 1988, PL 100–407, and the 1994 reauthorization of the Assistive Technology Act, PL 103–218), however, paved the way in a non-specific manner for assistive technology applications to be used to benefit children with disabilities in all arenas (Lewis et al 2012). So, by extension (although indirectly), the federal policy on assistive technology comes close to addressing adaptation in sports for children with disabilities.

Recreational pursuits

Most sporting and recreational activities can be adapted for children with SCI; however, not all of them have received research attention. This section describes a few of the more common recreational sports and activities.

Wheelchair Sports

Wheelchair sports are among the most popular of the adaptive sports. There are a number of options ranging from team sports such as wheelchair rugby, wheelchair basketball, wheelchair softball, wheelchair soccer, wheelchair power lifting, and wheelchair billiards to field events such as shot put, discus, and javelin, as well as track events such as wheelchair racing. Most of these sports require very specific adaptive equipment based on the needs of the child with SCI.

Wheelchair racing is a track sport and road races vary including 100m, 200m, and 400m; middle distances of 800m and 1500m; long distances of 5000m and 10 000m; and relay races of 4 × 100m and 4 × 400m. A number of marathons have adopted the wheelchair marathon as a mainstream event. Participants compete in specialized wheelchairs that allow them to reach speeds of up to 30km/hour.

In wheelchair rugby, two opposing teams play with four players from each team on the court at any time. Played indoors on a hardwood court with the same measurements as a basketball court, wheelchair rugby has rules adopted from and similar to basketball, ice hockey, and handball. Players use custom-made sports wheelchairs specifically designed for wheelchair rugby. Key features of the chair include a front bumper designed to help strike and hold an opposing player, and wings that are positioned in front of the main wheels to make the wheelchair more difficult to stop and hold. All wheelchairs are equipped with spoke protectors (to prevent damage to the wheels) and anti-tip devices.

Wheelchair basketball retains most of the major rules and the scoring system of basketball, along with a 10-foot basketball hoop and standard basketball court. The exceptions are the rules which have been modified for a wheelchair user. Similar to wheelchair rugby, wheelchair basketball requires a specific adaptive chair that is lightweight, with a footplate in the protection bar in the front.

In addition to wheelchair sports, hand cycling and watersports such as rowing, kayaking, sailing, waterskiing, and scuba diving are alternatives available for children with SCI interested in outdoor activities.

Snow Sports

Adaptive skiing can be an exciting and inspiring experience for adults and children with SCI. With proper equipment, training, and assistance, adaptive skiers can enjoy the downhill speeds of alpine skiing or the peaceful scenes experienced during Nordic skiing. Specific training and equipment, such as monoskis, bi-skis, and sit skis, are required to master the skill for independent skiing. Skiers with good upper extremity strength use outriggers, an adaptive version of forearm crutches with hinged mini skis attached at their bottom for balance and steering. Alpine sit skis have a molded fiberglass bucket-shaped seat attached on a frame over a ski or skis (Fig. 26.1). The skier's legs extend in the front, supported on the footrests. Sit skis are usually built with a shock absorber linking the frame and skis, and some are equipped with self-loading mechanisms to quickly change to a 'lift' position, which enables the skier to use a regular lift.

Nordic skiing is beginner-friendly and allows individuals with less trunk and limb control to enjoy the activity. A bucket seat is installed on a rigid frame with a pair of skis, which are narrower and longer than alpine skis. Compared with alpine skiing, Nordic skiing is less complicated owing to simpler equipment, gentler terrain, and no involvement of chair lifts. Individuals with good upper extremity strength can propel with fixed outriggers. Besides recreation, the propeling movement during Nordic skiing facilitates the activation of shoulder stabilization muscles and lower back muscles, which are very different from the muscles used to propel a manual wheelchair. This sport may help with the muscle strength of manual wheelchair users, helping to combat the effects from daily wheelchair propulsion (Nasuti and Temple 2010).

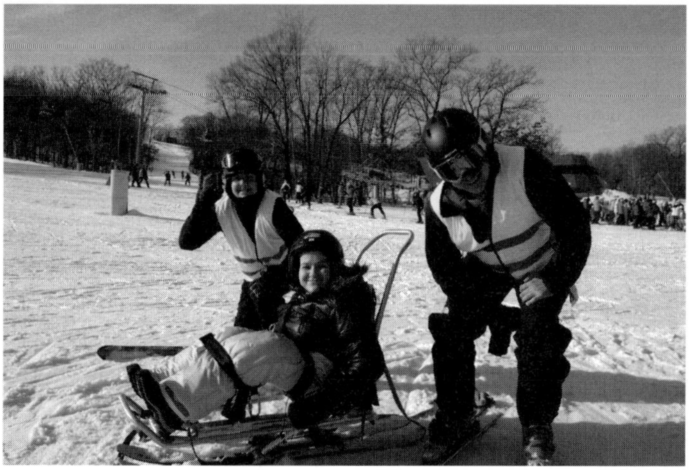

Fig. 26.1 Alpine sit skis with a molded bucket-shaped seat.

Exergaming

Video game playing, television watching, and computer use have been linked to sedentary behavior in all children and adolescents (Antle et al 2008). Screen time has the potential to decrease participation in sport, recreational activities, and physical activities, as well as increase social isolation (Dorman 1997). When used appropriately, however, exergaming (i.e. games which use technology that tracks body movement, e.g. cycling games) is a unique tool combining the motivational qualities of video game playing with physical activity. For children with SCI who may not be able to participate in standard forms of therapeutic or home exercise, exergaming may be an option to increase physical activity. Although not a replacement for physical or occupational therapy, many rehabilitation centers, schools, and out-patient physical therapy offices are incorporating exergaming as an adjunct to therapeutic or adaptive exercise. For example, children receiving home-based physical therapy may participate in a therapeutic exergaming regimen that can be carried out with family or friends. With the risks in mind, exergaming can enhance motivation and cooperation in therapeutic activities as well as physical activity participation. A watchful and wise choice of equipment with the right kind of game can make exergaming an excellent leisure activity.

Summary

There are several varieties of sports and recreational activities to support adequate play and aid in the growth and development of a child with SCI. With early facilitation, adequate training with the use of appropriate assistive and adaptive equipment can improve the health and quality of life of children with SCI.

REFERENCES

Antle B, Mills W, Steele C, Kalnins I, Rossen B (2008) An exploratory study of parents' approaches to health promotion in families of adolescents with physical disabilities. *Child Care Health Dev* 34: 185–93. doi: 10.1111/j.1365-2214.2007.00782.x

Brenes G, Dearwater S, Shapera R, LaPorte RE, Collins E (1986) High density lipoprotein cholesterol concentrations in physically active and sedentary spinal cord injured patients. *Arch Phys Med Rehabil* 67: 445–50.

Bult M, Verschuren O, Jongmans M, Lindeman E, Ketelaar M (2011) What influences participation in leisure activities of children and youth with physical disabilities? A systemic review. *Res Dev Disabil* 32: 1521–9. doi: 10.1016/j.ridd.201101.045

Clayton KS, Chubon RA (1994) Factors associated with the quality of life of long-term spinal cord injured persons. *Arch Phys Med Rehabil* 75: 633–8. http://dx.doi.org/10.1016/0003-9993(94)90184-8

Cooper RA (2012) Wheelchair research progress, perspectives, and transformation. *J Rehabil Res Dev* 49: 1–5. http://dx.doi.org/10.1682/JRRD.2011.10.0199

Dallmeijer AJ, van der Woude LH, van Kamp GJ, Hollander AP (1999) Changes in lipid, lipoprotein and apolipoprotein profiles in persons with spinal cord injuries during the first 2 years post-injury. *Spinal Cord* 37: 96–102. http://dx.doi.org/10.1038/sj.sc.3100776

Dorman S (1997) Video and computer games: effect on children and implications for health education. *J Sch Health* 67: 133–8. http://dx.doi.org/10.1111/j.1746-1561.1997.tb03432.x

Fernhall B, Heffernan K, Jae SY, Hedrick B (2008) Health implications of physical activity in individuals with spinal cord injury: a literature review. *J Health Hum Serv Adm* 30: 468–502.

Gorter JW (2009) Transition to adult-oriented health care: perspectives of youth and adults with complex physical disabilities. *Phys Occup Ther Pediatr* 29: 362–6. doi: 10.3109/01942630903222100

Ittenbach RF, Bruininks RH, Thurlow ML, McGrew KS (1993) Community integration of young adults with mental retardation: a multivariate analysis of adjustment. *Res Dev Disabil* 14: 275–90. http://dx.doi.org/10.1016/0891-4222(93)90022-C

Jacobs P (2009) Effects of resistance and endurance training in persons with paraplegia. *Med Sci Sports Exerc* 41: 992–7. doi: 10.1249/MSS.0b013e318191757f

Johnson K, Klaas S (2000) Recreation involvement and play in pediatric spinal cord injury. *Top Spinal Cord Inj Rehabil* 6: 105–9. doi: 10.1310/F7XL-F11-JU26-GFTK

Kehn M, Kroll T (2009) Staying physically active after spinal cord injury: a qualitative exploration of barriers and facilitators to exercise participation. *BMC Public Health* 9: 168. doi:10.1186/1471-2458-9-168

King G, Tucker M, Baldwin P, Lowry K, LaPorta J, Martens L (2002) A life needs model of pediatric service delivery: services to support community participation and quality of life for children and youth with disabilities. *Phys Occup Ther Pediatr* 22: 53–77.

Klaas S, Kelly E, Gorzkowski J, Homko E, Vogel C (2010) Assessing patterns of participation and enjoyment in children with spinal cord injury. *Dev Med Child Neurol* 52: 468–74. doi: 10.1111/j.1469-8749.2009.03552.x

Lewis A, Cooper R, Seelman K, Cooper R, Schein R (2012) Assistive technology in rehabilitation: improving impact through policy. *Rehabil Res Policy Educ* 26: 19–32. http://dx.doi.org/10.1891/216866512805000901

McGowan M, Roth S (1987) Family functioning and functional independence in spinal cord injury adjustment. *Paraplegia* 24: 357–65. http://dx.doi.org/10.1038/sc.1987.64

Martin Ginis K, Jörgensen S, Stapleton J (2012) Exercise and sport for persons with spinal cord injury. *PM R* 4: 894–900. doi: 10.1016/j.pmrj.2012.08.006

Mulligan H, Whitehead L, Hale L, Baxter G, Thomas D (2012) Promoting physical activity for individuals with neurological disability: indications for practice. *Disabil Rehabil* 34: 1108–13. doi: 10.3109/09638288.2011.631683

Muraki S, Tsunawake N, Hiramatsu S, Yamasaki M (2000) The effect of frequency and mode of sports activity on the psychological status in tetraplegics and paraplegics. *Spinal Cord* 38: 309–14. http://dx.doi.org/10.1038/sj.sc.3101002

Nash MS (2005) Exercise as a health-promoting activity following spinal cord injury. *J Neurol Phys Ther* 29: 87–103, 106. http://dx.doi.org/10.1097/01.NPT.0000282514.94093.c6

Nasuti G, Temple V (2010) The risks and benefits of snow sports for people with disabilities: a review of the literature. *Int J Rehabil Res* 33: 193–8. doi: 10.1097/MRR.0b013e32833638a5

Pachalski A, Pachalska MM (1984) Programme of active education in the psycho-social integration of paraplegics. *Paraplegia* 22: 238–43. doi:10.1038/sc.1984.40

Rimmer J (2008) Promoting inclusive physical activity communities for people with disabilities. *Pres Counc Phys Fit Sports Res Dig* 9: 1–8.

Rimmer J, Riley B, Wang E, Rauworth A, Jurkowski J (2004) Physical activity participation among persons with disabilities: barriers and facilitators. *Am J Prev Med* 26: 419–25. http://dx.doi.org/10.1016/j.amepre.2004.02.002

Shikako-Thomas K, Shevell M, Lach L et al; QUALA group (2013) Picture me playing-a portrait of participation and enjoyment of leisure activities in adolescents with cerebral palsy. *Res Dev Disabil* 34: 1001–10. doi: 10.1016/j.ridd.2012.11.026

Slater D, Meade M (2004) Participation in recreation and sports for persons with spinal cord injury: review and recommendations. *NeuroRehabilitation* 19: 121–9.

US Department of Education (2011) *Creating Equal Opportunities for Children and Youth with Disabilities to Participate in Physical Education and Extracurricular Athletics*. Washington, DC: Office of Special Education and Rehabilitative Services, Office of Special Education Programs.

Van Naarden Braun K, Yeargin-Allsopp M, Lollar D (2006) Factors associated with leisure activity among young adults with developmental disabilities. *Res Dev Disabil* 27: 567–83. http://dx.doi.org/10.1016/j.ridd.2005.05.008

Vargus-Adams J, Martin L (2011) Domains of importance for parents, medical professionals and youth with cerebral palsy considering treatment outcomes. *Child Care Health Dev* 37: 276–81. doi: 10.1111/j.1365-2214.2010.01121.x

Zebracki K, Anderson A, Chlan K, Vogel L (2010) Outcomes of adults with pediatric-onset spinal cord injury: longitudinal findings and implications on transition to adulthood. *Top Spinal Cord Inj Rehabil* 16: 17–25. doi: 10.1310/sci1601-17

Section 8 Research Priorities and Future Directions

27
BIOLOGICAL INTERVENTIONS AND CLINICAL TRIALS

George Ghobrial and James S Harrop

Introduction

The loss of neurologic function after traumatic spinal cord injury (SCI) is believed to be the product of several processes, which have been categorized into two broad groups. The first is the primary mechanical insult or traumatic injury owing to the mechanical compression of the spinal cord. The second is the biomechanical response that initiates at the site of injury in an anterograde and a retrograde fashion. This secondary mechanism of injury is believed to be the result of several processes. These include demyelination from apoptosis of the oligodendrocytes, changes in chemical gradients, hypoperfusion, excitatory apoptosis, and inflammatory responses, all of which further aggravate damage. Historically, many of the goals of treatment of SCI have focused on the utilization of pharmacologic therapies to try to limit secondary injury. In the future, with targeted cellular-based therapies, the treatment armamentarium will expand to include agents that replace absent cellular architecture in the post-injury state, restore the neural relay, or provide neuroprotection in the post-injury environment. Advances in the development of cellular stocks with committed glial and neural lineages are in the developmental phase for the replacement of lost neurons, astrocytes, and oligodendrocytes, and the repair of the disrupted axonal circuitry. Currently, the state of basic scientific research in this field holds promise for future treatments; however, the lack of medical and surgical systematic universal treatment processes and limited grading or outcome measures has hampered these efforts. Despite these limitations, there are several compounds that appear to show promise at the cellular level or in small animal traumatic SCI models in various aspects. A systematic approach to generating results that translate these promising preliminary or bench experiments to human trials is required. Unfortunately, one difficulty with basic scientific research is that, in clinical scenarios, the patients typically do not have the opportunity to receive medication before the injury, as in most patients they are spontaneous traumatic occurrences.

Potential clinical therapies need to show persistent prolonged benefits. The North American Clinical Trials Consortium has proposed a benchmark of 3 months after injury for a compound to demonstrate therapeutic benefit before it should be considered clinically relevant (Grossman et al 2012). Potential translational therapies should be reproducible across multiple injury models and between experimental models to account for the tremendous variability in forces and mechanisms of traumatic SCI.

Finally, any potential clinical therapy must demonstrate safety at clinically relevant doses. Another formidable barrier to translational clinical trials at present is the exceptional cost of performing a phase I study (Geisler 1998). Therefore, several investigators have utilized the transition of Food and Drug Administration (FDA)-approved medication for 'off-label' use in traumatic SCI trials.

Acute steroid administration in spinal cord injury

The acute use of steroids as a means for neuroprotection in SCI is surrounded by controversy, and even more so in the pediatric population, which lacks level I evidence to support its use. Indeed, all level I evidence is encountered in the adult population. The use of methylprednisolone for SCI first gained attention in 1984 in the results from the first National Acute Spinal Cord Injury Study (NASCIS) in a multicenter, randomized double-blind clinical trial evaluating the dose–response relationship of methylprednisolone (Bracken et al 1984). No clinical benefit was found with the use of methylprednisolone. It was not until 1990 that interest began to mount, when the second NASCIS comparing methylprednisolone with placebo found a slight benefit at 6 months after injury with fine touch and pinprick modalities (Bracken et al 1990). However, that benefit was lost at 1 year after injury. More attention was brought to NASCIS II in a post-hoc analysis that found a slight motor benefit at 1 year after injury (Bracken et al 1992). NASCIS III also did not find a statistical difference in outcomes. All three studies report the significantly higher rates of pneumonia, sepsis, and pulmonary embolism encountered in the methylprednisolone arm. A 2013 joint statement by the American Association of Neurological Surgeons and the Congress of Neurological Surgeons found insufficient evidence for its use, in lieu of the complication risks (Walters et al 2013). The suggestion of a benefit in tandem with medicolegal implications of not administering this drug has led to the practice of methylprednisolone use per NASCIS II protocol. One additional issue raised is the question of the benefit in a younger population, given the lack of level I evidence in this age group.

Non-steroidal anti-inflammatory drugs

Non-steroidal anti-inflammatory drugs (NSAIDs) have long been investigated for their potential role in reducing the inflammatory cascade that is prominent in secondary injury after traumatic SCI. Several preclinical or animal studies detailing their use have been reported (Kwon et al 2011). Unfortunately, the information is limited in clinical trials, since the majority of these studies used a pre-injury dosage protocol, such as medication being started before the injury, or medication given at or before the onset of the SCI.

More recent studies have tested ibuprofen as a treatment agent. Wang et al (2009) showed a statistically significant improvement in blood–brain barrier scores in a rat model of SCI at 7 weeks after injury after dosing the injured rats with continuous infusions of ibuprofen for 28 days. These results were significantly greater than both a saline control and a naproxen treatment group. In a second study, histologic examination demonstrated suppression of RhoA injury-induced activation. Histologic samples showed enhanced corticospinal and serotonergic sprouting caudal to the injury (Fu et al 2007).

Erythropoietin

Erythropoietin (EPO) is an endogenous glycoprotein hormone produced by interstitial fibroblasts in the renal parenchyma and whose activity regulates red blood cell production. This compound has also been well studied in neurologic injury models. Unfortunately, and similar to what is seen in the literature on NSAIDs, these studies are difficult to interpret and move into the clinical arena.

Histologically, EPO appears to have multiple mechanisms of action in the central nervous system, including both white and gray matter sparing, reduced apoptosis, and decreased inflammatory cytokine release. In two studies, there were statistically significant increases in measures of locomotion in rats treated with EPO at 30 to 60 minutes after injury with improvement consistent at 14 days and 6 weeks after injury (Gorio et al 2002, Boran et al 2005). Notably, these improvements were more apparent at lower doses of EPO. However, two more recent trials did not validate those histologic improvements with statistically significant improvement in motor function (Mann et al 2008, Pinzon et al 2008).

Glyburide

Glyburide is a sulfonylurea drug, known outside the USA as glibenclamide, typically used in the treatment of type 2 diabetes. It acts to inhibit sulfonylurea receptor 1 (SUR1), an adenosine triphosphate (ATP)-sensitive cation channel, causing a membrane depolarization which opens voltage gated calcium channels, allowing intracellular calcium to rise. This channel is transcriptionally upregulated in astrocytes after ischemic insult and becomes active when intracellular ATP is depleted, resulting in cytotoxic edema and cell death. Blockage of this channel mitigates these effects in vitro and a human study showed that the use of sulfonylureas in diabetics hospitalized with stroke was associated with better outcomes (Simard et al 2007).

There is a rapidly expanding understanding of the mechanism of action of glyburide, particularly with neurologic injuries. Simard and colleagues demonstrated that the use of glyburide treatment after traumatic SCI in a rodent model decreased intracord hemorrhage when measured by multiple assays compared with a vehicle control. Animals were tested at 1 and 7 days after injury and, in both cases, there was approximately a threefold decrease in lesion size in the sulfonylurea-treated animals.

Objective functional outcome measurements performed in this rodent population included spontaneous rearing, inclined plane scores, ipsilateral paw placement, and blood–brain barrier scores. In each case, the animals treated with glyburide demonstrated statistically significant improvements at 7 days and 6 weeks after injury ($p<0.05$). Human investigation with glyburide has not entered the investigational phase at this point.

Magnesium sulfate

Treatment with magnesium sulfate is currently FDA approved for the treatment of tetany in hypomagnesemia, as well as for pre-eclampsia and eclampsia in pregnant women. The neuroprotective mechanisms of magnesium are believed to be based on the ability of the chemical to disrupt the apoptotic process. In vitro studies demonstrate its blockade of intracellular calcium release via the *N*-methyl-D-aspartate receptor, as well as caspase-3 activity: an important step in the IP-3 messenger system that leads to membrane instability and ultimately apoptosis (Lee et al 2004). The administration of magnesium with a polyethylene glycol (PEG) formulation had a synergistic effect. PEG has been shown to stabilize cell membranes by fusion and sealing of cell membranes, restoring ion permeability, and enhancing compound action potentials (Kwon et al 2009).

Magnesium sulfate works against apoptosis with an interaction of the caspase-3 system, as shown by Solaroglu et al (2005). A single dose (600mg/kg) was given via the intraperitoneal route to rodents immediately after a weight drop spinal cord contusion, and histology was performed at 24 hours with a significant reduction in caspase-3 activity ($p<0.05$)

Recent studies have further demonstrated histologic efficacy in this PEG/magnesium formulation. Kaptanoglu et al (2003a) noted that a 600mg/kg intraperitoneal dose of magnesium sulfate given to rodents with acute traumatic SCI at the time of injury resulted in subcellular changes similar to the no-injury control group, and significantly better funcitonal outcomes with respect to saline-treated controls. Similarly, a larger study by Ditor et al (2007) also found statistically significantly smaller lesions after treatment with magnesium sulfate and PEG. However, a smaller rodent study by Wiseman et al (2009) reported no differences in lesion size 24 hours after acute traumatic SCI and administration of magnesium sulfate. This group also reported improved white matter sparing when they tested magnesium sulfate with and without concurrent methylprednisolone therapy (30.3% and 42.3%, respectively; $p<0.05$) when measured 10 minutes after injury, a finding confirmed by the Ditor group.

Kwon et al (2009) sought to reproduce and validate the Ditor study with a different injury mechanism. These authors reported that, at 6 weeks after acute contusion-based SCI by a 150kdyn impactor, the lesion size in the magnesium-treated group was reduced by 33% compared with the saline vehicle alone ($p=0.0139$) (Kwon et al 2009). It should be noted that the Kwon and Ditor studies both utilized a PEG and magnesium formulation that allowed a lower magnesium dose, which reportedly is tolerable in humans. The addition of PEG appears to have a synergistic effect with the magnesium so that, combined, there was a reduction of the traumatic SCI histology lesion volume by greater than 51% ($p<0.05$) (Kwon et al 2009).

Despite the improvements of histologic findings, these results did not uniformly translate into improved functional outcomes. Kwon reported that the addition of PEG to magnesium was necessary for significant improvements in motor scores; however, the Ditor study noted that PEG was not necessary for significant ambulatory results. Kaptanoglu et al (2003b) reported improved locomotion when magnesium sulfate alone was dependent on the time of delivery. Rodents that received magnesium in the early group, within 8 hours, had improved recovery after SCI compared with the 10- or 12-hour groups. The use of PEGylated magnesium in acute SCI entered its enrollment phase in 2014.

Minocycline

Minocycline is a broad-spectrum, second-generation tetracycline antibiotic medication primarily used for the treatment of skin infections, such as acne. It has been extensively examined as a neuroprotective agent because of its anti-inflammatory properties. Its ability to reduce neurologic injury is believed to be a result of the numerous interactions which impede the secondary injury cascade, including inhibition of caspase-1 and caspase-3 in the apoptosis pathway, inhibition of nitric oxide production, cyclooxygenase 2, and prostaglandin E_2 expression, reduction in microglia and macrophage activation, decrease in cytochrome c release, and decreased T-lymphocyte transmigration.

Studies on the effectiveness of minocycline as a neuroprotective agent for traumatic SCI vary markedly in methodology and dosing parameters. Festoff et al (2006) tracked hind limb motor function after injuring rodents with a controlled weight drop spinal cord contusion model and subsequently dosing them with minocycline versus tetracycline, an earlier generation medication in the tetracycline class. The minocycline-treated rats demonstrated a statistically significant improvement in functional outcome compared with control animals. Furthermore, histologic samples demonstrated a reduced number of apoptotic cells in the lesioned portion of the spinal cord, as well as those in adjacent segments when minocycline was utilized. Specifically, there was a decrease in caspase-3 expression compared with the control (53%, $p<0.04$) and this was further confirmed by measurement using reverse transcription polymerase chain reaction and of caspase-cleaved proteins. There was also a significant decrease in the microglial activation at the sites of injury, linked to a decrease in TNF-α, the inciting cytokine.

Stirling et al (2004) reported the effects of minocycline in a cervical dorsal columns transection rodent model compared with saline control treatments. The minocycline treatment over 48 hours after SCI significantly reduced the number of apoptotic oligodendrocytes by 37% distally and 47% proximally 14 days after injury, which correlated with the finding of statistically significantly improved lesion size ($p<0.01$). However, functional outcome at 14 days was mixed: some parameters improved, whereas others remained unaffected relative to the saline-treated group. Two recent studies by Saganova et al (2008) and Pinzon et al (2008), despite showing histologic improvements, illustrated no benefit in functional outcomes. A phase I study was performed in Canada, which illustrated no clinical benefit in the complete SCI populations, but there was a suggestion of a potential improvement in the patients with incomplete cervical SCI (Casha et al 2012). Owing to the encouraging initial clinical trial, a larger multicenter trial is being organized.

Progesterone

Progesterone is a female steroid hormone that effects and supports the menstrual cycle, pregnancy, gestation, and embryogenesis. However, several studies have shown its effect on the central nervous system, as a neurosteroid, acting through the GSK-β pathway and promoting myelination. As a pharmacologic agent for acute traumatic SCI, progesterone has been investigated in rodent sharp injury and contusion models. However, quantitative measures of success are lacking and no data were collected on long-term functional outcomes. The two contusion models had contradictory results, despite similar methodologies. Fee at al (2007) reported no histologic improvement in lesion sizes for progesterone-treated rodents (4–16mg/kg from 0.5–120h after injury). However, an earlier study by Thomas and colleagues reported significant histologically and functionally improvement at 6 weeks (Thomas et al 1999). For these reasons, progesterone has not gained favor for human clinical experimentation.

Estrogen

Estrogen is another female steroid hormone that effects and supports the menstrual cycle, pregnancy, gestation, and embryogenesis, which has been recently studied for its potential role in ameliorating traumatic SCI. However, of the eight studies involving estrogen and traumatic SCI, only one gave the estrogen after the traumatic injury occurred. All remaining studies preloaded the experimental rodents before the experimental SCI, limiting the usefulness of this experimentation in real-world applications. All the studies that noted behavioral results demonstrated stable or improved performance with estrogen treatment (Kwon et al 2011).

Nimodipine

Nimodipine is a dihydropyridine calcium-channel blocker that was originally developed as an antihypertensive agent. In the cardiovascular system, it decreases afterload through vasodilation of the arterial system. In the central nervous system, it has a particularly specific vasodilatory effect on the vessels by a mechanism that is not fully understood. Presently, this medication is widely employed in the prevention of vasospasm after subarachnoid hemorrhage.

The proposed nimodipine mechanism of action is through the prevention of excessive entry of calcium ions into cells and apoptosis, in addition to increasing post-traumatic spinal cord blood flow. Early studies focused on quantifying the potential for systemic hypotension induced by nimodipine. The literature is inconclusive on this topic, as most studies found that mean arterial pressures in nimodipine- and saline-treated animals were statistically similar (Pointillart et al 1993), but one study noted a transient but statistically significant decrease in mean arterial pressures at 60 minutes after administration (Guha et al 1987). In a similar trend, spinal cord blood flow was found to be similar between nimodipine- and saline-treated groups in most studies, with few exceptions. Pointillart and colleagues, in a large primate model, treated baboons over 8 days with nimodipine after acute traumatic SCI, and found increased spinal cord perfusion compared with the control group. The same study showed significant improvements in lesion length in both white and gray matter tracts (Pointillart et al 1993).

In the assessments of motor and neurologic recovery, studies are similarly mixed. Although there were some promising findings of motor improvement, none of the objective measurements of motor function demonstrated any statistically significant benefits of treatment with nimodipine. Nimodipine was tested in a 100-patient trial in 1996 with a 1-year follow-up. This study did not find a statistically significant neurologic benefit compared with a control group (Petitjean et al 1998), although proponents argue that the study was underpowered (Baptiste and Fehlings 2006).

Riluzole

Riluzole is an antagonist of the tetrodotoxin voltage-sensitive sodium channel, and it acts to reduce intracellular calcium and, secondarily, to prevent stimulation of glutamate receptors. It is currently used in the treatment of amyotrophic lateral sclerosis where it has been shown to prolong survival. Presently, eight studies have evaluated riluzole in a variety of animal models. As with other compounds, results and outcomes with riluzole vary widely, as dose timing and regimens were not standardized in these studies. Efficacy for neurologic recovery was found with doses of 5 to 8mg/kg and higher doses resulted in ataxia and lethargy.

Several studies have reported that riluzole significantly reduces lesion size and preserves greater numbers of neurons when administered after traumatic SCI in rodents compared with saline controls ($p<0.05$). Schwartz and Fehlings (2001), in a rodent histopathologic analysis, noted a significant increase in neuron cell quantity, volume, and axonal diameter in the riluzole treatment group at 7 weeks after injury. Nogradi and Vrbova (2001) further demonstrated that the numbers of all neurons and cholinergic cells were improved in the post-injury riluzole groups. This preservation effect was time dependent, as earlier treatment groups that were treated at days 5 and 10 after injury showed a greater effect than those treated at days 14 or 16.

The demonstrated effects of riluzole on other indicators of inflammation and oxidative stress were mixed. Various studies have found statistically significant decreases in lipid peroxidation levels, mitochondrial function, and glucose uptake compared with controls. Studies looking at glutamate uptake showed mixed results, with one study reporting a statistically significant reduction, while another reported that rates were unaffected. Several animal studies available in the literature have documented a delayed response in the improvement of motor scores or clinical function after treatment with riluzole. Across multiple studies, testing points at 2 hours to 3 weeks after injury showed no significant difference between control and riluzole-treated animals after SCI; however, studies by Schwartz and Fehlings (2001) and Nogradi and Vrbova (2001) demonstrated statistically significant improvements in multiple assessments of motor function, including blood–brain barrier scores, incline plane scores, and accelerating rotarod tests. This improved level of function was persistent in up to 3 months of testing. Other studies demonstrated statistically significant improvements in wrist dorsiflexion, and amplitude, duration, and latency of somatosensory evoked potentials in riluzole-treated rats. In some cases, recovery at 3 months closely approximated normal function.

Success with riluzole in human clinical trials was reported in phase I trials (Grossman et al 2014). Investigators administered 50mg by mouth or nasogastric tube twice a day for 14 days to patients predominantly with cervical American Spinal Injury Association impairment grades A–C SCI presenting within 12 hours, and a significant improvement was found. Although this study was designed for safety rather than efficacy, these early results are promising.

Targeted cellular-based therapies

Advances in both adult and embryonic stem cells, as well as various pathways of differentiation into neural stem cells, in recent decades have elevated the promise for future effective therapies in SCI, as they address the direct mechanical injury that results from trauma to the spinal cord. Perhaps these therapies, in conjunction with the proven success of pharmacologic treatments to limit secondary injury, may be combined into the most effective treatment strategy.

Administration of neural stem cells or neural progenitor cells that result from differentiation could simultaneously reconstitute the injured spinal cord architecture, reconnect spinal cord tracts, and promote plasticity; all three are needed to show improvement in locomotion.

Use of non-autologous cellular therapies requires high-dose immunosuppression, which arguably carries a considerable morbidity. Advances in induced pluripotent stem cell lines has allowed for the production of autologous neural lineages. However, current technology does not allow for this to be implemented in acute SCI.

The use of Schwann cells appears to be a logical means to this end, allowing for an autologous treatment for the restoration of axonal growth and remyelination. However, Schwann cells are limited, as they do not replace neural or glial lineages lost in the initial SCI. Schwann cells are typically harvested from a peripheral nerve that would confer limited morbidity, such as a sural or intercostal nerve. To date, limited case reports have experimented with delivery into the wound bed in the chronic injury environment of autologous Schwann cells (Saberi et al 2008). Guest and coinvestigators have realized the potential of this treatment, bringing this therapy from the bench to bedside, through an FDA-approved phase I safety study (Guest et al 2013).

Summary

Many compounds show promise to improve recovery in SCI when tested in the preclinical setting. Given the substantial expenditure of cost and effort required to translate a therapy from the preclinical setting to human use, some criteria are needed to identify the most promising therapies and promote their development in a systematic way. Initial studies are needed to demonstrate efficacy and mechanisms. Follow-up studies should attempt to identify therapeutic dosages and optimum times and methods of administration, while paying heed to the real-world conditions in which the treatment will be ultimately utilized.

Benefits should be persistent over weeks and should be demonstrated in a variety of animals and models to better mimic the variety of mechanisms present in trauma. Ideally, they should be validated repeatedly. To date, based on these criteria, among the many compounds being tested, five show particular promise, as identified by the North American Clinical Trials Consortium: glyburide, magnesium with and without the addition of polyethlene glycol, minocycline, nimodipine, and riluzole. Further testing is ongoing for all of these compounds.

Cellular therapies for SCI are in the earliest stages of investigation, and involve the implementation of neural stem cells and Schwann cells. With a growing number of FDA-registered clinical trials in 2014, it is expected that the efficacy of these therapies will be at the forefront of discussion.

REFERENCES

Baptiste DC, Fehlings MG (2006) Pharmacological approaches to repair the injured spinal cord. *J Neurotrauma* 23: 318–34. http://dx.doi.org/10.1089/neu.2006.23.318

Boran BO, Colak A, Kutlay M (2005) Erythropoietin enhances neurological recovery after experimental spinal cord injury. *Restor Neurol Neurosci* 23: 341–5.

Bracken M, Collins W, Freeman D et al (1984) Effects of methylprednisolone in acute spinal cord injury. *JAMA* 251: 45–52. doi:10.1001/jama.1984.03340250025015

Bracken M, Shepard M, Collins W et al (1990) A randomized, controlled trial of methylprednisolone or naloxone in the treatment of acute spinal-cord injury: results of the second National Acute Spinal Cord Injury Study. *N Engl J Med* 322: 1405–11. doi: 10.1056/NEJM199005173222001

Bracken M, Shepard M, Collins W et al (1992) Methylprednisolone or naloxone treatment after acute spinal cord injury: 1-year follow-up data. Results of the results of the second National Acute Spinal Cord Injury Study. *J Neurosurg* 76: 23–31. http://dx.doi.org/10.3171/jns.1992.76.1.0023

Casha S, Zygun D, McGowan MD, Bains I, Yong VW, Hurlbert RJ (2012) Results of a phase II placebo controlled randomized trial of minocycline in acute spinal cord injury. *Brain* 135: 1224–36. doi: 10.1093/brain/aws072

Ditor DS, John SM, Roy J, Marx JC, Kittmer C, Weaver LC (2007) Effects of polyethylene glycol and magnesium sulfate administration on clinically relevant neurological outcomes after spinal cord injury in the rat. *J Neurosci Res* 85: 1458–67. doi: 10.1002/jnr.21283

Fee D, Swartz K, Joy K, Roberts K, Scheff N, Scheff S (2007) Effects of progesterone on experimental spinal cord injury. *Brain Res* 1137: 146–52. http://dx.doi.org/10.1016/j.brainres.2006.12.024

Festoff BW, Ameenuddin S, Arnold PM, Wong A, Santacruz KS, Citron BA (2006) Minocycline neuroprotects, reduces microgliosis, and inhibits caspase protease expression early after spinal cord injury. *J Neurochem* 97: 1314–26. doi: 10.1111/j.1471-4159.2006.03799.x

Fu Q, Hue J, Li S (2007) Nonsteroidal anti-inflammatory drugs promote axon regeneration via RhoA inhibition. *J Neurosci* 27: 4154–64. doi: 10.1523/JNEUROSCI.4353-06.2007

Geisler FH (1998) Clinical trials of pharmacotherapy for spinal cord injury. *Ann N Y Acad Sci* 845: 374–81. doi: 10.1111/j.1749-6632.1998.tb09689.x

Gorio A, Gokmen N, Erbayraktar S et al (2002) Recombinant human erythropoietin counteracts secondary injury and markedly enhances neurological recovery from experimental spinal cord trauma. *Proc Natl Acad Sci USA* 99: 9450–5. doi: 10.1073/pnas.142287899

Grossman R, Toups E, Frankowski R, Burau K, Howley S (2012) North American Clinical Trials Network for the Treatment of Spinal Cord Injury: goals and progress. *J Neurosurg Spine* 17(Suppl 1): 6–10. doi: 10.3171/2012.4.AOSPINE1294

Grossman R, Fehlings M, Frankowski R et al (2014) A prospective, multicenter, phase I matched-comparison group trial of safety, pharmacokinetics, and preliminary efficacy of riluzole in patients with traumatic spinal cord injury. *J Neurotrauma* 31: 239–55. doi: 10.1089/neu.2013.2969

Guest J, Santamaria A, Benavides F (2013) Clinical translation of autologous Schwann cell transplantation for the treatment of spinal cord injury. *Curr Opin Organ Transplant* 18: 682–9. doi: 10.1097/MOT.0000000000000026

Guha A, Tator CH, Piper I (1987) Effect of a calcium channel blocker on posttraumatic spinal cord blood flow. *J Neurosurg* 66: 423–30. http://dx.doi.org/10.3171/jns.1987.66.3.0423

Kaptanoglu E, Beskonakli E, Okutan O, Selcuk Surucu H, Taskin Y (2003a) Effect of magnesium sulphate in experimental spinal cord injury: evaluation with ultrastructural findings and early clinical results. *J Clin Neurosci* 10: 329–34. doi: 10.1016/S0967-5868(03)00031-6

Kaptanoglu E, Beskonakli E, Solaroglu I, Kilinc A, Taskin Y (2003b) Magnesium sulfate treatment in experimental spinal cord injury: emphasis on vascular changes and early clinical results. *Neurosurg Rev* 26: 283–7. doi: 10.1007/s10143-003-0272-y

Kwon BK, Roy J, Lee JH et al (2009) Magnesium chloride in a polyethylene glycol formulation as a neuroprotective therapy for acute spinal cord injury: preclinical refinement and optimization. *J Neurotrauma* 26: 1379–93. doi: 10.1089/neu.2009.0884

Kwon BK, Okon E, Hillyer J et al (2011) A systematic review of non-invasive pharmacologic neuroprotective treatments for acute spinal cord injury. *J Neurotrauma* 28: 1545–88. doi: 10.1089/neu.2009.1149

Lee JS, Han YM, Yoo DS et al (2004) A molecular basis for the efficacy of magnesium treatment following traumatic brain injury in rats. *J Neurotrauma* 21: 549–61. doi: 10.1089/089771504774129883

Mann C, Lee JH, Liu J et al (2008) Delayed treatment of spinal cord injury with erythropoietin or darbepoetin – a lack of neuro-protective efficacy in a contusion model of cord injury. *Exp Neurol* 211: 34–40. doi: 10.1016/j.expneurol.2007.12.013

Nogradi A, Vrbova G (2001) The effect of riluzole treatment in rats on the survival of injured adult and grafted embryonic motorneurons. *Eur J Neurosci* 13: 113–18. doi: 10.1046/j.0953-816X.2000.01362.x

Petitjean ME, Pointillart V, Dixmerias F (1998) Medical treatment of spinal cord injury in the acute stage. *Ann Fr Anesth Reanim* 17: 114–22. doi: 10.1016/S0750-7658(98)80058-0

Pinzon A, Marcillo A, Pabon D, Bramlett HM, Bunge MB, Dietrich WD (2008) A reassessment of erythropoietin as a neuroprotective agent following rat spinal cord compression or contusion injury. *Exp Neurol* 213: 129–36. doi: 10.1016/j.expneurol.2008.05.018

Pointillart V, Gense D, Gross C et al (1993) Effects of nimodipine on posttraumatic spinal cord ischemia in baboons. *J Neurotrauma* 10: 201–13. doi: 10.1089/neu.1993.10.201

Saberi H, Moshayedi P, Aghayan H et al (2008) Treatment of chronic thoracic spinal cord injury patients with autologous Schwann cell transplantation: an interim report on safety considerations and possible outcomes. *Neurosci Lett* 443: 46–50. doi: 10.1016/j.neulet.2008.07.04

Saganova K, Orendacova J, Cizkova D, Vanicky I (2008) Limited minocycline neuroprotection after balloon compression spinal cord injury in the rat. *Neurosci Lett* 433: 246–9. doi: 10.1016/j.neulet.2008.01.041

Schwartz G, Fehlings MG (2001) Evaluation of the neuroprotective effects of sodium channel blockers after spinal cord injury: improved behavioral and neuroanatomical recovery with riluzole. *J Neurosurg* 94: 245–56.

Simard JM, Tsymbalyuk O, Ivanov A et al (2007) Endothelial sulfonylurea receptor 1-regulated NC Ca-ATP channels mediate progressive hemorrhagic necrosis following spinal cord injury. *J Clin Invest* 117: 2105–13. doi: 10.1172/JCI32041

Solaroglu I, Kaptanoglu E, Okutan O, Beskonakli E, Attar A, Kilinc K (2005) Magnesium sulfate treatment decreases caspase-3 activity after experimental spinal cord injury in rats. *Surg Neurol* 64(Suppl 2): S17–21. doi: 10.1016/j.surneu.2005.07.058

Stirling DP, Khodarahmi K, Liu J et al (2004) Minocycline treatment reduces delayed oligodendrocyte death, attenuates axonal dieback, and improves functional outcome after spinal cord injury. *J Neurosci* 24: 2182–90. doi: 10.1523/JNEUROSCI.5275-03.2004

Thomas A, Nockels R, Pan H, Shaffrey C, Chopp M (1999) Progesterone is neuroprotective after acute experimental spinal cord trauma in rats. *Spine* 24: 2134–8. http://dx.doi.org/10.1097/00007632-199910150-00013

Walters B, Hadley M, Hurlbert R et al; Congress of Neurological Surgeons (2013) Guidelines for the management of acute cervical spinal and spinal cord injuries: 2013 update. *Neurosurgery* 60(Suppl 1): 82–91. doi: 10.1227/01.neu.0000430319.32247.7f

Wang X, Budel S, Baughman K, Gould G, Song KH, Strittmatter SM (2009) Ibuprofen enhances recovery from spinal cord injury by limiting tissue loss and stimulating axonal growth. *J Neurotrauma* 26: 81–95. doi: 10.1089/neu.2007.0464

Wiseman DB, Dailey AT, Lundin D et al (2009) Magnesium efficacy in a rat spinal cord injury model. *J Neurosurg Spine* 10: 308–14. doi: 10.3171/spi.2009.10.4.308

28
NEUROLOGIC RECOVERY AND RESTORATIVE REHABILITATION

Dena R Howland, Shelley A Trimble and Andrea L Behrman

Case vignette

Kyle, a male aged 4 years 6 months, suffered a spinal cord injury owing to an accidental gunshot wound 16 months ago. The locomotor training occurred five times per week for 76 sessions. His initial lower extremity motor score (4/50) and the time since the injury (16 months) both supported the presumption that Kyle was unlikely to recover his walking ability. He used a manual wheelchair permanently for mobility and had received the best current standards for therapy and equipment including a standing frame, wheeled stander, and reciprocating gait orthosis. Initially, locomotor training involved 1 hour of step and stand retraining on the treadmill, with approximately 30 minutes of each, followed by attempts to walk on the ground using the principles of locomotor training (see Table 28.1). The locomotor training used with Kyle had three components: (1) intense *retraining* of the neuromuscular system, which occurs on the treadmill with partial body weight support and manual facilitation by trainers, (2) *transfer and assessment* of walking skills on the ground (off the treadmill), and (3) *daily life activities* to guide choices supporting continued application of locomotor training principles, training, and skill progression outside of the clinic, termed *community integration* (Harkema et al 2011). From sessions 1 to 33, with the exception of successful thoracic extension, Kyle did not volitionally contribute to movement during locomotor training. From session 22, an emphasis was placed on augmentation of hip flexor and tibialis anterior cues while standing in a diagonal stride position during weight shift to facilitate a flexor response. In session 29, a right leg step without cuing was seen. This 'spinal step' occurred on the ground after a facilitated left leg step. It was characterized by synergistic hip, knee, and ankle flexion and Kyle was not aware it had occurred. In session 33, after being placed in a diagonal stance position, Kyle initiated and took seven independent (no cuing), consecutive steps on the ground using a postural control walker for balance. After this, walking ability progressed daily up to the final session (76) when he could initiate and sustain independent mobility with a reverse rolling walking. Several months later, after returning home, Kyle entered kindergarten as a full-time ambulator with a walker. Lower extremity motor scores were unchanged from prelocomotor training (4/50) and did not reflect the significant change in capacity to generate steps, suggesting the significant contributions of the neural system below the level of the lesion to walking recovery in this child (Behrman et al 2008).

Introduction

There is little doubt that the central nervous system (CNS) is capable of significant plasticity. The evidence is clear that neural activity produced by experience can alter connections and have lasting effects. Although most extensively documented for learning and memory in adults (Buschkuehl et al 2012, Caroni et al 2012), the literature is rapidly expanding, showing that activity also can affect spinal circuitry (Edgerton and Roy 2009, Wolpaw 2010). Furthermore, plasticity is not a unique feature of the normal nervous system. Plasticity, in a number of systems, appears to correlate with, or has the potential to support, beneficial functional outcomes (Onifer et al 2011). Thus, the challenge for neuroscience and rehabilitation is to harness and drive plasticity toward end points that support desirable functional outcomes after spinal cord injury (SCI).

Neuroplasticity

Continually mounting evidence for therapeutically induced behavioral recovery after experimental SCIs in animal models provides a strong stimulus for the rapidly growing interest in, and push for, bench-to-bedside application for adults with SCIs (Kleitman 2004). Of particular interest are studies showing the effects of hind limb step training using a treadmill with animals that have anatomically complete spinal transections above the spinal centers innervating the hind limbs (Lovely et al 1986, Edgerton et al 2004, Ichiyama et al 2008, Courtine et al 2009, Rossignol and Frigon 2011, Rossignol et al 2011). Not only does stepping occur and improve in these animals with intensive training, but also improvements in functional performance are accompanied by changes at the circuitry (Courtine et al 2009) and molecular (Tillakaratne et al 2002, Wang et al 2006, 2009) levels. This work underlines the capacity of the spinal cord to produce basic stepping, independent of descending connections, and it shows that the specificity of the task appears to be key and intensive practice of non-task-specific activities may prevent desired task recovery and performance (Hodgson et al 1994, García-Alías G et al 2009). These findings provided the fundamental framework for locomotor training, which has become a standard of practice delivered to some adults with SCI across select sites throughout the Christopher and Dana Reeve Foundation NeuroRecovery Network (Harkema et al 2012a). Coupled with increasing evidence for training effects on neurotrophin expression (Gómez-Pinilla et al 2002), the possibility for promoting effective functional repair in the spinal cord with rehabilitation and other therapeutic modalities continues to gain more attention. Typically, advancements in the pediatric setting follow behind those made in research and clinical programs for adults. This is not surprising as the US SCI Model Systems are adult based, there are fewer children injured annually, and there are challenges associated with the inclusion of growing children in clinical trials.

Implications for rehabilitation

The emerging understanding of plasticity dramatically changes the way functional potential after SCI should be viewed and opens up opportunities for new rehabilitation paradigms. The current standard of care for rehabilitation of the patient with an SCI is based on the premise that the consequences of SCI (e.g. paralysis, weakness, sensory loss) may be recovered to some degree, but that compensatory strategies will be needed for mobility and function. Thus, patients with SCIs typically are taught and use compensatory movement strategies alone or in combination with adaptive devices to achieve some level of functional independence. Adaptive equipment used for upright postures and mobility has traditionally included static and passive standing frames and braces with walkers or crutches (see Chapter 22).

Although the intent of adaptive equipment is to enhance activity and function, it may be inconsistent with recovery-based approaches. The long-term effects of musculoskeletal inactivity and/or altered activity have an impact on more than just the nervous system. Immobility and a lack of active load bearing through the legs are correlated with multiple negative events including fractures, bone demineralization, osteopenia, and contractures (Giangregorio and McCartney 2006, Jiang et al 2006). Furthermore, the impact may be greater in children owing to ongoing skeletal growth and maturation processes (Vogel et al 2004, 2012, Parent et al 2011). Thus, one of the greatest challenges of rehabilitation, using a neurorecovery paradigm, is to determine how to best guide plasticity to maximize positive functional recovery and minimize dysfunction (Garraway et al 2011, Ferguson et al 2012a,b). The experiences that promote and drive changes in circuitry are key.

Based upon our knowledge of activity-dependent plasticity, the activity most engaged in (e.g. time, repetitions) will most strongly direct changes in, or maintenance of, synaptic connections. Thus, incorporating therapeutic elements into daily hours outside of therapy, in addition to during therapy, may more readily guide circuitry changes that will support greater neurorecovery. The critical threshold for tipping the balance toward change required for recovery or integration of a new skill is unknown and may even vary based upon the task. It is critical to appreciate the bidirectional relationship between plasticity and the desired activity or function. Activity drives plasticity and plasticity (circuitry modification) drives the behavior. This bidirectional relationship is well appreciated during nervous system development (Shatz and Stryker 1978, Yao and Dan 2005) and is critical for the continual shaping, refinement, and reinforcement of both the desired behavior and the underlying anatomical substrates.

Recovery-based rehabilitation is best designed when it promotes optimal CNS function in support of preserved, recovered, and new behaviors. The injured, remodeled, or essentially 'new' CNS after SCI (Edgerton et al 2004) is influenced not only by current experiences, but also by experiences before SCI. Although individuals injured as adults will have prior experience with all basic motor activities, a child may not. Dependent upon the child's age at the time of his or her injury, their CNS may or may not have prior experience, for example, with independent sitting, crawling, standing, reaching, walking, or running. We do not yet understand how experience or lack of experience might be important in choice or design of therapeutic approaches. Preliminary data from our group show that a lack of prior walking experience does not preclude development of walking after SCI (see Fig. 28.1) (Howland et al 2010, 2011).

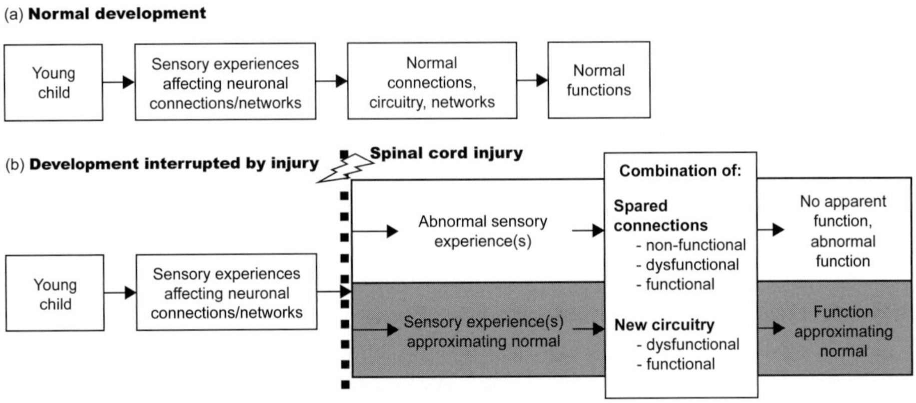

Fig. 28.1 Developmental flow chart comparing (a) normal development and (b) development interrupted by a spinal cord injury from an experience perspective. (a) During normal development, sensorimotor experiences influence and reinforce neural circuitry leading to the establishment of developmentally appropriate (typical) performances. (b) The extent of prior motor experiences varies across children with SCIs based upon their developmental motor status at the time of their injuries. This also means that the established circuitry varies. After injury, as is the case during any other time, sensory experiences guide circuitry formation, plasticity, and permanence. Unlike other times, the extent of abnormal sensory experiences is very high. These abnormal experiences support the alternative circuitry compared with that which underlies normal sensorimotor events. Thus, it is important to consider the type and quality of sensory and sensorimotor experiences the child has, as these will guide neural circuitry after injury, just as they do in the child with typical development.

Sensory input is a critical component of any motor performance. A sensation may not only be the trigger for movement, but also provide feedback about ongoing movement so that movement features can be adjusted to achieve and perpetuate successful performance. The CNS circuitries that are necessary for many lower extremity reflexes, as well as basic stepping, are located within the spinal cord and may be activated by sensory cues via the peripheral nervous system. Studies assessing the H-reflex and basic stepping performance clearly show that, by using peripheral sensory cues on the lower extremities, basic reflex and stepping patterns can be modified in the neurally intact and the isolated caudal spinal cords (Nielsen et al 1993, Chen and Wolpaw 1995, Rossignol et al 1996, Thompson et al 2009). These studies, along with others (Lovely et al 1990, De Leon et al 1998), also show that the spinal cord is trainable and provide the basis for clinical approaches, which initially target activation of the spinal cord below the level of the injury using sensory cues which activate cutaneous and subcutaneous receptors, in particular the mechanoreceptors.

Based on studies in rats and cats (Rossignol et al 2011) and humans (Nadeau et al 2010), the caudal spinal cord contains a central pattern generator for locomotion. The extensive network of interneurons that comprise the central pattern generator responds to, and organizes its activities based upon, sensory information. It then interacts with motor neurons to produce leg movements associated with walking (Fig. 28.2).

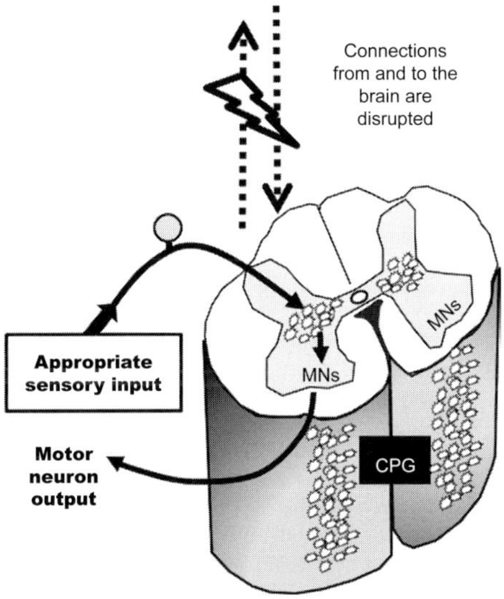

Fig. 28.2 After spinal cord injury owing to disruption of descending signals from the brain to the spinal cord to drive motor output, the intact sensory input from the periphery at the spinal cord level becomes even more critical for generating motor output. Sensory information from multiple sources (e.g. cutaneous, joint, muscle) enters the spinal cord through the dorsal roots to provide an ensemble of information about the state or activity of the individual. An interneuronal network (shown as white cells), which comprises the central pattern generator (CPG) for locomotion, lies within the gray matter of the spinal cord. This central pattern generator receives, integrates, interprets, and organizes this ensemble of sensory information into a 'meaningful' context. Based upon the interpreted context, information is sent forward to the motor neurons (MNs). The axons of these motor neurons form the ventral roots and then peripheral nerves, which innervate the muscles.

Based upon our knowledge of activity-dependent plasticity and the neural control of walking (Roy et al 2012), the current activity-based locomotor training approach was developed for adults (Behrman and Harkema 2000, Behrman et al 2005, Harkema et al 2011). The key aspect of this training approach is its application of intense, walking-specific sensory input and practice on a treadmill using an adjustable body weight support system to promote normal movement patterns of the trunk, pelvis, arms, and legs. The treadmill facilitates intense walking practice. The repetition that can be achieved is critical in facilitating and establishing the circuitry required to support walking (Hebb 1949, Cooke and Bliss 2006). Equally important is the ability to adjust body weight support (Harkema et al 1997), alter treadmill speed (Beres-Jones and Harkema 2004), and enhance other sensory inputs through manual cues (Ferris et al 2004, Galvez et al 2007) provided by trainers. Repetitive training with constant reassessment of the patient's neuromuscular capacity allows for daily adjustment of the sensory cues to continually challenge and promote the patient's capacity. Immediately after training on the treadmill, the locomotor training approach includes evaluation and practice of walking, standing, and sitting activities on the ground on a daily basis (see Fig. 28.3). Locomotor training is guided by four training principles (Table 28.1), which emphasize plasticity and activation of neural circuitry, including the central pattern generator, below the level of an SCI to achieve the primary goal of walking activity. These principles (Behrman and Harkema 2000, Behrman et al 2005, Harkema et al 2011) are designed to provide the appropriate sensorimotor ensemble for walking on the treadmill and on the ground.

TABLE 28.1
The four principles of locomotor training

Principle	Description
Maximize load bearing by the lower extremities, and minimize load bearing by the upper extremities	This principle is supported by reports of increased lower extremity electromyographic amplitudes as a result of increasing the weight through the legs in experimental animals and humans after SCI, as well as in able-bodied individuals during the stance phase of walking (Harkema et al 1997, Dietz et al 2002). An adjustable body weight support system allows modification of this important parameter as the neuromuscular system becomes capable of accepting more weight
Optimize the sensory cues for walking	Training at normal walking speed, typically ≥1.0m/s (2.2mph), enhances stepping. This element of the sensory experience modulates electromyographic frequency and amplitude in individuals with complete and incomplete SCI, as well as able-bodied individuals (Beres-Jones and Harkema 2004, Lünenburger et al 2006)
Optimize the kinematics for the trunk, pelvis, and extremities	Appropriate load bearing and hip extension promote, during select epochs of the step cycle, critical afferent input from joint receptors (proprioception), muscle spindles and Golgi tendon organs (muscle length), and the cutaneous receptors (skin surface) during upright posture. In particular, these cues are triggers for the transition from stance to swing of the same limb and swing to stance of the contralateral limb (Harkema et al 1997, 2011). Manual cuing (stretch/pressure) of key muscle tendons at appropriate points during the step cycle are used to enhance normal afferent inputs and should be graded as the system response increases
Maximize recovery strategies; minimize compensation strategies	To maximize recovery, strategies should promote receptor activation in spatial–temporal patterns similar to those used during normal movements. The goal is to foster more normal neural activity that supports a more normal sensorimotor experience. Promoting and approximating normal activity minimizes the use of compensatory strategies, particularly those that change task kinematics and decrease the motor output of the lower extremities, pelvis, and trunk (Visintin and Barbeau 1994). The choice of whether to use a device (e.g. orthosis or assistive device), the choice of device type, and how it is used all should be carefully made (see Fig. 28.3). For example, traditional walkers promote an anteriorly flexed posture, which prevents an upright trunk position and hip extension beyond neutral. These kinematic features diminish key sensory walking cues, including load bearing and maximal hip extension, important to normal walking. Thus, if using a walker, it is important to cue and train an upright posture to facilitate normal walking kinematics, as well as to maximize load bearing by the lower extremities. Alternatively, a postural control walker (positioned behind the patient with arm supports to each side) allows for a more upright posture

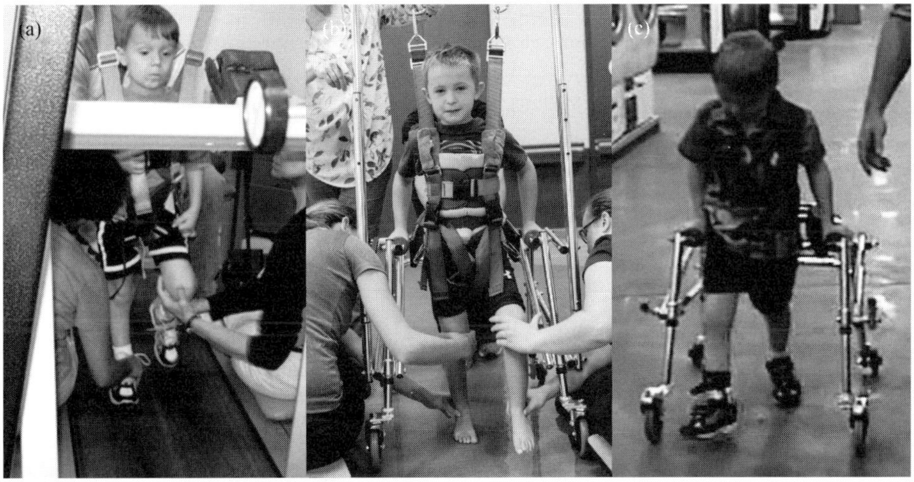

Fig. 28.3 Three components of locomotor training. (a) Intense retraining in the treadmill environment with partial body weight support and manual facilitation by trainers. (b) Transfer and assessment of skills on the ground (off the treadmill) introducing postural control walker and overhead support for greater ease in progressing speed of walker and assisting with load bearing while initiating steps. (c) Application of locomotor training principles within the home and community to increase the intensity of training and advance practical skills (e.g. walking in the hardware store was motivating for the child and included environmental challenges including negotiation of puddles in the parking lot, displays, and other individuals in the store). Photographs printed with consent.

Locomotor training in clinical practice

Translation of locomotor training into the clinical setting began formally in the USA around 2005 with the formation of the Christopher and Dana Reeve Foundation NeuroRecovery Network through a cooperative agreement with the Centers for Disease Control (Harkema et al 2012a). Several elements supported and continue to support this process. These include (1) standardized training for any sites interested; (2) within the network, standardized training, standardized outcome measures, annual competency evaluations for staff, and ongoing program evaluation; (3) publication of a locomotor training manual (Harkema et al 2011); (4) publications of data acquired across the network to demonstrate standardization of procedures (Morrison et al 2012), evaluate established and newly developed outcome measures (Behrman et al 2012), determine outcomes (Buehner et al 2012, Forrest et al 2012, Harkema et al 2012b), and identify longitudinal patterns of recovery (Datta et al 2012, Lorenz et al 2012) within the network compared with existing literature (Harkema et al 2012c). The current translation is effective not only in providing a new cutting-edge neurorecovery-based approach, but also in establishing a reimbursement mechanism as a clinical treatment using standardized codes (e.g. neuromuscular re-education). Although children represent only 5% of the population with SCI, the structure and framework used with adults in the NeuroRecovery Network may potentially provide a basis for this approach with children.

TABLE 28.2

Comparison of locomotor training approach to compensation-based approaches for achieving mobility

Feature	Locomotor training approach	Compensation-based approach
Expectation of recovery from physical rehabilitation	Expect neuromuscular recovery below the level of the lesion during acute and chronic periods after spinal cord injury and physical rehabilitation to impact rate, magnitude, and trajectory of overall recovery	Expect neuromuscular recovery during 'natural recovery' period <1y after spinal cord injury and rate diminishing with time with little expectation for physical rehabilitation to alter recovery trajectory
View of spinal cord	Target substrate that is responsive, adaptable, trainable, and can alter motor output	Not viewed as a target substrate for rehabilitation
Rehabilitation	Activate neuromuscular system below the level of the lesion through sensory cues followed by integration of voluntary control. Incorporate neuromuscular system above and below the lesion	Focus on spared, voluntary control of muscles above and below the level of the lesion to compensate for weakness and paralysis
Functional goals	Pre-injury movement patterns (closest approximation) to achieve functional goals and independence	Alternative movement strategies, e.g. momentum, leverage, substitution to accomplish functional goals
Use of compensatory devices	Minimize or eliminate use of assistive devices and braces. Assistive devices introduced after training the neuromuscular system. How the devices are used is consistent with locomotor training principles. Two devices may be introduced to achieve two different goals, e.g. endurance or independence	Assistive devices, mobility aids, and braces are provided early in the rehabilitation process to achieve mobility as the end goal and are permanently integrated
Sensory input	Focus on providing task-specific sensory experiences to retrain and activate the neuromuscular system and generate task-specific motor output	Focus on achieving trunk/pelvic/limb alignment and stabilization via equipment, mobility devices, bracing, or surgical intervention
Duration of training and type of sensory experience	Overall amount of time retraining the neuromuscular system increases as skills improve and targets consistency with normal (pre-injury) movement patterns. Training and promotion of locomotor training principles also occurs in the home and community with goals evolving relative to neuromuscular gains	Amount of time spent in wheelchair and/or using alternative mobility strategies, bracing, and assistive devices provides repetitive sensory experience often inconsistent with normal (pre-injury) movement patterns
Therapeutic effect	With training, expect therapeutic effect; thus, positive change in neuromuscular system and functional gains via activation of the system below the level of the injury with locomotor training as well as above	With rehabilitation, expect functional gains; however, no therapeutic effect (relatively permanent change in motor capacity). If device is removed (e.g. brace), function is diminished or lost

Adapted from Behrman et al (2006) with permission of the American Physical Therapy Association.

Priorities for research

Based on the existing literature, the broad research priorities for children with SCI should include (1) the development of pediatric-appropriate assessment tools across relevant domains that are sensitive for all SCI magnitudes and etiologies, (2) the use of common assessments across sites and studies for effective comparison of similar and different treatment approaches (locomotor training and others), (3) the assessment of activity-based approaches that are recovery focused, (4) the assessment of treatment effects across multiple systems, primary and secondary targets, and the domains of the International Classification of Functioning, Disability and Health, and (5) the assessment of immediate and long-term costs and benefits of treatment approaches.

Summary

Sufficient evidence from basic scientific research, developmental work, the adult spinal cord literature, and emerging work in children after SCI warrants a shift in our thinking regarding rehabilitation potential after pediatric-onset SCI. Research has shown (and continues to demonstrate) that the spinal cord is 'smart'. It can receive, integrate, and respond to sensory input during the practice of specific tasks (Roy et al 2012). Furthermore, specific tasks can be designed to produce a desired motor output, such as stepping and/or postural control, and then adjusted during training to promote further learning and refinement of that task. In summary, spinal circuitry has the capacity to learn, change, and promote development or restoration of complex motor behavior. These findings have led to the development of the activity-based locomotor training intervention (Behrman and Harkema 2007, Harkema et al 2011). Although in some instances rehabilitation will continue to rely on the use of compensation to achieve functional goals, physical rehabilitation should also be used as an agent for neurologic change and restoration of function after pediatric SCI. Table 28.2 provides a comparison of approaches for mobility: activity-based and compensation including expectations for outcomes, assumptions concerning plasticity, and clinical decision making. This is a new era in rehabilitation for adults and children with SCI. New expectations and possibilities for improved outcomes based on recovery and development of motor skills with age-appropriate performance as the reference point should be pursued.

Disclosure

The contents of this chapter do not represent the views of the Department of Veterans Affairs or the US Government.

REFERENCES

Behrman AL, Harkema SJ (2000) Locomotor training after human spinal cord injury: a series of case studies. *Phys Ther* 80: 688–700.

Behrman AL, Harkema SJ (2007) Physical rehabilitation as an agent for recovery after spinal cord injury. *Phys Med Rehabil Clin N Am* 18: 183–202. doi: 10.1016/j.pmr.2007.02.002

Behrman AL, Lawless-Dixon AR, Davis SB et al (2005) Locomotor training progression and outcomes after incomplete spinal cord injury. *Phys Ther* 85: 1356–71.

Behrman AL, Bowden MG, Nair PM (2006) Neuroplasticity after spinal cord injury and training: an emerging paradigm shift in rehabilitation and walking recovery. *Phys Ther* 86:1406–25. http://dx.doi.org/10.2522/ptj.20050212

Behrman AL, Nair PM, Bowden MG et al (2008) Locomotor training restores walking in a nonambulatory child with chronic, severe, incomplete cervical spinal cord injury. *Phys Ther* 88: 580–90. doi: 10.2522/ptj.20070315

Behrman AL, Ardolino E, Vanhiel LR et al (2012) Assessment of functional improvement without compensation reduces variability of outcome measures after human spinal cord injury. *Arch Phys Med Rehabil* 93: 1518–29. doi: 10.1016/j.apmr.2011.04.027

Beres-Jones JA, Harkema SJ (2004) The human spinal cord interprets velocity-dependent afferent input during stepping. *Brain* 127: 2232–46. doi: 10.1093/brain/awh252

Buehner JJ, Forrest GF, Schmidt-Read M, White S, Tansey K, Basso DM (2012) Relationship between ASIA examination and functional outcomes in the NeuroRecovery Network Locomotor Training Program. *Arch Phys Med Rehabil* 93: 1530–40. doi: 10.1016/j.apmr.2012.02.035

Buschkuehl M, Jaeggi SM, Jonides J (2012) Neuronal effects following working memory training. *Dev Cogn Neurosci* 2(Suppl 1): S167–79. Erratum in: *Dev Cogn Neurosci* 2: 291. doi: 10.1016/j.dcn.2011.10.001

Caroni P, Donato F, Muller D (2012) Structural plasticity upon learning: regulations and functions. *Nat Rev Neurosci* 13: 478–90. doi:10.1038/nrn3258

Chen XY, Wolpaw JR (1995) Operant conditioning of H-reflex in freely moving rats. *J Neurophysiol* 73: 411–15.

Cooke SF, Bliss TVP (2006) Plasticity in the human central nervous system. *Brain* 129: 1659–73. doi: 10.1093/brain/awl082

Courtine G, Gerasimenko Y, van den Brand R et al (2009) Transformation of nonfunctional spinal circuits into functional states after the loss of brain input. *Nat Neurosci* 12: 1333–42. doi: 10.1038/nn.2401

Datta S, Lorenz DJ, Harkema SJ (2012) Dynamic longitudinal evaluation of the utility of the Berg Balance Scale in individuals with motor incomplete spinal cord injury. *Arch Phys Med Rehabil* 93: 1565–73. doi: 10.1016/j.apmr.2012.01.026

De Leon RD, Hodgson JA, Roy RR, Edgerton VR (1998) Locomotor capacity attributable to step training versus spontaneous recovery after spinalization in adult cats. *Neurophysiology* 79: 1329–40.

Dietz V, Müller R, Colombo G (2002) Locomotor activity in spinal man: significance of afferent input from joint and load receptors. *Brain* 125: 2626–34. doi:10.1093/brain/awf273

Edgerton VR, Roy RR (2009) Activity-dependent plasticity of spinal locomotion: implications for sensory processing. *Exerc Sport Sci Rev* 37: 171–8. doi: 10.1097/JES.0b013e3181b7b932

Edgerton VR, Tillakaratne NJ, Bigbee AJ, de Leon RD, Roy RR (2004) Plasticity of the spinal neural circuitry after injury. *Annu Rev Neurosci* 27: 145–67. doi: 10.1146/annurev.neuro.27.070203.144308

Ferguson AR, Huie JR, Crown ED, Grau JW (2012a) Central nociceptive sensitization vs. spinal cord training: opposing forms of plasticity that dictate function after complete spinal cord injury. *Front Physiol* 3: 396. doi: 10.3389/fphys.2012.00396

Ferguson AR, Huie JR, Crown ED et al (2012b) Maladaptive spinal plasticity opposes spinal learning and recovery in spinal cord injury. *Front Physiol* 3: 399. doi: 10.3389/fphys.2012.00399

Ferris DP, Gordon KE, Beres-Jones JA, Harkema SJ (2004) Muscle activation during unilateral stepping occurs in the nonstepping limb of humans with clinically complete spinal cord injury. *Spinal Cord* 42: 14–23. doi: 10.1038/sj.sc.3101542

Forrest GF, Lorenz DJ, Hutchinson K et al (2012) Ambulation and balance outcomes measure different aspects of recovery in individuals with chronic, incomplete spinal cord injury. *Arch Phys Med Rehabil* 93: 1553–64. doi: 10.1016/j.apmr.2011.08.051

Galvez JA, Budovitch A, Harkema SJ, Reinkensmeyer DJ (2007) Quantification of therapists' manual assistance on the leg during treadmill gait training with partial body-weight support after spinal cord injury. *Conf Proc IEEE Eng Med Biol Soc* 4028–32. doi: 10.1109/IEMBS.2007.4353217

García-Alías G, Barkhuysen S, Buckle M, Fawcett JW (2009) Chondroitinase ABC treatment opens a window of opportunity for task-specific rehabilitation. *Nat Neurosci* 12: 1145–51. doi: 10.1038/nn.2377

Garraway SM, Turtle JD, Huie JR et al (2011) Intermittent noxious stimulation following spinal cord contusion injury impairs locomotor recovery and reduces spinal BDNFTrkB signaling in adult rats. *Neuroscience* 199: 86–102. doi: 10.1016/j.neuroscience.2011.10.007

Giangregorio L, McCartney N (2006) Bone loss and muscle atrophy in spinal cord injury: epidemiology, fracture prediction, and rehabilitation strategies. *J Spinal Cord Med* 29: 489–500.

Gómez-Pinilla F, Ying Z, Roy RR, Molteni R, Edgerton VR (2002) Voluntary exercise induces a BDNF-mediated mechanism that promotes neuroplasticity. *J Neurophysiol* 88: 2187–95. http://dx.doi.org/10.1152/jn.00152.2002

Harkema SJ, Hurley SL, Patel UK, Requejo PS, Dobkin BH, Edgerton VR (1997) Human lumbosacral spinal cord interprets loading during stepping. *J Neurophysiol* 77: 797–811.

Harkema SJ, Behrman AL, Barbeau H (2011) *Locomotor Training: Principles and Practice*. New York, NY: Oxford University Press. http://dx.doi.org/10.1093/acprof:oso/9780195342086.001.0001

Harkema SJ, Schmidt-Read M, Behrman AL, Bratta A, Sisto SA, Edgerton VR (2012a) Establishing the NeuroRecovery Network: multisite rehabilitation centers that provide activity-based therapies and assessments for neurologic disorders. *Arch Phys Med Rehabil* 93: 1498–507. doi: 10.1016/j.apmr.2011.01.023

Harkema SJ, Schmidt-Read M, Lorenz DJ, Edgerton VR, Behrman AL (2012b) Balance and ambulation improvements in individuals with chronic incomplete spinal cord injury using locomotor training-based rehabilitation. *Arch Phys Med Rehabil* 93: 1508–17. doi: 10.1016/j.apmr.2011.01.024

Harkema SJ, Hillyer J, Schmidt-Read M, Ardolino E, Sisto SA, Behrman AL (2012c) Locomotor training: as a treatment of spinal cord injury and in the progression of neurologic rehabilitation. *Arch Phys Med Rehabil* 93: 1588–97. doi: 10.1016/j.apmr.2012.04.032

Hebb DO (1949) *Organization of Behavior: A Neuropsychological Theory*. New York, NY: John Wiley.

Hodgson JA, Roy RR, de Leon R, Dobkin B, Edgerton VR (1994) Can the mammalian lumbar spinal cord learn a motor task? *Med Sci Sports Exerc* 26: 1491–7. doi: 10.1249/00005768-199412000-00013

Howland DR, Fox EJ, Tester NJ et al (2010) Responses to locomotor training and identification of functional long tracts in children with severe, chronic spinal cord injury. Society for Neuroscience, 40th Annual Meeting, San Diego, CA. 14 November 2010.

Howland DR, Fox EJ, Trimble S et al (2011) Robust walking response to locomotor training despite disparate SCI etiologies, ages, and chronicity in pediatrics. Society for Neuroscience, 41st Annual Meeting, Washington, DC. 13 November 2011.

Ichiyama RM, Courtine G, Gerasimenko YP et al (2008) Step training reinforces specific spinal locomotor circuitry in adult spinal rats. *J Neurosci* 28: 7370–5. doi: 10.1523/JNEUROSCI.1881-08.2008

Kleitman N (2004) Keeping promises: translating basic research into new spinal cord injury therapies. *J Spinal Cord Med* 27: 311–18.

Jiang SD, Dai LY, Jiang LS (2006) Osteoporosis after spinal cord injury. *Osteoporos Int* 17: 180–92. doi: 10.1007/s00198-005-2028-8

Lorenz DJ, Datta S, Harkema SJ (2012) Longitudinal patterns of functional recovery in patients with incomplete spinal cord injury receiving activity-based rehabilitation. *Arch Phys Med Rehabil* 93: 1541–52. doi: 10.1016/j.apmr.2012.01.027

Lovely RG, Gregor RJ, Roy RR, Edgerton VR (1986) Effects of training on the recovery of full-weight-bearing stepping in the adult spinal cat. *Exp Neurol* 92: 421–35. doi: 10.1016/0014-4886(86)90094-4

Lovely RG, Gregor RJ, Roy RR, Edgerton VR (1990) Weight-bearing hindlimb stepping in treadmill-exercised adult spinal cats. *Brain Res* 514: 206–18. doi:10.1016/0006-8993(90)91417-F

Lünenburger L, Bolliger M, Czell D, Müller R, Dietz V (2006) Modulation of locomotor activity in complete spinal cord injury. *Exp Brain Res* 174: 638–46. doi:10.1007/s00221-006-0509-4

Morrison SA, Forrest GF, VanHiel LR, Davé M, D'Urso D (2012) NeuroRecovery Network provides standardization of locomotor training for persons with incomplete spinal cord injury. *Arch Phys Med Rehabil* 93: 1574–7. doi: 10.1016/j.apmr.2011.06.041

Nadeau S, Jacquemin G, Fournier C, Lamarre Y, Rossignol S (2010) Spontaneous motor rhythms of the back and legs in a patient with a complete spinal cord transection. *Neurorehabil Neural Repair* 24: 377–83. doi: 10.1177/1545968309349945

Nielsen J, Petersen N, Ballegaard M, Biering-Sørensen F, Kiehn O (1993) H-reflexes are less depressed following muscle stretch in spastic spinal cord injured patients than in healthy subjects. *Exp Brain Res* 97: 173–6. doi: 10.1007/BF00228827

Onifer SM, Smith GM, Fouad K (2011) Plasticity after spinal cord injury: relevance to recovery and approaches to facilitate it. *Neurotherapeutics* 8: 283–93. doi: 10.1007/s13311-011-0034-4

Parent S, Mac-Thiong JM, Roy-Beaudry M, Sosa JF, Labelle H (2011) Spinal cord injury in the pediatric population: a systematic review of the literature. *J Neurotrauma* 28: 1515–24. doi: 10.1089/neu.2009.1153

Rossignol S, Frigon A (2011) Recovery of locomotion after spinal cord injury: some facts and mechanisms. *Annu Rev Neurosci* 34: 413–40. doi: 10.1146/annurev-neuro-061010-113746

Rossignol S, Chau C, Brustein E et al (1996) Locomotor capacities after complete and partial lesions of the spinal cord. *Acta Neurobiol Exp (Wars)* 56: 449–63.

Rossignol S, Frigon A, Barrière G et al (2011) Spinal plasticity in the recovery of locomotion. *Prog Brain Res* 188: 229–41. http://dx.doi.org/10.1016/B978-0-444-53825-3.00021-8

Roy RR, Harkema SJ, Edgerton VR (2012) Basic concepts of activity-based interventions for improved recovery of motor function after spinal cord injury. *Arch Phys Med Rehabil* 93: 1487–97. doi: 10.1016/j.apmr.2012.04.034

Shatz CJ, Stryker MP (1978) Ocular dominance in layer IV of the cat's visual cortex and the effects of monocular deprivation. *J Physiol* 281: 267–83.

Thompson AK, Chen XY, Wolpaw JR (2009) Acquisition of a simple motor skill: task-dependent adaptation plus long-term change in the human soleus H-reflex. *J Neurosci* 29: 5784–92. doi: 10.1523/JNEUROSCI.4326-08.2009

Tillakaratne NJ, de Leon RD, Hoang TX, Roy RR, Edgerton VR (2002) Tobin AJ. Use-dependent modulation of inhibitory capacity in the feline lumbar spinal cord. *J Neurosci* 22: 3130–43.

Visintin M, Barbeau H (1994) The effects of parallel bars, body weight support and speed on the modulation of the locomotor pattern of spastic paretic gait. A preliminary communication. *Paraplegia* 32: 540–53. doi:10.1038/sc.1994.86

Vogel LC, Hickey KJ, Klaas SJ, Anderson CJ (2004) Unique issues in pediatric spinal cord injury. *Orthop Nurs* 23: 300–8. http://dx.doi.org/10.1097/00006416-200409000-00004

Vogel LC, Betz RR, Mulcahey MJ (2012) Spinal cord injuries in children and adolescents. *Handb Clin Neurol* 109: 131–48. http://dx.doi.org/10.1016/B978-0-444-52137-8.00008-5

Wang Y, Pillai S, Wolpaw JR, Chen XY (2006) Motor learning changes GABAergic terminals on spinal motoneurons in normal rats. *Eur J Neurosci* 23: 141–50. doi: 10.1111/j.1460-9568.2005.04547.x

Wang Y, Pillai S, Wolpaw JR, Chen XY (2009) H-reflex down-conditioning greatly increases the number of identifiable GABAergic interneurons in rat ventral horn. *Neurosci Lett* 452: 124–9. doi: 10.1016/j.neulet.2009.01.054

Wolpaw JR (2010) What can the spinal cord teach us about learning and memory? *Neuroscientist* 16: 532–49. doi: 10.1177/1073858410368314

Yao H, Dan Y (2005) Synaptic learning rules, cortical circuits, and visual function. *Neuroscientist* 11: 206–16. doi: 10.1177/1073858404272404

29
ADVANCES IN IMAGING

Feroze B Mohamed, Scott H Faro and Nadia Barakat

Introduction

Several imaging modalities are currently being used to obtain diagnostic information in children with spinal cord injuries (SCIs). Among them, magnetic resonance imaging (MRI), computed tomography (CT) myelography, and plain radiography are the most widely used. MRI is a non-invasive imaging method that uses magnetic fields and radiofrequency waves and provides soft tissue contrast of the spinal cord and surrounding tissues within the spinal canal. On the other hand, CT is based on X-rays, provides excellent bone contrast, and is the first line of diagnostic imaging performed after a traumatic injury in both adults and children to evaluate for fractures and spinal subluxation. Subsequently, MRI is performed to evaluate for the presence of spinal cord compression, spinal cord edema and/or hemorrhage, epidural/subdural hemorrhage, prevertebral edema, and ligamentous injury. Although still not widely available, in addition to providing good structural information, MRI has evolved in recent years to provide functional characteristics of the spinal cord. This includes information such as diffusion of the water molecules within the spinal cord providing functional information of white matter based on diffusion tensor imaging (DTI), and neuronal activation sites within the gray matter of the spinal cord based on blood oxygenation level-dependent (BOLD) imaging. These functional neuroimaging biomarkers may potentially help us to understand the mechanisms of SCI and could guide and track the changes of new therapeutic procedures. This chapter will cover the current MRI-based methods used to capture structural and functional properties of the spinal cord and discuss challenges involved in MRI in pediatric spinal cord injury (SCI), and will finish with potential clinical applications of these techniques.

Structural magnetic resonance imaging

The current clinical diagnostic workup for SCI using MRI includes a variety of imaging pulse sequences. A pulse sequence is a general term used to describe a specific MRI technique typically used to obtain images using the MRI scanner. Typically, these pulse sequences generate images which are termed as T1-, T2-, proton density-, and T2*-weighted. These various MRI weightings produce images with various contrast characteristics based on the tissue type being imaged. In this section, we will discuss the MRI pulses that are generally used to capture structural information on the pediatric spinal cord and present a few case studies.

A sagittal fast spin echo (FSE) pulse sequence is typically used to obtain T1- and T2-weighted magnetic resonance images of the spinal cord. Clinically, if intramedullary or dural/subdural hemorrhage is suspected, an additional pulse sequence based on a gradient echo (GRE T2*) sequence is used in addition to the conventional FSE sequence. If any intramedullary edema/infarction of the spinal cord is suspected, then a T2-weighted inversion recovery pulse sequence is often used. Figure 29.1a shows an example of a sagittal reformation using CT of a 15-year-old male after an acute SCI, showing fractures of the C4 and C5 vertebral bodies with associated prevertebral soft tissue swelling. Figure 29.1b shows a sagittal FSE T2-weighted magnetic resonance image of prevertebral soft tissue swelling and acute swelling of the mid-cervical cord and associated increased intermedullary signal consistent with edema and cord contusion in the same case. Figure 29.2 shows an example of traumatic spinal cord transection in an 8-month-old female. Figure 29.2a shows fractures of the C2 and C3 vertebral bodies with associated prevertebral soft tissue swelling. Figure 29.2b is a sagittal FSE T2-weighted magnetic resonance image that shows similar findings as Figure 29.2a with poor cord definition and diffuse abnormal increased signal, which extends from the cervical medullary junction to C4, consistent with edema and extensive axonal injury, prevertebral soft tissue swelling, and distraction of C2 and C3. Figure 29.2c shows chronic changes of upper cervical kyphotic angulation deformity with heterogeneous mixed increased and decreased signal and loss of normal cord architecture, which extends from the cervical medullary junction to the C3, consistent with cord transection and hemosiderin of the same child. There is also adjacent

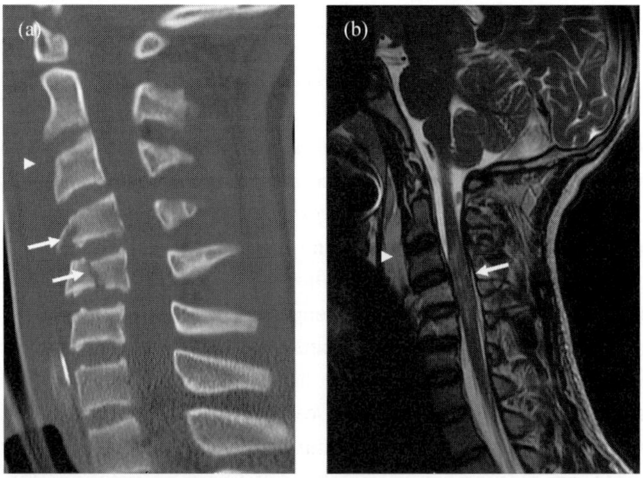

Fig. 29.1 (a) An example of a sagittal reformation of computed tomography of a 15-year-old male after an acute spinal cord injury, showing fractures of the C4 and C5 vertebral bodies (arrows) with associated prevertebral soft tissue swelling (arrowhead). (b) A sagittal fast spin echo T2-weighted magnetic resonance image of prevertebral soft tissue swelling (arrowhead) and acute swelling of the mid-cervical cord and associated increased intermedullary signal (arrow), consistent with edema and cord contusion. (Images courtesy of Tina Poussaint, MD.)

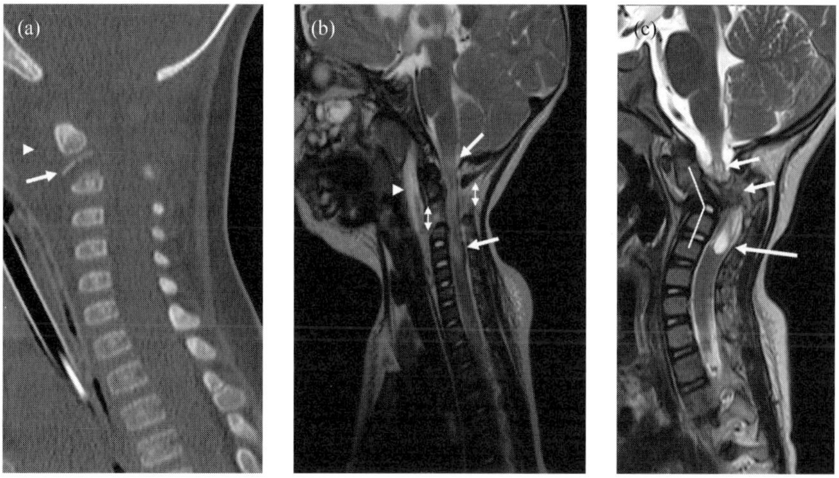

Fig. 29.2 An example of traumatic spinal cord transection in an 8-month-old female. (a) Fractures of the C2 and C3 vertebral bodies (arrow) with associated prevertebral soft tissue swelling (arrowhead). (b) A sagittal fast spin echo T2-weighted magnetic resonance image that shows similar findings to Figure 29.1 with poor cord definition and diffuse abnormal increased signal (arrows), which extends from the cervical medullary junction to C4, consistent with edema and extensive axonal injury, prevertebral soft tissue swelling (arrowhead), and distraction of C2 and C3 (double arrows). (c) Chronic changes of upper cervical kyphotic angulation deformity (angled lines) with heterogeneous mixed increased and decreased signal and loss of normal cord architecture (short arrows) which extends from the cervical medullary junction to the C3, consistent with cord transection and hemosiderin. There is also adjacent increased intermedullary signal at the C4 level, consistent with syringohydromyelia (long arrow). (Images courtesy of Tina Poussaint, MD.)

increased intermedullary signal at the C4 level consistent with syringohydromyelia. Figure 29.3 shows a sagittal FSE T2-weighted magnetic resonance image of an 11-year-old female with chronic SCI of the lower cervical spine, posterior spine fusion, and focal cord atrophy with low signal, consistent with hemosiderin and adjacent focal myelomalacia.

Functional magnetic resonance imaging

Recent years have seen a number of imaging methods based on MRI that generate functional measures in addition to diagnostic information obtained from conventional structural images. Of these, DTI and BOLD imaging have been researched since the early 2000s in their applicability to the human spinal cord (Clark and Werring 2002, Giove et al 2004, Feldman et al 2010, Cadotte et al 2011). The majority of these studies have been restricted to adult populations; however, there has been an increasing trend in expanding these state-of-the-art functional techniques to study children. Although a variety of spinal cord diseases have been studied using these methods, DTI in particular has found its niche in its applicability to study SCI. In the following sections, we will discuss the methodologies underlying these techniques, their strengths and weaknesses pertaining to studying SCIs, and current and future applications.

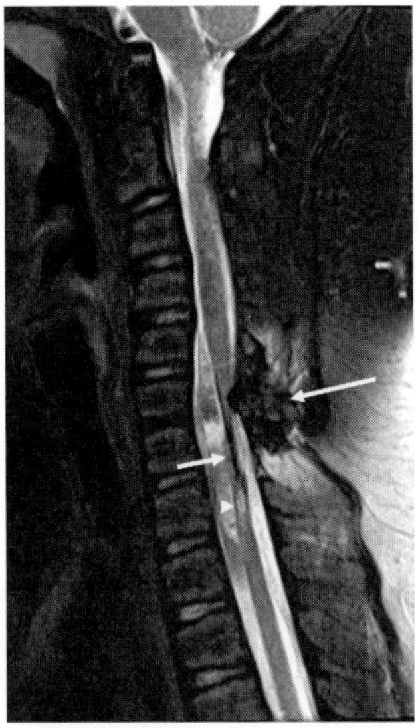

Fig. 29.3 A sagittal fast spin echo T2-weighted magnetic resonance image of an 11-year-old female with chronic spinal cord injury of the lower cervical spine, posterior spine fusion (long arrow), and focal cord atrophy with low signal (short arrow), consistent with hemosiderin and adjacent focal myelomalacia (arrowhead).

Diffusion tensor imaging

Diffusion tensor imaging is a relatively new non-invasive MRI technique that quantifies the diffusion of water molecules in directions parallel and transverse to the axis of neuronal axons. Water is located intracellularly as part of the axoplasm, and extracellularly in small amounts owing to the dense packing of axons. Anisotropic diffusion occurs when water molecular displacement is not similar in all directions. In an axon, water molecules move further, on average, along the axonal length than across. The dense characteristics of the axon may seem to present a barrier to water diffusion perpendicular to the axon; however, several studies have ruled out the role of neurofilaments and microtubules in axonal anisotropy (Beaulieu 2002). These studies examined large diameter axons, 300µm, where water molecules do not encounter a membrane barrier. A typical diffusing water molecule travels a distance of about 5 to 11µm within a diffusion time of 40ms. Results from these studies showed that, in the absence of membrane barriers, diffusion is isotropic, even if molecules encounter neurofilaments and microtubules (Beaulieu and Allen 1994a,b, Takahashi et al 2002, Johansen-Berg and Behrens 2013). These studies eliminated the role of neurofilaments and microtubules in the observed axonal anisotropic diffusion. The other two structures believed to contribute to the restriction of movement of water molecules are the axonal membrane and the myelin sheath. In the intact spinal cord, the axons and myelin sheaths in the white matter are oriented longitudinally; thus, water diffusion typically occurs in this direction. In gray matter, this type of axonal organization is lacking. Thus, DTI has the ability to differentiate between white and gray matter, quantify directionality of the white matter tracts, provide quantification of three-dimensional water diffusivity, track healthy nerve tissue within white matter, and assess structural damage of the cord. DTI has the potential to fill the void left by conventional MRI and the International Standards for Neurological Classification of Spinal Cord Injury

(ISNCSCI) (American Spinal Injury Association 2003) in the assessment of damage to white matter tracts within the spinal cord (Cheran et al 2011, Mulcahey et al 2011). For example, DTI can reveal the precise location of the injury, which conventional MRI often fails to show. Parameters generated from DTI data may provide new metrics in the evaluation of individuals with SCI and improve accuracy in the classification of injury severity. DTI can also be used to extract different bundles of white matter tracts in the spinal cord for analyzing motor and sensory functions separately. DTI has the potential to become a reliable and valid method to evaluate and classify the neurologic consequence of SCI.

There are several diffusion parameters or indices that are extracted from these DTI measurements that reflect certain aspects of the white matter biological characteristics. The most prominent of these terms are defined below. Mean diffusivity, measured in mm^2/s, refers to the average displacement of the water molecules within the white matter. Radial diffusivity (often referred to as λ_T) and axial diffusivity (often referred to as λ_L), both of which are also measured in mm^2/s, represent the diffusivities perpendicular and parallel to the white matter tracts, respectively (LeBihan et al 2001, Ellingson et al 2008a,b). The degree of anisotropy in spinal cord white matter can also be measured. A high index of anisotropy is indicative of a healthy white matter structure. Fractional anisotropy is a ratio from 0 to 1 that represents the degree to which diffusion is anisotropic. High fractional anisotropy (highly anisotropic) values indicate that diffusion is greater in one direction than in other directions, whereas low fractional anisotropy (highly isotropic) values indicate diffusion is relatively equal in all directions. In the healthy spinal cord, fractional anisotropy values are high, reflecting the movement of water molecules along longitudinal spinal tracts. In contrast, in the injured cord, fractional anisotropy values are low owing to the breach in the longitudinal tracts allowing for diffusivity in multiple directions (Ellingson et al 2008a,b, Barakat et al 2011). There are various other DTI indices one can derive from this imaging method, but their clinical significance is still under investigation.

Various technical factors limit the use of DTI for the spinal cord (Kharbanda et al 2006, Figley and Stroman 2007) and, until recent work by Mohamed et al (2011) and Barakat et al (2012), its use in the pediatric population has been presumed to be too challenging (Rosenberg et al 1997, Malisza et al 2010). The small cord volume of children (approximately 1cm in diameter) yields a low signal-to-noise ratio of the measured diffusion signal. Physiological parameters such as cerebrospinal fluid pulsation and blood flow can produce prominent ghosting artifacts and degrade image quality. The thoracic spinal cord specifically is subject to more respiratory and cardiac movements, which cause image blurring and increased or decreased signal intensity. Different tissue interfaces (bone, soft tissue, or fluid) can create susceptibility artifacts. These artifacts are unique to MRI and present in areas where there are more than one medium present (e.g. air/tissue) and cause distortion in the magnetic field. Additionally, in pediatric imaging in particular, the possibility of increased movement of the participant makes obtaining accurate and reproducible DTI parameters challenging. Moreover, in children, the presence of metal such as teeth braces and spinal instrumentation pose unique challenges.

Artifact-reducing techniques can be employed to overcome some of these challenges. Cardiac gating and respiratory compensation can be used to reduce artifacts from physiological parameters. These techniques typically increase the imaging time and can be cumbersome to implement, particularly in children. In general, sedation may be difficult to achieve in children and some may wake up before the examination is complete. Thus, fast, reliable, and high-resolution imaging is needed to image children with SCIs.

Currently, the MRI pulse sequences of choice for DTI are echo planar imaging-based designs. These MRI pulse sequences offer short acquisition times, which reduce motion-related artifacts. However, they are highly sensitive to susceptibility artifacts and eddy-current distortions (Clark and Werring 2002). These distortions can cause geometric deformities in the images thus reducing the accuracy of DTI measures. Recent work using reduced field-of-view imaging sequences showed significant reduction in geometric distortions when imaging the spinal cord (Wilm et al 2007, Saritas et al 2008, Finsterbusch 2009). This approach takes advantage of the small diameter spinal cord morphology and applies a relatively small rectangular field of view to the area of interest. In addition to pulse sequence choice, correcting motion-related artifacts is an important step in data analysis and can improve image quality. Artifact-reduction techniques can be applied during data acquisition, which may increase imaging time, or at the post-processing stage (Middleton et al 2014), where the impact of additional imaging time is not present.

Figure 29.4 shows cervical spinal cord images of a healthy child obtained with the inner field-of-view pulse sequence (Barakat et al 2012). High spatial resolution diffusion tensor images were obtained with this pulse sequence. Minimal eddy-current distortions and

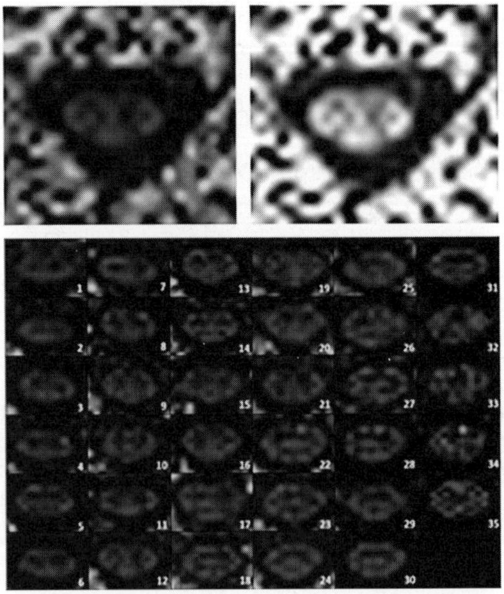

Fig. 29.4 Cervical spinal cord images of a healthy child obtained with the inner field-of-view pulse sequence. Axial fractional anisotropy map (top left) and grayscale fractional anisotropy map (top right) along the 35 cervical slices of a healthy participant (bottom). A color version of this figure is available in the color plate section.

distinctive delineation of gray and white matter structures were observed in most slices. In the axial fractional anisotropy color images of the spinal cord, the H-shaped gray matter can be clearly localized within the surrounding white matter. These results are consistent throughout the transverse slices of the cervical spinal cord and are being demonstrated for the first time in the pediatric spinal cord.

Figure 29.5a–d shows two examples of DTI fractional anisotropy color maps along with their T2-weighted magnetic resonance images in a healthy participant (a and b) and a patient with SCI (c and d). Figure 29.5b,d shows the reconstructed sagittal anisotropy maps in which the spinal cord white matter is well delineated from the surrounding cerebrospinal fluid. It is worth noting that, in fractional anisotropy color maps, blue, green, and red color components correspond to the superior–inferior, anterior–posterior, and left–right directions, respectively. Reducing the imaging field-of-view enabled high-resolution acquisition of the pediatric cervical spinal cord without pronounced geometric distortions. Figure 29.5d shows the reconstructed sagittal anisotropy map in a patient with SCI. This patient had an injury at the C5 level. One can clearly observe the focal thinning of the spinal cord in both T2-weighted and fractional anisotropy images. These fractional anisotropy maps can be used

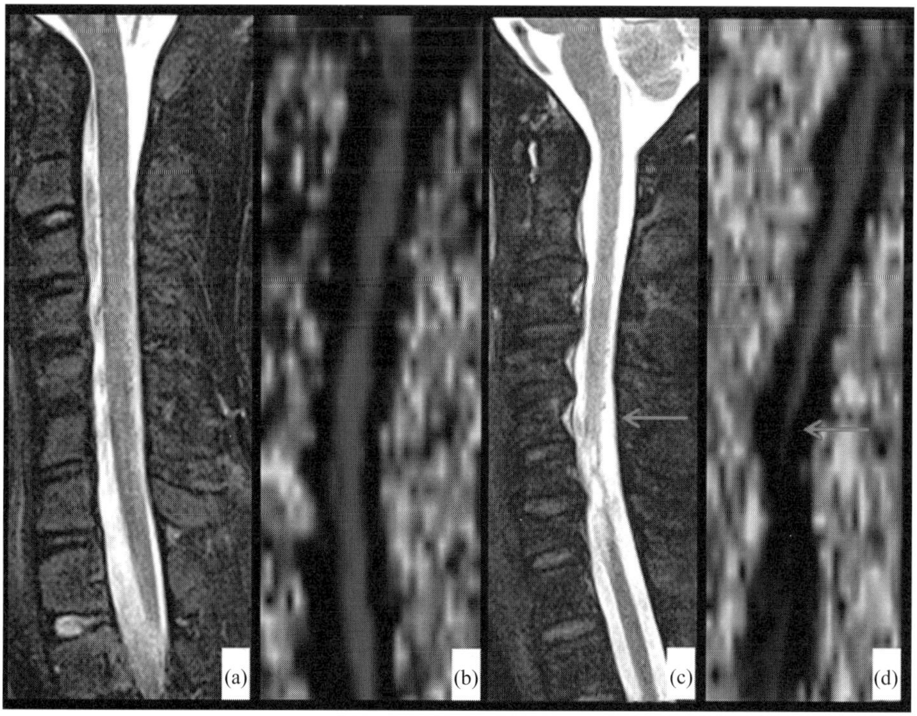

Fig. 29.5 Midline sagittal T2-weighted magnetic resonance image and fractional anisotropy color map of a healthy participant (a, b) and a patient with spinal cord injury (c, d). Arrow represents level of injury (C5). A color version of this figure is available in the color plate section.

to qualitatively observe the cord and evaluate the nature of the cord above and below the injury level. However, the DTI data measured can be used to provide quantitative information about the injury as well.

Quantitative diffusion tensor imaging characteristics of healthy patients and those with spinal cord injury

A recent study has shown DTI indices in a healthy pediatric group (25 children) (Barakat et al 2012). The authors reported a mean (SD) using fractional anisotropy of 0.50 (SD 0.11), axial diffusivity of 0.97 (SD 0.20) × $10^{-3}mm^2/s$, radial diffusivity of 0.41 (SD 0.13) × $10^{-3}mm^2/s$, and mean diffusivity of 0.59 (SD 0.15) × $10^{-3}mm^2/s$. This study has also shown reproducibility of these values by imaging the children twice. Moderate to strong test–retest reliability of DTI parameters values across all levels of the cervical spinal was reported. The interclass correlation coefficients (ICC) and their 95% confidence intervals (CI) were as follows: fractional anisotropy (ICC=0.87, CI 0.78–0.97), and axial diffusivity (ICC=0.97, CI 0.92–0.99). These data provide evidence in support of DTI as a reproducible technique and have characterized DTI for the healthy pediatric cervical cord. These values were somewhat different from DTI measures obtained from adult populations (Ellingson et al 2008a,b, Cheran et al 2011). The same group measured DTI indices in 10 children with SCI and showed a mean (SD) using fractional anisotropy of 0.30 (SD 0.10), axial diffusivity of 1.07 (SD 0.28) × $10^{-3}mm^2/s$, radial diffusivity of 0.73 (SD 0.25) × $10^{-3}mm^2/s$, and mean diffusivity of 0.85 (SD 0.26) × $10^{-3}mm^2/s$. Figure 29.6 shows group differences in DTI measurements between the healthy participants and patients with SCI. These results showed significantly lower fractional anisotropy and higher diffusivity values (mean diffusivity, axial diffusivity, and radial diffusivity) in patients with SCI than the comparison group ($p<0.05$).

Additionally, the DTI results of one representative patient were compared with the averaged results of healthy participants (Barakat et al 2012). In these graphs (Figure 29.7), the arrow points to the MRI level of injury. The differences in diffusion measurements are detected particularly around the lesion site. However, these differences were not limited to lesion sites but were also observed at regions remote from the injury site. These results were consistent across the patient population (Barakat et al 2012) and have shown that DTI values remote to the injury level differ from normative values and differ between complete and incomplete lesions (Barakat et al 2012). Similar findings of changes in the diffusivity values have been shown in acute (Cheran et al 2011) and chronic SCI (Petersen et al 2012) adult populations. These findings might suggest both axonal degeneration and demyelination of the ascending and descending neuronal pathways in the spinal cord.

Clinical correlations of diffusion tensor imaging in children with spinal cord injury

In another study (Mulcahey et al 2013), the correlation of DTI values with values from the ISNCSCI and MRI was examined to evaluate the strength of DTI as a clinical biomarker to evaluate spinal cord damage. The mean and standard deviation values for DTI parameters were calculated based on the measurements from DTI of each individual. Mean values were compared by groups using analysis of variance for repeated measures. Mean values were also compared by region of the cord at the ISNCSCI motor and MRI levels with regions remote

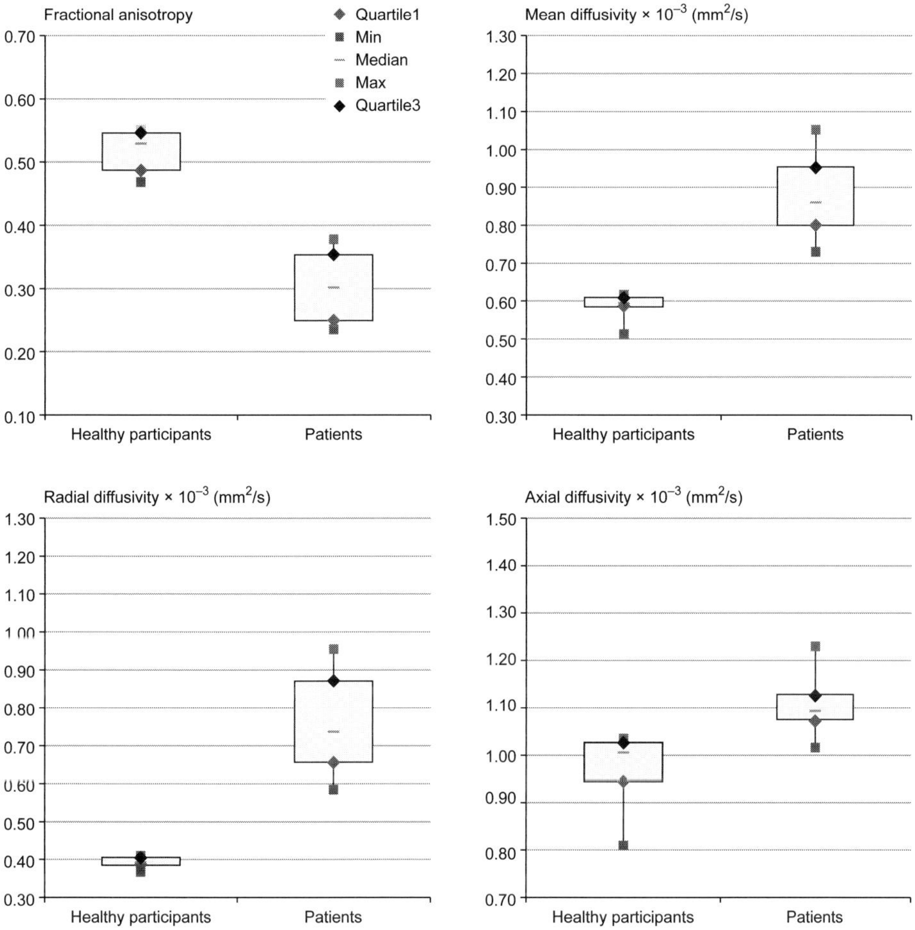

Fig. 29.6 Box plots of diffusion tensor imaging parameters averaged in the groups of healthy participants and patients. 'Quartile 1' and 'Quartile 3' represent the 25th and 75th centiles, respectively.

from motor and MRI level of injury. This study showed that DTI values differ not only between uninjured and injured cords but also between complete and incomplete injuries. This finding is clinically relevant, as the ability to distinguish between complete and incomplete injuries in children using the clinical examination is difficult and, when performed, yields high false-positives (suggesting injury is incomplete when it is actually complete). The authors also showed that, compared with radiologist examination of conventional T1- and T2-weighted magnetic resonance images, DTI values have shown good correlation with the clinical measures. Fractional anisotropy had a statistically significant correlation with all clinical values, with the exception of anal contraction and total pinprick. They claim that DTI appears to be superior to conventional MRI in correlation with the clinical examination, for quantifying the degree of white matter integrity, and potentially for monitoring the effects of therapy in SCI.

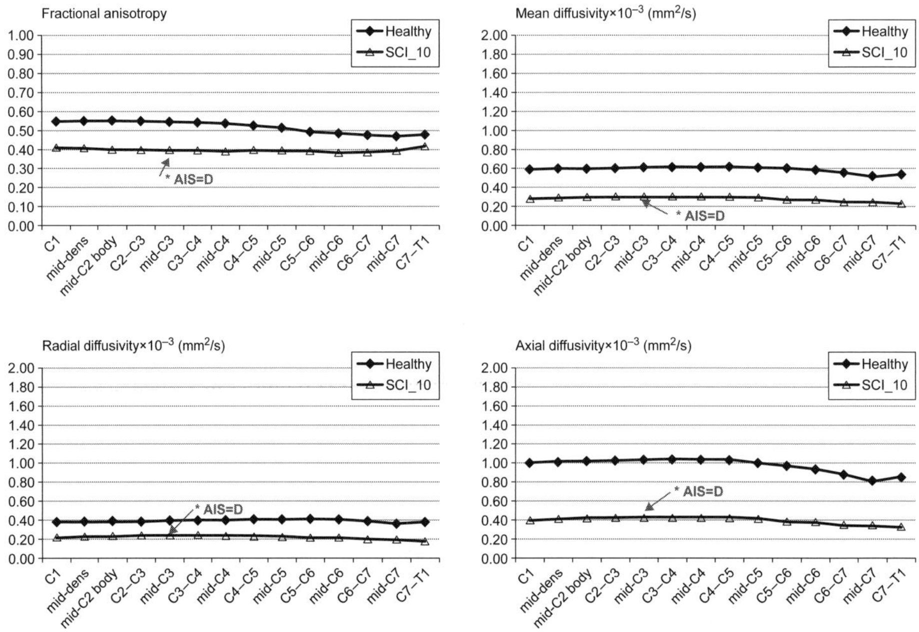

Fig. 29.7 DTI parameters from a patient with mid-C3 magnetic resonance imaging level of injury (arrows) and American Spinal Injury Association Impairment Scale (AIS) grade D, compared with averaged results of healthy participants. *=p<0.05.

Blood oxygenation level-dependent imaging

Functional MRI based on BOLD imaging is an indirect method of measuring neuronal activation (Ogawa et al 1990). This method has been used extensively to study brain functions and, to a lesser extent, the spinal cord (Stroman et al 1999, Madi et al 2001). Brain activity, as represented by synaptic firings, is associated with increased energy demands, which, under normal conditions, are satisfied by way of oxidative glucose metabolism. At the onset of brain activity in a particular region, local feeding arterioles dilate, increasing blood flow in downstream capillaries. Although at the no-stimulus baseline all capillaries are already perfused, regional brain activity increases blood flow through the capillaries in an immediate vicinity of active neurons. The amount of oxygen brought by this influx is in excess of what is consumed through oxidative glucose metabolism. As a result, the overall fraction of oxygenated hemoglobin is increased. In the configuration with bound oxygen, ferrous iron of the heme molecule changes its conformation and becomes progressively more diamagnetic (less paramagnetic) as more oxygen molecules bind. Diamagnetism of oxygenated hemoglobin (oxyhemoglobin) imparts reduced magnetic susceptibility when placed in the magnetic field of an MRI scanner and thus shows an increase in MRI signal. This method is called BOLD imaging and is being used to study various brain functions as well as spinal cord activations. BOLD functional MRI has been used in pediatric populations by researchers for the purpose of classifying the severity of SCI in children (Krisa et al 2013).

The signal of BOLD imaging, however, is low in the spinal cord and an alternative method to observe the activation in the spinal cord directly, called signal enhancement by extravascular water protons (SEEP), was first proposed by (Stroman et al 2001). SEEP contrast is based on changes in tissue water content that arise from the increased production of extracellular fluid and the swelling of neurons and glial cells at sites of neuronal activity. Because the dominant sources of MRI signals in biological tissues are water and lipids, an increase in tissue water content is reflected by a local increase in MRI signal intensity. These two methods can be potentially used to study populations with SCI.

Future of neuroimaging in pediatric spinal cord injury

There are several new imaging methods and protocols that have been explored in adult SCI populations but are under study in pediatric populations (Freund et al 2012). Quantitative measurement of cross-sectional spinal cord volume changes have been studied by various investigators in chronic adult SCI populations (Cohen-Adad et al 2011, Lundell et al 2011). These research studies have reported a decline of up to 30% in the cross-sectional spinal cord volume in images of patients with SCI obtained with MRI, presumably owing to spinal atrophy. These findings are very interesting, as they demonstrate the relationship between disability owing to SCI and spinal cord atrophy. Recent developments in the high-resolution imaging of the spinal cord with reduced field-of-view structural imaging will enable better resolution of characteristics of gray and white matter tissues. This will facilitate the use of computer segmentation methods for accurate classification and volumetric analysis of the injured cord.

The primary application of SEEP today has been functional MRI of the spinal cord because the bone/tissue interfaces around the spinal cord cause poor image quality with conventional functional MRI methods. A recent paper using SEEP on adults, involving 20 comparison participants, nine patients with American Spinal Injury Association Impairment Scale (AIS) grade BCD SCI, and six patients with AIS E SCI, has shown evidence for spinal plasticity in patients with incomplete SCI, and these plastic changes are evident in those who fully recover from their injury (Cadotte et al 2012).

Since the early 2000s, there has been a steady increase in the development of techniques to study brain function: methods to observe volumetric changes in the white and gray matter of the brain, techniques to measure cortical surface area and thickness (voxel-based morphometry) (Ashburner and Friston 2000), as well as methods to quantify cortical thinning (voxel-based cortical thinning). These methods have been shown to be effective in quantifying brain morphologic changes in various brain disorders. Recently, studies have shown the relationship between spinal cord dysfunction and changes in brain structures. Reduction in the volumes of white matter and volumetric changes in gray matter have been observed in the denervated leg region of the primary motor and sensory cortices (Freund et al 2011). Furthermore, magnetization transfer imaging and diffusion kurtosis imaging techniques that can provide sensitive and specific markers of white matter pathology are being explored. In the years to come, one can envision these advanced imaging tools and measurements being used to study children with SCI.

REFERENCES

American Spinal Injury Association (2003) *International Standards for the Neurological Classification of Spinal Cord Injury*. Chicago, IL: American Spinal Injury Association.

Ashburner J, Friston K (2000) Voxel-based morphometry – the methods. *Neuroimage* 11: 805–21. doi: 10.1006/nimg.2000.0582

Barakat N, Hunter L, Finsterbusch J et al (2011) Diffusion tensor imaging of the pediatric spinal cord using an inner-FoV EPI pulse sequence in normals and patients with SCI. *Proc Annu Meet Int Soc Magn Reson Med* 19: 400.

Barakat N, Mohamed F, Hunter L et al (2012) Diffusion tensor imaging of the normal pediatric spinal cord using an inner-FoV EPI sequence. *Am J Neuroradiol* 33: 1127–33. doi: 10.3174/ajnr.A2924

Beaulieu C (2002) The basis of anisotropic water diffusion in the nervous system? A technical review. *NMR Biomed* 15: 435–55. doi: 10.1002/nbm.782

Beaulieu C, Allen PS (1994a) Determinants of anisotropic water diffusion in nerves. *Magn Reson Med* 31: 394–400. doi: 10.1002/mrm.1910310408

Beaulieu C, Allen PS (1994b) Water diffusion in the giant axon of the squid: Implications for diffusion-weighted MRI of the nervous system. *Magn Reson Med* 32: 579–83. doi: 10.1002/mrm.1910320506

Cadotte DW, Wilson JR, Mikulis D, Stroman PW, Brady S, Fehlings MG (2011) Conventional MRI as a diagnostic and prognostic tool in spinal cord injury: a systemic review of its application to date and an overview on emerging MRI methods. *Expert Opin Med Diagn* 5: 121–33. doi: 10.1517/17530059.2011.556111

Cadotte DW, Stroman P, Bosma R, Mikulis DJ, Nugaeva N, Fehlings MG (2012) Visualizing plasticity and altered neuronal signaling in the injured human spinal cord with fMRI. *Neurosurgery* 71: E558. http://dx.doi.org/10.1227/01.neu.0000417734.16924.ec

Cheran S, Shanmuganathan K, Zhuo J et al (2011) Correlation of MR diffusion tensor imaging parameters with ASIA motor scores in hemorrhagic and nonhemorrhagic acute spinal cord injury. *J Neurotrauma* 28: 1881–92. doi: 10.1089/neu.2010.1741

Clark CA, Werring DJ (2002) Diffusion tensor imaging in spinal cord: methods and applications – a review. *NMR Biomed* 15: 578–86. doi: 10.1002/nbm.788

Cohen-Adad J, El Mendili MM, Lehericy S et al (2011) Demyelination and degeneration in the injured human spinal cord detected with diffusion and magnetization transfer MRI. *NeuroImage* 55: 1024–33. doi: 10.1016/j.neuroimage.2010.11.089

Ellingson BM, Ulmer JL, Kurpad SN, Schmit BD (2008a) Diffusion tensor MR imaging in chronic spinal cord injury. *Am J Neuroradiol* 29: 1976–82. doi: 10.3174/ajnr.A1272

Ellingson BM, Ulmer JL, Kurpad SN, Schmit BD (2008b) Diffusion tensor MR imaging of the neurologically intact human spinal cord. *Am J Neuroradiol* 29: 1279–84. doi: 10.3174/ajnr.A1064

Feldman HM, Yeatman JD, Lee ES, Barde L, Gaman-Bean S (2010) Diffusion tensor imaging: a review for pediatric researchers and clinicians. *J Dev Behav Pediatr* 31: 346–56. doi: 10.1097/DBP.0b013e3181dcaa8b

Figley CR, Stroman PW (2007) Investigation of human cervical and upper thoracic spinal cord motion: implications for imaging spinal cord structure and function. *Magn Reson Med* 58: 185–9. doi: 10.1002/mrm.21260

Finsterbusch J (2009) High-resolution diffusion tensor imaging with inner field-of-view EPI. *J Magn Reson Imaging* 29: 987–93. doi: 10.1002/jmri.21717

Freund P, Weiskopf N, Ward NS et al (2011) Disability, atrophy and cortical reorganization following spinal cord injury. *Brain* 134: 1610–22. doi: 10.1093/brain/awr093

Freund P, Curt A, Friston K, Thompson A (2012) Tracking changes following spinal cord injury: insights from neuroimaging. *Neuroscientist* 19: 116–28. doi: 10.1177/1073858412449192

Giove F, Garreffa G, Giulietti G, Mangia S, Colonnese C, Maraviglia B (2004) Issues about the fMRI of the human spinal cord. *Magn Reson Imaging* 22: 1505–16. doi: 10.1016/j.mri.2004.10.015

Johansen-Berg H, Behrens TE (eds) (2013) *Diffusion MRI: From Quantitative Measurement to In Vivo Neuroanatomy*. 2nd Ed. San Diego, CA: Academic Press.

Kharbanda HS, Alsop DC, Anderson AW, Filardo G, Hackney DB (2006) Effects of cord motion on diffusion imaging of the spinal cord. *Magn Reson Med* 56: 334–39. doi: 10.1002/mrm.20959

Krisa L, Middleton D, Faro S, Calhoun CL, Mohamed FB, Mulcahey MJ (2013) Cerebral activation during the test of spinal cord injury severity in children: an FMRI methodological study. *Top Spinal Cord Inj Rehabil* 19: 121–8. doi: 10.1310/sci1902-121

Le Bihan D, Mangin JF, Poupon C et al (2001) Diffusion tensor imaging: concepts and applications. *J Magn Reson Imaging* 13: 534–46. doi: 10.1002/jmri.1076

Lundell H, Barthelemy D, Skimminge A, Dyrby T, Bieringsorensen F, Nielsen J (2011) Independent spinal cord atrophy measures correlate to motor and sensory deficits in individuals with spinal cord injury. *Spinal Cord* 49: 70–5. doi: 10.1038/sc.2010.87

Madi S, Flanders AE, Vinitski S, Herbison GJ, Nissanov J (2001) Functional MR imaging of the human cervical spinal cord. *Am J Neuroradiol* 22: 1768–74.

Malisza KL, Martin T, Shiloff D, Yu DCT (2010) Reactions of young children to the MRI scanner environment. *Magn Reson Med* 64: 377–81. doi: 10.1002/mrm.22438

Middleton DM, Mohamed FB, Barakat N et al (2014) An investigation of motion correction algorithms for pediatric spinal cord DTI in healthy subjects and patients with spinal cord injury. *Magn Reson Imaging* 32: 433–9. doi: 10.1016/j.mri.2014.01.020

Mohamed FB, Hunter LN, Barakat N et al (2011) Diffusion tensor imaging of the pediatric spinal cord at 1.5T: preliminary results. *AJNR Am J Neuroradiol* 32: 339–45. doi: 10.3174/ajnr.A2334

Mulcahey M, Samdani A, Gaughan J et al (2011) Diffusion tensor imaging in pediatric spinal cord injury: preliminary examination of reliability and clinical correlation. *Spine* 37: E797–803. doi: 10.1097/BRS.0b013e3182470a08

Mulcahey MJ, Samdani AF, Gaughan JP et al (2013) Diagnostic accuracy of diffusion tensor imaging for pediatric cervical cord. *Spinal Cord* 51: 532–7. doi:10.1038/sc.2013.36

Ogawa S, Lee TM, Kay AR, Tank DW (1990) Brain magnetic resonance imaging with contrast dependent on blood oxgenation. *Proc Natl Acad Sci USA* 87: 9868–72. http://dx.doi.org/10.1073/pnas.87.24.9868

Petersen JA, Wilm BJ, Von Meyenburg J et al (2012) Chronic cervical spinal cord injury: DTI correlates with clinical and electrophysiological measures. *J Neurotrauma* 29: 1556–66. doi: 10.1089/neu.2011.2027

Rosenberg DR, Sweeney JA, Gillen JS et al (1997) Magnetic resonance imaging of children without sedation: preparation with simulation. *J Am Acad Child Adolesc Psychiatry* 36: 853–9. doi: 10.1097/00004583-199706000-00024

Saritas EU, Cunningham CH, Lee JH, Han ET, Nishimura DG (2008) DWI of the spinal cord with reduced FOV single-shot EPI. *Magn Reson Med* 60: 468–73. doi: 10.1002/mrm.21640

Stroman PW, Nance PW, Ryner LN (1999) BOLD MRI of the human cervical spinal cord at 3 Tesla. *Magn Reson Med* 42: 571–6. doi: 10.1002/(SICI)1522-2594(199909)42: 3<571::AID-MRM20>3.0.CO;2-N

Stroman PW, Krause V, Malisza KL, Frankenstein UN, Tomanek B (2001) Characterization of contrast changes in functional MRI of the human spinal cord at 1.5 T. *Magn Reson Imaging* 19: 833–9. doi: 10.1016/S0730-725X(01)00409-X

Takahashi M, Hackney DB, Zhang G et al (2002) Magnetic resonance microimaging of intraaxonal water diffusion in live excised lamprey spinal cord. *Proc Natl Acad Sci USA* 99: 16192–6. doi: 10.1073/pnas.252249999

Wilm BJ, Svensson J, Henning A, Pruessmann KP, Boesiger P, Kollias SS (2007) Reduced field-of-view MRI using outer volume suppression for spinal cord diffusion imaging. *Magn Reson Med* 57: 625–30. doi: 10.1002/mrm.21167

INDEX

Notes

Page references in *italics* refer to material in figures, those in **bold** refer to tables, and those followed by 'b' refer to boxes. *vs* indicates a comparison or differential diagnosis. Abbreviations used: DTI, diffusion tensor imaging; MRI, magnetic resonance injury; SCI, spinal cord injury; TBI, traumatic brain injury.

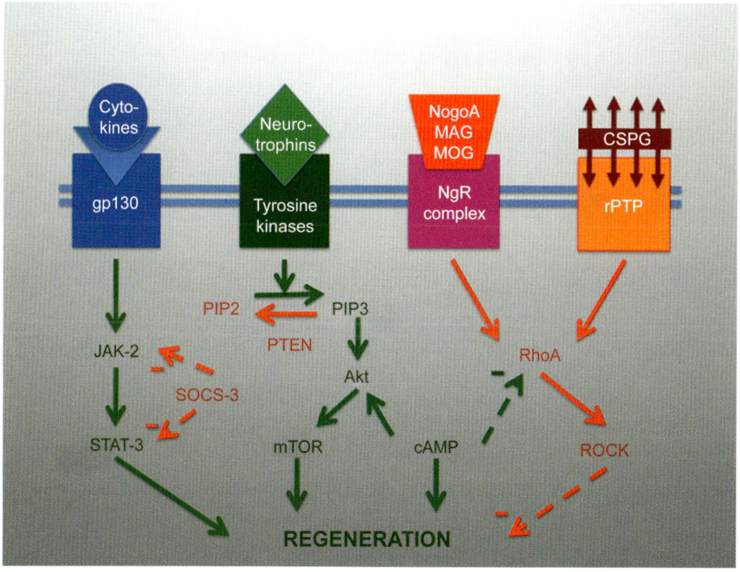

Plate 5.3 See page 77 for full legend.

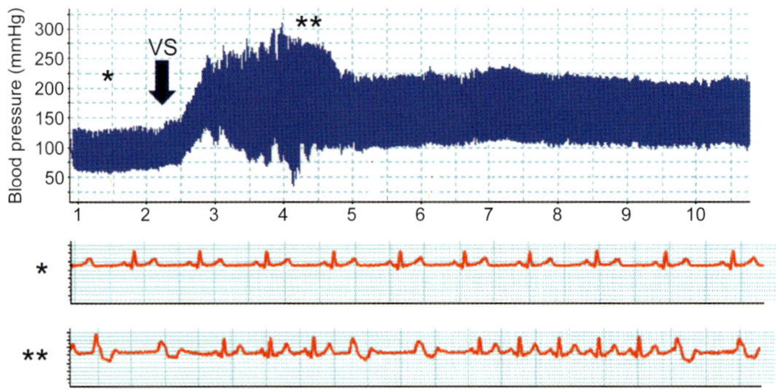

Plate 13.2 See page 188 for full legend.

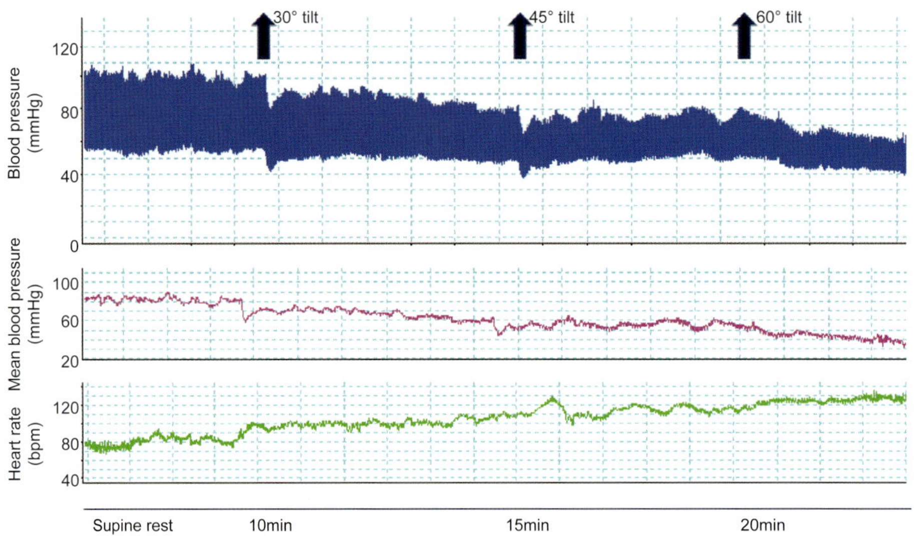

Plate 13.3 See page 190 for full legend.

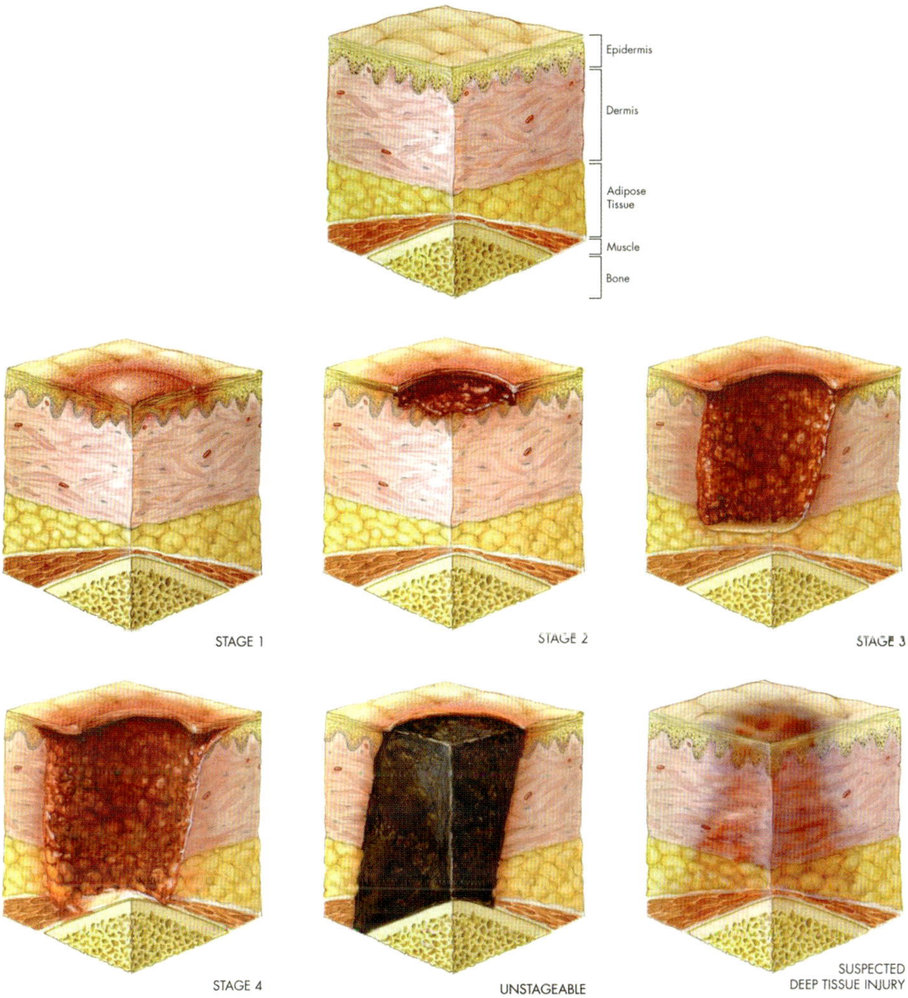

Plate 15.1 See pages 220–221 for full legend.

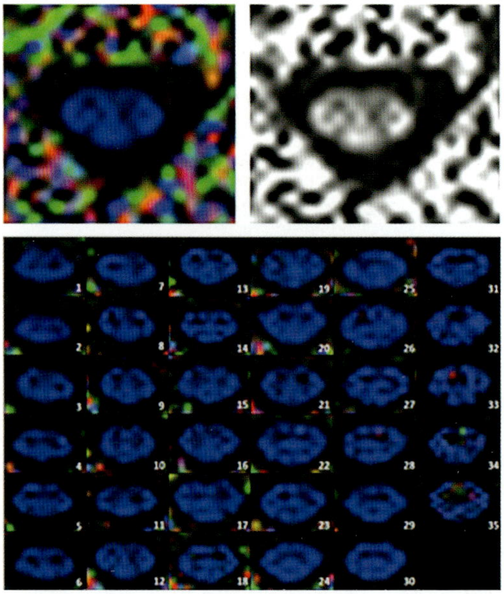

Plate 29.4 Cervical spinal cord images of a healthy child obtained with the inner field-of-view pulse sequence. Axial fractional anisotropy map (top left) and grayscale fractional anisotropy map (top right) along the 35 cervical slices of a healthy participant (bottom).

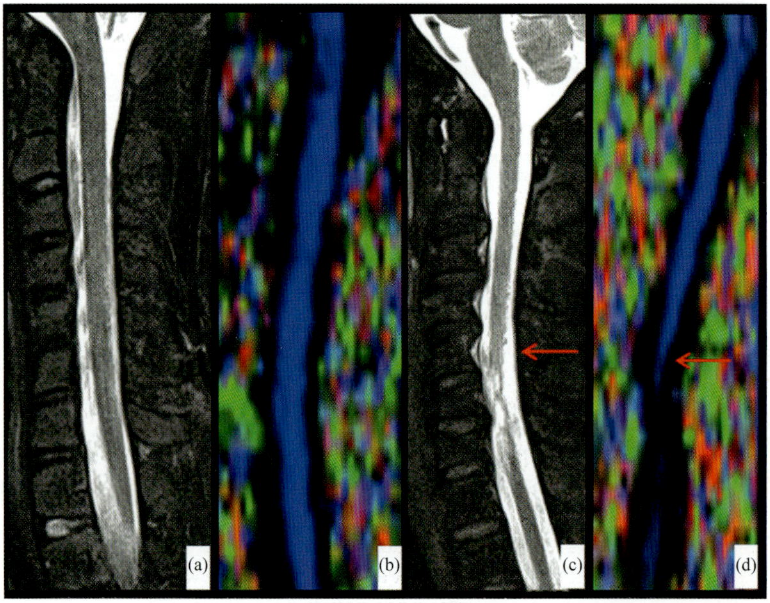

Plate 29.5 Midline sagittal T2-weighted magnetic resonance image and fractional anisotropy color map of a healthy participant (a, b) and a patient with spinal cord injury (c, d). Arrow represents level of injury (C5).

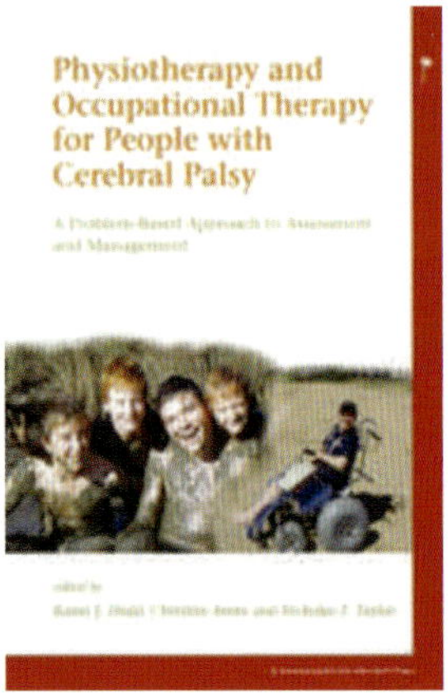

Physiotherapy and Occupational Therapy for People with Cerebral Palsy
Karen J. Dodd, Christine Imms, Nicholas F. Taylor (Editors)

A practical guide from Mac Keith Press
2010 ▪ 320pp ▪ softback ▪ 978-1-898683-68-1
£29.95/ €36.00 / $41.99

This book is a practical resource for physiotherapists and occupational therapists who support people with cerebral palsy, helping them to solve the problems with movement and other impairments that so often accompany cerebral palsy, so that they can be more active and better able to participate in roles such as study, work, recreation and relationships.

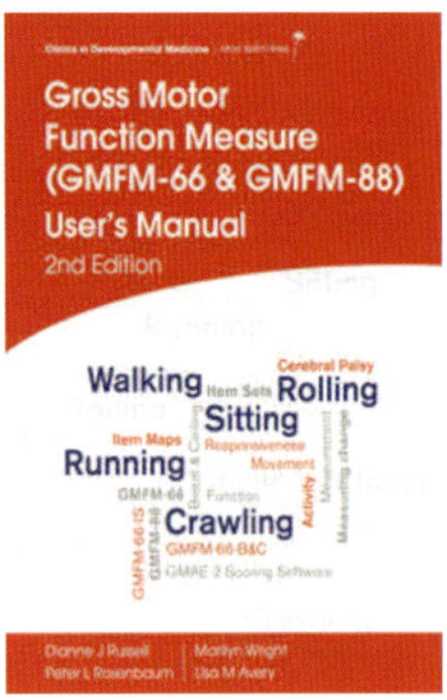

Gross Motor Function Measure (GMFM-66 and GMFM-88) User's Manual, 2nd Edition
Dianne J. Russell, Peter L. Rosenbaum, Marilyn Wright, Lisa M. Avery

Clinics in Developmental Medicine
2013 ▪ 304pp ▪ spiral-bound softback ▪ 978-1-908316-88-2
£70.00 / €84.00 / $115.00

The Gross Motor Function Measure (GMFM) has become the best evaluative measure of motor function designed for quantifying change in the gross motor abilities of children with cerebral palsy. The new version of the scoring programme has now been released, and includes two abbreviated methods of estimating GMFM-66 scores using the GMFM-66-Item sets and the GMFM-66-Basal & Ceiling. This new edition builds on the wide success of the first edition.

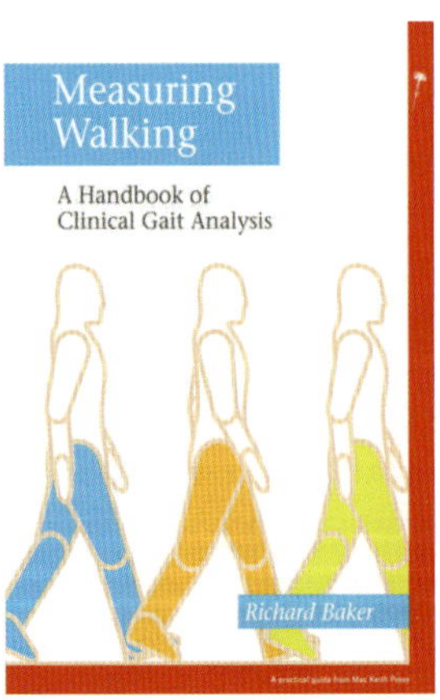

Measuring Walking: A Handbook of Clinical Gait Analysis
Richard Baker

A practical guide from Mac Keith Press
2013 ▪ 248pp ▪ softback ▪ 978-1-908316-66-0
£49.95 / €60.60 / $84.95

This book is a practical guide to instrumented clinical gait analysis covering all aspects of routine service provision. It reinforces what is coming to be regarded as the conventional approach to clinical gait analysis. Data capture, processing and biomechanical interpretation are all described with an emphasis on ensuring high quality results. There are also chapters on how to set up and maintain clinical gait analysis services and laboratories.

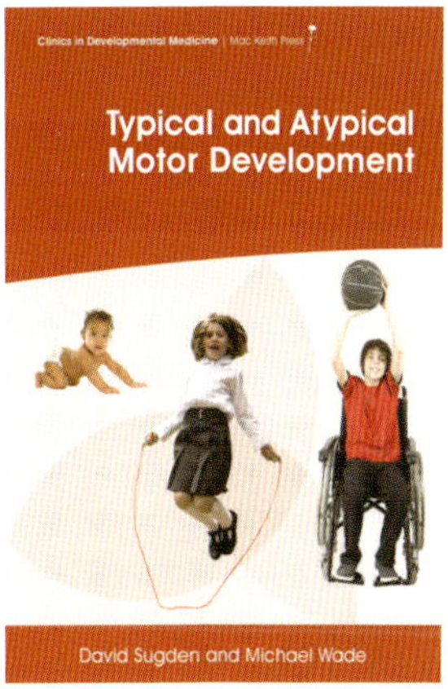

Typical and Atypical Motor Development
David Sugden and Michael Wade

Clinics in Developmental Medicine
2013 ▪ 400pp ▪ hardback ▪ 978-1-908316-55-4
£145.00 / €180.00 / $234.95

Sugden and Wade, leading authors in this area, comprehensively cover motor development and motor impairment, drawing on sources in medicine and health-related studies, motor learning and developmental psychology. A theme that runs through the book is that movement outcomes are a complex transaction of child resources, the context in which movement takes place, and the manner in which tasks are presented.

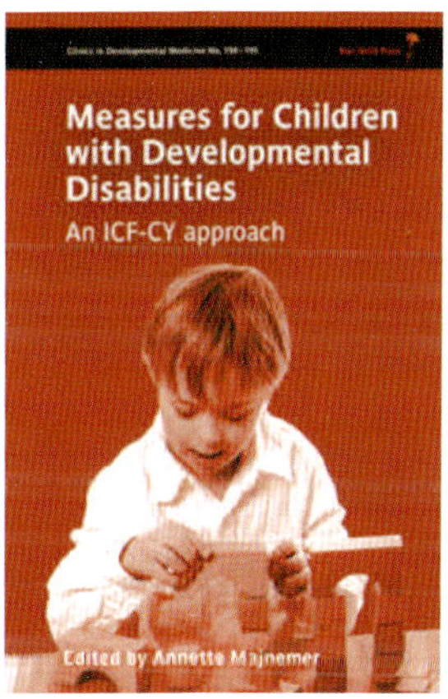

Measures for Children with Developmental Disabilities An ICF-CY approach
Annette Majnemer (Editor)

Clinics in Developmental Medicine No 194-195
2012 ▪ 552pp ▪ hardback ▪ 978-1-908316-45-5
£154.00 / €184.80 / $235.00

This title presents and reviews outcome measures across a wide range of attributes that are applicable to children and adolescents with developmental disabilities. It uses the children and youth version of the International Classification of Functioning, Disability and Health (ICF-CY) as a framework for organizing the various measures into sections and chapters. Each chapter coincides with domains within the WHO framework of Body Functions, Activities and Participation, and Personal and Environmental Factors.

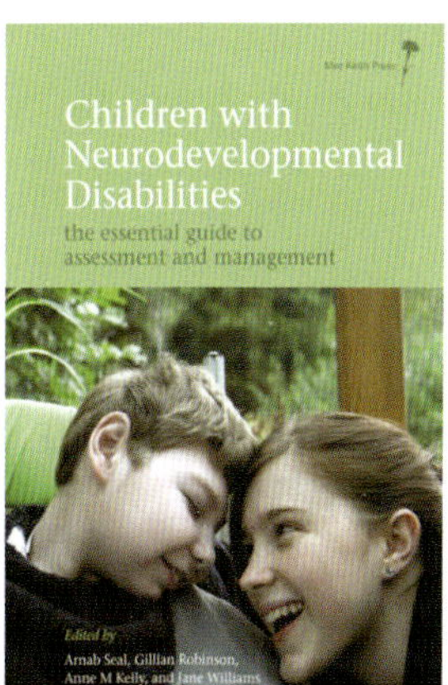

Children with Neurodevelopmental Disabilities: the essential guide to assessment and management
Arnab Seal, Gillian Robinson, Anne M. Kelly and Jane Williams (Editors)

2013 ▪ 744pp ▪ softback ▪ 978-1-908316-62-2
£65.00 / €78.00 / $99.95

A comprehensive textbook on the practice of paediatric neurodisability, written by practitioners and experts in the field. Using a problem-oriented approach, the authors give best-practice guidance, and centre on the needs of the child and family, working in partnership with multi-disciplinary, multi-agency teams. It provides a ready reference for managing problems encountered in the paediatric clinic.

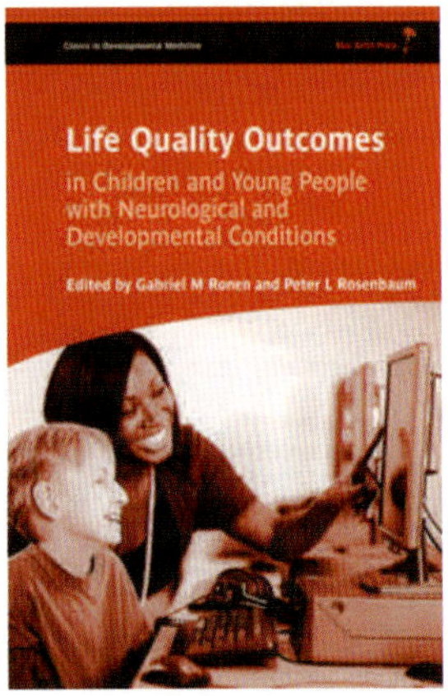

Life Quality Outcomes in Children and Young People with Neurological and Developmental Conditions

Gabriel M. Ronen and Peter L. Rosenbaum (Editors)

Clinics in Developmental Medicine
2013 ▪ 394pp ▪ hardback ▪ 978-1-908316-58-5
£95.00 / €120.70 / $149.95

Healthcare professionals need to understand their patients' views of their condition and its effects on their health and well-being. This book builds on the World Health Organization's concepts of 'health', 'functioning' and 'quality of life' for young people with neurodisabilities: it emphasises the importance of engaging with patients in the identification of both treatment goals and their evaluation. Uniquely, it enables healthcare professionals to find critically reviewed outcomes-related information.

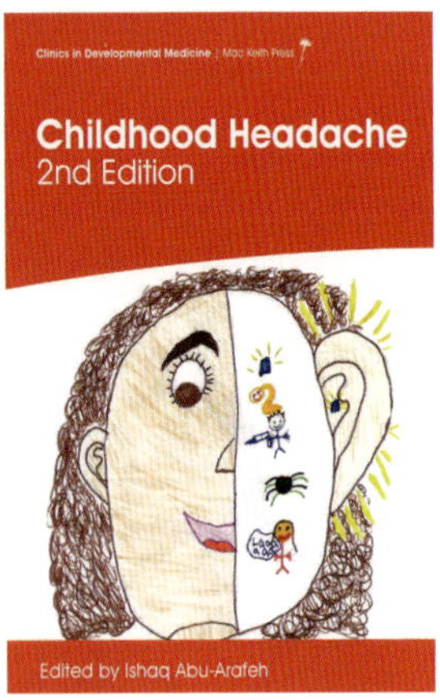

Childhood Headache, 2nd Edition

Ishaq Abu-Arafeh (Editor)

Clinics in Developmental Medicine
2013 ▪ 352pp ▪ hardback ▪ 978-1-908316-75-2
£95.00 / €115.20 / $154.95

Headache is a common problem which has a significant impact on children's quality of life. *Childhood Headache* is a comprehensive source of knowledge and guidance to practising clinicians looking after children with headache that includes many clinical examples to illustrate the difficulties in diagnosis or options for treatment. It is also a resource for researchers who are looking for a full analysis of the published studies.

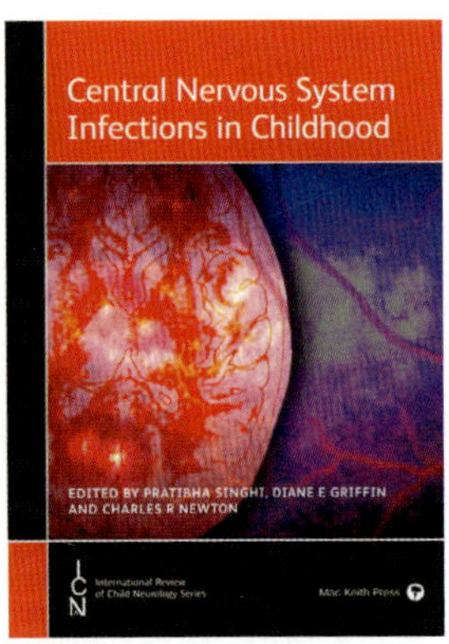

Central Nervous System Infections in Childhood

Pratibha Singhi, Diane E. Griffin and Charles R. Newton (Editors)

International Review of Child Neurology Series
2014 ▪ 390pp ▪ hardback ▪ 978-1-909962-44-6
£95.00 / €115.20 / $159.95

This title has been developed with the International Child Neurology Association to provide information on common CNS infections.
It covers almost all CNS infections commonly seen in children across the world in both developed and resource poor countries. It provides a concise, state of the art overview of viral, bacterial, tubercular, fungal, parasitic and many other infections of the CNS. The book is intended to be of practical use to residents, physicians, paediatricians and paediatric neurologists across the globe.